A HISTORY OF MEDICINE

*

A HISTORY OF MEDICINE

HENRY E. SIGERIST

I

PRIMITIVE AND ARCHAIC MEDICINE

*

OXFORD UNIVERSITY PRESS
New York Oxford

Oxford University Press
Oxford New York Toronto
Delhi Bombay Calcutta Madras Karachi
Petaling Jaya Singapore Hong Kong Tokyo
Nairobi Dar es Salaam Cape Town
Melbourne Auckland

and associated companies in
Beirut Berlin Ibadan Nicosia

First published in 1951 by Oxford University Press, Inc.,
200 Madison Avenue, New York, New York 10016

First issued as an Oxford University Press paperback, 1967

Reissued 1987

Publication No. 27
Historical Library
Yale Medical Library

The Library of Congress has catalogued the
first printing of this title as follows:
Sigerist, Henry Ernest, 1891-1957.
A history of medicine. New York, Oxford University Press,
1951-61.
2 v. illus., ports., maps. 24 cm. (Publication / Historical Library, Yale Medical Library ; no. 27) (v. 2: Publication / Department of the History of Medicine, Yale University ; no. 38)
Includes bibliographies.
Contents: v. 1. Primitive and archaic medicine.—v. 2. Early Greek, Hindu, and Persian medicine.
1. Medicine—History. I. Title. II. Series: Publication (Yale Medical Library, Historical Library) ; no. 27. III. Series: Publication (Yale University. Dept. of the History of Medicine) ; no. 38.
R131.S533 610.9 51-9041
Vol. 1 ISBN 0-19-500739-5(pbk.)
Vol. 2 ISBN 0-19-505079-7(pbk.)

2 4 6 8 10 9 7 5 3 1

Printed in the United States of America

To the Memory of

KARL SUDHOFF

WILLIAM H. WELCH

HARVEY CUSHING

whose Teachings and Encouragement
made this Work possible.

*

Preface

When Henry Sigerist succeeded to the chair of Karl Sudhoff and the directorship of the Institut für Geschichte der Medizin at Leipzig in 1925, he had already formulated in his mind an idea for a history of medicine, global in scope. In subsequent years, after he had come to occupy William H. Welch's chair in the history of medicine at Johns Hopkins University, the plan for this history was further clarified—one that would place medicine in the broad setting of general history and give some indication of the vast role played by the medical sciences among the forces which have determined the progress of mankind.

No such history of medicine has ever before been attempted. The *Handbuch* of Puschmann, edited by Neuburger and Pagel, and the histories of Neuburger, Sudhoff-Pagel, Castiglioni, and Garrison, excellent in their way, were not designed to give the comprehensive scope that is envisaged in the present undertaking. Dr. Sigerist is probably the only living scholar who has both the training and the vision to approach the development of medicine on this vast scale. Having acquired a solid classical education, a medical degree, training in historiography, and an impeccable knowledge of the modern tongues of Western Europe and the English-speaking world and the cultures they represent, he has also devoted several years to the study of Oriental languages and, more recently, to Russian.

During his fifteen years in the United States he traveled to the Soviet Union, to India, and to South Africa, as well as making frequent visits to England and the Continent, and he became so much in demand as a lecturer and consultant that no time was available for the project that he had come to look upon as his major life work. It was with rare fortitude, therefore, that Henry

Sigerist at the very height of his popularity made the decision to give up active work with students and colleagues, which he so much enjoys, and to give his entire time to writing the history of medicine, now envisaged as an eight-volume work. At the age of fifty-six he retired from his chair at Johns Hopkins University and went to live in the hamlet of Pura on Lake Lugano. There, in the idyllic surroundings of a Swiss-Italian villa not unlike that of Fracastoro on Lake Garda, with vineyard and lake before him and behind him the hills that have inspired many another scholar—there at the crossroads of the learned world, Henry Sigerist is making one of the greatest contributions to the scholarship of our time.

When he retired from Johns Hopkins, Yale University was proud to make Dr. Sigerist a Research Associate with professorial rank on indefinite leave of absence, but with the hope that he would from time to time return to the United States to give us the benefit of his inspiring leadership. The progress of his great work is, however, the all-important thing, now and in the future. He has graciously dedicated his history to the memory of Karl Sudhoff, William Welch, and Harvey Cushing, who, in their several ways, did so much to enrich the history of medicine to which Henry Sigerist has in his turn dedicated his own talents and energies.

When invited to write the preface to this ambitious undertaking, I eagerly accepted because of the opportunity thus afforded to express the gratitude of scholars everywhere for what Henry Sigerist has given us—the many publications from Leipzig, the *Bulletin of the History of Medicine* (now in its twenty-fourth volume), his Hopkins monograph series, innumerable books and papers—and, above all, for the warm personal stimulus which will ever be the inspiration of the youngest student and the most accomplished scholar. He gives us the modern credo of humanism.

John F. Fulton

Historical Library
Yale University
Autumn, 1950

*

Contents

*

List of Illustrations

*

Foreword

The present book is the result of more than twenty-five years of research and teaching. Ever since it was my privilege to assist Karl Sudhoff in the preparation of his *Kurzes Handbuch der Geschichte der Medizin,* I had resolved to write a history of medicine that would approach the subject from a somewhat different angle. I was well aware, however, that many years of study would be needed before I could think of undertaking such a task. My career took me to many lands, and at times my work seemed to be far remote from my original plan. And yet I never lost sight of it and always kept it in mind. Every book and every paper I wrote was meant to be a preparatory study, and many of my lecture and seminar courses were given not only for the benefit of students but to fill some gap in my knowledge or to review a period or a set of problems about which I had doubts. Field work in social medicine carried out in many countries seemed to have no connection whatever with my historical studies; yet after every such tour I knew that I had a deeper understanding of the workings of history.

I had intended to begin writing this book in 1941, that is, when I was to be fifty years of age. By that time, I thought, I should have gained sufficient knowledge and experience and should have a fair chance of completing the project without neglecting my academic duties. When the time came, however, America was at war, and it was out of the question to undertake a task of such magnitude. And when the war was over, time was getting short and to my great sorrow I realized that I should have to make a choice between an academic job that I loved and a scholarly project for which I had been preparing for so many years.

It took me two years to make a final decision. I had spent most of my life in universities, first as a student, then for twenty-six years as a teacher and as head of the best institutes of the history of medicine in Europe and America. I had lived in close touch with students, many of whom had become my closest friends. I knew how difficult it would be for me to relinquish the academic atmosphere. On the other hand, I felt a strong obligation to write the book which I thought was needed, which was to be at once a synthesis and a starting point for further research, and with which I would try to set a new pattern of medical historiography. But I was fully aware that this was possible only if I could be relieved of academic routine work.

The decision was made when Yale University considered my project important enough to be subsidized, and to that end appointed me Research Associate, with the freedom to work where I pleased, and with a salary large enough to make it possible for me to devote all my time to the task. The funds were contributed by Mr. and Mrs. John Hay Whitney, together with the Helen Hay Whitney Trust, the William S. Paley Foundation, Mrs. Harvey Cushing, Mr. Henry K. Cushing, Mrs. Vincent Astor, Mrs. Barbara Cushing Mortimer, Mr. Edward R. Murrow, and Mr. S. S. Spivak. To all of them, as well as to the Board of Permanent Officers of the Yale School of Medicine, I am deeply grateful for generous support and much encouragement.

The task of writing such an eight-volume work is gigantic. The basic texts may have been read critically many times, but when it comes to writing about them, they must be read again. I studied fourteen languages in order to be able to consult the original texts, but I find that one cannot master all tongues equally well at the same time, and for every volume I have to engage in preparatory language studies. This explains why my progress was not as rapid as I had hoped.

Another difficulty is presented by the fact that the book is addressed to historians as well as to physicians. This means that I am obliged to make statements that are obvious to historians but not to physicians, and vice versa. A history of medicine is always both, a medical book and a history book. One has to take a middle way, and while this is not fully satisfactory to the writer, it has the advantage that it makes the book accessible to young students and also to laymen interested in the subject.

The present volume suffered many interruptions. I began writing it during a summer vacation on the campus of Cornell University, continued it at odd moments at Johns Hopkins University, and finished it in the Swiss village where I have established my residence. It deals with the beginnings of medicine. The methodological introduction may seem rather long, but an eight-volume work requires a statement of policy, particularly when an attempt is made to break with certain traditions and to proceed along new paths. Primitive medicine is timeless and could have been discussed in the last volume as well as in the first, but it seemed more logical to have it here because it has many elements in common with the medical systems of ancient civilizations. Folk medicine, however—that strange mixture of primitive views and reminiscences of scientific systems of the past—will be treated later, as it recapitulates the entire history of medicine.

I am well aware that medicine developed at an early date not only in Egypt and Mesopotamia but also in India and China, and it would be justifiable to include the history of early Indian and Chinese medicine in this volume. To do so, however, would burden the volume with too many civilizations and too many repetitions, since archaic medicine is much the same, or at least very similar, everywhere. The earliest Indian and Chinese medical texts that we possess are, moreover, decidedly younger than those of Egypt and Mesopotamia; another important difference lies in the fact that Egyptian and Babylonian medicine completed their course long ago, while ancient Indian and Chinese medicine are still fully alive and are practiced today on millions of people. India's medical systems will be presented in our second volume, those of China in the third.

Some readers may be astonished that I did not include a chapter on Jewish medicine as reflected in the Old Testament. This could have been done very well, since the medicine of the Hebrews was strongly influenced by both Mesopotamia and Egypt. I decided to postpone this chapter, however, because I want it to serve as a link between the Ancient Orient and the Middle Ages, when Jewish influence was strongly felt in the East as well as in the West.

In the preparation of this volume I was helped by so many colleagues that I cannot possibly name all of them. However, I wish to express my deeply felt gratitude particularly to the members of my former staff at the Johns Hopkins Institute of the History of Medicine, Owsei Temkin, Ludwig Edelstein, Erwin H. Ackerknecht, and Genevieve Miller, with whom I discussed the problems of this book for many years, who read the manuscript as a whole or in parts, and who improved it with valuable suggestions.

So far as the illustrations are concerned, I am greatly indebted to the Wellcome Historical Medical Museum in London and to its director, Dr. E. Ashworth Underwood, who supplied me, in the most liberal way, with excellent photographs from the rich holdings of this unique museum. I am also much indebted to Dr. Karl Reucker of the Ciba Corporation in Basle, one of our foremost experts in medical iconography, who very kindly helped me with advice and with pictures.

Dr. John F. Fulton, Sterling Professor of Physiology at Yale University and Chairman of the Advisory Board of the Historical Library, Yale Medical Library, was a constant source of encouragement, and I am most grateful to him for his generous preface.

I made use of many libraries and I regret that I cannot name all the librarians who gave me much of their time, helped me with bibliographic references, and supplied me with books, photostats, and microfilms. However, I wish to mention especially Dr. Sanford Larkey, of the William H. Welch Medical Library in Baltimore; Dr. Claudius F. Mayer, of the Army Medical Library in Washington; Morris C. Leikind, of the Library of Congress in Washington; Madeline Stanton, of the Historical Library, Yale Medical Library; and last but not least, my daughter, Erica E. Sigerist, at present librarian at the World Health Organization in Geneva, who helped me in establishing my workshop in Switzerland and took a very active part in the preparation of this book.

For secretarial services I wish to thank Hope Trebing, my secretary of many years in Baltimore, and Claire Bacher, who also shared with me the burden of proofreading.

And, finally, I am much indebted to the following publishers, museums, and societies for the permission to quote or to use illustrations from their works: The University Presses of Cambridge, Chicago, Illinois, Oxford, Yale; Ciba Aktiengesellschaft, Basle; J. M. Dent & Sons Ltd., London; Houghton Mifflin Company, Boston; Luzac & Company Ltd., London; Macmillan & Co. Ltd., London; Librairie Maloine, Paris; Methuen & Co. Ltd., London; Ejnar Munksgaard, Copenhagen; Editions Payot, Paris; J. C. B. Mohr (Paul Siebeck), Tubingen; Routledge & Kegan Paul Ltd., London; Smithsonian Institution, Bureau of American Ethnology, Washington; Southwest Post Card Co., Albuquerque; Charles C Thomas, Springfield, Ill.; the Viking Fund, Inc., New York; the British Museum, London; the Metropolitan Museum of Art, New York; Pitt Rivers Museum, Oxford; the Wellcome Historical Medical Museum, London; the Royal Asiatic Society, London; the Royal Society of Medicine, London.

Henry E. Sigerist

Pura, Switzerland
30 *June* 1950

I. INTRODUCTION

*

1. The Historical Approach to Medicine

The history of medicine is at the same time a very old and a very young field of study. In the beginning of the nineteenth century ancient medicine was still alive. For over two thousand years ancient medical writings had been consulted as authorities, or at any rate as sources of information. In 1804 Laënnec, the inventor of the stethoscope, one of the great pioneers of modern clinical medicine, wrote his inaugural dissertation, *Propositions sur la doctrine d'Hippocrate relativement à la médecine pratique,*[1] a thesis in which he compared views and methods of Hippocrates with those of his teacher, Xavier Bichat, and in which he stressed the superiority of the Hippocratic theory of fevers.

In the School of Medicine of the University of Paris, reorganized during the Revolution in 1794 as L'Ecole de Santé, the Director was required to give courses in Hippocratic Medicine and Rare Cases. In 1811 after the death of the first Director and Dean, A. Thouret, the courses were abolished as being unnecessary, since all professors were teaching Hippocratic medicine.[2] Editions and translations of ancient medical writers were published primarily for the benefit of medical students and practitioners. It was for them that Albrecht von Haller had prepared his *Artis Medicae Principes*[3] published from 1768 to 1774. And as late as 1839 Emile Littré in the preface to the first volume of his monumental edition and translation of the works of Hippocrates wrote that his purpose was to make the Hippocratic writings available to physicians in such a way that they might be read and understood like a contemporary book.[4] When Charles Daremberg, twelve years later, began the publication of a collection of Greek and Latin medical writers, he undertook it for students of medical history,[5] and the *Corpus Medicorum Graecorum* was launched in the beginning of our century by philologists for philologists.[6]

Thus we see that until about a hundred years ago the history of medicine was primarily medicine. The approach to the past was not a critical, historical one, but was medical. Books were read for their content irrespective of the period in which they had been written. Of course, attempts were made at all times to trace medical developments. Ancient and medieval writers often speculated about the origins and early beginnings of the healing art. The medical views of the various schools were listed. In the Renaissance when people were particularly interested in individual achievements, biographies of prominent physicians and bibliographies of their works were written. The bio-bibliographical approach has remained very popular to this day. At the end of the seventeenth century and in the beginning of the eighteenth a Frenchman, Daniel Le Clerc, an Englishman, J. Friend, and a German, J. H. Schulze, each wrote a history of medicine. Their books had a profound influence on the historiography of medicine, and together with Kurt Sprengel's great *Versuch einer pragmatischen Geschichte der Arzneykunde* (1792-1803) they established a pattern that has been followed ever since.[7] In their hands, the history of medicine was primarily history, but to the great majority of medical men it remained part of the theory of medicine, the experience of the preceding generations that had to be assimilated if progress was to be achieved.

This attitude toward the past of medicine changed radically in the second half of the nineteenth century when a new medical science developed and progress was achieved such as never before. The past seemed dead. To the average physician the history of medicine appeared as the history of errors. Nothing could be learned from it; to study it, to read the ancient writers, was a waste of time. Science was worshiped and the best minds turned to the laboratory with great enthusiasm.

Yet this very generation of medical scientists was trained in the humanities. The French lycée, the German gymnasium, Oxford and Cambridge, Harvard and Yale remained centers of humanistic studies. A physician might become a pathologist or bacteriologist, but he still could read Greek and Roman writers in their original language. And at that time many doctors read the classics of medicine not in order to learn how to treat pneumonia or to reduce a dislocated shoulder, but as historical documents in order to know what the Greeks, the Romans, the people of the Renaissance had done to protect and restore their health and what ideas had been guiding their actions. The physicians' attitude toward the past now was primarily historical.

At the same time the scope of historical and philological studies was broadened considerably. History was no longer limited to the story of dynastic quarrels, of wars and treaties of peace; it became the history of civilization, the history of man, living and working in groups, producing food and commodities, conquering nature, endeavoring to interpret and understand the world, re-creating it in art and literature. Philologists, and among them the classical philologists first, no longer limited themselves to the study of literary, historical, and philosophical writings but bravely attacked mathematical, biological, and medical texts.

Thus, in the second half of the nineteenth century the history of medicine became a critical, historical discipline in which historians, philologists, philosophers, and physicians collaborated. In this as in other historical disciplines, an enormous amount of work was devoted to the preparation of critical editions of basic sources. C. G. Kühn's edition of Galen, published in 22 volumes from 1821 to 1833, was anything but critical; it was chiefly a compilation from Renaissance editions. Salvatore De Renzi, from 1852 to 1859, printed in his *Collectio Salernitana*, none too critically, whatever texts he could find in manuscripts, including sometimes texts that had no connection whatever with the school of Salerno. But at the same time Charles Daremberg began the publication of the works of Oribasius and based his text on all manuscripts available. Work on the *Corpus Medicorum Graecorum* began with a survey of manuscripts and the publication of a catalogue.[8]

The moment medical history had become primarily an object of historical research, increased attention was paid to periods that had been neglected in the past, such as the Middle Ages, because they had no particular appeal to the medical reader. Medicine progressed relatively little in the thousand-year period of the Middle Ages, but to the historian it is important to know how ancient medicine was transmitted in East and West, what diseases affected people in the Middle Ages, what was done to preserve and restore health, what place Greek medical theories held in the philosophical systems of the period, and upon what foundations the Renaissance built.

Medical history, without any doubt, is first of all history, a historical discipline like the history of philosophy, the history of art, or the history of music. It therefore has the general methods of historical research in common with all other historical disciplines. But it is a special history and therefore different from all others, with problems and methods of its own.

It is one of the youngest historical disciplines in the modern sense of the word, and still has very few centers of research and training. The first research institute in Europe was founded in 1905 at the University of Leipzig by Karl Sudhoff, and the first research institute in America was created by William H. Welch at the Johns Hopkins University in 1929. Most medical historians were not trained in the field but acquired their knowledge of historical research methods in some other discipline—general history, sociology, classical or Oriental philology, history of literature, art, or some other historical field. It seems, therefore, desirable to give at this point a brief outline of the methodology of medical history in order to clarify our thought and for the benefit of students entering the field.[9] Even students of well-established disciplines such as the history of art feel from time to time the need of reasserting their position and of reassessing their methods.[10]

It would be a mistake to assume that medical history today is a concern of historians and philologists alone and of no interest to physicians. Medical history is medicine also, today as it was in the past. We shall have to demonstrate this. Several generations of philologists and historians have made valuable contributions to the field. They did most of the spade work, made sources available, and, by looking at medicine from outside, brought in interesting points of view. It seems to me, however, that today more than ever there is need also for medical interpretations and evaluations of the past of medicine.

THE PROBLEMS

When we consult the past of medicine, what do we want to know? We obviously want to discover what medicine was like at a given time, in a given place. But we must first agree upon what we mean by medicine.

There are people who consider medicine whatever the physician does. He who is not a physician is a layman and what he does cannot be medicine. This is a very narrow interpretation and one that certainly does not hold true in historical studies. Today we have a legal definition of the physician. A physician is an individual who has a license to practice medicine, a license issued to him by an authority, usually the state, upon his having demonstrated that he possesses the minimum knowledge in the field required by that authority. Similarly we have licensed dentists, pharmacists, registered nurses, and other recognized medical personnel.

But in antiquity, who was a physician and who not? Who before the nineteenth century was a dentist? The great majority of all cases of illness, moreover, even today, are never seen by a physician. They are treated by the patient himself or by his relatives. And this self-treatment may be according to principles of the scientific medicine of the time. It may be dictated by commercial interests, by advertisements, or it may be folk-medicine pure and simple. But why should this important aspect be omitted from a historical study?

The scope of medicine is so broad that it includes, under any circumstances, infinitely more than the physician's actions. The task of medicine may be outlined under the following four headings:

1. Promotion of health
2. Prevention of illness
3. Restoration of health
4. Rehabilitation

Medical history, therefore, will study health and disease through the ages, the conditions for health and disease, and the history of all human activities that tended to promote health, to prevent illness, and to restore the sick, no matter who the acting individuals were.

The medical historian consulting the past will first endeavor to find out what health conditions were in a given society at a given time. Was there much illness or little? What diseases prevailed? Did people die young or did many of them live to a ripe old age? It may be impossible to answer these questions, but we must raise them and must try to find answers to as many as possible.

We know that general health conditions are determined primarily by two factors, geography and economics. We realize that knowledge of a country's geography is as important for the study of medical history as it is for the study of political and economic history. The standard of living of a population, on the other hand, is also responsible to a large extent for the incidence of illness, and from the very beginning we understand the necessity for the medical historian to be thoroughly familiar with the economic and social conditions of the society he is studying.

The individual's illnesses are the result of heredity and environment, and while there is little we can find about the history of hereditary disposition to disease, it is relatively easy to obtain a picture of the physical and social environment in which men lived in different periods of history. We must know how people lived, the rich and the poor, the master and the slave; under what conditions they produced food and commodities, what their housing was, their nutrition, their recreations. We have to borrow heavily from archaeology. The history of disease is of such basic importance that we shall devote a special introductory chapter to the discussion of its problems.

Once we know what the health and disease conditions were in a given country at a given time, we want to know what was done to maintain and promote health and to prevent illness. All peoples acted toward that end consciously or unconsciously. Here we have to consult the history of religion and the history of education. All ancient people had a strongly developed concept of purity. He who entered the temple and appeared in the presence of his god had to be pure; it was a spiritual concept. On the temple of Asclepios in Epidauros was written: 'Pure must be he who enters the fragrant temple; purity means to think nothing but holy thoughts.' [11]

But this spiritual purity had to be documented physically and he who entered the temple had to be washed and dressed in spotless linen. Thus the spiritual, religious concept of purity undoubtedly had great hygienic consequences, which we shall discuss in detail when we come to the Mosaic Code.

Physical education, athletics, and sports were at all times powerful measures in the promotion of health, in the development of a concept of positive health as a joyful attitude toward life. It was the educational ideal much more than medical considerations that determined the status of physical education—in Athens, for instance, the fact that it was included in the *enkyklios paideia.* Large-scale measures of public health, on the other hand, the building of aqueducts, the drainage of swamps, housing projects for large groups of people, can be expected only where there was a state power strong enough to carry out such measures.

The history of hygiene and public health must be approached from two different angles.[12] The more the people knew about the cause, nature, and mechanism of a disease, the more effectively they could interfere in its course and the better they were prepared to prevent it. The history of hygiene and public health, of preventive medicine at large, will therefore always reflect the history of medical science. But medical knowledge must be applied in order to become effective, and whether it was possible to apply such knowledge to the prevention of disease depended on a great variety of non-medical factors: a society's attitude toward the human body, its valuation of health and disease, the religious and philosophical factors that we mentioned before, quite apart from social and economic factors that determined whether hygiene was limited to a small upper class or was shared by large groups of the population, and whether a country could afford public-health institutions or not.

When health has broken down, disease takes hold of an individual. At all times, man reacted against disease and endeavored to restore health, with magic and prayer; by encouraging the use of certain foods and forbidding others; by prescribing vegetable, animal, and mineral substances not usually consumed as food and therefore considered drugs; by heating, cooling, rubbing the parts; by cutting with the knife or burning with the cautery. In other words, we study the history of therapy, of magical, religious, and rational treatments, of dietetic, pharmacological, physical, surgical, and also psychological therapy.

We soon find that the physician's actions originate from two sources, experience and theory. Experience teaches that a special drug or a special treatment are effective, although it may not be possible to explain their action. The knowledge of such a treatment is passed on from father to son, from master to pupil, from one generation to another. It serves the purpose, helps in restoring health, and some day science may suddenly be able to explain it.[13]

On the other hand we find that many actions are the result of views held by physicians and others on the origin and nature of disease. The tendency was always to remove the cause of disease, *causa remota cessat effectus.* And it obviously made a great difference whether disease was considered the result of possession by an evil spirit, punishment for sin by the benevolent deity, a disturbance in the balance of hypothetical humors, or atoms, or in the balance of physical and chemical forces.

Thus we are interested not only in the physician's actions but in the ideas that were guiding him. We study the magical, religious, philosophical, theological, and scientific systems of medicine. Here we investigate not the craft of medicine but its theory; not the practice of medicine, but medical science. We make no evaluations because every theory was correct until it was superseded when more knowledge was gained. Nothing could be more foolish in comparing ancient theories with ours than to call progressive what corresponds to our views, and primitive what is different.

When we investigate the history of medical doctrines, endeavoring not to judge but to understand them, we must try to forget our present medical theories for a moment and place ourselves into the position of the naïve observer. We remember the symptoms of a given disease, pneumonia, malaria, epilepsy[14]—diseases with outspoken symptoms—and we try to find out how the physicians of different periods saw them, what they thought of them, how they evaluated them, and what views they formed on the nature of disease on the basis of their observations and using the concepts of thought available at the time. We must keep in mind the fact that ideas are the result of the entire material and cultural structure of a given period. They are linked up and interwoven with the general philosophy of the time, and nobody can think beyond the framework of his world—or if he does, in his own time he is without influence and following. Long before Copernicus, Aristarchus described the heliocentric system, but Ptolemy's views prevailed.

Medical theories always represent one aspect of the general civilization of a period, and in order to understand them fully we must be familiar with the other manifestations of that civilization, its philosophy, literature, art, music. We soon find that a common denominator, a general trend or style, may be found in all of them. A study of the history of art is particularly enlightening in such investigations because art, being spontaneous, usually expresses a new trend first. A new philosophy, a new attitude of man toward his fellow man and toward the world at large, is frequently felt by the artist before it is formulated in words, and he expresses it in the choice of his subjects and in the style of his creations long before the scientist, who must build upon the accumulated experience of the past, can do it. Thus a study of Michelangelo, Tintoretto, or Bernini may give us a clue for a better understanding and more correct historical interpretation of William Harvey.[15]

If we attempt to see the theories of medicine as products of their time, in their cultural setting, then we understand the religious character of Babylonian medicine. We understand why the Greek physicians interpreted the phenomena of health and disease in philosophic terms. In such light a theory like that of the four humors does not appear fantastic; it was the logical product of the philosophic structure of its time, and besides a very workable theory. We understand why medieval doctors thought in terms of theology and why a new medicine based on the natural sciences developed in the West from the Renaissance on. We understand the significance of the anatomical movement that took place in Europe at the time of the Renaissance, a movement the East never experienced.[16]

This may be the place to discuss briefly the problem of the contribution of the individual to the making of medical history. Medical history, like history at large, is always made by individuals, and just as there have been great philosophers, statesmen, poets, painters, and musicians, there have been great doctors, men of genius, who made discoveries and inventions, paved new ways, became the founders of schools, and are universally worshiped as benefactors of mankind. This is as it should be, because mankind owes a debt of gratitude to the men who contributed to its liberation from the bonds of disease and also because every profession needs heroes, inspiring examples for young people to follow.

History remembers many names and has forgotten many. A strange process of selection takes place. Doctors who were very popular during their lifetime, who had their portraits painted by famous masters and had large-sized engravings made from them, may be completely forgotten today, and when we have to catalogue such a portrait we may have great difficulty in finding out who the man was. Others remained or became famous after their death. They all had to appear before the tribunal of history. Historians, with the advantage of being able to look at events from a distance, examined, interpreted, and evaluated their lives and work.

Some men are remembered as scientists for the lasting contributions they made to medical science, men such as Vesalius, Harvey, Morgagni, Pasteur. Others are remembered not for their discoveries and inventions but because they were great doctors, because in the people's opinion they came closest to the medical ideal of their time, men such as Sydenham, Boerhaave, Osler. Every society has an ideal physician in mind whose characteristics are determined primarily by the social and economic structure of that society and the technical means available to medicine at that time.

Interpretations and evaluations change, and this is why there is no such thing as a 'definitive history.' Brutus appeared to some as a ruthless murderer, to others as a liberator from tyranny. And similarly Paracelsus was sometimes looked upon as a magician and quack and sometimes as a physician of genius.

Nobody will deny the great significance of the part played by the individual in the making of medical history, but we should also remember that the individual is to a large extent the product of his environment. At all times there are potential heroes and villains, potential men of genius. It is the structure of the society in which they live and the historical moment that determine whether they will be able to develop their genius and to what end they will apply it.

We must also keep in mind that discoveries are usually not made by one man alone, but that many brains and many hands are needed before a discovery is made for which one man receives the credit. The very popular hunting for 'Fathers' of every branch of medicine and every treatment is, therefore, rather foolish; it is unfair not only to the mothers and ancestors but also to the obstetricians and midwives.

Vesalius undoubtedly made a great contribution to science and medicine when he published his *De humani corporis fabrica libri septem* in 1543. But he had important precursors; he had a helper in his artist Van Kalkar. The whole period was oriented toward anatomy, and if Vesalius had not completed his manuscript in 1542, Giovanni Battista Canano might have finished his own book.

When William Harvey, in 1628, described the circulation of the blood, he announced an important physiological discovery and, at the same time, inaugurated a method of research, the experimental method with a quantitative approach. Again, he had precursors; the lesser circulation was known if not fully appreciated; his teacher, Fabricius of Acquapendente, had described the valves of the veins. Harvey left a gap in his demonstration because he had not seen the capillaries that Malpighi described later. The whole period was thinking in terms of motion and was experimenting. Harvey had the good luck of having attacked a problem that could be solved with the means available at the time. His contemporary, Santorio, was working along exactly the same lines, experimentally and quantitatively, spending part of his life on scales; but his problem was human metabolism, a problem that could not be solved before chemistry was more advanced.

This does not mean that Vesalius and Harvey should not be given the credit they so richly deserve. They made great and lasting contributions that nobody else had made. Their personalities and work, however, should be studied and appraised in their own setting. Even if we do not accept Hippolyte Taine's theories integrally, we must admit, nevertheless, that the point at which a man lived in space and time, the environment, and the historical moment are of extraordinary importance. A man of the gifts and training of William H. Welch, living as he did from 1850 to 1934, would in all probability have been one good pathologist among many others if he had lived in Germany or some other Western European country. In the United States, at this particular historical moment, he became infinitely more, one of the great organizers of scientific medicine in the country.

I do not mean that we should waste our time speculating what a man would have done if he had lived in another country at another time; this would be a most futile game. What I do mean is that we must never study the individual and his work in isolation but must investigate the forces that acted on him, that shaped his destiny and his creations. The individual then appears as the exponent of these forces, as the representative of a trend, of a school, or of a period. It is possible to trace the development of medical thought in a series of biographies if we are careful in the selection of truly representative individuals.[17]

The history of medicine, however, is infinitely more than the history of the great doctors and their books. Medical science is important, but is wasted unless its findings are applied on a large scale. We should have a completely wrong picture of French medicine in the early nineteenth century if we limited our studies to the great accomplishments of a few clinicians of genius in some Paris hospitals. We must also try to find out what medical services the peasant in the village, the coal miner in the factory town, the millworker in the suburb of the cities received at that time.

It is important for a country to have distinguished medical scientists working in great research centers, because research is the source spring that feeds all other activities. But it is equally important for a country to have a high standard for general practitioners, men who apply the teachings of the great scientists. We therefore must pay much attention to the history of the rank-and-file doctor and of the other medical workers.

We must always keep in mind that medicine is not a natural science, either pure or applied. Methods of science are used all the time in combating disease, but medicine itself belongs much more to the realm of the social sciences because the goal is social.[18] Medicine, by promoting health and preventing illness, endeavors to keep individuals adjusted to their environment as useful and contented members of society. Or by restoring health and rehabilitating the former patient, it endeavors to readjust individuals to their environment. There are other causes of social maladjustment than disease, and other human activities such as education or the administration of the law are directed toward the same end as medicine. They are all very closely interrelated, and medicine actually is but one link in a chain of social-welfare institutions. Our approach to the history of medicine, therefore, cannot be broad enough.

The social character of medicine is also the result of the fact that in all medical actions there are always two parties involved: the medical corps, in the broadest sense of the word, and society; or, in its simplest form, physician and patient, whereby, however, the two meet not only as individuals but also as members of society with obligations toward it.[19]

In consulting the past of medicine, we are interested not only in the history of health and disease, of the physician's actions and thoughts, but also in the social history of the patient, of the physician, and of their relationship. What was the position of the sick man in the various societies? What did disease mean to the individual, how did it affect his life? While there is a good deal of literature on the history of the physician,[20] the history of the patient has been rather neglected.[21] Yet it is very important. The challenge to medicine is different in a society that takes no interest in the sick individual from what it is in one that feels a strong obligation toward him.

The history of the physician has sometimes been distorted when it was written by doctors who had not sufficient historical training and, therefore, were inclined to project present conditions into the past. A conservative historiography sometimes tried to prove that the task of medicine, the physician's profession, and his relation to the patient, had always been the same, in order to demonstrate that there was no reason why there should be any change now or in the future. It goes without saying that such a view is wrong. The task of medicine has broadened considerably in the course of time; the social and economic structure of society has changed, and as a result the social position of the physician, the conditions of his life and work have changed considerably. It obviously made a great difference whether the doctor was a sorcerer, priest, craftsman, cleric, or a scientifically trained social worker; whether he was economically independent from his patients or whether he had to sell his services on the open market to whoever was able to buy them.

We shall have to study these conditions, including medical education and physicians' organizations, guilds, vocational and scientific societies. And we obviously shall not limit ourselves to the physician, but shall extend our studies to cover the history of all medical workers, legitimate and illegitimate.

Not only are we interested in what the physician did to protect and restore health but we want to know under what conditions he acted. Where were patients treated? In the streets, in the homes, in temples, or in hospitals? How easily available were medical services in the cities, in the country? What was the cost of medical care? Was it such that only the rich could afford a doctor? If this was the case, what medical care, if any, was available to the poor?

We shall also pay attention to the precautions a society took in order to protect itself against misuse of the physician's power. At all times society needed the physician and therefore permitted him to possess all the power that the exercise of his profession required. The physician has free access to drugs that through ignorance or malice may become poisons. Physical, chemical, and biological forces of great potency are placed freely into his hands. He enters all homes on the virtue of his profession, is entrusted with secrets the patient would not divulge to anyone else, and which gives him power over the people. From the time of Hammurabi, society tried to protect itself by setting standards for the physician's behavior: by making him liable for damage, in requiring him to prove that he possessed a definite amount of knowledge. This is an aspect of medical history that must not be neglected.

We shall also study the various attempts of society to organize medical services. For a long time, health and disease were considered a private matter of the individual, and it was left to him to seek medical aid if he wished to do so and could afford it. But even in antiquity there were certain groups of people whose health was considered of such importance that the community assumed responsibility for it. This was particularly the case with conscripted armies, and military medicine is perhaps the earliest form of organized medical services. In Buddhist India and the Christian West, compassion and charity were the driving forces of medical organization, and from the time of the late Middle Ages the principle of mutual insurance was applied to the provision of medical care, until the protection and restoration of health became a public service to which the citizen was entitled. The history of these organized services is a very important aspect of the general picture.

Thus the history of medicine is a much broader subject today than it was formerly. Today when we consult the past of medicine we study the history of the various human societies in their social and economic structure and in their struggle against disease. We want to know what their health problems were and what they did to promote health, to prevent illness, to restore health, and to rehabilitate the sick. Furthermore we want to know who the chief actors in this drama were, what they did individually, and what thoughts guided their actions.

THE METHODS

We have discussed what we want to find out when we consult the past of medicine, and we must now examine the various methods we must employ in order to obtain answers to the many questions raised.

The history of medicine, as we said before, is a historical discipline, and the historian of medicine, therefore, proceeds in the beginning like the general historian.[22] He wants to reconstruct an aspect of the past—something that does not exist any more—and in order to know about it he looks for *sources.* What is a historical source?

While taking a walk in the country I find a stone. If this stone does not show any trace of human influence but has merely been washed into my path by the rains, it is of no interest to the historian. It may be an object of scientific research to the mineralogist. It may be a historical record to the geologist who studies the history of the earth. But then the history of the earth, like the history of the universe, or the history of plants and of animals is commonly assigned to the realm of science, and by history proper we mean the history of men living and acting in groups.

My stone, then, becomes a historical source the moment it shows the slightest trace of human influence: a drawing, a sculpture, a few letters carved in, or merely the fact that it has been cut by an instrument. This inert stone has assumed significance to me in that it tells me about something that human beings did in the past. My first task is to describe it as accurately as possible, just as a scientist would describe an object of nature. I shall not only describe it in words but shall have it photographed, and my intention is to make this source available to other historians.

The second task is a strictly historical one and consists of dating the source. I shall try to locate my stone as accurately as possible in time and space. The dating of historical records is sometimes extraordinarily difficult, and history has developed a number of auxiliary disciplines with which the historian must be familiar, such as paleography, the history of ancient writing, and many others. Chronology is the iron foundation of all historical work. It is somewhat out of fashion because the time is not far past when historians were mere chroniclers, and it certainly is more interesting to interpret historical events than to list and classify them. But every interpretation presupposes an accurate dating of sources.

Once I have described and dated my stone, I am faced with a third and most important task, interpreting it as a historical source. What has been done to that stone at a given moment by a human being, and what does it mean? Here I have to mobilize all my sagacity and specialized knowledge. If the signs I perceive on the stone are letters, I must be a paleographer, epigrapher, linguist, or philologist in order to be able to read and understand the text. If they are religious symbols, I must be familiar with the history of religion, and if they are the playful drawing of an artist, I must know art and its history.

This stone is a direct source. What I am holding in my hand is the very object that another individual hundreds, perhaps thousands, of years ago held in his hands when he worked on it. We are two men facing each other, the one who in the past created the document and I, the historian, trying to understand what he did and what he meant by doing it.

The historians of art are the most fortunate of all historians because they work primarily with direct sources and investigate the original creations of artists of the past. A building, a sculpture, a painting, and an engraving are the same today as they were when they were created, and the historian need not consult literature about them but can examine them directly.[23] They may still be serving the purpose for which they were made; and although the choice of subject and the style of a work of art are determined by the period, yet the appeal may be the same today as it was in the past. It is easy for us to see the pyramids of Egypt, and they are as impressive today rising out of the desert as they appeared to previous generations. It is infinitely more difficult to find, reconstruct, and understand ancient Egyptian medicine.

We have direct sources in medical history also. In studying the history of disease we do not depend on literary sources exclusively. We may examine skeletons and mummies for pathological lesions, and the following chapter will show what important results have been obtained by such a method. In these investigations we are applying methods of science to the solution of historical problems.

Another very important group of direct sources consists of the physician's tools. Here we are examining the instruments and apparatuses with which doctors actually worked at a given time. We can handle them as they did, and ascertain what results may be obtained by their use. The history of medicine is to a large extent the history of its tools; this is particularly true in the case of surgery and the surgical specialties. New and improved tools permitted new and more successful operations, and new ideas in surgery called for new instruments. It goes without saying that the history of the surgical instrument is closely related to and must be studied in relation to the general history of technology.[24]

In every field of medicine, scientific and practical, we find such direct sources that throw important light on early developments. Anatomical preparations, such as the wax preparations of Mascagni preserved in Florence and Vienna, are important sources, and so are early physiological apparatuses that can be found in the attics of most European physiological institutes. The history of the microscope from the primitive instruments of Galileo and Leeuwenhoek to the electron microscope of today forms the backbone of the history of pathology during the last few centuries. The history of clinical medicine is inconceivable without the history of its diagnostic instruments: from the thermometer and pulsilogium of Santorio to the stethoscope of Laënnec, the ophthalmoscope of Helmholtz, and the many instruments devised to explore the cavities of the body and make them accessible to the physician's eye, and finally to Roentgen's x-rays.

The chief difficulty we encounter with this kind of source is that the number of objects preserved is not very large and that they are scattered all over the world. An obsolete medical book is still kept in the library; it may be removed to the attic or to the basement but is rarely destroyed. An obsolete surgical instrument, however, is discarded and the metal used perhaps for some other purpose. Books are collected systematically in libraries but medical objects are not; they are the despised stepchildren of museums. Some medical institutions, schools, hospitals, societies, and libraries possess collections of objects, but they are as a rule haphazard, merely containing whatever was presented to that institution. There are very few museums covering the field of medical history systematically and in which the objects are identified and catalogued expertly so that they can be used for purposes of research. Yet there is no doubt that every country should make an effort to have at least one such museum that could serve as a repository for the medical objects of that country and as a center of historical research.[25]

Another group of direct sources is represented by such antiquities of public health as aqueducts, pipe lines, fountains, thermae, and other means of supplying cities with water for drinking and bathing purposes; constructions for the disposal of sewage such as the *cloaca maxima* in Rome; and, of course, hospitals. Many European hospitals can be traced back to the Middle Ages or, at least, to the Renaissance; many are seventeenth- or eighteenth-century structures.

Such material, again, is widely scattered and should, therefore, be collected in photographs. A photograph will obviously never replace the study of the original object, but a photographic index of the antiquities of medicine with references to existing literature would be extraordinarily valuable.

Thus we see that in medical history we have direct sources also, but not many. Most of the questions we raise cannot be answered by examining these alone. If we want to know the incidence of malaria on the Aegean Islands in the fifth century B.C., what was done to combat the disease, and what ideas were guiding the physicians, or if we want to know what influence Vesalius's work had on the development of medicine, we have to consult indirect sources. We do not see the facts or events. All we can hope for is to read about them. We see them in a mirror, the mirror of literature—one that is never quite accurate. We are no longer two individuals facing each other, not I and the man who once suffered from malaria, or the one who treated malaria patients; between us is a third individual, the one who wrote about malaria patients and their treatment. Before I can ascertain the facts, I must find the mirror that reflects them and must decide whether this mirror gives a correct picture or a distorted one.

The chief source of medical history is literature: books, pamphlets, broadsides, articles in journals, inscriptions, and other literary documents. We consult first of all the medical literature in which medical workers wrote about their observations, experiences, ideas, and actions. As we shall see in this volume, the medical literature can be traced far back. Prescriptions and incantations were often long and complicated and, therefore, not easy to remember; yet they lost their virtue unless they were applied literally. Hence they were recorded in writing at an early date, and in all ancient civilizations medical texts are found among the oldest literary documents preserved.

During approximately 4500 years preceding the era of printing, medical like other books were transmitted in manuscript copies. The original that the physician or, under his dictation, a scribe had written was soon lost, and copies were made from copies. Medical books were not written for literary enjoyment but for highly practical purposes, like cookery books or manuals of engineering; and it is easy to understand that the doctor who owned such a book and used it in his practice made changes in it. He added recipes and observations of his own and canceled others that he disliked. Copies were made from such an amended book, and once the process had been going on for a number of centuries it might easily happen that dozens of manuscripts of the same book were very different from one another and from the original book.[26]

I mention this in order to stress that the medical books of antiquity and of the Middle Ages, even more than other books, require an enormous amount of philological work before their content can be fully and safely evaluated. At a time when the poets, philosophers, and other writers of antiquity were available in critical editions, medical texts still had to be used in reprints from Renaissance editions, and many medieval texts have not been published even yet.

The Greek and Roman medical literature preserved is limited and it should therefore be possible to have it published in new critical editions in the near future. The *Corpus Medicorum Graecorum,* launched in 1901 at the first meeting of the International Union of Academies and finally entrusted to the Prussian Academy of Science, is about half a century old by now but is far from being finished. Its completion is perhaps the most urgent project of medical history. It should be extended so as to include collections of fragments and important Latin, Arabic, Syriac, and Hebrew translations.[27]

Similarly the *Corpus Medicorum Latinorum,* published under the auspices of the Puschmann Foundation at the University of Leipzig,[28] could profitably be extended so as to include the anonymous and pseudonymous Latin medical literature of the early Middle Ages that consists almost exclusively of classical material.

The project of a much-needed *Corpus Medicorum Arabicorum* has been discussed repeatedly [29] but without any success, and the plan of a *Corpus of Medieval Scientific Literature in Latin* suggested by Lynn Thorndike [30] did not even reach the stage of discussion.[31] Even if it is not yet necessary to apply fully the strict rules of classical philology to the editing of Oriental texts,[32] there is no doubt that we need better editions of the Arabic medical writers than we possess today. Most Oriental printings are inadequate and besides, many important texts have so far not been printed at all.

The mere preparatory work for a *Corpus Medicorum Arabicorum*, the compilation of a catalogue of manuscripts, comparable to that of H. Diels, would be of great value. A collection of medieval Latin medical writers while undoubtedly highly desirable is probably not quite so urgent. The works of the more important writers were printed during the Renaissance in editions that are far from perfect, to be sure, but the tradition was so much shorter than in the case of ancient books that texts, as a rule, did not deteriorate quite so much. The chief task here will be to publish texts that have not been printed so far and to do this whenever possible in editions based on all extant manuscripts.

Editors of difficult texts in ancient and Oriental languages should make it a rule to add a translation into a modern language to their edition. A translation is an interpretation and no one knows a text more intimately than its editor, who has pondered over every word so that his interpretation should be of particular value.

Our literary sources are supplemented by pictorial sources. From the time of Aristotle biological and medical books were sometimes illustrated. The ancients felt as we do that certain things can be expressed much more clearly in a picture than in words. For thousands of years the identification of plants presented enormous difficulties, as long as there was no uniform and generally accepted nomenclature, and every country and region used different names. Herbals, therefore, were frequently illustrated, and these plant pictures are an interesting source of botanical and pharmacological lore. Similarly, surgical, obstetrical, and later, of course, anatomical books were often illustrated; and in anatomy from the time of the Renaissance pictures were at least as important as texts. With the development of pathological anatomy the demand for illustrations became very great in that field also. Skin diseases are very difficult to describe in words, and colored pictures will reproduce them much more accurately. Many of the new diagnostic methods could not have been developed without the co-operation of artists. What the physician's eye saw through the ophthalmoscope, uroscope, gastroscope, and similar instruments had to be pictured in atlases for didactic purposes, and such pictures are therefore very revealing sources.

When we study the history of individuals who played a part in medicine we are anxious to see them, and we search for portraits. A man's appearance is part of his personality, like his autograph. But if a portrait is to be helpful in our understanding of a man's character, it must be a good portrait, that is, one made from nature by a good artist. Today we have photographs which we know are all made from nature, but there are good and bad photographs also. An interesting new kind of source is being created today by having talking moving pictures made of prominent men. Indeed these films recall an individual in an extraordinarily realistic way, and we wish we had such records of Vesalius or Harvey. Every medical institution of any standing should make it a point to build up a film archive of its distinguished members.

In our historical investigations, medical books represent our chief sources, but we shall also have to consult a great many non-medical books and documents. Such works as Pepys' diary, the memoirs of St. Simon, the letters of Madame de Sévigné are full of information on various illnesses and their treatments as seen from the patient's angle. They tell us better than medical books what disease meant to the individual and how it affected his life. Works of fiction reflect events and views of the time. No physician has ever given a better picture of the plague-ridden city than Boccaccio gave in the introduction to his *Decameron*. The novels of Emile Zola reflect the great influence exerted by the new experimental physiology in a most impressive way.

Medicine is so broad, reaching as it does into every field of human activity and thought, that according to the problem we are trying to solve we may have to consult any type of literature, political manifestoes, law codes, commercial accounts as well as prayer books. And the same applies to pictures and other works of art. Paintings and statues of saints in churches may to us be important sources to the history of the plague.[33] Pictures made without any medical intent, by reflecting the customs of the time, become revealing documents that tell us how physicians dressed or what the leper's costume was; they permit us to look into the sick room, into the room of the woman in childbirth, into the doctor's office, the apothecary's shop, or the barber's bathhouse. We thus obtain information on subjects that are rarely discussed in the literature.

There is, finally, another group of sources that we sometimes may consult profitably, although it must be done with great caution: I refer to the oral tradition. We must remember that oral tradition plays a very important part in the transmission of medicine because so much in it is τέχνη, craft. The physician works not only with his brain but with his hands, in some periods more, in others less; [34] he must not only be learned but skilful. It is very difficult, however, if not impossible, to learn techniques, the proper use of one's hands, or to acquire skills from books. The surgeon at all times learned his craft while serving a master as apprentice. This is the case even today. Surgery was transmitted primarily in a practical way from master to pupil and often from father to son. In certain periods the surgeon was a craftsman who had no general education and was unable to read and write. Thus it may happen that we have no written records of surgery for centuries, but it would be wrong to conclude that there was no surgery at all during such a period. Then, suddenly may come a time when surgeons are university graduates, as was the case in thirteenth-century Italy. These educated surgeons wrote books and we find it difficult to trace the source of their knowledge, which may very well have been the oral tradition.

Ancient traditions are still alive today in many countries. We often forget that our modern scientific medicine reaches only a relatively small group of people; over half the population of the world has no share in it. In India the overwhelming majority of close to 400 million people receive medical services from indigenous practitioners who treat their patients either according to the principles of Ayurvedic or ancient Hindu medicine, or according to the teachings of Unani or Graeco-Arabic medicine, or some other ancient or medieval system. Conditions are very similar in China and other Asiatic countries where the old medical classics are still alive and ancient and medieval medicine is practiced on hundreds of millions of people. The classics of Arabic medicine are still read and followed in Mohammedan countries of North Africa and the Near East.

In such countries we can study the history of medicine not only from books but from life.[35] We can watch the physician of old while he examines or treats a patient and while he compounds his drugs. We can listen to the teacher interpreting the classics and commenting on them. Such studies, however, must be carried out cautiously and critically. We must be aware that not all that an indigenous practitioner does is old. Traditions have not remained pure; some elements of modern medicine have always been taken over, consciously or not.

The same is true for another source that we may have to consult occasionally, medical folklore, or folk medicine. We mentioned before that many patients do not consult a doctor but treat themselves, either because their illness is a minor one, or because no physician is available, or because they cannot afford him or have no confidence in him, whatever the reason may be. We find that particularly among peasant populations old practices and beliefs have persisted with incredible tenacity, surviving the centuries and millennia. Religious and magical treatments are performed unashamedly today following the same ritual that prevailed thousands of years ago, not only in Africa but in Europe and America.

Folk medicine is a big hodgepodge in which primitive lore is blended with reminiscences of views and practices of academic medicine of the past. As a source of medical history it has little value on account of its total lack of chronology, but its study is interesting because it permits us to watch old practices and thus helps us in understanding the past.

In trying to reconstruct an aspect of the past of medicine, we look for sources and investigate them. We act very much like an attorney prosecuting a criminal case. He too wants to reconstruct a historical happening and he is looking for every bit of evidence he can find, direct or indirect, objects connected with the crime, or depositions of witnesses. However, he has the great advantage that the event he wants to reconstruct occurred in the immediate past, in a society of which he himself is a member, while the process we are studying may have taken place hundreds or thousands of years ago, in a totally different world.

Like the attorney we hunt for evidence, for sources. They may be scarce, and in this volume the scarcity of sources will be our chief difficulty. We shall have to mobilize every scrap of evidence and shall have to be very careful not to draw too far-reaching conclusions from the scanty material available.

In some cases, the sources are so scarce that it is impossible to solve a problem. It would be very interesting to know whether cholelithiasis, the gallstone disease, was frequent in antiquity or whether it is a disease of a later civilization caused perhaps by changed nutritional habits. Ruffer mentions having seen one gall bladder that 'undoubtedly contained biliary calculi'; [36] there are a few, very few, passages in Greek medical literature that might be interpreted, although not necessarily, as referring to gallstones; while beginning in the fifteenth century there is plenty of evidence for the incidence of the disease in Europe.[37] It would be wrong to conclude from the lack of sources that the disease was extremely rare in antiquity. There are no sources because there were no systematic dissections of human cadavers with the exception of a short period in Alexandria, most of the literature of which is lost. The disease appeared and seemed to become frequent when autopsies were performed in increasing number, that is, from the fifteenth century on. In other words, this is a problem that cannot be solved with certainty because of lack of sources.

The closer we come to our own time, the more numerous sources are; and in investigating a problem we may be so overwhelmed by the aggregate of sources available that we must make a selection, concentrating our attention on some and discarding others as unimportant. Let us assume that we want to find out what health conditions were in the industrial population of England in the first half of the nineteenth century. The sources are immeasurable and we could spend a lifetime doing nothing but reading them; at the end we should be so confused that we should not know the answer to our question. We must, therefore, make an intelligent selection of sources, not spend years reading every newspaper of the period, every annual report of every factory and the case histories of every hospital, but begin, for example, by analyzing vital statistics, then studying reports to the government, such as that of Chadwick,[38] physicians' monographs, like that of Thackrah,[39] and similar documents. Gradually we shall begin to see the answer to our question, in outline first, but every new source adds color to the picture, and when we have reached the point at which new sources merely confirm what we have found so far, we shall know that we have been on the right track and that the analytical part of our task is nearing completion.

The scientist may charge that by selecting sources we introduce an arbitrary element into our investigation and proceed very unscientifically. This may be true, but the scientist, after all, proceeds in a very similar way. He too selects his problem. When he experiments he asks nature questions just as we put questions to our sources. In animal experiments, he creates artificial conditions and observes how the organism reacts to them. There is a personal, more or less arbitrary element in every human investigation whether scientific or historical.

Once we have found sources that may answer our questions, we analyze and investigate them; and we do so from two different points of view, philological and medical, although the two cannot be separated. A Greek medical book is Greek literature, prose as a rule, sometimes verse. We examine it in respect to form and content. We must date it, determine its authorship, the dialect and style in which it was written, and the literary genre to which it belongs. It obviously makes a difference whether the text is a monograph, a student's notebook, or a medical lecture addressed to a lay audience. We are interested in the school from which this book came, in the general philosophy it reflects, but, being historians of medicine, we are interested first of all in its medical content, and in order to understand and evaluate it we need medical as well as historical knowledge.

It would be very difficult to interpret Galen's anatomical writings correctly without having a rather extensive knowledge of anatomy. How could we identify diseases without knowing them, how evaluate the efficacy of a treatment unless we had medical experience? It is very difficult to visualize an operation unless one has performed it or at least seen it performed. We must always keep in mind what we mentioned once before, namely, that the history of medicine is, first of all the history of a τέχνη, of a craft. While most historical disciplines study events that happened once or creations that are unique, medical history, like the history of other crafts, agricultural and industrial, examines skills, techniques, practical achievements. There is no doubt that Hippocrates and Paracelsus were unique, that every physician was unique, that every book they wrote was unique; but we examine the Hippocratic writings not only as literary documents and a manifestation of fifth-century Greece, but because we want to know what diseases were plaguing the Greeks at that time and what the physicians did to promote health, to prevent illness, and to restore health.

We want to know more: we want to know whether they did a good job or not, whether their observations were correct and their treatments efficacious. Nothing but the medical interpretation of sources will tell us this. Special methods have been devised to this end: a treatment or an operation may be repeated today; [40] the efficacy of an ancient drug may be tested in experiments.[41]

Medical knowledge alone would not permit us to interpret ancient sources correctly. Physicians reading the early classics without historical knowledge have made gross mistakes just as philologists did who had historical but no medical training. The mere nomenclature presents serious difficulties. The meaning of current terms, such as 'diet' or 'diathesis,' changed in the course of time. As long as the concept of disease was different from ours the grouping of symptoms was different.

Thus we see that the interpretation of historical sources of medicine is a difficult analytical process that requires wide experience and profound knowledge, philological as well as general historical and medical.

THE WRITING OF MEDICAL HISTORY

Driven by some insatiable intellectual curiosity, by an overpowering living interest, we have set out to consult the past of medicine, to revive and re-create some of its aspects. We have been hunting for sources, have found them, have analyzed and grouped them. We started out with a vague idea that we used as a working hypothesis. This might have been the conventional view of the subject, one that we shared with many other people, one, however, that left us dissatisfied; so we decided to try to come closer to the truth. Or it was an idea of our own that guided us in our search, but one that we were ready to sacrifice at any time if our findings showed that we were wrong.

As our work proceeded and we examined our sources, we found some of our views confirmed while others had to be amended. The vague picture with which we started out slowly acquired outlines and color. We interrogated the sources until they revealed their secrets, and gradually from separate elements a synthesis was formed in us. Events, people, theories of the past were resuscitated. Now that we know of them, to us they are alive and we experience them. Whatever is alive, every experience, wields influence, an influence that in the beginning does not reach beyond ourselves because we alone know about it. But now, our task as historians is to share our experience with others, to make the result of our labors available to others. To this end we must formulate our experience, the picture of the past that became alive in us and we found to be truthful. We must put it into words, thus giving it literary form. The historical investigator becomes a writer of history, and the writing of history is a creative process, is art.

Like every artistic creation a book of history has a strong personal note. The historian cannot create freely as the poet does. The subject of his narrative is given to him, and the methods of historical research impose an iron discipline upon his imagination. Nevertheless, it is *my* experience that I am passing on, *my* interpretation of history, what *I*, as a result of *my* labors, have come to consider the truth. This is why so much depends on the personality of the historian. The work of a historian of genius will have tremendous persuasive power, while the work of a mere craftsman will pass away without any repercussions.

Lucian was right when he said of history ἔχει τι ποιητικόν,[42] it has a creative element, and this is just the reason why history, the picture we carry in us of our past, is a powerful instrument of life. It determines our actions to a much greater degree than we commonly assume. Benedetto Croce justly begins his treatise on historiography with the proposition that 'every true history is contemporary history,'[43] because it is a living contemporary interest that drives a man to consult the past. This statement may need some explanation.

Like the poet and the philosopher the historian lives as a member of society, and if he is true to his task, aware of his responsibilities, like them he will not stand aloof but on the contrary live in close touch with his fellow men, taking an active part in their struggles, sharing their hopes and fears, their joys and sorrows. The poet is the heart and voice of the group, who spontaneously expresses its emotions and thus stirs, elates, and inspires it. The philosopher is its intellect; he thinks and formulates what others only vaguely feel and puts it into a system. And once the aspirations of the group are formulated and systematized they become conscious and exert a tremendous influence by guiding the people in their actions. The philosophers are the most powerful makers of history. There would be no United States without the philosophers of the eighteenth-century Enlightenment, no Soviet Union without Karl Marx. The historian, similarly, is the memory of the group. He too feels very keenly with the society of which he is a member, and driven by a contemporary living interest he sets out to consult the past and to re-create it in his writings.[44] In doing this he gives the nation its conscience, or, as J. Huizinga so beautifully put it, 'History is the spiritual form under which a culture gives itself an account of its past.'[45] His work is related to that of the philosopher although it is more limited. Every situation in which we find ourselves is the result of certain historical developments and trends of which the people as a rule are not aware. Through historical analysis we are able to make these developments and trends conscious, and as a result a situation that seemed confused becomes clear all of a sudden. We understand it, can face and discuss it openly, and act more intelligently than we could before.

What is true for the historian at large applies to the historian of medicine also. The historian of medicine is a physician, trained in the research methods of history, who takes an active part in the life of his time and is in close touch with the medical problems of his time.[46] He never is a narrow specialist who perceives only limited aspects of medicine, but he tries to see medicine as a whole, not only from the point of view of the medical profession but of society as well. Driven by a contemporary living interest he sets out to consult and re-create the past of medicine.

This, however, means that medical history is not only history but medicine as well, part of the theory of medicine. If general history is an instrument of life in general, then medical history is an instrument of medical life. The picture a physician has of the past of his profession exerts a distinct influence on his thinking and therefore on his actions as well. Traditions always put obligations on us.

It is obvious that a doctor can treat a patient suffering from pneumonia or syphilis or any other disease successfully without any knowledge of general or medical history. The only history he must know is that of his patient. The moment, however, when we plan an anti-venereal disease or anti-tuberculosis campaign, or medical services for rural districts, or whatever it may be—the moment, in other words, when we address our efforts not to a single individual but to a group—we need more historical knowledge. The success or failure of our efforts may well depend on whether we have a correct appreciation of the many social, economic, political, religious, philosophical, and other non-medical factors that determine the situation, an appreciation that we may acquire only as the result of historical analysis.

Medical history teaches us where we came from, where we stand in medicine at the present time, and in what direction we are marching. It is the compass that guides us into the future. If our work is not to be haphazard but to follow a well-laid plan, we need the guidance of history, and it is not by accident that all great medical leaders were fully aware of the value of historical studies.

It is a sheer waste of effort to oppose powerful social trends. Historical analysis reveals that these trends are not accidental but the result of the whole economic and social structure of a given society. We can influence developments and can take an active part in shaping the future—there is no reason for fatalism—but we can do so only in certain directions. And history tells us what these directions are.

From all that has been said, it becomes apparent that medical historians like historians at large have a great responsibility. The writer of a biography re-creates a man. Our present medical students did not know William Osler or William H. Welch. To them Osler is the man whom Harvey Cushing pictured,[47] Welch what Simon and James Thomas Flexner made him.[48]

There are quacks among the historians of medicine, and their actions are just as pernicious as those of other quacks. History must be true. True history is always fruitful while pseudo-history is destructive. It is difficult to approach a problem objectively, but whoever refuses to submit to the discipline imposed upon him by the methods of historical research, whoever writes history uncritically or frivolously, or to prove a thesis, acts like a pseudo-scientist who fakes laboratory reports.

Summing up, we can say that medical history is not only the concern of history, not only an attempt to produce a more complete picture of the history of civilization, but that it is medicine as well, an approach to the problems of medicine. And the medical historian, while serving the truth as a historian, is endeavoring to contribute to the progress of medicine.

NOTES

1. A facsimile edition of Laënnec's own copy, which he had annotated, was published in Paris in 1923.
2. A. Prévost, *La Faculté de médecine de Paris, ses chaires, ses annexes et son personnel enseignant, de* 1794 *à* 1900, Paris, 1900; A. de Beauchamp, *Enquêtes et documents relatifs à l'enseignement supérieur. XXVIII, Médecine et pharmacie. Projets de lois,* 1789-1803; A. Corlieu, *Centenaire de la faculté de médecine de Paris* (1794-1894), Paris, 1896.
3. In 11 volumes including works of Hippocrates, Aretaeus, Alexander, Caelius Aurelianus, Celsus, and Rhazes. In the preface to vol. I Haller makes the characteristic statement: 'Medicis veteribus morborum cognitio potius major fuerit, quam nuperis; eorum signa et praesagia nunquam accuratius, quam a Graecis artis parentibus tradita sunt. Nam etiam post elapsa viginti secula nemo solertiam Hippocratis aut contempsit, aut superavit. Si quisquam nuperorum medicamentorum usu eo sene superior fuit, nemo certe in morborum historia eum acquavit, si communis peritorum sensus audiri potest.' Haller's purpose in preparing a new edition was *veterum medicorum usum discentibus faciliorem reddere.*

4. *Œuvres complètes d'Hippocrate*, I, ix: 'Mon but a été de mettre les œuvres hippocratiques complètement à la portée des médecins de notre temps, et j'ai voulu qu'elles pussent être lues et comprises comme un livre contemporain.'
5. *Collection des médecins grecs et latins, publiée sous les auspices du Ministère de l'Instruction Publique, conformément au plan approuvé par l'Académie des Inscriptions et Belles Lettres et par l'Académie de Médecine.* Only two medical writers were published in this collection, Oribasius (1851-76) and Rufus of Ephesus (1879). The series is dedicated to E. Littré, and in the preface Daremberg states: 'La *Collection des Médecins grecs et latins* doit son origine au désir de répandre parmi les médecins le goût des études historiques et philologiques et de fournir en même temps, pour la constitution de la science, des notions essentielles, mais tombées presque entièrement dans l'oubli.'
6. In a preface to *Die Handschriften der antiken Ärzte*, II. Teil, Berlin, 1906, H. Diels described the origin of the *Corpus Medicorum Graecorum.* No medical man was ever consulted in the matter. There was never any question of translations into a modern language or modern commentaries to the texts, although translations were permitted in the case of Arabic texts.
7. A short sketch of the history of medical historiography is given in Appendix I.
8. H. Diels, *op. cit.*, I. Teil, 'Hippokrates und Galenos,' Berlin, 1905; II. Teil, 'Die übrigen griechischen Ärzte ausser Hippokrates und Galenos,' Berlin, 1906; erster Nachtrag, Berlin, 1908; the catalog lists also Latin, Syriac, Arabic, and Hebrew translations.
9. I have discussed principles and methods of medical history several times in the past, usually at decisive points of my career, first in an inaugural address at the University of Zurich, 'Aufgaben und Ziele der Medizingeschichte,' *Schweiz. med. Wschr.*, 1922, 3:318-22; then in an inaugural address at the University of Leipzig, 'Die historische Betrachtung der Medizin,' *Arch. Gesch. Med.*, 1926, 18:1-19; again a few years later in a paper read before the Eighth International Congress of Medical History in Rome in 1930, 'Probleme der medizinischen Historiographie,' *Arch. Gesch. Med.*, 1931, 24:1-18; and finally in a lecture to the New York Academy of Medicine, 'The History of Medical History,' *Milestones in Medicine,* New York and London, 1938, pp. 163-84. In an open letter to George Sarton, 'The History of Medicine and the History of Science,' *Bull. Inst. Hist. Med.*, 1936, 4:1-13, I tried to show that the history of medicine is not a mere chapter in the history of science but has intrinsic problems of its own.
10. See, e.g. Heinrich Wölfflin, *Kunstgeschichtliche Grundbegriffe,* Munich, 6th ed., 1923; or Josef Strzygowski, *Die Krisis der Geisteswissenschaften vorgeführt am Beispiel der Forschung über bildende Kunst,* Vienna, 1923.
11. ἁγνὸν χρὴ ναοῖο θυώδεος ἐντὸς ἰόντα
ἔμμεναι· ἁγνεία δ' ἐστὶ φρονεῖν ὅσια.
In Porphyrius, *De abstinentia,* II, 19, and also Clemens Alexandrinus, *Stromateis,* V, 1, 13.

12. I developed this idea in a Sedgwick Lecture at the Massachusetts Institute of Technology, 'The Philosophy of Hygiene,' *Bull. Inst. Hist. Med.*, 1933, 1:323-31.
13. Thus, e.g. sunlight was used as a healing agent for centuries; rickets was treated with ultra-violet rays. To the 'scientific' physician this was a mere superstition because until the vitamins were discovered and it was found that sunlight changes the ergosterol of the skin into vitamin D he could not explain the results.
14. See Owsei Temkin, *The Falling Sickness, a History of Epilepsy from the Greeks to the Beginnings of Modern Neurology*, Baltimore, 1945.
15. H. E. Sigerist, 'William Harveys Stellung in der europäischen Geistesgeschichte,' *Arch. f. Kulturgesch.*, Leipzig, 1928, 19:158-68; also 'The Historical Aspect of Art and Medicine,' *Bull. Inst. Hist. Med.*, 1936, 4:271-97.
16. H. E. Sigerist, 'Die Geburt der abendländischen Medizin,' *Essays on the History of Medicine presented to Karl Sudhoff*, Zurich, 1924, pp. 185-205.
17. I once tried to do this, see *Grosse Ärzte*, Munich, 1932 (*The Great Doctors*, New York and London, 1933).
18. See H. E. Sigerist, 'The Social Sciences in the Medical School,' *The University at the Crossroads*, New York, 1946, pp. 127-42; Bernhard J. Stern, *Social Factors in Medical Progress*, New York, 1927; *Society and Medical Progress*, Princeton, 1941; *American Medical Practice in the Perspective of a Century*, New York, 1945.
19. Hans Freyer, 'Der Arzt und die Gesellschaft,' *Der Arzt und der Staat*, Leipzig, 1929.
20. J. H. Baas, *Grundriss der Geschichte der Medizin und des heilenden Standes*, Stuttgart, 1876 (*Outlines of the History of Medicine and the Medical Profession*, New York, 1889); Hermann Peters, *Der Arzt und die Heilkunde in der deutschen Vergangenheit*, Leipzig, 1900; Norman Moore, *The Physician in English History*, Cambridge, 1913; E. D. Baumann, *De dokter en de geneeskunde*, Amsterdam, 1915; Arthur Selwyn-Brown, *The Physician throughout the Ages*, Boston, 1938; Kate Campbell Hurd-Mead, *A History of Women in Medicine*, Haddam, Conn., 1938; and many others.
21. H. E. Sigerist, 'Die Sonderstellung des Kranken,' *Kyklos*, 1929, 2:11-20.
22. E. Bernheim, *Lehrbuch der historischen Methode*, 5th and 6th ed., Leipzig, 1908, and his short *Einleitung in die Geschichtswissenschaft*, Leipzig, 1912; C. V. Langlois and C. Seignobos, *Introduction aux études historiques*, 4th ed., Paris, 1909 (*Introduction to the Study of History*, London, 1912); C. Seignobos, *La Méthode historique appliquée aux sciences sociales*, Paris, 2nd ed., 1909; J. H. Vincent, *Historical Research*, New York, 1911; F. M. Fling, *The Writing of History: An Introduction to Historical Method*, New Haven, 1920; W. Bauer, *Einführung in das Studium der Geschichte*, Tübingen, 2nd ed., 1928.
23. Literary documents may be consulted profitably in order to find out under what circumstances a work of art was created and other similar facts, but such information is not necessary for the esthetic evaluation of the artistic creation.
24. Unfortunately this has rarely been done; see e.g. C. J. S. Thompson, *The History and Evolution of Surgical Instruments*, New York, 1942, or

V. Møller-Christensen, *The History of the Forceps,* Copenhagen and London, 1938, books that are useful repertories but can hardly be called histories.

25. See Appendix III where an attempt has been made to list some of the chief collections of medico-historical objects.
26. A good example of such a practical text that underwent many characteristic changes in the course of the centuries is to be found in 'The Herbal of Pseudo-Apuleius' (ed. E. Howald and H. E. Sigerist, *Corpus Medicorum Latinorum* IV, Leipzig and Berlin, 1927).
27. The *CMG* has occasionally included Arabic and Latin translations when the Greek original was lost, but since translations played a very important part in the history of medicine, and since there are no critical editions available of most of them, it would be very desirable, for philological and historical reasons, to have at least the most important translations included.
28. The widow of the Viennese historian of medicine, Theodor Puschmann (1844-99), left her fortune amounting to about half a million marks to the University of Leipzig as a foundation 'for the promotion of scholarly research in the field of medical history.' The *Puschmann-Stiftung* was formally established 1 January 1905. Small as the amount was—according to American standards—it permitted the creation of a chair of medical history, the Leipzig Institute of the History of Medicine, a journal, a series of monographs, and the *Corpus Medicorum Latinorum.* See *Mitt. Gesch. Med. Naturw.,* 1905, 4:226-7, and following issues.
29. Particularly in the Academy of the History of Science, which from 1930 on had a special Committee for Studies in Arabic Science.
30. 'Prospectus for a Corpus of Medieval Scientific Literature in Latin,' *Isis,* 1930, 14:368-84.
31. These failures are easy to understand when we remember that we live in a world in which research in the humanities, as in any other cultural field not of immediate practical value, is haphazard, planless, and poorly supported financially.
32. Perfectionism has more than once frustrated attempts to edit much-needed Arabic and other Oriental texts. At the present stage of development we can hardly expect perfect texts, but the edition of an important or unknown text, even if it is based on only one or a few good manuscripts, can render invaluable services.
33. See H. E. Sigerist, 'Sebastian-Apollo,' *Arch. Gesch. Med.,* 1927, 19:301-17.
34. B. Farrington, 'Vesalius on the Ruin of Ancient Medicine,' *The Modern Quarterly,* 1938, 1:23-8.
35. H. E. Sigerist, 'The Need for an Institute of the History of Medicine in India,' *Bull. Hist. Med.,* 1945, 17:113-26.
36. Marc Armand Ruffer, *Studies in the Paleopathology of Egypt,* Chicago, 1921, p. 50.
37. G. Muleur, *Essai historique sur l'affection calculeuse du foie depuis Hippocrate jusqu'à Fourcroy et Pujol* (1801-1802), Paris, 1884.
38. E. Chadwick, *Report on the Sanitary Condition of the Labouring Population of Great Britain,* London, 1843.

39. C. T. Thackrah, *The Effects of the Principal Arts, Trades, and Professions, and of Civic States and Habits of Living, on Health and Longevity* . . . London, 1831.
40. I remember Professor Meyer-Steineg in Jena once telling me that he had performed a surgical operation using nothing but ancient instruments or replicas of them.
41. Thus Marguerite Baur tested the efficacy of *spongia somnifera* in animal experiments, *Janus,* 1927, 31:170ff.
42. Quoted from B. Croce, *Theory and History of Historiography,* London, 1921, p. 187.
43. Ibid. p. 12.
44. Arnold J. Toynbee in his extremely stimulating book, *A Study of History* (London, 1934, vol. I, p. 6f.), points out that the historian frequently selects his subject not for its importance but for the wealth and availability of source material. This is true for the mere craftsman but not for the creative historian.
45. J. Huizinga, *Wege der Kulturgeschichte,* Munich, 1930.
46. Karl Sudhoff was a general practitioner until he was fifty years old; Max Neuburger was a neurologist; Charles Singer worked in cancer research in his early days and was an army physician during the First World War. I myself was an army doctor during that war and since then have been active in social medicine.
47. Harvey Cushing, *The Life of Sir William Osler,* London, New York, etc., 1925, 2 vols. (new edition in 1 vol., 1940).
48. Simon Flexner and James Thomas Flexner, *William Henry Welch and the Heroic Age of American Medicine,* New York, 1941.

*

2. Disease in Time and Space

The history and geography of disease are the foundation of all medico-historical work. Indeed, it is the incidence of illness in general and of special diseases in particular that constitutes the health problems of a society. And if we wish to understand the reactions of that society against its diseases we must know of them. In every volume of this work we shall, therefore, have to discuss various aspects of the distribution of disease in time and space. Here in the beginning, however, in an introductory way we must raise and try to answer a few general problems of the history of disease and discuss briefly a few general principles of historic-geographical pathology.

The first question that comes to mind is that of the origin of disease. How old is the phenomenon 'disease'? Is it as old as life itself or is it the result of civilization? Was there a time when everyone lived to a ripe old age and died the physiological death of old age, or was man at all times fettered by the bonds of disease, and if so, to what extent and by what diseases?

THE ANTIQUITY OF DISEASE: PALEOPATHOLOGY

Speculation on the subject leads us to the assumption that disease must be as old as life itself. Why? Because disease is nothing else but life, life under changed circumstances, as Virchow defined it.[1] It is obvious that man at all times suffered accidents that caused wounds and fractures of bones,[2] and we may safely assume that the organism through its innate healing power endeavored to overcome the lesion and to restore the disrupted continuity of its parts.

The human organism is able to adapt itself to widely differing environmental conditions, and we can live safely in the tropics and in the arctic, at sea level and in high altitudes. There can be no doubt, however, that at all times there must have been chemical, physical, or biological stimulations acting on the organism that exceeded its adaptability so that its reactions were no longer physiological but pathological; reactions that to the observer would appear as symptoms of disease. It is also very likely that the phenomenon of parasitism must be very old. All through nature we see plants and animals living at the expense of one another, and there is no reason for the assumption that parasitism might be a recent development.

It is obvious, however, that we cannot be satisfied with a mere speculative answer to the important question of the antiquity of disease and we must try to solve the problem objectively. It can be done because one organ system, that of the bones, survives the centuries and millennia; and bones have been preserved not only of early historic and prehistoric man but also of prehistoric animals.

Since most basic forms of disease manifest themselves in the bones, we should be able to draw far-reaching conclusions from our findings. Bones will not tell us directly whether pneumonia or pleurisy occurred at an early date but they will reveal whether there was such a pathological mechanism as inflammation at that time. And if the bones reacted against certain lesions with inflammation, we are justified in assuming that other organs did too.

Fossil bones early attracted the attention of naturalists. Felix Platter, in the sixteenth century, thought he was describing an early giant human race while he was writing about bones of a fossil elephant,[3] and similarly the Zurich naturalist, J. J. Scheuchzer, in the eighteenth century, depicted bones of a giant salamander that he thought to be the remnants of a man who had been drowned in the Biblical flood.[4]

In 1761 Giovanni Battista Morgagni published his *De sedibus et causis morborum per anatomen indagatis libri quinque,* the foundation stone of pathological anatomy, and in 1774, that is at a time when the new pathology was still in its infancy, the German minister and naturalist E. J. C. Esper described the femur of a cave bear with a considerable tumor that he thought to be an osteosarcoma,[5] which, however, was later found to be the callus following a fracture.[6] Esper himself gave a picture of the broken pelvis of a Pleistocene mammal that had healed with formation of a good-sized callus.[7]

Beginning at this time fossil bones showing pathological changes were described more frequently, by Goldfuss,[8] Cuvier,[9] Clift,[10] and particularly von Walther, who discussed eleven diseased bones of Pleistocene cave bears and lions; [11] also by Schmerling, who examined Belgian material,[12] and by Mayer, who in 1854 reviewed the existing literature on the subject and added the description of twenty-four bones of cave bears and lions with pathological lesions.[13]

With Rokitansky and Virchow, pathological anatomy in the middle of the nineteenth century became the iron foundation of medicine, and since Virchow was not only a pathologist but a distinguished anthropologist as well, he as a matter of course paid much attention to the pathology of fossil bones.[14] From the middle of the century on, anthropologists and paleontologists were equally interested in the subject, and the number of publications increased considerably.[15] In our time, 'the science of the diseases which can be demonstrated in human and animal remains of ancient times' became a special field of investigation, very aptly named *Paleopathology*,[16] one to which various distinguished scientists devoted their life work, notably the American anatomist and anthropologist, Roy L. Moodie,[17] who in 1923 published the first comprehensive book on the subject.[18] Monographs had been written before, but their scope was usually limited to a discussion of the materials of a given country or collection,[19] while Moodie's book covered the entire field, analyzing and presenting the work of the predecessors and adding the author's many original observations. The book greatly stimulated studies in paleopathology. Moodie himself from 1923 to the time of his death in 1934 contributed valuable papers and monographs.[20] An American pathologist, Herbert U. Williams,[21] worked along similar lines, and we shall have to say more about his studies when we discuss the antiquity of syphilis. In 1930 a French army physician, Léon Pales, published a monograph which like that of Moodie covers the entire field. This is the most recent comprehensive presentation of the subject, a well-organized, thoughtful book with a most valuable bibliography.[22]

Paleopathology began with the examination of bones. Bones and teeth are still the most important materials we possess, because they have been preserved in relatively large numbers, from far remote periods and from various sections of the globe. The early investigators could not do more than examine bones macroscopically, and while certain bone lesions are so characteristic the diagnosis cannot be missed, others are rather ambiguous. Bones buried in the earth for centuries are, moreover, exposed to the action of roots, rodents, and bacteria, as a result of which erosions or other changes may appear that look like pathological lesions.

Today it is possible to examine the histology of fossil bones with the microscope. The bone is fixed in formaldehyde and then is decalcified, whereupon sections are made, stained, and embedded in celloidin. Other sections may be made by grinding.[23] The microscopic examination permits a much more precise diagnosis than would be possible otherwise. But by far the greatest technical advance was made when radiology began to be used in the examination of anthropological and paleontological materials. In 1925 the Field Museum of Natural History in Chicago established a Division of Roentgenology, thus inaugurating a new departure in museum practice and technique. Moodie, who in 1923 had only a few x-rays in his book, and rather poor pictures at that, was able to publish in 1931 *Roentgenologic Studies of Egyptian and Peruvian Mummies* from the Field Museum [24] with superb x-ray photographs that revealed many disease conditions. The roentgenological examination, moreover, has the great advantage that it permits the investigator to examine bones without destroying them and to inspect mummies without unwrapping them.

We just mentioned mummies and it is time to discuss this other rich source of ancient pathological evidence. From no other country have so many remains of deceased mankind come down to us as from Egypt. Climate, soil, religious beliefs, burial customs, all contributed toward the earth's preserving what had been entrusted to it. The examination of skeletal remains for pathological lesions was undertaken at the end of the last century by R. Fouquet [25] and ten years later, on a much larger scale, by G. Elliot Smith and F. Wood Jones, who measured and investigated thousands of skeletons from Nubia.[26] They found many evidences of disease within the limitations imposed by the material, which consisted of bones exclusively.

G. Elliot Smith, who examined and catalogued the royal mummies in Cairo [27] and devoted a great deal of work to a study of mummification,[28] was fully aware of the fact that the microscopic examination of mummified tissues would yield important results, and he occasionally turned over parts of organs to his medical friends.[29] One of them, Marc Armand Ruffer, a brilliant and lovable medical administrator, professor of bacteriology in the Cairo Medical School, developed the methods for examining mummies and became one of the foremost pioneers in the field of paleopathology. From 1909 to the time of his tragic death in 1917,[30] he wrote a series of splendid papers, most of which were collected after his death and published as a volume under the title, *Studies in the Paleopathology of Egypt*,[31] one of the great classics of the subject.

In order to appreciate what we may expect from a histological examination of mummies, we must be familiar with the Egyptian methods of embalming. This is the more necessary because medical historians for a long time assumed that the custom of embalming the dead resulted in a profound knowledge of human anatomy.

We possess two ancient descriptions of the Egyptian process of embalming, one by Herodotus (5th century B.C.) and one by Diodorus Siculus (1st century B.C.). The best we can do is to quote a few passages from them. Herodotus tells us[32] that embalming was practiced as a special craft and that three methods, varying in thoroughness and price, were in use in his time. The costliest was the following:

> First they draw out the brain with an iron hook, at least part of it, the rest they extract by injecting drugs. Next, they make a cut along the flank with a sharp knife of Ethiopian stone and remove all the intestines, whereupon they cleanse the cavity rinsing it thoroughly with palm wine and, in turn, with pounded aromatics. After this they fill the belly with pure ground myrrh and cassia and all sorts of other spices, except frankincense, and sew it up again. Having done this they embalm the body placing it in natron for seventy days. It is not permissible to embalm it for a longer space of time. When the seventy days are passed they wash the corpse and wrap the whole of it in bandages of fine linen cloth, smeared over with gum, which the Egyptians generally use instead of glue. It is then returned to the relatives who enclose it in a wooden case made in the shape of a man. Having fastened the case, they keep it safe in a sepulchral chamber upright against the wall. This is the most costly method of embalming the dead.
>
> Those who choose the middle way, desirous to avoid extravagant costs, are prepared as follows: Syringes are filled with cedar oil which is then injected into the dead man's belly. No incision is made nor are the bowels removed, but the oil is injected through the anus and is prevented from returning, whereupon they embalm the body for the prescribed number of days. On the last day they allow the oil they had injected to escape, and such is its power that it brings out the inner parts and bowels all dissolved. The natron has eaten away the flesh and so nothing is left of the dead body but the skin and the bones. Having done this, they return the body without taking any further trouble.
>
> The third method of embalming used by the poorer people is as fol-

lows: They cleanse the belly with a purge, embalm the body the seventy days and then return it to be taken away.

Four and a half centuries later Diodorus gave a similar description of the process of embalming.[33] He too knew of three classes of burial and wrote that the cost of the first was one talent of silver, of the second twenty minae, while the third was very cheap indeed. Unlike Herodotus, however, he did not describe the methods in any detail and seems to have had only a vague knowledge of them, as becomes easily apparent from the following passage:

> The so-called embalmers are held worthy of every honor and consideration. They associate with priests and enter the temple without hindrance as pure people. When they have gathered to treat the body after it has been cut open, one of them thrusts his hand through the cut into the cavity and takes everything out except kidneys and heart; another cleanses every single intestine rinsing it with palm wine and aromatics. In general, they treat the whole body for over thirty days, first with cedar oil and some other substances, then with myrrh and cinnamon and spices which have the faculty not only of preserving it a long time but also of rendering it fragrant.

These undoubtedly are important documents, but we must keep in mind that both are very recent, written at a time when Egyptian civilization had completed its course and old traditions were continued by the force of inertia and not necessarily in their pure form. If we wish to know what methods of embalming were used a thousand or two thousand years before Herodotus, we must dissect and analyze mummies from these periods. This was done by Thomas J. Pettigrew as early as 1834,[34] and in more recent time by G. Elliot Smith and his co-workers, and by many others.[35] While the methods of embalming varied to a certain extent in the various centuries and the process was more or less elaborate according to the rank of the deceased, the principle remained much the same. First the organs were removed from the body,[36] whereupon body and organs were kept for seventy days in a pickling solution, the νάτρον of Herodotus.[37] After that time the organs were sprinkled with sawdust of aromatic woods, shaped roughly so that they would resume more or less their original form, wrapped tightly in linen, and thoroughly dried. The organs were then either kept in canopic jars or, as was the custom during the XXIst Dynasty, put back into the cavities of the body.[38] Whatever space was left was filled with sawdust, linen, or mud. The wound was left open, or covered with a plate, or infrequently closed with a ligature and the whole body was then enveloped in bandages. This was the basic and relatively simple process; the rest was decoration, which in the case of a king could assume considerable proportions.[39]

Whatever method was used in particular, there are two general conclusions that we may draw. One is that the custom of embalming did not provide opportunities for anatomical studies. The organs were extracted through a relatively small opening in a rough and brutal manner. They are frequently found mutilated; and the embalmers, moreover, were uneducated craftsmen. They had some anatomical knowledge to be sure, the same kind of knowledge that the butchers and cooks had, or the priests who sacrified animals to the gods, but not more.

The other conclusion we may draw is that the organs of mummies are preserved well enough to permit microscopic examination. To that end the mummified tissues must be softened, they must be restored to original size and consistency, and artificial coloring matter must be extracted. Ruffer found that he had best results when he placed tissues in a stock solution containing alcohol 30 cc., water 50 cc., 5 per cent carbonate of soda solution 20 cc.[40] We can well imagine what his feelings must have been when for the first time he saw the striation of voluntary muscular fibers and the nuclei of cells from the body of an individual who had died eight thousand years before.[41]

Mummies have been found not only in Egypt but also in America, notably in Peru, and as early as 1904 an American anthropologist, H. H. Wilder, described methods for the examination of dried tissues.[42] The experience gained with the rich Egyptian material was a stimulus and benefited American archaeology. The pathology of pre-Columbian America, however, belongs to a totally different period of history, and will therefore be discussed in a later volume of this book.

To the examination of bones and mummies we must add a third method that may sometimes be used when the others fail, namely, the interpretation of early works of art.[43] It is not an ideal method because works of art are indirect sources, the interpretation of which is often difficult and very uncertain, and because the early material available is very limited. But we have recourse to it to fill in gaps taking advantage particularly of the rich findings of Egyptian archaeology.

The question now arises: What are the results of paleopathology? Examining human and animal remains of early historic and prehistoric times, do we find evidences of disease? If so, of what diseases? And how far back can we trace a disease? We shall survey the field briefly, beginning with the diseases of bones, articulations, and teeth, and adding observations made on other organs such as have been preserved in Egyptian mummies.

Beginning with *disturbances in development and metabolism*, we find that deformations are not rare in our material. A deformity of the skull attributed to hydrocephalus was found in an Egyptian mummy of the Roman period. It was that of an individual of about thirty years of age whose brain condition had also caused a partial hemiplegia as evidenced by the atrophy of the bones of the left side.[44] Spina bifida usually causes the early death of the newborn infant but cases of occult open spine are found in adults, and Pales has described an open sacrum from neolithic France.[45] He also found in the same Collection Prunières at the Muséum in Paris a neolithic femur of an individual who in all probability suffered from a congenital dislocation of the right hip.[46] Talipes equinovarus or congenital club foot was no rarity in Egypt. Siphtah, one of the kings of the XIXth Dynasty, had one,[47] and individuals affected with this deformity have been depicted frequently on the walls of tombs.[48]

Dwarfs in ancient Egypt have been the subject of a number of studies. They were then popular with the courts just as they were in Rome, in the Middle Ages, and in the Renaissance. Most of them were not cretins but intelligent little fellows, witty and strong. They owed their condition to a strange disease of still unknown origin, chondrodystrophia fetalis or achondroplasia, a disease of the cartilage during fetal life as a result of which the endochondral ossification stops while periosteal bone formation continues. Such infants are born, therefore, with very short legs and arms but large skulls and normal muscles. An excellent example of the kind was Chnoum Hotep, whose limestone statuette was found at Sakkara. He lived at the time of the Vth Dynasty, held an important position at court, being 'Chief of the Perfumes' or 'Head of the Wardrobe,' and must have acquired wealth and prestige because his tomb was one of the finest in a very exclusive burial ground. There can be no doubt about the diagnosis, because the features and the expression of the face are highly characteristic. There are records of many more such achondroplastic dwarfs but not all of them succeeded in making so brilliant a career. It seems that their chief occupation in the household of an Egyptian nobleman was the care of pet animals and the care and making of jewelry.[49] Dwarfism of a different kind seems to be evidenced by a skull of the XVIIIth Dynasty that Seligman diagnosed as being that of a cretin.[50]

At this place, we may mention a disease first described in 1876 by Paget as osteitis deformans, now usually referred to as Paget's disease. It is a disease of mature and old age and is characterized by a thickening and at the same time softening of the bones of the extremities and of the skull, with resulting typical deformities, leontiasis of the skull, and bent extremities. In 1929 Pales described a neolithic femur from the Lozère which macroscopically and in x-ray pictures shows the characteristic features of Paget's disease.[51]

Atrophy of the bone due to old age, senile osteoporosis, cannot be called a disease. It is a normal occurrence and is, therefore, frequently encountered in ancient remains. Its degree permits the investigator to determine the age of a skeleton. Atrophy may also result from pressure. Elliot Smith found numerous skulls with strange, large symmetrical depressions of the parietal bone. The fact that these skulls invariably belonged to Egyptians of the upper classes led him to the assumption that the deformity might have been caused by the pressure of heavy wigs.[52] A rather strange symmetrical osteoporosis, notably of the parietal and frontal bones of the skull but extending often to the occipital and sometimes also to the temporal bones and sphenoids, has been found frequently in American skulls, and Williams made a special study of it without being able, however, to determine the nature of this condition.[53]

It is not limited to American material but has also been described as occurring in skulls of neolithic France,[54] Egypt, and particularly Nubia,[55] as well as a few other places,[56] although never to the extent in which it occurred in America and notably Peru. It affected all ages but chiefly young individuals. Syphilis [57] and rickets [58] were thought to be responsible for this condition, but it is also possible that it was due to pressure. Wood Jones thought of pressure caused by the carrying of heavy jars. But for thousands of years, all over the Near East women have carried heavy weights on their heads, apparently without osteoporosis's being caused. Williams thought 'that the pressure produced on the occiput of the Indian baby resting on a head board would tend to create a venous hyperemia in the parietal and frontal regions, the venous outlets for the posterior region being impeded.' Such a hyperemia combined with other factors could cause osteoporosis and would be responsible for its localization.

Another disease that affects young children and leaves definite marks in the bones is *rickets.* There is very little evidence for the occurrence of the disease in prehistoric and early historic times. Not a single body has ever been found in Egypt that could have been diagnosed with any certainty as having been affected with rickets, although the number of children's bodies preserved is large.[59] There are a few wall paintings representing bowlegged individuals that may be interpreted as an indication of rickets,[60] and the mummy of a baboon examined by Poncet,[61] but this is about all.[61a] Hrdlička was very outspoken in declaring that rickets was unknown in pre-Columbian America.[62] This lack of evidence is not astonishing when we remember that rickets is a deficiency disease that develops when children are not sufficiently exposed to the ultraviolet rays of the sun, under the influence of which vitamin D is formed. In Egypt as well as in tropical America, young children were kept nude most of the time and there was no lack of sunshine. Rickets is primarily a disease of the city slums and of the North. It is not astonishing, therefore, that Carl Fürst found traces of the disease in neolithic bones of Denmark and Norway.[63]

The counterpart of rickets in adults, particularly women, is *osteomalacia,* a disease that usually begins during pregnancy and like rickets leads to a decalcification of the bones with resulting deformities. The cause of the disease is different from that of rickets and is still rather uncertain. Fossil bones of various animals, a cave bear,[64] a quaternary carnivore,[65] and even one from the Eocene,[66] have been found that are unusually light, poor in calcium, and show deformities that suggest osteomalacia. The changes, however, are not characteristic enough to warrant a definite diagnosis. It is impossible, on the other hand, not to recognize the symptoms of *acromegaly,* a disease caused by increased activity of the anterior lobe of the pituitary body. Greatly enlarged bones of the face, hands and feet with exostoses, combined in many cases with gigantism, provide a very typical picture. A case of neolithic acromegaly from Switzerland has been described by O. Schlaginhaufen,[67] but his diagnosis has been contested and must remain uncertain since it is based on the examination of an incomplete femur only.

So far we have discussed diseases with anatomical changes in the bones that are due primarily to disturbances of development or of metabolism. We now must examine another group of diseases that may also affect the bones and must be considered basically as *defenses of the body against injury.* The human body is constantly exposed to a great variety of physical, chemical, and biological injuries. It is invaded by plant and animal parasites, which live and thrive at its expense. But nature has endowed it with powerful defensive forces. It is able to ward off foreign bodies, to destroy parasites, to repair wounds. Paleopathological studies are particularly important in this field because it is generally assumed that these defense mechanisms have been developed and perfected gradually,[68] and it would be interesting if we were able to ascertain at what point of development they first occurred and in what form.

The human body has a number of physiological mechanisms available for its protection. Bad food is ejected from the stomach through vomiting. Sneezing and coughing protect the respiratory tract from foreign substances. But the human body possesses in addition a number of pathological mechanisms that begin to act once an injury has taken place. The chief mechanisms of this type are inflammation, fever, the production of immunity, and repair. In examining ancient human and animal remains, we must discard fever, which does not leave any anatomical changes behind. The production of immunity is also difficult if not impossible to trace. Immunity is bound to the blood and we could think that enough of it might be preserved in mummies to permit serological tests. Experiments have been made in an attempt to obtain precipitation and anaphylactic reactions,[69] but the results have been far from satisfactory. We must remember that Egyptian bodies were kept in brine for a long period of time so that the mummies contained scarcely any dried blood.[70] Williams recommended that serological tests be undertaken on mummies that have not undergone the process of embalming and have only been dried, but recent investigations inaugurated by W. C. Boyd and L. G. Boyd have demonstrated the possibility of determining blood groups in Egyptian mummies from muscular and bony tissue.[71]

Thus the only defense reactions we may expect to find in bones and mummies are inflammation and repair. We are justified in expecting them because if the injury was serious enough both processes cause permanent and characteristic changes in the anatomical structure.

In the bone, inflammation may have its seat in the periosteum or in the marrow. In the first case the disease is called *periostitis*,[72] in the latter *osteomyelitis*. If the inflammation resides in the marrow of the spongious parts of the bone, the name *osteitis* is frequently used. The disease may begin in the periosteum and spread to the marrow or vice versa, so that after a while the whole bone is involved. It is no exaggeration to say that the great majority of all pathological changes found in early human and animal bones are the result of inflammatory processes.

Periostitis is often caused by an injury such as a blow. In minor acute cases the periosteum merely thickens, but if the process becomes chronic a periostitis ossificans develops. The periosteum produces new bone, which adheres to the surface of the old bone, and as a result the normally smooth surface appears rough and rugged. Many such bones have been found, in Egypt,[73] in neolithic Europe,[74] in remains of cave bears,[75] and, much earlier, in the arm bones of a mosasaur from the Cretaceous of Kansas.[76]

Osteomyelitis, too, seems to have been a frequent occurrence not only in man but in fossil animals. Moodie described a posterior dorsal spine of a Permian reptile, probably Dimetrodon, that shows signs of a fracture that was followed by osteomyelitis.[77] The microscopic examination revealed the characteristic cavities which during the animal's life were undoubtedly filled with pus. It is interesting to encounter the disease at such an early period of the history of the earth, long before the advent of man. Osteomyelitis today is always caused by bacterial infection—by staphylococci, as a rule, but other bacteria, the pneumococcus, the typhoid bacillus and others may likewise be responsible. The bacteria either invade the marrow directly, as in the case of an infected compound fracture, or they are carried through the bloodstream from some primary focus of infection. It is not astonishing that the early reptiles suffered fractures, but it is noteworthy that some of these fractures led to conditions that today we know to be the result of infection.

Osteomyelitis has also been found in bones of Pleistocene animals, the bison,[78] the cave bear,[79] and various carnivores.[80] It existed in ancient Egypt[81] and in neolithic Europe.[82] The mastoid disease, an osteitis that occurs as a complication of the inflammation of the middle ear, was frequent in Egypt and Nubia[83] and also occurred in pre-Columbian America.[84]

We now must discuss a group of chronic inflammatory diseases that affect the joints, and include the various types of arthritis deformans or spondylitis deformans, as the disease is called when it is localized in the spinal column. Etiology and pathogenesis are not too clear even today, and every pathologist seems to have his own theory and nomenclature.[85] This obviously is not the place to enter into a critical discussion of modern theories, particularly since isolated ancient bones are hardly a fit object for sharp differential diagnoses. Suffice it to say that we are using here the term arthritis deformans generically, meaning a group of chronic diseases of the joints of different origin, in the course of which the joints become enlarged, produce new bone, thus creating deformities, and with a tendency to ankylosis, a condition under which the joint has become completely rigid.

The arthritic diseases are today among the most disabling and crippling diseases,[86] and paleopathology teaches us that this was the case thousands and millions of years ago. Under the most varied climates, under the sun of Egypt, in the caves of neolithic France, in the mountains of Peru, people of all ages, but particularly people of mature and old age, suffered atrocious pains in their joints and felt their spine, their hip, or knee stiffening gradually until they could hardly move. They were crippled and helpless unless their neighbors attended to them. The material is so vast that we cannot possibly list all of it and therefore we will merely point out a few examples.

Numerous cases of arthritis and particularly spondylitis have been found in Egypt, from Nubia to the Delta, from 4000 B.C. to the Roman era.[87] Men of all races, Egyptians, Negroes, Asiatics, were equally subject to the disease. There has been much speculation why it was so prevalent in Egypt. Climate, mode of living, 'dabbling in the water of the Nile,'[88] have been held responsible. Explanations changed with the theory that happened to be fashionable at a given time. Today it is believed that many cases of arthritis develop from a primary infectious focus, following a tonsillitis or a dental infection. The Egyptians suffered from pyorrhea, to be sure, and certainly had tonsillitis at times, as well as other infections, but so have other nations. Everybody, everywhere, suffers frequently from minor infections, and we should admit that we still know very little about the etiology of arthritis.

In neolithic Europe also the disease was by no means rare, and bones with arthritic changes have been described particularly from France,[89] England, Germany, and the Scandinavian countries.[90] The disease can be traced back to paleolithic remains[91] and still further back to some of the earliest known human skeletons of the Neanderthal race.[92]

Arthritis deformans, moreover, was one of the early diseases to occur frequently in animals. Moodie, who collected the available evidence, described arthritic deformations in dinosaurs, in mosasaurs, in Eocene mammals, in a Miocene crocodile, a Pliocene camel, and in Pleistocene mammals.[93] The disease was so persistently found in remains of cave bears that a special name was coined for it, i.e. 'cave gout,' the *Höhlengicht* of Virchow.[94] Chronic arthritis is still a frequent disease of wild animals.[95]

Inflammation, as we know it, is a defense reaction of the organism to an injury that, as a rule, is caused by bacteria or at any rate by pathogenic micro-organisms. If this is true today and if we find in bones of fossil animals and early man the same anatomical changes that we see develop in inflammatory diseases today, we may be justified in assuming that the causative agent was the same then as it is now. In other words we have good reasons to believe that bacteria caused the osteomyelitis of the Peruvian reptile and the periostitis of the mosasaur, which we mentioned before. But again we should prefer to see these bacteria rather than merely conjecture about their existence.

Bacteria have been found in very early rocks; as a matter of fact, they are among the earliest forms of organic life. Walcott described a micrococcus he discovered in Algonkian rocks [96] that looks very much like bacteria we know today. Renault's classical studies on the micro-organisms of coal [97] revealed the existence of numerous types of bacteria, from the Devonian to the Jurassic, in petrified feces of fishes and reptiles, in stomach content, in the teeth and jaws of fossil vertebrates. Ruffer was able to demonstrate gram-positive and gram-negative bacteria in Egyptian mummies.[98]

The interpretation of these early bacteria presents considerable difficulties. Were they parasitic or not, pathogenic or not? Very few species of bacteria are pathogenic, and there is no reason at all for assuming that those early pre-Cambrian micro-organisms or those found in coal did in any way cause diseases, even if some of the latter may have been parasitic. Some may have been bacteria carrying out the normal and important function of decay. In the case of mummies it is almost impossible to decide whether bacteria found in a dried tissue had invaded the individual while he was alive or whether they developed later in the mummy. Nevertheless, in view of the fact that the mechanism of inflammation was apparently the same in fossil animals, prehistoric and early historic man, as it is in animals and man today, and that bacteria did occur at all and even before the Cambrian period, we may be permitted to conclude that the injury that caused inflammation was due to infection then as it is now.

The inflammatory diseases we have discussed so far were not specific, that is, they were diseases that could be caused by different agents. But then there are specific inflammations caused by one species of bacteria and no other. Such a disease is *tuberculosis.* We know that it occurred in Greek and Roman antiquity and in ancient India. Did it occur earlier and when do we encounter it for the first time?

Tuberculosis of the lungs has never been found in Egyptian mummies, but the number of lungs examined so far is exceedingly small. Tuberculosis, however, also attacks the bones and joints where we should be able to trace the disease more easily. The tuberculous osteomyelitis usually begins in one of the short bones or in the ends of the long bones. It spreads, attacks the joints, softens and destroys the bone, and thus causes deformities. When it is localized in the spine, it may destroy a number of vertebrae, whereupon the spine caves in under the weight of the body with the result that the patient becomes a hunchback. Percival Pott described the disease in 1779 [99] and it was subsequently named after him.

A number of bones, Egyptian and Nubian, with deformities that seemed almost certainly due to tuberculosis, were described by Derry and others.[100] Still, one was never quite sure. There was no hope of finding tubercle bacilli because they disappear rapidly after the patient's death. All the more important became a mummy that was investigated and described by Elliot Smith and Marc Armand Ruffer in 1910.[101] It is the mummy of a young man, a priest of Ammon who lived under the XXIst Dynasty (*c.*1000 B.C.). A chronic inflammatory process had destroyed the first lumbar and the lower three or four dorsal vertebrae. An angular curvature had resulted, the deformity of Pott's disease. Now, a characteristic feature of this process is that the tuberculous material burrows under the sheath of the psoas muscle and causes an abscess there. Our authors found in their mummy signs of a far-reaching destruction of the right psoas muscle and also found that a cavity had developed between muscle and bone. This makes the diagnosis as certain as such a diagnosis can be.

In the light of this evidence we feel much more confident in considering Derry's skeletons as tuberculous, and the disease actually seems to have occurred in Egypt as early as the predynastic period, before 3000 B.C. It probably was not rare. In a cemetery near Dakka on the Nile, ten predynastic skeletons were unearthed, four of which showed the signs of Pott's disease. In one tomb were both husband and wife who had succumbed to the 'white plague.' Another tomb contained the skeletons of two adult males and of a boy of nine years of age. One adult and the boy had typical destructions of the spine.[102] We also feel justified in diagnosing a statuette from the predynastic period found in the desert near Assuan as representing a case of Pott's disease.[103] Not only is the hump characteristic, but the highly emaciated body with the outstanding ribs points to tuberculosis. What contributing factors were responsible for the occurrence of the disease, poor living conditions, hard labor, malnutrition, or whatever it may be, is a matter of speculation. The material is too scanty to permit any conclusions.

While it seems quite certain that tuberculosis did plague the Egyptians from the earliest times on, we still feel uncertain about neolithic Europe. A number of bones have been considered tuberculous, particularly by French anthropologists,[104] but they have all been contested at some time or other. The only material I know of that may be considered evidence for neolithic tuberculosis is the skeleton of a young adult found at Heidelberg and described by Bartels.[105] The spine shows an almost complete destruction of the fourth and fifth dorsal vertebrae with resulting kyphosis and some scoliosis. This may well be Pott's disease, as Bartels thought, but even this case has been contested, and so able a paleopathologist as Williams expressed doubts and felt that the destruction might be the result of an impacted fracture.[106] Yet it would be very interesting to know whether tuberculosis did occur at this early time. With the material available at present, however, the question has to be left open.

Everybody agrees that tuberculosis did occur in the ancient Mediterranean world, but the antiquity of another specific disease, *syphilis*, presents one of the most controversial problems in the whole history of disease. For centuries historians and physicians have been debating, with good arguments on both sides, whether syphilis was indigenous to America and was brought to Europe by the sailors of Christopher Columbus, whereupon it would have spread to other continents, or whether the disease existed in Europe before the end of the fifteenth century, and possibly since remote antiquity. The question is obviously very important in the case of a disease that is contagious, renders people seriously ill for a long time, and has dire social consequences. This is not the place to discuss the whole controversy over the origin of syphilis,[107] and we must limit ourselves to its paleopathology, from which we might expect results, since syphilis, like tuberculosis, manifests itself in the bones. The difficulty is that while some syphilitic changes in the bone are highly characteristic, others are not. Most typical are the changes caused in the skull by a gummatous periostitis and osteitis; bone is destroyed and new bone is formed with the result that the surface of the skull is uneven, bumpy, of a 'worm-eaten' appearance. Whoever has seen such a skull will never forget it. But then there are other non-gummatous syphilitic inflammations of the skull and of the long bones that produce a thickening of the bone, osteophytes, scars in the marrow, changes that are not characteristic enough to warrant a diagnosis of syphilis with certainty. Matters are complicated still more by the fact that yaws, a tropical disease, produces changes extraordinarily similar to those of syphilis.

Many bones from various countries and periods have at some time or other been described as being syphilitic. In 1932 Herbert U. Williams published an enlightening survey of the entire material, and his conclusions are most convincing.[108] The present status of the problem is briefly as follows:

Ruffer repeatedly wrote that no evidence of syphilis had ever been found in Egypt,[109] and this was confirmed by Elliot Smith and the other investigators of Egyptian material. The erosions of the predynastic skull of Roda that Lortet and Gaillard considered to be syphilitic[110] were found to have been caused post mortem by rodents or beetles.[111] A femur and tibia described by Michaelis[112] might be syphilitic, although not necessarily, but their origin is not quite certain. They were in the Hunter Collection of the Royal College of Surgeons in London and were supposedly Nubian, dating from around 1000 B.C., but their history also is not too well known. If syphilis had existed in ancient Egypt, evidence of it would have been found not in one but in many bones. Elliot Smith alone examined over 25,000 Egyptian skulls, and thousands were examined by other investigators, but not one syphilitic skull was found. I think that the Egyptian material that has been scrutinized so far is large enough to permit the conclusion that syphilis was nonexistent in that country—a fact that is very important. Syphilis has in many respects the character of a tropical disease. If it had occurred in antiquity in Mediterranean Europe, it would have occurred in Egypt also; it would probably have come to the West from Egypt or via Egypt. If the disease had plagued the Egyptians, it would undoubtedly have spread from there to Palestine, Mesopotamia, and Crete; the Greek mercenaries of Psammetich would have brought it home, because syphilis, once it has a foothold in a country, does not remain there but travels with man and his urge, with the prostitute that follows the armies, without any respect for political boundaries or class barriers.

A number of bones from neolithic and even paleolithic France have been described as syphilitic, and for a while every French anthropologist was finding syphilitic material. The fashion was started by J. Parrot,[113] for whom every sign of rickets and every dental erosion were sure symptoms of congenital syphilis. Recently the French material was reviewed carefully by Pales,[114] by Williams,[115] by Jeanselme, who was a very able syphilologist and a keen student of history,[116] with the result we should expect after what we have learned from Egypt, namely, that the evidence it presented was negative or at least inconclusive. The very few long bones that might be interpreted as showing syphilitic changes are museum pieces of uncertain origin, and not a single skull has been found with the characteristic symptoms of dry caries.

Much material, on the other hand, has been unearthed in America, long bones and particularly skulls, in the diagnosis of which all investigators agreed. The chief difficulty with American anthropological material lies in dating it accurately, and while some syphilitic bones may be post-Columbian there can hardly be any doubt that many others must be pre-Columbian. Another complicating factor that must be kept in mind is that yaws also occurred in Central America. We shall review the entire American material and discuss the problem of the origin and epidemiology of syphilis critically in some other connection.

Inflammation is a defense reaction of the organism against injury, and if the injury has caused the destruction of tissue the body will immediately begin to produce new tissue in order to repair the damage. New growth takes place which is not the normal growth of the child, but growth in response to a pathological stimulus. In the case of minor injuries, e.g. of the skin, the repair may be so perfect that no visible trace of the lesion remains. If, however, the destruction was deep or had affected highly differentiated tissues, the organism, unable to regenerate the destroyed parts, will merely patch up the defect with connective tissue, producing a scar.

When a bone is fractured new bone is generated at both ends by the periosteum and the endosteum—the connective tissue of the marrow. The new tissue thus produced meets, hardens, and a callus is formed that holds the broken ends together. It is obvious that fractures occurred in animals and man at all times as a result of accidents or fights, and if the healing mechanism was the same then as we know it today, we should be able to find many bones with calluses. Many such bones have indeed been excavated all over the world. The oldest known callus is probably that of a Permian reptile that suffered a fracture of the radius.[117] From then on, throughout the entire history of the animal world, we find the evidence of fractures, some of which healed well with a small and regular callus, while others were infected, took a long time to heal, and produced a large and rugged callus or sometimes even a pseudarthrosis, a false joint, as occurred in an American bison described by Moodie.[118]

With the advent of man we again have a long series of fractured bones from every period, healed through formation of a callus. The precursor of man, Pithecanthropus, even had an exostosis on its left femur that has been considered by some the result of a fracture.[119] Evidence of fractures was found in skeletons of the Neanderthal race,[120] of paleolithic[121] and, of course, in increasing number of neolithic man.[122] Many specimens have also been described from Egypt.[123] There would be no point for us to list the existing material, since nobody doubts that fractures did occur and not rarely at that. What we are interested in is to know that the human and animal body, as far back as we can trace them, possessed the faculty of repairing injuries as we know it today.

There is one last group of diseases that we must discuss briefly, the *tumors*. It is the most puzzling group because the etiology of these diseases is still unknown. We can well understand the intentions of the body in the case of defense reactions and repair mechanisms. We can also grasp the significance of disturbances of development or metabolism. But why should a group of cells all of a sudden begin to grow independently, without respect for the organism as a whole, and live at its expense like a parasite? Or even worse, in the case of malignant tumors, why should such a growth destroy its host and in so doing destroy itself? There must be a principle involved that still escapes our understanding.

The tumor material preserved from prehistoric and early historic periods is very small. In the case of benign tumors, osteomata, we often find it difficult to decide whether an exostosis is a tumor or the end result of an inflammatory process. The earliest tumor that is considered an osteoma of which I know, is one found in a mosasaur and described by Moodie and Abel.[124] Two others, both affecting neolithic femurs, were described by Pales.[125] And as to malignant tumors, Elliot Smith and Dawson found several cases of what they considered osteosarcomata, one in a femur, two in humerus bones of the Vth Dynasty of Egypt.[126] Ruffer described a large tumor of a pelvis found in the catacombs of Kon el-Shougata, in Alexandria (A.D. *c.*250).[127] The tumor was highly vascularized, and *per exclusionem* Ruffer diagnosed it as being probably an osteosarcoma.

This is about all the early tumor material we have. What does its rarity mean? Does it mean that tumors, particularly malignant growths, are the late result of civilization? Yes and no. There is no doubt that more people die of cancer today than in the past because more people live longer than formerly and thus reach the age when a predilection for cancer develops, the years of maturity and old age. This is indirectly the result of civilization. On the other hand, we know that cancer and other tumors did occur in antiquity because we have a great deal of literary evidence for it,[128] although we have no way of finding out how frequent such diseases were. The rarity of prehistoric and early historic bones with tumors may actually mean that these diseases were rare, either because people died young or for some other reason. Or, it may also be that bones are not the best possible material to answer such a question. It is striking that cancer has never been found in any Egyptian mummy,[129] but again we must remember that the number of mummies of which the soft parts have been examined in any way systematically is not large.

The bones are not the only organ that survives the centuries and millennia. Still harder are the teeth, and thousands of early teeth have been preserved either loose or still in the jaws to which they belonged. As dentistry, a proud daughter of medicine, became highly emancipated, the paleopathology of teeth and jaws became a science of its own, *paleodontology;* Roy L. Moodie was Professor of Paleodontology for a while at the University of Southern California. Since J. R. Mummery's famous study on the relation of dental caries in the ancient inhabitants of Great Britain and aboriginal races to food and social conditions, published in 1870,[130] the literature on the subject has become very considerable, with many contributions from American authors.[131] This interest in the early pathology of teeth is not merely antiquarian but has very practical reasons. Dentistry is, like psychiatry, a discipline that deals with a small number of disease entities of which very little is known; hence the obvious need to consult the experience of other fields such as anthropology, geography, archaeology, or history.

Beginning with *pyorrhea alveolaris,* we can state without hesitation that this condition occurred at all times in men, and it was found even in a few fossil animals,[132] although animals suffer much less from dental diseases than humans. On the subject of pyorrhea, all investigators agree. It was described from early specimens of the Neanderthal race by Hans Virchow,[133] Baudouin,[134] and Martin.[135] In addition to pyorrhea, some of these early teeth showed considerable erosion due undoubtedly to the coarseness of the food, and some also had deposits of tartar. The symptoms of pyorrhea and of abscesses of the roots were found in late paleolithic [136] and neolithic material [137] and, very frequently, in Egypt.[138] There has been some speculation about the relation between pyorrhea and arthritis as evidenced by early skeletons, and, as a matter of fact, there are some in which the symptoms of both diseases can be demonstrated. The most famous example is probably the paleolithic skeleton of the Chapelle-aux-Saints, in France.[139] But as a rule the material available does not permit any conclusions. Neither can it be said that pyorrhea develops particularly in individuals of arthritic constitution, as some French investigators believed,[140] nor is a diseased tooth necessarily the portal of entrance for arthritic infection.

While there is a consensus of opinion concerning the antiquity of pyorrhea, it seems very uncertain at what time *caries* first made its appearance. The frequency of the disease undoubtedly increased from earlier to later periods with developing civilization. There is no evidence that it occurred in fossil and early paleolithic man. A very few cases have been described from the later paleolithic period. One concerns a skeleton found at Libos in France attributed to the Aurignacien by G. Astre, who described one tooth as showing signs of caries.[141] Another was a brachycephalic skull from Nagysáp in Hungary, examined by von Lenhossék.[142]

It is always dangerous to draw far-reaching conclusions from a few isolated specimens, particularly since we must always consider the possibility of error in the dating of the material.[143] Astre's skeleton was found very close to neolithic remains although in a deeper layer, and he himself stated that 'the caries was very little developed and affected an extremely worn and physiologically very old organ.' The date of von Lenhossék's skull is not too certain either. His theory that dental caries was a kind of epidemic disease brought from Asia to Europe by brachycephalic invaders at the end of the paleolithic period is witty but unfounded.

While it is possible, though doubtful, that caries first appeared toward the end of the paleolithic period, it was certainly present and not rare all over neolithic Europe.[144] Various attempts have been made to estimate the frequency of the disease. These statistics do not mean too much because the material is limited, but they are interesting nevertheless. Thus Mummery, investigating English material, found the following incidence of caries: [145]

Among 68 neolithic dolichocephalic skulls	2 cases	2.94 per cent
Among 32 skulls of the Bronze Age	7 cases	21.87 per cent
Among 59 Yorkshire early dolichocephalic skulls	24 cases	40.67 per cent
Among 44 ancient miscellaneous skulls	9 cases	20.45 per cent
Among 143 skulls of the Roman period	41 cases	28.67 per cent
Among 76 Anglo-Saxon skulls	12 cases	15.78 per cent

Fifty years later, von Lenhossék made a similar statistical analysis based on the examination of about 1000 skulls from Central Europe.[146] He rather arbitrarily assumed, which Mummery had not done, that every tooth lost during an individual's lifetime was lost as a result of caries, and counting in such a way he obtained extremely high percentage figures:

1st century [A.D.]	85 per cent
4th century	83 per cent
13th century	86 per cent
Recent skulls	90 per cent

Studies on French neolithic skulls revealed an incidence of about 3 or 4 per cent of dental caries,[147] and in Egypt the disease was very rare in the predynastic period but became more frequent with developing civilization, particularly among the wealthy classes. Elliot Smith examined the skulls of 500 aristocrats of the Old Kingdom buried at the Giza pyramids and found that among them 'tartar formation, dental caries and alveolar abscesses were at least as common as they are in modern Europe today.' He continues: 'And at every subsequent period of Egyptian history one finds the same thing—the wide prevalence of every form of dental disease among the wealthy people of luxurious diet, and the relative immunity from it among the poorer people who lived mainly on a coarse, uncooked diet.' [148] These observations have been confirmed by other investigators, and therefore it seems that caries became frequent among the common people of Egypt quite late, at the time of the Ptolemies and still more in the Byzantine period.[149]

Having discussed the diseases of bones and teeth we must now briefly review the evidence of diseases found in the soft organs of Egyptian mummies. This will not permit us to trace a pathological reaction beyond the fourth millennium B.C., but the results are important nevertheless. Thus it is rather surprising to hear that *arteriosclerosis* was not at all rare in ancient Egypt. We still know very little about the etiology of this disease but we like to relate it to the strain of modern life. Yet the Egyptians suffered from it too. King Merneptah, the Pharaoh of the Hebrew Exodus, whom we mentioned before in another connection, had arteriosclerosis of the aorta,[150] and Ruffer was able to demonstrate the disease in a number of mummies from the XVIIIth to the XXVIIth Dynasties as well as in later Greek and Coptic mummies.[151] The embalmer usually removed the aorta and the larger blood vessels, but sometimes bits of the aorta were left behind, and in some mummies the arteries of arms and legs were found intact. The microscopic examination of calcified arteries revealed the same pictures that we find in modern material today: atheromata, atheromatous patches, and ulcers, more or less completely calcified. With x-rays, it is possible to demonstrate the disease in mummy packs, and Moodie found a good example of such a case among the material of the Field Museum in Chicago.[152]

Although the lungs of mummies are very much shriveled, various diseases have been traced. Thus Ruffer described a case of advanced *anthracosis* in a mummy of the XXth Dynasty, the body of an individual who must have lived in a smoke-laden atmosphere.[153] Another mummy of the same period showed unmistakable signs of *pneumonia*. The alveoli of both lungs were filled with cells, in many of which nuclei could still be recognized. It was a case of pneumonia at the stage of hepatization.[154] In one lung of a later mummy from the Greek period, Ruffer found patches of inflammation in the upper part while the lower part was consolidated. In the lung and liver he found bacilli that looked like those of plague. If he had found a bubo, in addition, he would have diagnosed this as a case of plague.[155] Pleural adhesions, symptoms of *pleurisy*, were observed in various mummies by Elliot Smith and Dawson[156] and by Wood Jones.[157]

As to diseases of the urinary system, Ruffer referred to the congenital atrophy of the right kidney of a mummy he examined and to multiple abscesses in the kidneys of another mummy of the XVIIIth to XXth Dynasty with well-staining gram-negative bacilli.[158] He also described three vesical calculi found by Flinders Petrie in a predynastic skeleton.[159] Further cases of vesical calculi and three of kidney stones were discussed by Elliot Smith and Dawson.[160] The most important discovery in this connection was made by Ruffer, who in 1909 saw in the kidneys of two mummies of the XXth Dynasty (1250-1000 B.C.) large numbers of calcified eggs of *Schistosomum haematobium* located mostly among the straight tubules.[161] The Bilharzia disease [162] caused by this fluke worm is today still the curse of Egypt [163] and of other large sections of Africa. The parasite has a complicated life cycle. After having lived in various species of water snails it invades individuals through the skin in the form of cercariae. In the human body it matures in the veins and the eggs are carried into various tissues where they cause far-reaching destructions, particularly in the urinary tract. One common symptom of the disease, hematuria, the discharge of blood with the urine, is mentioned in Egyptian medical papyri, as we shall see later, but hematuria can occur also in the course of other diseases. The fact that Bilharzia eggs have been found in mummies proves that the disease was indigenous to Egypt three thousand years ago.

As we said before, no trace of venereal disease was ever found in Egypt, but the young princess Hehenit of the XIth Dynasty had a vesico-vaginal fistula, which was probably the result of protracted labor to which she succumbed, as she had an abnormally narrow pelvis.[164] The Egyptian remains, shriveled and parched as they are, tell the vivid story of many such tragedies: of the Coptic Negress who died in childbirth and was buried with the head of the fetus still wedged in her narrow pelvis. She had been a cripple all her life because her right sacro-iliac joint was missing, but crippled as she was, she had been abused and the result was her death.[165] Or the young girl from Nubia who was pregnant and had been beaten so that her hands and feet were broken and she finally died of a fractured skull.[166]

Few diseases of the gastro-intestinal tract have been described, possibly because these organs did not preserve too well. Elliot Smith, however, saw adhesions caused by chronic appendicitis.[167] He found gallstones in a mummy of the XXIst Dynasty,[168] the only case observed in ancient Egyptian material so far. Prolapse of the intestines was seen in several mummies as was also prolapse of the vagina.[169] A case of gout that occurred in the body of an early Christian was discussed in detail by Elliot Smith and Dawson.

Much has been written about poliomyelitis in ancient Egypt, the chief document to which reference is usually made being the funeral stele of a priest of the XVIIIth Dynasty.[170] The muscles of his right leg are highly atrophied, the leg is shortened and a pes equinovarus developed. He walked with difficulty and needed a stick. The Pharaoh Siphtah had a similar deformity of the foot, the origin of which is unknown.[171] A predynastic skeleton now in the Museum of the University of Pennsylvania was described by J. K. Mitchell, who found that the left femur was 8.2 cm. shorter than the right. A stick was found buried with the skeleton.[172] All these cases may very well be testimonies of infantile paralysis, but at the same time we must admit that such a diagnosis cannot be more than a guess because the same type of deformity is also caused by other diseases of the nervous system.

There is no doubt that Egypt was repeatedly visited by devastating epidemics. The Bible, as we shall discuss in detail later, is not the only literary source to the subject. It is very difficult, however, to decide in a given case what the epidemic disease actually was,[173] and some direct sources would, therefore, be very welcome. The difficulty is that bodies are not embalmed in times of great wars and epidemics, when large numbers of people die simultaneously. The material made available so far is very scanty. We have already mentioned the case that might have been one of plague, according to Ruffer. He examined another mummy, of the XXth Dynasty, the skin of which was 'the seat of a peculiar vesicular or bulbous eruption which in form and general distribution bore a striking resemblance to that of smallpox.[174] It is obvious that one such mummy does not prove the existence of smallpox in the neighborhood of Deir el-Bahri around 1100 B.C., but every case is important and must be registered and fully described because some day the number of cases may be large enough to permit definite conclusions. This is also true of the single case of leprosy found so far, mentioned by Smith and Derry [175] and pictured by Smith and Dawson.[176] We should also like to have direct evidence of malaria, which today is rather widespread in the Fayoum. Ruffer found enlarged spleens in several mummies, a condition that in the East is usually the result of malaria.[177]

What does paleopathology teach us? Speculating about the origin of disease, we thought that it must be as old as life itself because it is life, a manifestation of life, the reaction of a living organism to abnormal stimuli. Paleopathology basically confirms our assumption. While it is not possible to find the evidence of disease in the earliest known fossils of invertebrates, yet we saw that not only did man at all times for tens of thousands of years suffer from many kinds of ailments, but animals, millions of years before the advent of man, were also plagued with disease.

A result of paleopathological studies that seems to me still more important is that we find that disease occurred at all times in the same basic forms. Whether the bones we discussed were human or animal bones, whether they were neolithic or paleolithic, Eocene or Permian, we always found the same types of disease, disturbances of development and of metabolism, inflammation and repair, new-growth and true tumors, the same forms of disease that we can observe today. This shows that the animal organism at all times had only a very limited number of mechanisms available with which it reacted against lesions.

This observation, however, leads to another important conclusion. Pathologists like to tell us that the human organism developed and perfected its defense reactions in the course of time. MacCallum, for instance, speaking of defense mechanisms in general and of repair in particular, says: 'It is a mechanism like the others (viz. inflammation, fever, immunity production) which seems to have been perfected through long generations toward a rather complex end, for not only does it repair gaps in the tissue but it is protective in the sense that it brings about the encapsulation of any noxious material and prevents its further influence upon the neighboring tissues.'[178] Paleopathology, however, teaches us that these mechanisms are not the prerogative of man perfected through long generations, but that animals, millions of years ago, possessed them as well and perhaps even in much greater perfection. Indeed, we find that the lower an organism is in the evolutionary scale, the greater its defense and repair mechanisms are. A plant completely cut off near the ground is regenerated entirely from the roots. A hydra may be cut into two, three, or four pieces and each part will grow into an entire organism, as Trembley found as early as 1744. The earthworm can regenerate head and tail, and even amphibia still have the faculty of regenerating limbs and tails. How imperfect a mechanism is man's patching up of a defect with connective tissue! That man was able to survive and to attain the position he holds in nature is due to the fact that he was endowed with a larger brain and greater intelligence, which enabled him through long generations to perfect not his natural but artificial defense mechanisms, to direct and increase the natural healing power of the body with artificial means, learning to use physical, chemical, and biological forces to that end.

Paleopathology is a very interesting field that calls for the close co-operation of anthropologists, archaeologists, pathologists, and historians. Its popularity in the years between 1910 and 1930 dropped off considerably, probably because no new startling results were obtained. New findings seemed merely to confirm the old ones. Yet, these studies should be continued. There are still many unsolved problems; many old findings need confirmation. The collections of our museums should be searched systematically for pathological conditions, and every mummy should at least be x-rayed as a matter of routine.

PROBLEMS OF THE HISTORY AND GEOGRAPHY OF DISEASE

Paleopathology is one aspect of the large complex of studies devoted to the problem of disease in time and space, an important but a limited one. It investigates the earliest manifestations of disease, but, since the material available is very scanty, cannot possibly trace the history of a given disease. All it can do is to ascertain that a disease did occur at a certain time, in man or animals, at a certain point of the globe where the evidence was found. The geographical coverage too is sketchy and haphazard. We saw that Egypt for a number of reasons proved to be an unusually fertile ground for such studies. France yielded much material, particularly for the neolithic period. The North American continent was rich in fossil bones of early vertebrates, and we shall see that for a much later period Peru with its mummies provides also a wealth of material. But we have no knowledge whatever of the early incidence of illness in large sections of the globe.[179]

The main conclusion drawn from paleopathological studies, namely that the phenomenon of disease is very old and that disease always occurred in the same basic forms, is extremely important but obviously does not mean that the incidence of illness was the same everywhere and at all times. We know, on the contrary, that the incidence of illness varies a great deal from country to country and from period to period, and we wish to know what these variations in time and space have been and what factors have caused them.

People observed very early that some diseases were peculiar to certain countries or regions and speculated about the relation between climate, soil, water, air and the diseases that afflicted the inhabitants. The early classic of the genre is the Hippocratic treatise, *On Airs Waters Places,*[180] a book that had a very practical purpose in a country where most physicians were itinerant practitioners. It purported to teach the doctor who came to a place unknown to him what kind of people and diseases he might expect, judging from the environment in which they lived.[181] The Hippocratic *Epidemics,* particularly Books I and III,[182] are a good example of medico-geographical raw materials, a physician's notes on weather conditions and diseases he had observed. The theory that epidemics were the result of cosmic or telluric influences, that a certain *genius loci* was essential for the genesis of an epidemic, led to a very extensive investigation of geographical conditions, and for many centuries the epidemiological literature had a strong historical-geographical bias.

In the Renaissance, Paracelsus never tired of postulating the necessity of studying disease conditions in foreign countries. He lived what he preached, traveled all over Europe and the Near East, and when accused of being a man without a residence he answered in the fourth of his famous *Defensiones,* pointing out that 'diseases wander hither and thither throughout the breadth of the world, and stay not in one place. If a man wish to recognise many diseases, let him travel: if he travel far, his experience will be great and he will learn to recognise many things.' [183] 'How can a good Cosmographus grow in the chimney corner, or a Geographus?' The physician, however, 'should be a Cosmographus: not to describe how the countries wear their trousers, but to attack more bravely what diseases they have.' [184]

Stronger than a reformer's voice were economic forces that impelled European medicine to study the diseases of foreign lands. Every country is interested first of all in its own diseases, but when a country extends its frontiers overseas and becomes a colonial power, it automatically finds itself exposed to foreign diseases and is forced to act in order to protect its colonists and, ultimately, the homeland. And since the voyages of discovery and the creation of colonial empires took place in the sixteenth and seventeenth centuries, i.e. in a period of scientific awakening, foreign diseases were studied not only for obvious practical reasons but also to satisfy the intellectual curiosity of the early explorers, some of whom were doctors, who described the *cosas maravillosas* of the new colonies. A wealth of novel experiences was gained. The geography of disease broadened tremendously once European countries had a foothold in the tropics, where so many diseases thrive. Reports were either the naïve observations of travelers or regular medical monographs like that early classic of tropical medicine, *De Medicina Indorum,* published around 1642, the work of a Dutch physician who had lived in Indonesia.

The great colonial powers, Spain, Portugal, England, and Holland, were primarily interested in these studies, and for several centuries most of the contributions to the knowledge of exotic diseases came from them. And thereafter whenever a country had colonial aspirations it immediately documented a marked interest in medical geography and set up schools, hospitals, and research institutions for the study of tropical diseases.[185] This happened in France in the early nineteenth century, in Germany late in the same century, in Italy in the twentieth century.

Similarly, whenever a population migrated from one part of its country to another, settling and developing sparsely populated regions, problems of medical geography became acute. Thus Daniel Drake explored the medical topography of the Mississippi Valley, realizing that it was to become the melting pot of the nation.[186]

Or when a large country such as Russia became aware of its responsibilities toward the health of its people and realized how unexplored the country was medically, then again it felt the need for medico-geographical studies. This happened in Russia in 1864 when Zemstvo medicine was established, which brought medical services to the rural population. In 1865 the *Annals of Legal Medicine and Public Health* [187] was founded, followed in 1870 by a serial publication on medical topography; [188] for a number of years the Medical Society of Kazan devoted most of its activities to these problems.[189]

Efforts to prevent the spread of epidemics from country to country and to control them ultimately on a world-wide scale represent another line of development that called imperatively for geographic studies. A beginning was made in the Middle Ages after the Black Death, the pandemic of plague of 1348-9, when Ragusa first, and later one port after another, quarantined incoming vessels that had been in plague-infested countries. This required a system of medical intelligence: countries began to be vitally interested in the health and disease conditions of other regions, and it became the duty of diplomatic representatives to report to their home offices about epidemics. From 1664 on England required a bill of health from all ships coming from Turkey and Egypt. When the Suez Canal was opened in 1869, it was made a filter to catch diseases that threatened Europe from the East. The Sanitary Maritime and Quarantine Board of Egypt was established in 1892. And finally in our own century great world organizations were created for medical intelligence and international co-operation in the field of public health: the Pan-American Sanitary Bureau in 1902, the Office International d'Hygiène Publique, in Paris in 1909, the Health Section of the Secretariat of the League of Nations in 1921, with its head office in Geneva and an Eastern Bureau in Singapore, and finally the World Health Organization of the United Nations. All these organizations and many smaller ones that cannot be named here,[190] being international in outlook, greatly activated studies in the geography of disease.

Studies in tropical medicine, medical intelligence, and similar activities do not yet constitute a geography of disease but provide materials for one. Attempts to produce a synthesis were made repeatedly in the eighteenth and nineteenth centuries, particularly in Germany and France. It may seem strange that Germany should have taken a special interest in these studies at a time when the country was not unified but consisted of thirty odd states, most of which were very small, but it was a result of, among other factors, the universalism so prevalent in eighteenth-century Germany, which reflected itself in the world-historical outlook of Herder. And we must also remember that Germany produced the man who undoubtedly was the greatest geographer of the early nineteenth century, Alexander von Humboldt.

A small-town practitioner, Leonhard Ludwig Finke,[191] published at Leipzig, 1792-5, a work in three volumes entitled, *Versuch einer allgemeinen medicinisch-praktischen Geographie, worin der historische Theil der einheimischen Völker- und Staaten-Arzeneykunde vorgetragen wird.* He had never traveled but he compiled his treatise from all the books of travelers and foreign physicians he could obtain. His approach to the subject was closely related to and undoubtedly influenced by the views of Johann Peter Frank, the greatest hygienist among his contemporaries. Frank, in his great book, *System einer vollständigen medicinischen Polizey,*[192] had studied the life of man in his physical and social environment from the moment of conception to the moment of death and had investigated the influence of environmental factors, physical and social, on health; he had taught how and under what conditions the individual should live in order to maintain health and prevent illness. Finke also pictured the life of man in his physical and social environment, but it was the life of man in Italy, in China, and other foreign countries. He discussed the diseases from which people suffered in various countries, the physical and social conditions responsible for them, and also the treatments being used and the conditions of medical practice. It was an interesting and sound approach. The only trouble was that Finke, having no foreign experience of his own, used good and bad sources indiscriminately.

Finke had a few predecessors, although none had the ambition to be as comprehensive as he was.[193] During the following century he had many successors, some of whom approached the problems from the pathological angle, studying diseases under various geographic conditions[194]—sometimes using cartographic methods to illustrate the distribution of a disease in space;[195] to others, who pictured conditions in a given locality, a city, a region, a country, a continent, or the world, geography was the starting point. Some limited their studies to the diseases of an area,[196] while others included all medical aspects encountered in that area, thus presenting a medical topography or on a larger scale, a medical geography as Finke had done.[197]

By far the most successful and popular book of the kind in the second half of the nineteenth century, one that is still consulted today, was the *Handbuch der historisch-geographischen Pathologie* by August Hirsch. First published in two volumes in 1860 to 1864, it was completely revised and considerably enlarged for a second edition, which was issued in three volumes, 1881 to 1886, from which an English translation was made by Charles Creighton.[198] Hirsch's book is remarkable not only for the overwhelming amount of information and literary references it contains, which make it unsurpassed even today, but also for the fact that it combines the history and geography of disease—in other words, it traces a disease entity in time and space.

In the second half of the nineteenth century quite a number of more or less comprehensive books on medical geography and geographical pathology were available, and in addition some very fine studies on the history of certain diseases—particularly epidemic diseases—had been written.[199] Every geography contained some historical considerations and, as a matter of fact, what Finke himself had had in mind was to write ultimately the medical history of mankind. Every history of a disease, on the other hand, included geographical data, particularly in the case of epidemic diseases, because disease does not occur in a vacuum and epidemics move along the highways of traffic. Hirsch, however, was the man who combined the two approaches in a most fortunate way and in so doing developed a method for the investigation of disease that was intended to supplement the experience gained in clinic and laboratory. He set a pattern that was widely followed. In 1878 the brothers Heinrich and Gerhard Rohlfs, both physicians and one of them a geographer also, founded the *Deutsches Archiv für Geschichte der Medicin und medicinischen Geographie.* 'Critical historical research,' they said in the preface, 'sets in when experiments and the senses prove to be inadequate,' and 'who could deny that medical geography has the closest ties with the history of medicine?' Rohlfs' *Archiv* was discontinued in 1885, but in 1896 a new journal was founded in Holland, *Janus, Archives internationales pour l'histoire de la médecine et pour la géographie médicale,* which after fifty years is still being published. Professor Stokvis in a preface to the first volume wrote,

> Medicine is in a period of development of which we the contemporaries cannot grasp the full significance. But one thing is obvious, namely, that what we lack is no longer facts, observations, experiments, new treatments; it is rather the philosophy of medicine that is going astray. It is all too apparent that carried away we too much neglect the lessons of medicine of all times and peoples, that in the great family of medical sciences the history of medicine and medical geography are no longer considered full members with an authoritative voice but rather ladies in attendance who merely serve to add glamor on festive occasions.

How justified the complaint was and how much the new journal contributed to the turning of the tide that actually took place in the new century will not be examined here.

It was important that Hirsch and his successors emphasized the need for studies not only in the geography but also in the history of diseases. These are very difficult studies: direct sources are scarce and almost all our knowledge is derived from literary documents. Diseases with striking and characteristic symptoms, such as epilepsy,[200] some forms of malaria, and a few others, can be recognized without too much difficulty in ancient texts, but when we read of continuous fevers with vague symptoms, loss of appetite, headaches, occasional diarrheas, we find it practically impossible to decide what diseases were meant. The very concept of disease changed a great deal in the course of time, as we shall see in every volume of this book. Today we think in terms of well-defined disease entities, but this is a relatively recent development and previously symptoms were grouped differently. Many of our present entities are characterized chiefly by the agent that causes them. Thus we know that the nose can be destroyed by an ulcerative process, which may be syphilis, yaws, or tuberculosis. Today we may be unable to diagnose a clinical case without laboratory tests. How then could we decide which disease was meant in a verbal description or picture made hundreds or thousands of years ago, even if it came from a very keen observer? There are, moreover, diseases the symptoms of which are such that they cannot be described in words so that the reader will recognize them with any degree of certainty. I am thinking particularly of diseases of the skin. Some have highly characteristic symptoms but others have not. An eruption, a rash, macules, pustules, ulcers occur as symptoms of very different diseases.[201] Difficulties are presented also by symptoms that may just as likely be caused by an organic disease as by a neurosis.

And yet in spite of all difficulties we must investigate the history of diseases and pursue these studies as deeply as possible, because they are important in many respects. The history of disease, as we said before, is the starting point of all medico-historical research, and for this reason we emphasize it so strongly here, in the beginning of this book. We cannot understand or appraise a physician's actions unless we know what diseases he was fighting. They set the task to the doctor; they were the challenge, and this obviously was different on an Aegean island in the fifth century B.C. than it was in a Benedictine abbey north of the Alps, in the ninth century of the Christian era. We must be familiar with the history of disease also in order fully to understand certain medical theories. At first sight it may seem strange that in one such theory the spleen, an inconspicuous organ, was given the rank of one of the four cardinal organs, seat of the black bile, one of the four cardinal humors. It is not so strange when we know that the theory was elaborated in a region of endemic malaria, where splenomegaly was very frequent, where people had greatly enlarged spleens that could be felt through the skin more easily even than the liver.

Knowledge of the history of disease is necessary also for a deeper understanding of the history of civilization in its various aspects, because there have always been manifold interrelations between civilization and disease. With developing civilization, man learned to protect the body against many potential injuries and also learned to perfect and direct the defense and repair mechanisms of the organism, just as he learned to increase and direct the fertility of the soil when he developed agriculture. But civilization, by removing man from the natural rhythm of life, by creating new and artificial conditions, often produced new causes of disease. Nutrition, clothing, housing, all designed to protect man against environmental injuries, have also, when inadequate or wrongly approached, caused illness, even created new diseases. So has the ever increasingly differentiated process of production. Industry raised the material standard of life and in so doing improved health conditions, but at the same time new health hazards and new diseases were created. Disease always had economic consequences, and economic factors on the other hand were largely responsible for the incidence and social distribution of illness. Disease greatly affected man's position in society, a position that changed considerably in the course of time according to a society's evaluation of health and disease. We need not go far back in history to remember how man's social life was influenced, and actually still is, in a particular way by such diseases as leprosy, tuberculosis, and venereal and mental diseases.

Disease has influenced the course of history, economic, social, and political, has devastated entire countries, has stopped wars, wiping out victor and victim. It presented a challenge to religion, philosophy, and science, which were called upon to interpret disease and to give man power over it. And finally in literature and art, man re-creating life could not and did not ignore the phenomena of disease.[202]

Studies in the history of disease have a certain importance also as a method of modern pathology. In ancient Alexandria there developed a medical school, the followers of which called themselves Empiricists. Their chief doctrine was that the primary causes of disease are too obscure to be elucidated and that the physician must rely entirely on experience and observation. His chief source of knowledge was his own experience, but man's life is short and observations made in a lifetime are but a few. Therefore, they said, you must profit not only from your own experience but from that of others as well. The doctors of the past, our medical ancestors, were not fools. They saw and experienced a great deal and they tell us about it in their books. The doctor, therefore, in order to supplement his own experience must study the medical literature and not only that of his own days but the old books as well.[203]

This is to a certain extent true today too. If we wish to have a complete account of the character and nature of a disease, we shall not be satisfied with knowing it as it presents itself to us today, but we must study its history also. As a matter of fact, we are doing this constantly even without being aware of it. The clinical case history is justly called a 'history' because it gives a biographical account of a patient with particular emphasis on his ailments past and especially present. All hospital records are historical documents although they may cover only a very short period. When we speak of the mortality of a disease having decreased by 3 per cent during the last five years, we make a historical statement although we may be doing it in the same spirit as M. Jourdan, who spoke in prose without being aware of it. If we broaden our outlook and are not satisfied with studying a disease over a period of a few years only but investigate its history over a long period of time, our results will be the more reliable.

Historical investigations are indispensable in studying epidemic diseases where the time factor is so important. Pandemics of influenza occur once in a generation, and hardly any physician has experienced more than two of them. It is certainly interesting to know that the history of influenza can be traced far back, to the Middle Ages, and that it came over the world regularly once every thirty or forty years and caused much the same physical and psychological symptoms. Further it is important to know that many diseases have changed in their character. Syphilis, which is a chronic disease today, was much more acute in Europe at the end of the fifteenth and in the beginning of the sixteenth centuries; scarlet fever was much more malignant a few decades ago.

In spite of the great discoveries of bacteriology, there are still many unsolved problems in the field of epidemiology. We know the bacillus that causes plague, know how it is transmitted from rodents to man, and how an epidemic spreads along the highways of traffic. Yet we do not know why Europe was devastated by two pandemics of plague in the sixth and fourteenth centuries but experienced no serious outbreak of the disease during the intervening eight hundred years, although Europe had very close and intimate contacts with the Orient during the Crusades. We do not know why the sweating sickness that befell the European continent, coming from England in the winter of 1528-9, missed France and the southern European countries, and yet reached serious proportions in the Germanic countries.[204] There are factors in the origin of epidemics that still escape our detection, and careful historical studies covering long periods might prove enlightening.[205]

The incidence of illness changes constantly. In the economically advanced countries the acute infectious diseases and tuberculosis, which used to constitute the major causes of death, are in the background today and the majority of people die from chronic diseases of mature and old age: from diseases of heart, circulation, kidneys, and from cancer. We must be aware of these changes because we have to adapt our actions to the changing constellation of diseases. As long as acute infectious and communicable diseases dominate the scene, they will be opposed by general public-health measures, quarantine, sanitation, immunizations, and similar measures; while the chronic diseases of wear and tear call for individual services of general practitioner and specialist, preventive and curative, and the major organizational task at such a stage is to make all such services easily available to all the people. We must be aware not only of the changed incidence of illness but of the economic, social, and medical factors that caused it, and this is possible only through careful historical analysis.

The incidence of illness changes not only in time but also in space. Certain diseases are bound to certain localities and the same disease may appear in a different character in different places. Pneumonia in Madrid in the late winter months is a much dreaded disease that kills people in a few days. We know that it is iodine deficiency that makes goiter an endemic disease in the Alps, in the mountains of the Caucasus, in the northern provinces of Argentina.[206] But we do not know yet why stone diseases are more frequent in one locality than in another, why gastric ulcers are rare where stone diseases are frequent, and vice versa. We do not know why cancer of the breast occurs more often in some regions than in others. The fact that primary carcinoma of the liver is not rare in the Bantu of South Africa while it is not frequently found in white people may be due to racial factors, but what these factors are we do not know.[207]

These considerations bring us back to the geography of diseases. After a period of great vogue in the nineteenth century, these studies came somewhat into disrepute, for various reasons. One was the discovery of bacterial infection. Indeed, the discovery that diseases are caused by specific micro-organisms and that such a disease will never, without any exception, develop unless its micro-organism is present, was of such tremendous significance that it tended to overshadow all other factors that might have been considered and led to a somewhat oversimplified view. Whenever man, it was said, on any point of the globe swallows sufficient cholera bacilli, he develops cholera. The old ideas about cosmic-atmospheric-telluric influences were thrown overboard. Why then study geographic factors? Cholera undoubtedly will never break out without bacilli, but nobody can deny that there is a geography of cholera. It would be very easy to demonstrate it in the form of maps, and it would not be difficult either to show why cholera has disappeared from the economically advanced West while it is still endemic in India and China.

Another reason why medico-geographical studies became somewhat discredited was that the previous work had in many ways been too ambitious, attempting a synthesis before the materials were available. As early as 1880, the great American sanitarian, John Billings, criticized conditions when he said:

> In medical topography as a science there has been little advance for a thousand years, and so long as present methods are pursued, no great additions to our knowledge in this direction can be expected. Vague generalities and opinions must be replaced by specific information and from square miles we must come down to square feet. The result which we now have can best be compared to those obtained by the young chemist who made an analysis of a rat—putting the entire animal into his crucible.[208]

In order to remedy the situation in his own country and to obtain accurate information about health and medical conditions in the various localities, Billings, while he was president of the American Public Health Association in 1880, drew up a questionnaire that was to be submitted to all cities and towns of 5000 or more inhabitants. The plan was well meant, but the questionnaire included over 400 questions and it would have required a monograph to answer them fully and conscientiously, more than could be expected from about 325 communities. It is no wonder the plan was never carried out.[209]

And so at the beginning of our century systematic studies on the geography of diseases were at a rather low ebb. There were exceptions, such as Clemow's book published in the Cambridge Geographical Series in 1903,[210] and tropical medicine greatly profited by the discoveries of bacteriology. But as a whole, geographical studies were not popular with pathologists or pathological studies with geographers, and some of the best books on Human Geography hardly mention the geography of diseases or devote only a few pages to it.[211]

Yet just at that time, the world was beginning to become smaller because new intercontinental railway lines, faster ships, and the airplane were bridging the continents and reducing distances considerably. In the First World War soldiers from all continents were thrown together and found themselves living and fighting in all sections of the world under geographical conditions utterly foreign to them. East Indians brought to Europe died from tuberculosis in large numbers. Malaria played havoc with allied troops in Macedonia and the Near East, and after the war epidemics such as the world had not seen since the Middle Ages swept large sections of the globe.

Studies in the geography of diseases were given increased attention [212] and a number of remarkably wrong starts were made. In 1929 M. Askanazy, Professor of Pathology at the University of Geneva, founded the *International Society of Geographical Pathology*. Askanazy came from Königsberg in East Prussia, where he had observed diseases that had been brought from outside, like leprosy and scleroma and other parasitic diseases that were endemic as a result of the local custom of eating raw fish.[213] When he came to Switzerland he found goiter and a high incidence of cirrhosis of the liver, in short a totally different constellation of diseases, and he became very interested in geographic problems. The new society held its first international conference in Geneva in 1931. It was entirely devoted to the disease entity 'cirrhosis of the liver,' and was attended by delegates from twenty-four countries. A second conference took place at Utrecht in 1934 on the subject of gastric ulcer. A third conference was held at Stockholm in 1937, at which anemia was discussed. Two years later the war broke out, interrupting the activities of the society which as a whole had not been very successful. The mistake had been that the society had been built on a much too narrow foundation. Askanazy had originally announced that the geographical analysis of the causes of a disease must include the investigation of 'climate, soil, food, customs, general civilization, economic status, and hygiene.' Actually the society consisted primarily of professors of pathology and pathological anatomy who came together from various countries to compare the findings of their autopsy rooms. Such an approach can provide some interesting statistical data and can contribute to a clarification of concepts but is certainly not the proper method to develop a geography of diseases or geographical pathology, a subject that requires the close co-operation of workers from many different fields.[214]

Another abortive attempt was made, in the United States, when the Division of Medical Sciences of the National Research Council appointed a Committee on Survey of Tropical Diseases. It is strange that tropical medicine and medical geography at large were neglected in a country that reaches very close to the tropics, one that has tropical diseases, a great variety of climates, and from which great contributions to tropical medicine had been made in the past. One would have expected strong Schools of Tropical Medicine and specialized hospitals for the treatment of patients and the study of tropical diseases. Actually what little interest there was, was concentrated in the Army, in the U.S. Public Health Service, and in a few foundations. But to all these groups tropical medicine was merely a side line. There were, however, people, physicians and others, who felt strongly that an effort should be made to develop these studies. When the Second World War began with Japan's invasion of Manchuria in 1931 and gradually spread from one continent to another, it soon became apparent that knowledge of the diseases of foreign countries was not a luxury but an eminently practical matter which soon might prove to be of vital importance.

In 1929 there was hope that a philanthropist might endow the study of tropical medicine with a fund of $40,000,000. This hope, like so many others in the cultural field, was shattered by the economic depression, and the National Research Council appointed the committee mentioned before, with Dr. Earl Baldwin McKinley as Director of Studies. In 1935 he published with the help of twenty scientists a very disappointing book under the ambitious title *A Geography of Disease.*[215] As the title indicates, it was not limited to tropical diseases but included 'other diseases' as well. The book is arranged according to countries and very naïvely lists the answers to a questionnaire, indicating what diseases occur in what country, with approximate statistics if available. No attempt was made to analyze or interpret the figures. For every country there is a brief introduction giving facts regarding its socio-economic background, but unfortunately these introductions are full of mistakes.[216] The last section of the book consists of 'summaries of selected diseases, with special articles,' in which the world geography of syphilis is given two pages. The whole book is called a 'preliminary survey,' preliminary to what we do not know, because nothing more happened before it became obvious that the United States would be involved in the war.

Much broader in its approach, much more forceful, and very dangerous was a movement that developed in Nazi Germany and went under the barbaric name of *Geomedicine.*[217] Geomedicine is a department of geopolitics, a science that goes back to the German geographer F. Ratzel, although the term was coined by the Swedish political scientist R. Kjellén. Ratzel defined political geography as the science that studies the distribution of political power over the surface of the earth and its determination by form, soil, climate, and similar factors.[218] Kjellén took these concepts over from geography and adapted them to the field of political science. He coined the term geopolitics in a study on the frontiers of Sweden and developed it in a book on the state as a living organism.[219] This was at the time when the ideology of Nazism was being elaborated in Germany, and geopolitics was taken over eagerly and developed to political ends by General Haushofer and his co-workers. In their hands geopolitics became 'applied political geography,' or the 'science of the geographic determination of political processes,'[220] and ultimately it was to prepare and justify Germany's conquest of the world.

Once geopolitics was accepted, other disciplines became conscious of geography and began to play with maps. A German jurist, Langhans-Ratzeburg, established the field of 'Geo-jurisprudence,'[221] and medicine with its long tradition of geographical studies obviously could not stay behind, particularly not since it was to play an important part in coming events. And so geomedicine was launched in 1931 by Heinz Zeiss, a German hygienist who had traveled widely, been loaned from the University of Hamburg to the Soviet Union for a number of years, and given an important chair at the University of Berlin when Hitler came into power.[222] Zeiss has developed his program in a number of papers and has outlined the task in about the following way:

Geomedicine is much more than the geography of diseases or geographical pathology because it is concerned not only with diseases but with medicine, that is the maintenance and restoration of health and the prevention of disease in various areas. It is not medical geography, which, according to Zeiss, is 'the branch of geography which endeavors to investigate and to explain the effects of geographical space, of the earth and its vital manifestations on man, animal, and plant.'[223] It is not geography but medicine, a branch of medicine that has the following three major tasks:

1. Creation of geographic and cartographic means of information as geomedical methods. Preparation of medico-geographic and geomedical maps and atlases to replace the utterly inadequate maps and atlases previously published.

2. Co-operation, practical and theoretical, between physicians, veterinarians, and botanists on one side and geographers, meteorologists, agronomists, entomologists, and geologists on the other side, to elucidate the connection between weather, soil, climate, and the outbreak of acute infectious diseases among men, animals, and plants. Possibly, prediction of outbreaks of acute illnesses by geomedical weather stations.

3. Geomedicine to develop as prognosis, since it is just as dynamic as geopolitics, while political and medical geography decidedly have static qualities. Geomedicine, in other words, is interested in static matters only in so far as it contributes to the cognizance of the dynamism of disease. And

> while geopolitics puts into the hands of the statesman the weapons required for the present and future security of the state, geomedicine will enable the physicians—and among them particularly the physicians in public service and hygienists—whose function it is to protect the people's health, to draw the attention of the statesmen to momentary and still threatening health hazards, the combatting of which represents a political measure that is significant in internal as well as foreign policy.

Geomedicine, to put it more simply, was geographical medicine attached to the band wagon of Nazi geopolitics with a political purpose that was not clearly expressed in Zeiss's early publications but was implied in his teachings and was never denied by the members of his school. This purpose obviously was to provide medical arguments for Nazi Germany's claims to 'living space' (*Lebensraum*) and at the same time to provide medical information that would make Germany's conquest of foreign lands safe. In its early days geomedicine had a strange appeal abroad to people who were not familiar with the Nazi mentality, and Fielding H. Garrison in America hailed it as a 'new science in gestation.'[224] It took some time and all the horrors of war before the true character of this 'new science' was recognized.[225]

The global character of the Second World War forced every country to engage in studies of geographic medicine, and the divisions of medical intelligence of every army worked feverishly to gather the medical information that their armed forces required for successful military operations. And since the war brought many troops to the tropical belt, tropical medicine was cultivated as never before. Under the pressure of events much of the work was hurried and materials were collected, not always too critically, from every possible source.[226] It is to be expected that the interest in these studies will continue now that the war is over. If there is one thing that people should have learned, it is that peace and war are indivisible, that every war must necessarily assume a global character in our machine age and no nation can live in splendid isolation. Military medical authorities of every country will therefore be forced to maintain their international outlook. But so will the civilian health services at a time when air transportation is circling the globe. Nations may distrust, misunderstand, or even hate each other, but the new technology welds them together inexorably and creates a solidarity under which they will thrive or perish together.

Summing up and looking into the future, I think we must try to have a clear view of the basic problems these studies must attempt to solve, and it seems to me that we are dealing with two main groups of studies each of which shows two different basic approaches.

Subject of the first group is the *history and geography of disease.* We have established disease entities characterized by etiology, pathogenesis, anatomical form and seat, symptoms and course—entities such as cholera, plague, pneumonia, or gastric ulcer. To the experience of clinic and laboratory we add the study of a given disease in time and space. We want to know when it was first observed and where, what its character and incidence were at a given time and place and, if they changed, why they changed.[227] We trace a disease all over the world and examine the physical and social factors responsible for it. We are not satisfied with the knowledge that cholera still occurs in India; we want to know why it is found there while it has disappeared from all the Western countries. We are aware of the fact that cholera is caused by a bacillus, usually water-carried, and that the status of general sanitation is therefore very important. But there are other factors of a totally different nature which must be considered, such as the pilgrimages and other religious events which in India bring large masses of people together, and where a great deal of water is consumed. If cholera breaks out, the pilgrims carry the disease all over the land. We know that fresh fruit and vegetables prevent scurvy. The climatic conditions of a country are therefore important, and scurvy is by nature more likely to occur in the far North than in the temperate or hot zones. However, in this as in other similar diseases a great variety of other non-physical factors are just as important: transportation that brings fresh food to the cities, methods of preservation such as canning or freezing, and, last but not least, the price of food. In other words, we cannot be broad enough in these studies and may have to borrow from many other fields.

This approach is basically pathological and it embraces studies in *historical and geographical pathology.* We investigate one disease after another in time and space. This is what August Hirsch did in his once classical book. Sixty years have passed since its second edition came out, and during that time pathology has progressed a great deal and so has the history of medicine. A new book of this type should be written some day, but before it can be done we should have a series of monographs, each one devoted to the history and geography of a single disease with each one supplemented by an atlas.[228] The material would be overwhelming in the case of plague, leprosy, malaria, and similar diseases; it would be much more difficult of access in the case of pneumonia; and in the history and geography of gastric ulcer we may have to limit ourselves to the last few decades. But we should at least make an attempt to cover the whole field as thoroughly as possible.

The history and geography of disease may be approached also

with the accent not on disease but on geography. In such a case the primary object of our studies will not be plague or cholera but a geographic entity, Italy, Iran, India, or the desert, the steppe,[229] the Arctic. We study the physical, biological, and political geography of such a unit and its diseases in relation to them. Such a study must not be static but dynamic, that is historical. The physical geography has in all probability not changed, at least not perceptibly, during the last few thousand years, and the changes in its fauna and flora were probably not considerable either. But what have changed a great deal in all circumstances are the economic, social, and political conditions, and they always exert a strong influence on the incidence of illness. Numerous books have been written along this line of thought and more will undoubtedly come out. This is particularly necessary for economically backward countries that have not yet made a complete inventory of their diseases. Before this is done, they cannot expect to put their health services on a sound basis.

These studies, although also concerned with disease, are primarily geographical and may be called studies in *historical and pathological geography.*

The second group of studies deals not with disease alone but with medicine, that is with health and disease and all human activities that tend to promote and restore the one and prevent the other. Its field of research is the *history and geography of medicine,* or medicine in time and space. And here again the accent may be laid either on medicine or on geography. We may be interested primarily in *historical and geographical medicine*—that is, in the development and present status of medicine as a whole or of certain of its aspects over wide sections of the globe[230]—or geography becomes our starting point and we investigate all aspects of medicine, past and present, in a given country or other geographic unit,[231] thus engaging in studies of *historical and medical geography.*[232]

There are no sharp borderlines between these groups and it is equally obvious that geographical studies need not necessarily be combined with historical ones. It will soon be found, however, that the historical analysis greatly contributes to the clarification of present conditions.

NOTES

1. *Leben unter veränderten Bedingungen;* see R. Virchow, 'Die Einheitsbestrebungen in der wissenschaftlichen Medicin,' *Gesammelte Abhandlungen zur wissenschaftlichen Medicin,* 2nd ed., Hamm, 1862, p. 33. Before him Bichat gave a similar definition.
2. Adolph Schultz has shown that fractures occur frequently among wild monkeys and that a relatively large percentage of these fractures heals spontaneously with good functional result. This observation is important because it reminds us that we must be cautious in interpreting bones of prehistoric man and must not necessarily assume that every well-healed fracture is the result of surgical intervention. See Adolph H. Schultz, 'Notes on Diseases and Healed Fractures of Wild Apes, and Their Bearing on the Antiquity of Pathological Conditions in Man,' *Bull. Hist. Med.,* 1939, 7:571-82.
3. Felix Platter (1536-1614), professor at Basle, author of *De corporis humani structura et usu libri III,* Basle, 1583.
4. J. J. Scheuchzer (1672-1733), *Homo diluvii testis,* Zurich, 1726; see Rudolf Wolf, *Biographien zur Kulturgeschichte der Schweiz,* Zurich, 1858, 1:214f.
5. E. J. C. Esper, *Ausführliche Nachrichten von neuentdeckten Zoolithen unbekannter vierfüssiger Thiere,* Nuremberg, 1774, 14 plates.
6. [F. J. Carl] Mayer, 'Über krankhafte Knochen vorweltlicher Thiere,' *Nova Acta Leopoldina,* 1854, 24 (pt. ii):673-89.
7. *Loc. cit.*
8. August Goldfuss, *Die Umgebungen von Muggendorf,* Erlangen, 1810.
9. G. Cuvier, *Recherches sur les ossemens fossiles,* Paris, 1820.
10. 'On Some Fossil Bones Discovered in Caverns in the Limestone Quarries of Oreston. By Joseph Whidbey . . . to Which Is Added a Description of the Bones by William Clift,' *Phil. Tr. Roy. Soc.,* London, 1823, pt. I: 78-90, 12 plates.
11. Philip Fr. von Walther, 'Über das Alterthum der Knochenkrankheiten,' *J. f. Chir. u. Augenhlk.,* 1825, 8: 1-16.
12. P. C. Schmerling, 'Description des ossemens fossiles, à l'état pathologique, provenant des cavernes de la province de Liège,' *Bull. Soc. Géol. de France,* 1835, 2nd ser. 7:51-61.
13. See note 6.
14. His many publications on the subject are listed in J. Schwalbe, *Virchow-Bibliographie,* 1843-1901, Berlin, 1901, pp. 51ff.
15. They are listed in Moodie (note 18) and Pales (note 22).
16. Name and definition were given by Sir Marc Armand Ruffer, see note 30.
17. Roy Lee Moodie (1880-1934), Ph.D. University of Chicago, 1908; from 1914 to 1928 teaching anatomy and engaged in research in various positions at the University of Illinois, College of Medicine, Chicago. Professor of Paleodontology, College of Dentistry, University of Southern California,

1928-34; Paleopathologist, Wellcome Historical Medical Museum, London, 1929-34; see *Who Was Who in America,* Chicago, 1943, vol. I.

18. *Paleopathology, an Introduction to the Study of Ancient Evidences of Disease,* Urbana, University of Illinois Press, 1923, 567 pp., 117 plates. The same year Moodie published a short, more popular book, *The Antiquity of Disease,* The University of Chicago Press, 1923, The University of Chicago Science Series, 148 pp., 36 illus. (All references to Moodie are to this work unless indicated otherwise.)
19. So, e.g. Jules Le Baron, *Lésions osseuses de l'homme préhistorique en France et en Algérie,* Paris, 1881, which was based on the anthropological material of the Musée Broca and the Muséum at Paris.
20. See Appendix IV.
21. Herbert Upham Williams (1866-1938), M.D. University of Buffalo, 1889; M.D. University of Pennsylvania, 1891; Professor of Pathology and Bacteriology, Medical Department, University of Buffalo, 1894-1938; see *Who Was Who in America,* Chicago, 1943, vol. I. His chief general paper on the subject was a survey, 'Human Paleopathology, with Some Original Observations on Symmetrical Osteoporosis of the Skull,' *Arch. Pathol.,* 1929, 7:839-902, 18 illus. For his papers on syphilis see note 108.
22. *Paléopathologie et pathologie comparative,* Paris, 1930, 352 pp., 63 plates. The bibliography includes 660 titles. It is the most complete bibliography of paleopathology to the year 1930. In Appendix IV we have listed the chief literature published after that date. (All references to Pales hereafter are to this work unless indicated otherwise.)
23. Most investigators have described the methods they used; see e.g. Pales, 'La Paléopathologie; matériaux et méthodes de recherche,' *Procès-verbaux Soc. Linnéenne de Bordeaux,* 1929, vol. 81; Pales, loc. cit. pp. 17-30; Williams, loc. cit. pp. 845-7; see also Moritz Weber, 'Schliffe von mazerierten Röhrenknochen und ihre Bedeutung für die Unterscheidung der Syphilis und Osteomyelitis von der Osteodystrophia fibrosa, sowie für die Untersuchung fraglich syphilitischer prähistorischer Knochen,' *Beitr. z. path. Anat. u. z. allg. Path.,* 1927, 78:442-511, 47 illus., 1 plate.
24. Field Museum of Natural History, Anthropology, Memoirs, vol. III. Chicago, 1931, 66 pp., 76 plates. In an editor's note, p. 9, Berthold Laufer mentions the foundation of the new Division of Roentgenology. The first x-rays of mummies were made in 1898, only a few years after Roentgen's discovery, by Flinders Petrie (*Deshasheh,* 15th memoir of the Egypt. Explor. Fund, London, 1898, plate 37). In 1903 Elliot Smith x-rayed a royal mummy (*Cat. gén. antiqu. égypt. Musée Caire,* 1912, no. 61051-61100). In 1906 A. Baessler examined Peruvian mummies with x-rays (*Peruanische Mumien. Untersuchungen mit X-Strahlen,* Berlin, 1906, 15 plates). In 1913 Bertolotti, x-raying mummies for the presence of jewelry, found an anatomical abnormality ('Une Vertèbre lombaire surnuméraire complète chez une momie égyptienne de XIe dynastie. Trouvaille radiographique,' *Nouv. Iconogr. Salpêtrière,* 1913, 26:63-5, 1 plate). See the excellent study of Frans Jonckheere, *Autour de l'autopsie d'une momie. Le scribe royal Boutehamon,* Bruxelles, 1942, a book which gives a thorough description of all the methods employed in the examination of mummies.

25. In an Appendix to J. de Morgan, *Recherches sur les origines de l'Egypte*, Paris, 1897.
26. 'Report on Human Remains,' *The Archaeological Survey of Nubia. Report for 1907-08*, Cairo, 1910, II:1-375, atlas with 49 plates.
27. 'The Royal Mummies,' *Catalogue général des antiquités égyptiennes du Musée du Caire*, Cairo, 1912, vol. 59.
28. 'A Contribution to the Study of Mummification in Egypt, with Special Reference to the Measures Adopted during the Time of the XXIst Dynasty for Molding the Form of the Body,' *Mém. présentés à l'Inst. Egypt.*, Cairo, 1906, 5:1-53, 19 plates; with W. R. Dawson, *Egyptian Mummies*, London and New York, 1924.
29. This was the case with the aorta of King Merneptah, the Pharaoh of the Hebrew Exodus, that Elliot Smith sent to the Royal College of Physicians in London. The examination of the mummy revealed that the Pharaoh was not drowned in the Red Sea but died as a rather corpulent old man, with few teeth and little white hair left and with an arteriosclerotic aorta; see G. Elliot Smith, 'The Unwrapping of Pharaoh,' *British Med. J.*, 1908, pt. I:342-3; S. G. Shattock, 'Microscopic Sections of the Aorta of King Merneptah,' *Lancet*, 1909, 1:319. Long before that time J. N. Czermack had examined mummies with the microscope (*Beschreibung und mikroskopische Untersuchung zweier ägyptischer Mumien*, Prag, 1852, reprinted from *Sitzungsb. Ak. Wiss. Math.-naturw.* Cl., Wien., 1852, vol. IX), but his example had not been followed until the beginning of the present century.
30. Sir Marc Armand Ruffer (1859-1917), born in Lyon, France, educated at Brasenose College, Oxford, studied medicine at University College, London, became a student of Pasteur and Metchnikoff. In 1891 he was appointed the first Director of the British Institute of Preventive Medicine, resigned the post after having suffered an accident while testing diphtheria serum, went to Egypt, became Professor of Bacteriology at the Cairo Medical School in 1896, President of the Sanitary Maritime and Quarantine Council of Egypt (1901-17), served on the Indian Plague Commission, was head of the Egyptian Red Cross at the outbreak of World War I. Invited to reorganize the sanitary services of Greece, he went to Salonika in 1916 and on his return in the spring of 1917 his boat was torpedoed and he was drowned at sea; see F. H. Garrison's memorial notice in *Ann. Med. Hist.*, 1917, 1:218-20. His bibliography of 74 publications from 1888 to 1920 is in *Studies in the Paleopathology of Egypt*, pp. xvii-xx.
31. Edited by Roy L. Moodie, University of Chicago Press, 1921. 372 pp., 71 plates.
32. Herodotus, II, 85-8.
33. Diodorus Siculus, I, 91.
34. *A History of Egyptian Mummies and an Account of the Worship and Embalming of the Sacred Animals by the Egyptians. . . .* London, 1834 (with 10 plates by G. Cruikshank).
35. Loc. cit. note 18; also R. Fouquet, 'Note pour servir à l'histoire de l'embaumement en Egypte,' *Inst. Egypt., séance du 6 mars 1896;* K. Sudhoff, 'Aegyptische Mumienmacher-Instrumente,' *Arch. Gesch. Med.*, 1911,

5:161-71, 2 plates; W. R. Dawson, 'A Bibliography of Works Relating to Mummification in Egypt, with Excerpts, Epitomes, Critical and Bibliographical Notes,' *Mém. Inst. Egypte,* 1929, 13:1-49. K. Sethe, 'Zur Geschichte der Einbalsamierung bei den Aegyptern,' *Sitz. Ber. Berl. Ak. Wiss.,* 1934, pp. 211-39.

36. At the time of the XXIst Dynasty the heart was usually left in the body. It also sometimes happened that a kidney was left behind. See Ruffer, *Studies in the Paleopathology of Egypt,* pp. 57, 81.

37. There has been much speculation about the nature of this *natron.* Natron is the name for the natural soda found in Egypt which contains sodium carbonate, sodium chloride, sodium sulphate with additions of clay and calcium carbonate. Some investigators have thought the brine that was used contained nothing but common salt. See Ruffer, pp. 60f., 87f.; also, A. Lucas, 'Preservative Materials Used by the Ancient Egyptians in Embalming,' *Survey Dep. Paper 12,* Cairo, 1911; 'The Use of Natron by the Ancient Egyptians in Mummification,' *J. Egypt. Archaeol.,* 1914, 1:119-23.

38. Except the female genital organs which were not returned; see Ruffer, p. 59. About the history of canopic jars, see L. Dor, '*L'Evolution des vases canopiques depuis leur origine jusqu'à l'époque romaine,*' Thèse de l'Ecole du Louvre, Paris, 1938.

39. H. Carter, *The Tomb of Tutankhamen,* London, 1927, vol. II.

40. Op. cit. p. 64f.

41. Ibid. p. 12f.

42. Wilder kept the tissues in a 1-3 per cent solution of potassium hydroxide for from 12 to 48 hours until they had about reassumed their normal volume. He then placed them in water for a while and finally hardened them in a 3 per cent solution of formaldehyde; see 'The Restoration of Dried Tissues, with Especial Reference to Human Remains,' *Am. Anthrop.,* 1904, N.S. 6:1-17.

43. The relations between medicine and art, and particularly works of art as sources of medical history have been studied very extensively by Charcot and his co-workers, notably Paul Richer. In 1888 they launched a serial publication devoted to the subject, *Nouvelle Iconographie de la Salpêtrière;* an index of the first 18 volumes was published in 1903, *L'Oeuvre médico-artistique de la Nouvelle Iconographie de la Salpêtrière.* A number of valuable monographs came from the same school, such as, Charcot and Paul Richer, *Les Démoniaques dans l'art,* Paris, 1887, and *Les Difformes et les malades dans l'art,* Paris, 1889; Paul Richer, *L'Art et la médecine,* Paris, n.d. [1902]. In Germany these studies were cultivated particularly by Eugen Holländer, who in all his books discusses the early evidence of disease, *Die Medizin in der klassischen Malerei,* Stuttgart, 1903; *Die Karikatur und Satire in der Medizin,* Stuttgart, 1905; *Plastik und Medizin,* Stuttgart, 1912; see also H. E. Sigerist, 'The Historical Aspect of Art and Medicine,' *Bull. Inst. Hist. Med.,* 1936, 4:271-96.

44. D. E. Derry, 'A Case of Hydrocephalus in an Egyptian of the Roman Period,' *J. Anat. Physiol.,* 1913, 47:436-58.

45. Loc. cit. p. 35 and plate I, fig. 2.

46. Loc. cit. p. 35 and plate II.
47. According to G. Elliot Smith, who examined the mummy ('The Royal Mummies,' loc. cit. plate 62); Ruffer (p. 178) concurred with the diagnosis; while H. C. Slomann attributed the deformity to poliomyelitis, 'Contribution à la paléo-pathologie égyptienne,' *Bull. et mém. Soc. d'Anthrop. de Paris,* 1927, ser. 7, 8:81-6. About club foot, see also Margaret A. Murray, *The Tomb of Two Brothers,* Manchester, 1910, p. 42f., plate 14, fig. 14.
48. Ruffer, p. 42, plate IX.
49. See Ruffer's essay, 'On Dwarfs and Other Deformed Persons in Egypt,' op. cit. pp. 35-48, plates VII-XI, where further literature on the subject is mentioned. A predynastic statuette of a dwarf was described recently by F. Jonckheere, 'Le Bossu des Musées Royaux d'art et d'histoire de Bruxelles,' *Chronique d'Egypte,* 1948, 23:24-35, 3 fig.
50. C. G. Seligman, 'A Cretinous Skull of the Eighteenth Dynasty,' *Man,* 1912, 12:17-18.
51. Pales, 'Maladie de Paget préhistorique, avec note additionelle du Professeur R. Verneau,' *L'Anthropologie,* 1929, 39:263-70, 4 illus.; see also Pales, *Paléopathologie* . . . p. 45ff., and plates IV-VI. About the skull of the mummified baboon from Egypt considered to show symptoms of Paget's disease, see ibid. p. 47ff. Pales thinks that it is rather a case of goundou.
52. Loc. cit. note 26.
53. *Arch. Path.,* 1929, 7:850ff.
54. Pales, p. 250f.
55. B. Adachi, 'Die Porosität des Schädeldaches,' *Ztschr. f. Morph. u. Anthrop.,* 1904, 7:373-8, where the author discusses and pictures an ancient Egyptian skull and one of a Dyak; F. Wood Jones, loc. cit. (note 26), p. 203.
56. Pales, pp. 248-58.
57. Jules Parrot, 'Les Lésions osseuses de la syphilis héréditaire,' *Tr. Path. Soc. London,* 1879, 30:339-50.
58. See the pictures of David Hansemann, *Die Rachitis des Schädels,* Berlin, 1901; Williams' comment loc. cit. (note 21).
59. Wood Jones, loc. cit.
60. Ruffer (p. 43) had no doubt about the occurrence of rickets in Egypt but based his assumption entirely on wall paintings.
61. In Lortet and Gaillard, 'La Faune momifiée de l'ancienne Egypte et recherches anthropologiques,' *Arch. d. Mus. d'Hist. nat. de Lyon,* 1903-9, vol. 8, mém. 2; vol. 9, mém. 2; vol. 10, mém. 2.
61a. F. Proskauer thought that the skull deformations found in the family of Ikhnaton were due to rickets, but this is very uncertain; see his 'Zur Pathologie der Amarnazeit,' *Zschr. ägypt. Sprache,* 1932, 68:114-19.
62. *Handbook of American Indians,* Washington, D. C., Bureau of American Ethnology, Bull. 30, pt. I, 1907.
63. C. M. Fürst, *När de döda vittna,* Stockholm, 1920. The fact that rickets is unknown among Eskimos of the Arctic is the result of their diet, which is rich in vitamin D.

64. O. Abel, 'Neuere Studien über Krankheiten fossiler Wirbeltiere,' *Verhandl. d. zool. botan. Ges. Wien*, 1924, 73:104.
65. von Walther, 'Über das Alterthum der Knochenkrankheiten,' *J. d. Chir. u. Augenhlk.*, 1825, 8:1-16.
66. Moodie, pp. 252f., 268, plate LI.
67. *Die menschlichen Skeletreste aus der Steinzeit des Wauwilersees (Luzern) und ihre Stellung zu andern anthropologischen Funden aus der Steinzeit*, Zurich, 1925, pp. 154-5.
68. E.g. W. G. MacCallum, *A Text-book of Pathology*, Philadelphia and London, 1940, 7th ed., pp. 142ff.
69. P. Uhlenhuth and O. Weidanz, 'Die biologischen Methoden im Dienste der anthropologischen Forschung, mit besonderer Berücksichtigung der Untersuchungen von ägyptischem Mumienmaterial und von Mumien aus dem "Bleikeller" im Bremer Dom,' *Ztschr. f. Morph. u. Anthrop.*, 1914, 18:671-716; J. Meyer, 'Über die biologische Untersuchung von Mumien-Material vermittelst der Präzipitinreaction,' *Münch. med. Wschr.*, 1904, 51:663-4; H. U. Williams, 'Gross and Microscopic Anatomy of Two Peruvian Mummies,' *Arch. Path.*, 1927, 4:26-33.
70. Ruffer, examining hundreds of specimens, never found red blood corpuscles and was never able to get blood reactions, loc. cit. p. 56.
71. H. U. Williams, 'Human Paleopathology,' *Arch. Path.*, 1929, 7:890. It is interesting to note, however, that embalming does not necessarily destroy certain faculties of the cell. Thus O. Steppuhn and X. Utkina-Ljubowzova were able to find proteolytic cell enzymes in Egyptian mummies; they found such enzymes also in fossil mammoths, *Biochem. Ztschr.*, 1930, 226:237-42. It is also possible to determine the blood group to which a mummified individual belonged; W. C. Boyd and L. G. Boyd did it with muscular tissue, see 'An Attempt to Determine the Blood Group of Mummies,' *Proc. Soc. Exp. Biol.*, 1934, 31:671; 'Blood Grouping Tests on 300 Mummies,' *J. Immunology*, 1937, 32:307; 'Les Groupes sanguins chez les anciens Egyptiens,' *Chronique d'Egypte*, 1937, 12:41-4; L. C. Wyman and W. C. Boyd, 'Blood Group Determinations of Prehistoric American Indians,' *Am. Anthrop.*, 1937, 39:583-92; P. B. Candela succeeded in determining the blood group from bony tissue, 'Blood Group Reactions in Ancient Human Skeletons,' *Am. J. Physical Anthrop.*, 1936, vol. 31, no. 3; 'Blood Group Determinations upon Minnesota and New York Skeletal Material,' *Am. J. Physical Anthrop.*, 1937, vol. 32, no. 1.
72. The Greek adjective ending -ῖτις attached to the name of an organ designates an inflammation of the organ. This is a mere convention which, however, has by now been generally accepted. It is bad taste to attach a Greek ending to a Latin word, and such terms as appendicitis are barbarisms. Since there is a good Greek word for the appendix, namely ἀπόφυσον, apophysitis would have been the correct designation of this disease. Physicians who discover new diseases should always consult with a philologist before making up a name that may shock their contemporaries and subsequent generations.
73. Wood Jones, *passim*.

74. Pales, p. 187f.
75. O. Abel, loc. cit., and Moodie, p. 276, plate LV.
76. Moodie, pp. 172, 202, plate XXXIV.
77. Ibid. pp. 130, 150, 244f., plates XV, XXI.
78. Ibid. p. 218, plate XLII.
79. R. Virchow, 'Knochen vom Höhlenbären mit krankhaften Veränderungen,' *Ztschr. f. Ethnol.*, 1895, 27:706-8.
80. Moodie, 'Pleistocene Examples of Traumatic Osteomyelitis,' *Ann. med. Hist.*, 1926, 8:413-18, 6 figs.
81. Ruffer, p. 163.
82. Pales, p. 190.
83. Elliot Smith and W. R. Dawson, *Egyptian Mummies*, New York, 1934, p. 160.
84. H. U. Williams, 'Human Paleopathology,' *Arch. Path.*, 1929, 7:869.
85. See e.g. Russel L. Cecil, *The Diagnosis and Treatment of Arthritis*, New York, 1936; R. T. Monroe, *Chronic Arthritis*, New York, 1939.
86. See R. Pemberton, *Arthritis and Rheumatoid Conditions*, Philadelphia, 1929. R. Pemberton and E. G. Peirce, 'A Clinical and Statistical Study of Chronic Arthritis, Based on 1100 Cases,' *Am. J. Med. Sc.*, 1927, 173:31-46.
87. Chief sources for Egypt are Wood Jones, *Bull. Archaeol. Survey Nubia*, 1908, no. 2, and an excellent study by Ruffer and A. Rietti, 'On Osseous Lesions in Ancient Egyptians,' *J. Pathol. Bacteriol.*, 1912, 16:439-65, reprinted in Ruffer, loc. cit. pp. 93-126.
88. Wood Jones (note 26), 2:273.
89. Le Baron, loc. cit.; A. Rouillon, *Lésions osseuses pathologiques de la Vendée*, Paris (thesis), 1923; P. Raymond, 'Les Maladies de nos ancêtres à l'âge de la pierre,' *Aesculape*, 1912, 2:121-3, and many others.
90. Carl Fürst, op. cit.
91. Verworn, Bonnet, and Steinmann, *Der diluviale Menschenbefund von Obercassel bei Bonn*, Wiesbaden, 1919.
92. M. Boule, 'L'Homme fossile de la Chapelle-aux-Saints,' *Ann. de Paléont.*, 1911, 6:109-72; 1912, 7:18-56, 85-192; 1913, 8:172; K. Gorjanović-Kramberger, 'Anomalien und pathologische Erscheinungen am Skelett des Urmenschen aus Krapina,' *Korresp. Bl. d. deutsch. Gesell. f. Anthrop. Ethnol. u. Urgesch.*, 1908, 39:108-12.
93. See Moodie's chapter, 'Deforming Arthritides in the Early Vertebrates,' pp. 161-221.
94. R. Virchow, 'Beiträge zur Geschichte der Lues,' *Dermat. Ztschr.*, 1896, 3:4.
95. Herbert Fox, 'Chronic Arthritis in Wild Animals,' *Trans. Am. Phil. Soc.*, 1939, N.S. 39 [pt. ii]:73-148.
96. C. D. Walcott, 'Pre-Cambrian Algonkian Algal Flora,' *Smithson. Misc. Coll.*, 1914, 64 [no. 2], no. 2271; 'Discovery of Algonkian Bacteria,' *Proc. Nat. Acad. Sc.*, 1915, 1:256ff.
97. Bernard Renault summed up his investigations in 'Microorganismes des combustibles fossiles,' *Bull. Soc. Ind. minérale à Saint-Etienne*, 1899, sér. 3, 13:865-1161; 1900, 14:5-159, with atlas.
98. Ruffer, loc. cit. p. 16.

99. Percival Pott (1714-88), distinguished British surgeon at St. Bartholomew's Hospital, *Remarks on That Kind of Palsy of the Lower Limbs Which Is Frequently Found to Accompany a Curvature of the Spine . . .* London, 1779.
100. *Archeol. Survey of Nubia, Bull.,* 3:32; 4:20, 26; 5:21-2.
101. Grafton Elliot Smith und Marc Armand Ruffer, 'Pott'sche Krankheit an einer ägyptischen Mumie aus der Zeit der 21. Dynastie (um 1000 v. Chr.),' *Zur historischen Biologie der Krankheitserreger,* Heft 3, Giessen, 1910. With an introduction by Karl Sudhoff. Reprinted without the introduction in Ruffer, op. cit. pp. 3-10.
102. Derry, loc. cit.
103. Schrumpf-Pierron, 'Le Mal de Pott en Egypte 4000 ans avant notre ère,' *Aesculape,* 1933, 23:295-9.
104. Discussed critically by Pales, pp. 227ff.
105. Paul Bartels, 'Tuberkulose (Wirbelkaries) in der jüngeren Steinzeit,' *Arch. f. Anthrop.,* 1907, N.F. 6:243-55.
106. *Arch. Pathol.,* 1929, 7:870.
107. This will be done in vol. IV of this book.
108. Herbert U. Williams, 'The Origin and Antiquity of Syphilis: the Evidence from Diseased Bones. A Review with Some New Material from America,' *Arch. Pathol.,* 1932, 13:779-814, 931-83; 'The Origin of Syphilis: Evidence from Diseased Bones. A Supplementary Report,' *Arch. Dermat. Syphil.,* 1936, 33:783-7.
109. Ruffer, loc. cit. pp. 29, 94, 313.
110. L. C. Lortet, *Bull. Soc. Anthrop. Lyon,* 1907, 26:211ff.; and Gaillard, *Arch. Mus. Hist. Nat. Lyon,* 1909, 3rd ser., p. 42.
111. Williams, *Arch. Path.,* 1932, 13:802.
112. L. Michaelis, 'Vergleichende mikroskopische Untersuchungen an rezenten, historischen und fossilen menschlichen Knochen,' *Veröffentl. a. d. Kriegs- und Konstitutionspathologie,* no. 24, Jena, 1930, vol. 6, no. 1.
113. Jules Parrot (1829-83), 'Les Lésions osseuses de la syphilis héréditaire,' *Tr. Path. Soc. London,* 1879, 30:339-50.
114. Loc. cit. p. 192ff.
115. See note 108.
116. E. Jeanselme, 'Histoire de la syphilis,' *Traité de la syphilis,* Paris, 1931, 1:10ff.
117. Moodie, pp. 116ff., plate XIV.
118. Ibid. p. 129f., plate XXIV.
119. E. Dubois, 'Über die Hauptmerkmale des Femur von Pithecanthropus erectus,' *Anthrop. Anz.,* 1927, 4: 131-46; Williams, *Arch. Path.,* 1929, 7:861f.
120. A. Hrdlička, 'The Most Ancient Skeletal Remains of Man.' *Rep. Smithsonian Inst. for 1913,* 1914, p. 520; Karl Gorjanović-Kramberger, *Der diluviale Mensch von Krapina in Kroatien,* Wiesbaden, 1906; 'Anomalien und pathologische Erscheinungen am Skelett des Urmenschen von Krapina,' *Korresp. Bl. d. Deutsch. Ges. f. Anthrop. u. Urgesch.,* 1908, 39: 108-12; Arthur Keith, *The Antiquity of Man,* 2nd ed., London, 1925, p. 417.

121. Verworn, Bonnet, and Steinmann, *Der diluviale Menschenbefund von Obercassel bei Bonn,* Wiesbaden, 1919.
122. Pales, pp. 77ff.
123. Wood Jones, loc. cit. He also found skeletons of 100 men who in Roman times had been executed in Nubia by hanging and showed characteristic fractures, *Brit. Med. J.*, 1908, 1:736-7.
124. Moodie, p. 170, plate xxxix; O. Abel, 'Neuere Studien über Krankheiten fossiler Wirbeltiere,' *Verhandl. d. zool. botan. Ges. Wien,* 1924, 73:104.
125. Loc. cit. p. 263f.
126. Elliot Smith and W. R. Dawson, *Egyptian Mummies,* New York, 1924, p. 157.
127. M. A. Ruffer and J. Graham Willmore, 'A Tumor of the Pelvis Dating from Roman Times (A.D. 250) and found in Egypt,' *J. Path. Bact.*, 1914, 18:480-84; reprinted in Ruffer, *Studies in the Paleopathology of Egypt,* pp. 179-83.
128. Jacob Wolff, *Die Lehre von der Krebskrankheit von den ältesten Zeiten bis zur Gegenwart,* Jena, 1907.
129. Smith and Dawson, loc. cit. p. 157.
130. *Tr. Odontol. Soc. Great Britain,* 1870, N.S. 2:7-80.
131. See Appendix IV for the literature from 1930 on.
132. Moodie, pp. 221ff.
133. Hans Virchow, 'Die Unterkiefer von Ehringsdorf . . .' *Ztschr. f. Ethnol.*, 1915, 47:446ff.
134. M. Baudouin, 'La Polyarthrite alvéolaire à l'époque paléolithique,' *Sem. Méd.*, 1912, 32:170-71; see also J. Choquet, 'La Polyarthrite alvéolo-dentaire de l'homme de la Chapelle-aux-Saints,' *Verhandl. des V. Internat. Zahnärztl. Kongresses,* Berlin, 1909, 1:57-93.
135. Henri Martin, 'L'Homme fossile moustérien de la Quina (Charente),' *Bull. Soc. Préhist. de France,* séance du 27 juin 1912, p. 489; 'La Mandibule d'adulte de la Quina ne présente pas de trace de carie,' ibid. 28 nov. 1912.
136. H. U. Williams, pp. 42ff.
137. Pales, p. 108.
138. See Ruffer's splendid 'Study of Abnormalities and Pathology of Ancient Egyptian Teeth,' *Am. J. Phys. Anthrop.*, 1920, 3:335-82, 8 plates; reprinted in *Studies in the Paleopathology of Egypt,* pp. 268-321.
139. See note 92.
140. Thus Baudouin and Rouillon, see Pales, p. 109.
141. G. Astre, 'Les Hommes fossiles de Libos. Un squelette aurignacien stratigraphiquement inclus dans la terrasse monastirienne," *Bull. Soc. Hist. Nat. Toulouse,* 1925, 53:53-91, 3 figs., 4 plates.
142. M. von Lenhossék, 'Die Zahnkaries einst und jetzt,' *Arch. f. Anthrop.*, 1919, N.F. 17:44-66.
143. Thus the skulls described by A. de Quatrefages and E. T. Hamy (*Crania ethnica, 1re partie: Races humaines fossiles,* Paris, 1882), long considered evidence of paleolithic caries and quoted as such by Ruffer (p. 291f.) were later proved to be neolithic. See Pales, p. 99.

144. A good survey is P. Bouvet, *Lésions dentaires de l'homme préhistorique,* Paris (thesis), 1922.
145. See note 130.
146. See note 142.
147. J. Ferrier, 'Considérations sur les mâchoires et les dents d'un ossuaire de la pierre polie,' *Rev. Stomatol.,* 1912, 19:11-18; also 'Etude sur les dents temporaires recueillies dans un ossuaire néolithique à Vendrest,' ibid. 1913, 20:171-8; Bouvet, loc. cit.; Spalikowski, 'Les Dents des Normands dans la préhistoire et à l'époque contemporaine,' *L'Anthrop.,* 1897, 8:205; P. Raymond, 'Note sur la carie dentaire à l'époque préhistorique,' *Bull. Soc. Préhist. de France,* 1904, 1:243-6.
148. *Archeol. Survey of Nubia,* 1907-8, 2:281.
149. K. H. Thoma, 'Oral Diseases in Ancient Nations and Tribes,' *J. Allied Dent. Soc. New York,* 1917, 12:327; see also Ruffer, loc. cit.
150. S. G. Shattock, 'Microscopic Sections of the Aorta of King Merneptah,' *Lancet,* 1909, 1:319.
151. M. A. Ruffer, 'Remarks on the Histology and Pathological Anatomy of Egyptian Mummies,' *Cairo Scient. J.,* 1910, 4:3-7; 'On Arterial Lesions Found in Egyptian Mummies (1580 B.C.-A.D. 525),' *J. Pathol. Bacteriol.,* 1911, 15:453-62, reprinted in *Studies of the Paleopathology of Egypt,* pp. 11-17, 20-31.
152. Roy L. Moodie, see note 24.
153. Ruffer, p. 15.
154. Ibid.
155. Ibid. pp. 15-16.
156. *Egyptian Mummies,* p. 160.
157. *Archeol. Survey of Nubia,* vol. 2.
158. Loc. cit. p. 17.
159. Loc. cit. p. 11f.
160. Loc. cit. p. 156.
161. 'Note on the Presence of "Bilharzia haematobia" in Egyptian Mummies of the Twentieth Dynasty (1250-1000 B.C.),' *British Med. J.,* 1910, 1:16; reprinted in *Studies in the Paleopathology of Egypt,* pp. 18-19.
162. Named after the German physician Theodor Bilharz who died in Cairo in 1862.
163. See e.g. F. C. Madden, *Bilharziosis,* New York, 1907; A. Rosenstein, *Contribution à l'étude étiologique et prophylactique de la schistosomiase humaine (bilharziose),* Paris, 1925.
164. Observation of Douglas E. Derry, reprinted by Williams, *Arch. Path.,* 1929, 7:893.
165. D. E. Derry, *Bull. Archeol. Survey of Nubia,* 1908, no. 3.
166. *Bull. Archeol. Survey of Nubia,* 1908, no. 2, p. 55.
167. *Egyptian Mummies,* p. 160.
168. Ibid. p. 156.
169. Wood Jones, loc. cit.
170. O. Hamburger, 'Un Cas de paralysie infantile dans l'antiquité,' *Bull. Soc. Franç. Hist. Méd.,* 1911, 10:407-12; H. C. Slomann, 'Contribution à la paléo-pathologie égyptienne,' *Bull. et mém. Soc. d'Anthrop. de Paris,* 1927,

8:62ff.; see also H. Ranke, *Istar als Heilgöttin in Ägypten,* Egypt Exploration Soc., Studies presented to F. L. Griffith, London, 1932, pp. 412-18.

171. Elliot Smith, *The Royal Mummies,* Cairo, 1912, plate 62; Slomann, loc. cit., attributed this deformity to poliomyelitis also.
172. John K. Mitchell, 'Study of a Mummy Affected with Anterior Poliomyelitis,' *Trans. Ass. Am. Phys.,* 1900, 15:134-6; G. H. Rolleston described an English neolithic skeleton in which the left humerus was 3.25 cm. and the left radius 2 cm. shorter than the corresponding bones of the right arm; he attributed the condition to poliomyelitis, *J. Anthrop. Inst. Great Britain and Ireland,* 1878, 7:377ff.
173. Even then when it was described by so brilliant an observer as Thucydides.
174. M. A. Ruffer and A. R. Ferguson, 'An Eruption Resembling that of Variola in the Skin of a Mummy of the Twentieth Dynasty (1200-1000 B.C.),' *J. Pathol. Bacteriol.,* 1911, 15:1-3; reprinted in *Studies in the Paleopathology of Egypt,* pp. 32-4; see also p. 175f.
175. *Bull. Archeol. Survey of Nubia,* 1909, no. 6.
176. *Egyptian Mummies,* p. 160, fig. 66-7.
177. Loc. cit. p. 150f.
178. W. G. MacCallum, *A Text-book of Pathology,* 7th ed., 1940.
179. This is particularly true of Asia and of Africa south of the Sahara. In countries where ancient religions are still alive and particularly where ancestor worship is strong the examination of the content of graves is difficult. B. Adachi, a Japanese pathologist trained in Germany, was one of the few Asiatic scientists to undertake studies in paleopathology. Some excellent work on paleodontology was done in South Africa. See bibliography in Appendix IV.
180. The most convenient edition for the reader to consult is that in the Loeb Classical Library, which has the Greek text and an English translation by W. H. S. Jones; Hippocrates, I, 70ff.
181. See L. Edelstein, *Peri Aëron und die Sammlung der Hippokratischen Schriften,* Berlin, 1931.
182. Hippocrates, I, 146ff.
183. 'Seven Defensiones, the Reply to Certain Calumniations of His Enemies,' translated by C. Lilian Temkin, *Four Treatises of Theophrastus von Hohenheim Called Paracelsus,* Baltimore, 1941, p. 26.
184. Ibid. pp. 25, 27.
185. H. Harold Scott, *A History of Tropical Medicine,* 2nd ed., London, 1942, 2 vols.
186. Daniel Drake, *A Systematic Treatise, Historical, Etiological and Practical, on the Principal Diseases of the Interior Valley of North America, as They Appear in the Caucasian, African, Indian and Esquimaux Varieties of Its Population,* vol. I, Cincinnati, 1850; vol. II, Philadelphia, 1854.
187. Medical jurisprudence and public health were frequently combined in the 19th century and the French *Annales d'hygiène publique et de médecine légale,* founded in 1829, served as a model to other countries.
188. See e.g. P. Peskov, *Meditsinskaya statistika i geografiya,* Kazan, 1874.
189. See Obshchestvo vrachei g. Kazani, *Trudy, Dnevnik; Zapiski.*

190. Such as, for instance, the International Health Division of the Rockefeller Foundation. The international health movement will be discussed in detail in a later volume of this book.
191. See L. L. Finke, 'On the Different Kinds of Geographies, but Chiefly on Medical Topographies, and How To Compose Them,' translated by George Rosen, *Bull. Hist. Med.*, 1946, 20:527-38.
192. Published from 1779 to 1819 in 6 parts, 8 vols.
193. The preceding works were mostly monographs in which an attempt was made to correlate certain endemic diseases with climatic factors, such as, e.g. Friedrich Hoffmann, *A Dissertation on Endemial Diseases; or Those Disorders Which Arise from Particular Climates, Situations, and Methods of Living*, London, 1746; or Johann Friedrich Cartheuser's *De morbis endemiis libellus*, Frankfurt a. d. O., 1771. See Arne Barkhuus, 'Medical Geographies,' *Ciba Symposia*, 1945, 10:1997-2016; also: Gerhard Voigt, *Die medizinischen Topographien in Deutschland bis zum Ende des 18. Jahrhunderts*, Diss. Berlin, 1939.
194. F. Schnurrer, *Geographische Nosologie, oder die Lehre von den Veränderungen der Krankheiten in den verschiedenen Gegenden der Erde, in Verbindung mit physischer Geographie und Natur-Geschichte des Menschen*, Stuttgart, 1813; A. Mühry, *Die geographischen Verhältnisse der Krankheiten, oder Grundzüge der Noso-Geographie in ihrer Gesammtheit und Ordnung und mit einer Sammlung Thatsachen dargelegt*, Leipzig, 1856, 2 vols.; Henri-Clermond Lombard, *Traité de climatologie médicale, comprenant la météorologie médicale et l'étude des influences physiologiques, pathologiques et thérapeutiques du climat sur la santé*, Paris, 1877-80, 4 vols.; M. Nielly, *Eléments de pathologie exotique*, Paris, 1881; L. Poincaré, *Prophylaxie et géographie médicale des principales maladies tributaires de l'hygiène*, Paris, 1884; A. Davidson, *Geographical Pathology*, Edinburgh and London, 1892, 2 vols.
195. Berghaus, *Physikalischer Atlas*, 7. Abteilung: Anthropogeographie no. 2, Planiglob zur Übersicht der geographischen Verbreitung der vornehmsten Krankheiten, denen der Mensch auf der ganzen Erde ausgesetzt ist, Gotha, 1848; H. C. Lombard, *Atlas de la distribution géographique des maladies*, Paris, 1880; A. Bordier, *La Géographie médicale. Cartes explicatives*, Paris, 1884.
196. Studies on the diseases of single areas are so numerous that we cannot possibly attempt to list them. The earlier literature will be found in the *Index-Catalogue of the Library of the Surgeon-General's Office, U.S. Army*, under Geography, Topography, Climate, and under names of countries and places.
197. T. E. Isensee, *Elementa nova geographiae et statistices medicinalis*, Berlin, 1833; J. Ch. M. Boudin, *Essai de géographie médicale ou étude sur les lois qui président à la distribution géographique des maladies, ainsi qu'à leurs rapports topographiques entre elles. Lois de coïncidence et d'antagonisme*, Paris, 1843; *Traité de géographie et de statistique médicales et des maladies endémiques*, Paris, 1857, 2 vols.; H. Schweich, Zwei Abhandlungen zur practischen Medicin, I. *Einleitung in die medicinische Geo-*

graphie, Kreuznach, 1852; C. F. Fuchs, *Medicinische Geographie*, Berlin, 1853; E. Laurent, *Géographie médicale*, Paris, 1905.

198. August Hirsch, *Handbook of Geographical and Historical Pathology*, London, The New Sydenham Society, 1883-6, 3 vols. The English edition has an excellent index that the German has not.

199. Such as, e.g. the classical monographs of J. F. K. Hecker on the history of plague, sweating sickness, dancing mania, etc., which were collected by A. Hirsch and published under the title, *Die Grossen Volkskrankheiten des Mittelalters*, Berlin, 1865; H. Haeser, *Historisch-pathologische Untersuchungen*, Dresden-Leipzig, 1839-41, 2 vols.

200. O. Temkin, *The Falling Sickness, a History of Epilepsy from the Greeks to the Beginnings of Modern Neurology*, Baltimore, 1945.

201. It is quite instructive to read modern clinical histories of dermatological cases written by hospital physicians with specialized training. Even in such modern documents written after a disease entity had long been established, it is almost impossible to make a diagnosis with any certainty from the mere description. It is easily realized how much greater the difficulties are when the description was written centuries ago in different nomenclature and at a time when the disease entity had not yet been established.

202. I have discussed these problems in a series of Messenger Lectures at Cornell University, published under the title, *Civilization and Disease*, Ithaca, 1943.

203. A brief summary of the doctrine is given in Celsus, prohoem. 27ff. The fragments of the School were collected by Karl Deichgräber, *Die griechische Empiriker Schule. Sammlung der Fragmente und Darstellung der Lehre*, Berlin, 1930.

204. Herbert Senf, 'Ein kartographischer Beitrag zur Geschichte des englischen Schweisses,' *Kyklos*, 1930, 3:273-91, 8 maps.

205. See the very stimulating books of Major Greenwood, *Epidemics and Crowd-Diseases, an Introduction to the Study of Epidemiology*, London and New York, 1937; and *Epidemiology, Historical and Experimental*, Baltimore, London, Oxford, 1932. In the preface to the latter Greenwood correctly says: 'I have long been convinced not only that the history of ideas is an essential part of the education of both public health officers and laboratory workers, but that we must try to study the ideas of our predecessors *sympathetically*. Because some remote predecessor held opinions very different from ours, it does not follow that his work was unimportant while to have anticipated some doctrine now held to be true is not a proof of greatness.'

206. 'El bocio endémico en las provincias del norte,' *Bol. San.*, Buenos Aires, 1938, 2:673-94, 696-701, 702-8.

207. See the publications of C. Berman in: *South Afr. J. Med. Sc.*, 1940, 5:54-72, 92-109; 1941, 6:11-26, 145-56.

208. Quoted from Fielding H. Garrison, 'Geomedicine: A Science in Gestation,' *Bull. Inst. Hist. Med.*, 1933, 1:5.

209. Fielding H. Garrison, *John Shaw Billings, a Memoir*, New York and London, 1915, pp. 161-2.

210. Frank G. Clemow, *The Geography of Disease*, Cambridge, 1903.

211. The geography of disease is not mentioned at all in P. Vidal de la Blache's splendid book, *Principes de géographie humaine*, Paris, 1922, but this may be owing to the fact that it was published from an unfinished manuscript after the author's death. Ellsworth Huntington in his *Principles of Human Geography*, 5th ed., New York [1943], has a few paragraphs on 'Climate in relation to health and energy' (p. 70) and on 'Migration of disease' (p. 480). Jean Brunhes, *Human Geography, an Attempt at a Positive Classification, Principles and Examples*, trans. by T. C. Le Compte, ed. by Isaiah Bowman and Richard Elwood Dodge, Chicago and New York, 1920, mentions the geography of diseases (pp. 576-7) and states that there is such a science 'because there is certainly a geography of insects, acarians, rodents, etc., which transmit such diseases as malaria, yellow fever, or cholera. The connection between the natural environment and man is established through a small living being which must itself first be studied.' The impression is created that there was a geography of parasitic diseases only, but there is doubt that other environmental factors determine the geography of other diseases, factors that are known e.g. in the case of goiter but still unknown in the case of other diseases.

212. But by no means everywhere. In 1932 I approached several American foundations and tried to interest them in a research project devoted to the history and geography of diseases, but without any success. A few years later when the war broke out there was a sudden and urgent demand for medical geography. See H. E. Sigerist, 'Problems of Historical-Geographical Pathology,' *Bull. Inst. Hist. Med.*, 1933, 1:10-18. In 1944 the American Geographical Society decided to prepare an Atlas of Diseases, see *Geogr. Rev.*, 1944, 34:642-52.

213. M. Askanazy, *Comptes rendus de la première conférence internationale de pathologie géographique, Genève*, 8-10 *octobre* 1931, Genève [1932], p. 26.

214. The Society invited several medical historians to join its Committee but never listened to their recommendations. If it had, it might have been reminded of Billings's remark that we should come down from square miles to square feet. Indeed the thorough investigation—medical, social, economic, historical—of a disease in a limited area might have yielded greater results than studies limited to pathological anatomical findings on a large scale.

215. Published as a supplement to *The American Journal of Tropical Medicine*, Washington, D. C. The George Washington University Press, 1935, 495 pp.

216. E.g. under Union of South Africa (p. 103) we read: 'Owing to variation in the laws regarding registration of births and deaths no reliable figures exist. However, in 1930, there were 47,534 births and 17,415 deaths among the Europeans and 56,277 births and 45,211 deaths among the non-Europeans.' The total population of South Africa is given as 'about 8,000,000,' the European population is 'estimated at 1,859,400.' In other words, it sounds as if the European birth rate were about three times higher than the non-European one, which is of course nonsense.

217. Barbaric because it is one of those awful combinations of Greek and Latin, and also sounds unpleasant because of its Nazi origin.
218. F. Ratzel, *Politische Geographie*, Leipzig, 1897.
219. Rudolf Kjellén, *Der Staat als Lebensform*, 4th ed., Berlin, 1924.
220. Haushofer, Obst, Lautensach, Maull, *Bausteine zur Geopolitik*, Berlin, 1928; Hennig, *Geopolitik*, Leipzig, 1929; Schmidt-Haack, *Geopolitischer Typenatlas*, Gotha, 1929; see also the journal, *Zeitschrift für Geopolitik*, since 1924.
221. Langhans-Ratzeburg, 'Geographische Rechtswissenschaft,' *Zschr. f. Geopolitik*, 1928, 5:89-98, 160-77, 265-72; 'Begriff und Aufgaben der geographischen Rechtswissenschaft,' *Zschr. f. Geopolitik*, Beiheft 2, 1928.
222. Zeiss is the author of numerous historical papers dealing primarily with epidemic diseases in Russia. Of his papers dealing with geomedicine one of the most important is: 'Notwendigkeit einer deutschen Geomedizin,' *Zschr. f. Geopolitik*, 1932, 9:474-84. During the war he published: *Seuchen-Atlas.* Herausgegeben im Auftrag des Chefs des Wehrmachtssanitätswesens von Oberstabsarzt Prof. Dr. H. Zeiss. 1.-9. Leiferung.Gotha, 1942-5.
223. This and the following from H. Zeiss, 'Geomedizin (geographische Medizin) oder medizinische Geographie,' *München. med. Wschr.*, 1931, 78:198.
224. Fielding H. Garrison, 'Geomedicine: A Science in Gestation,' *Bull. Inst. Hist. Med.*, 1933, 1:2-9.
225. See the very good analysis and final remarks of Arne Barkhuus, 'Geomedicine and Geopolitics,' *Ciba Symposia*, 1945, 6:2017-20.
226. Medical officers of the U.S. Army (J. S. Simmons, T. F. Whayne, G. W. Anderson, H. MacL. Horack, and collaborators) published in 1944 the first volume of a *Global Epidemiology, a Geography of Disease and Sanitation,* covering India and the Far East and the Pacific area (Philadelphia, London, Montreal, 1944, 504 pp.). It is good, but necessarily sketchy, and will have to be expanded considerably in later editions on the basis of field work. Since conditions change rapidly, new revised editions of such books must be issued every few years.
227. A beautiful study along this line is Erwin H. Ackerknecht, 'Malaria in the Upper Mississippi Valley, 1760-1900,' *Bull. Hist. Med.*, Supplement 4, Baltimore, 1945, 142 pp., 6 maps.
228. This is what I recommended for a number of years in addition to a much-needed journal that would serve as a clearing house; see *Bull. Inst. Hist. Med.*, 1933, 1:18.
229. See the fine study of Max H. Kuczynski, *Steppe und Mensch. Kirgisische Reiseeindrücke und Betrachtungen über Leben, Kultur und Krankheit in ihren Zusammenhängen*, Leipzig, 1925. The author, who is now active in Peru, is undoubtedly the most gifted and most successful writer in this field. See his recent books: *La vida en la Amazonía peruana; observaciones de un médico*, Lima, 1944; *Estudios médico-sociales en minas de Puno,* Lima, 1945; with C. E. Paz Soldán, *La Selva peruana,* Lima, 1939.
230. The present book is to a certain extent such a study in that it pictures the history of medicine in Egypt, Babylonia, Greece, Rome, etc.

231. See H. E. Sigerist, *Amerika und die Medizin*, Leipzig, 1933 (*American Medicine*, New York, 1934); *Socialized Medicine in the Soviet Union*, New York and London, 1937 (Spanish trans. *La medicina socializada en la Unión Soviética*, La Habana, 1944). *Medicine and Health in the Soviet Union*, New York, 1947.

232. The term 'geomedicine' should be dropped. There is no need for it and it is never sound to continue the use of a terminology with which the minds of millions of people have been poisoned even when the old terms are given new meanings.

II. PRIMITIVE MEDICINE

I: DISTURBANCES IN DEVELOPMENT

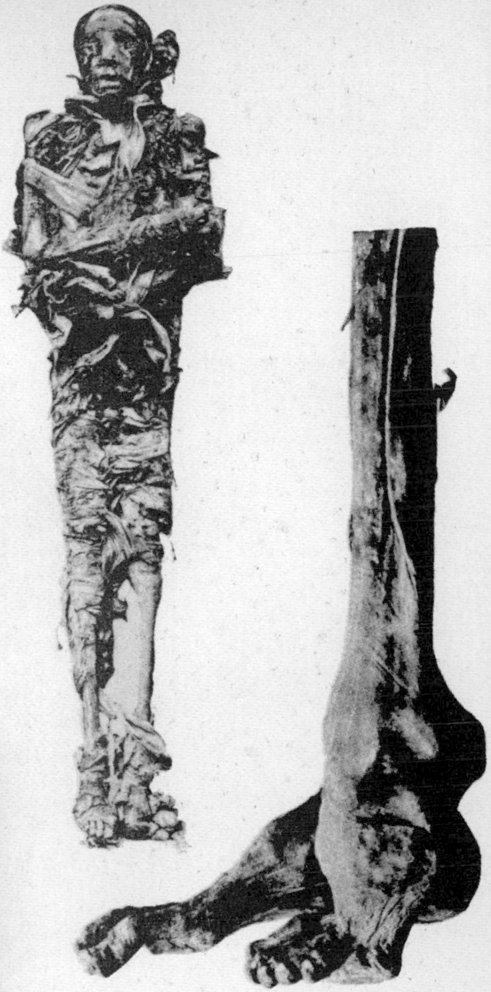

1 and 2: Congenital clubfoot of Pharaoh Siphtah, XIXth Dynasty. From G. Elliot Smith, *The Royal Mummies,* Catalogue du Musée du Caire, 1912, plate LXII.

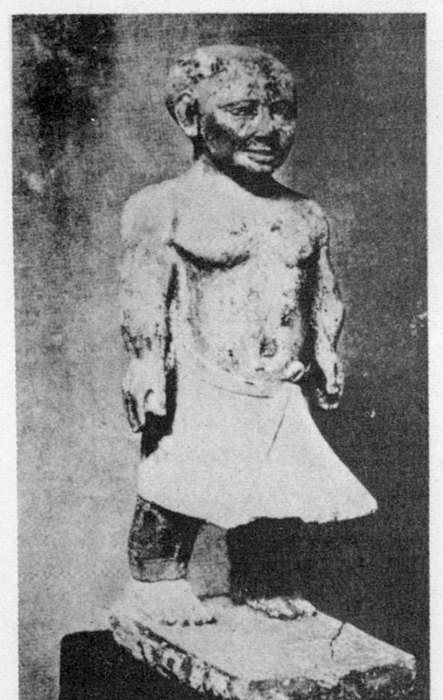

3: Achondroplastic dwarf, Chnoum-Hotep, Vth Dynasty. From Marc Armand Ruffer, ***Studies in the Paleopathology of Egypt,*** University of Chicago Press, 1921, plate VII.

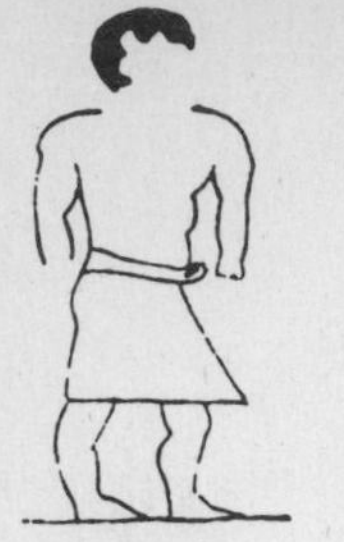

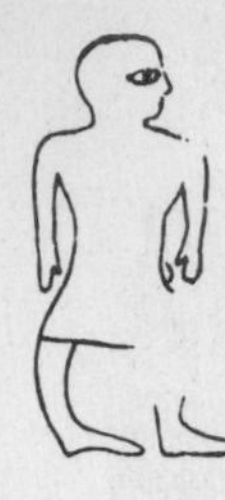

4: Rickety (?) dwarfs. Egyptian wall paintings. The bowlegs suggest the possibility of rickets. From Ruffer, plate IX.

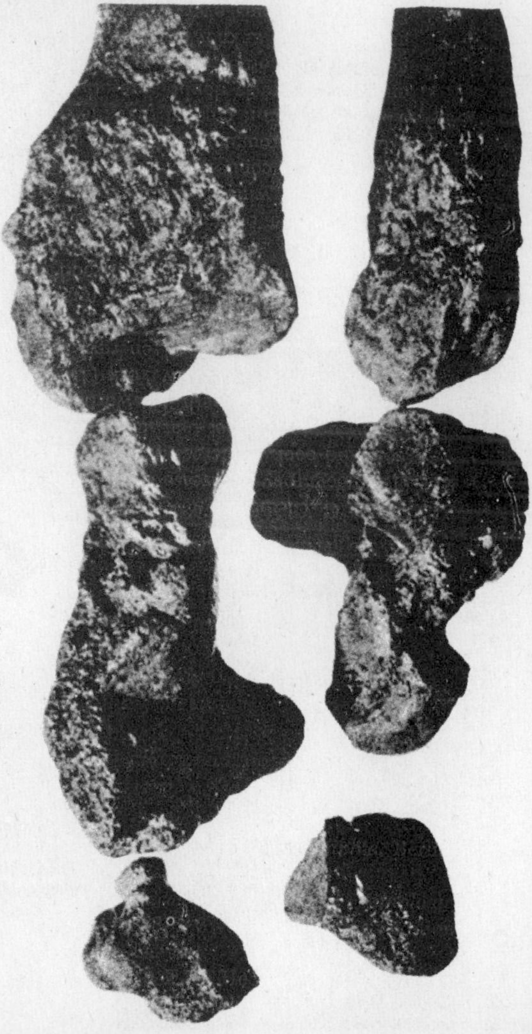

II: DISTURBANCES IN METABOLISM

5: Eocene Osteomalacia. Lower ends of tibia and fibula with tarsal bones of Limnocyon potens. The diagnosis is suggested by the considerable exostoses but is by no means certain. From Roy L. Moodie, *Paleopathology*, University of Illinois Press, Urbana, Ill., 1923, plate LI.

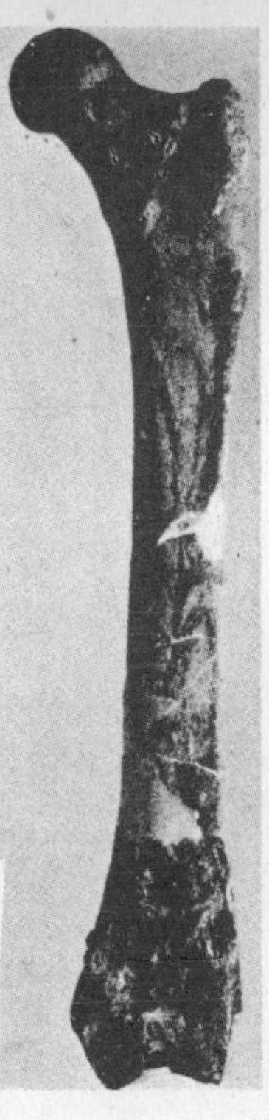

6: Osteoperiostitis. Right femur of cave bear from Cumberland Cave, Md. From Moodie, plate LV.

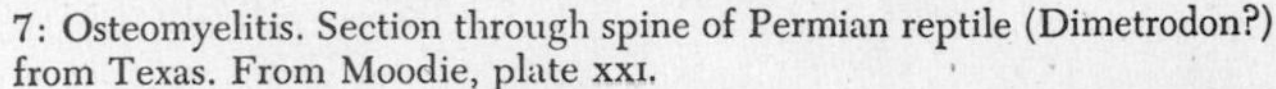

7: Osteomyelitis. Section through spine of Permian reptile (Dimetrodon?) from Texas. From Moodie, plate XXI.

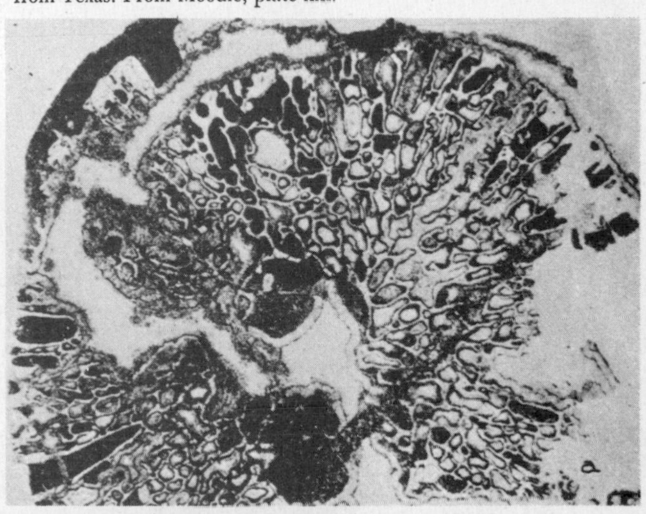

III: INFLAMMATION

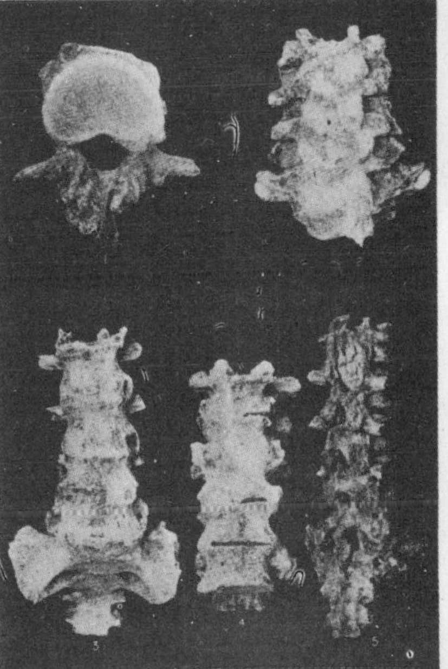

8: Spondylitis deformans, from skeleton of IIIrd Dynasty. From Ruffer, plate XXIII.

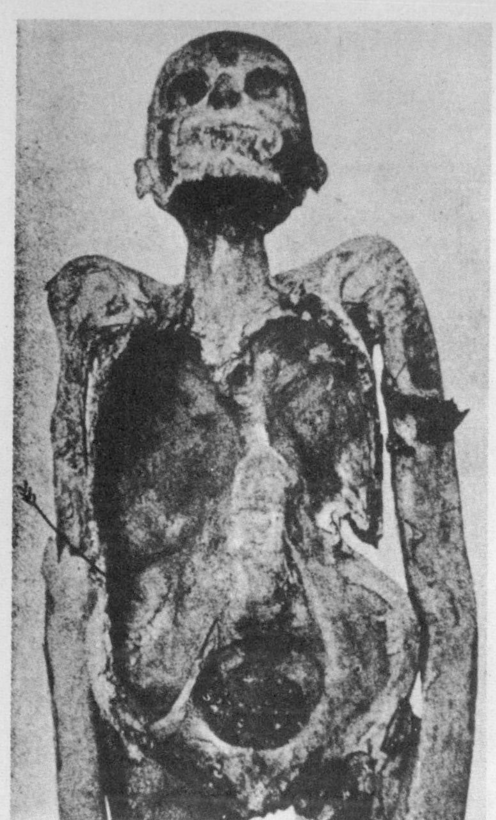

IV: TUBERCULOSIS

9: Pott's disease. Mummy of priest of Ammon, XXIst Dynasty, showing destruction of the spinal column and at the point of the arrow a large psoas abscess. From Ruffer, plate 1.

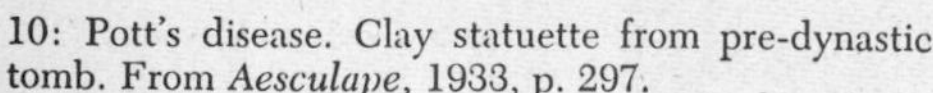

10: Pott's disease. Clay statuette from pre-dynastic tomb. From *Aesculape,* 1933, p. 297.

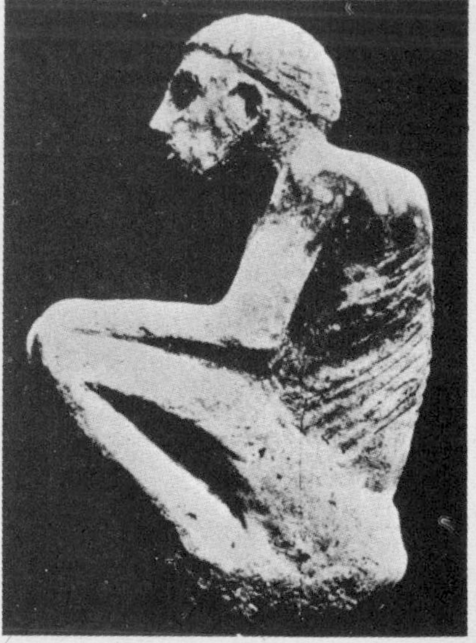

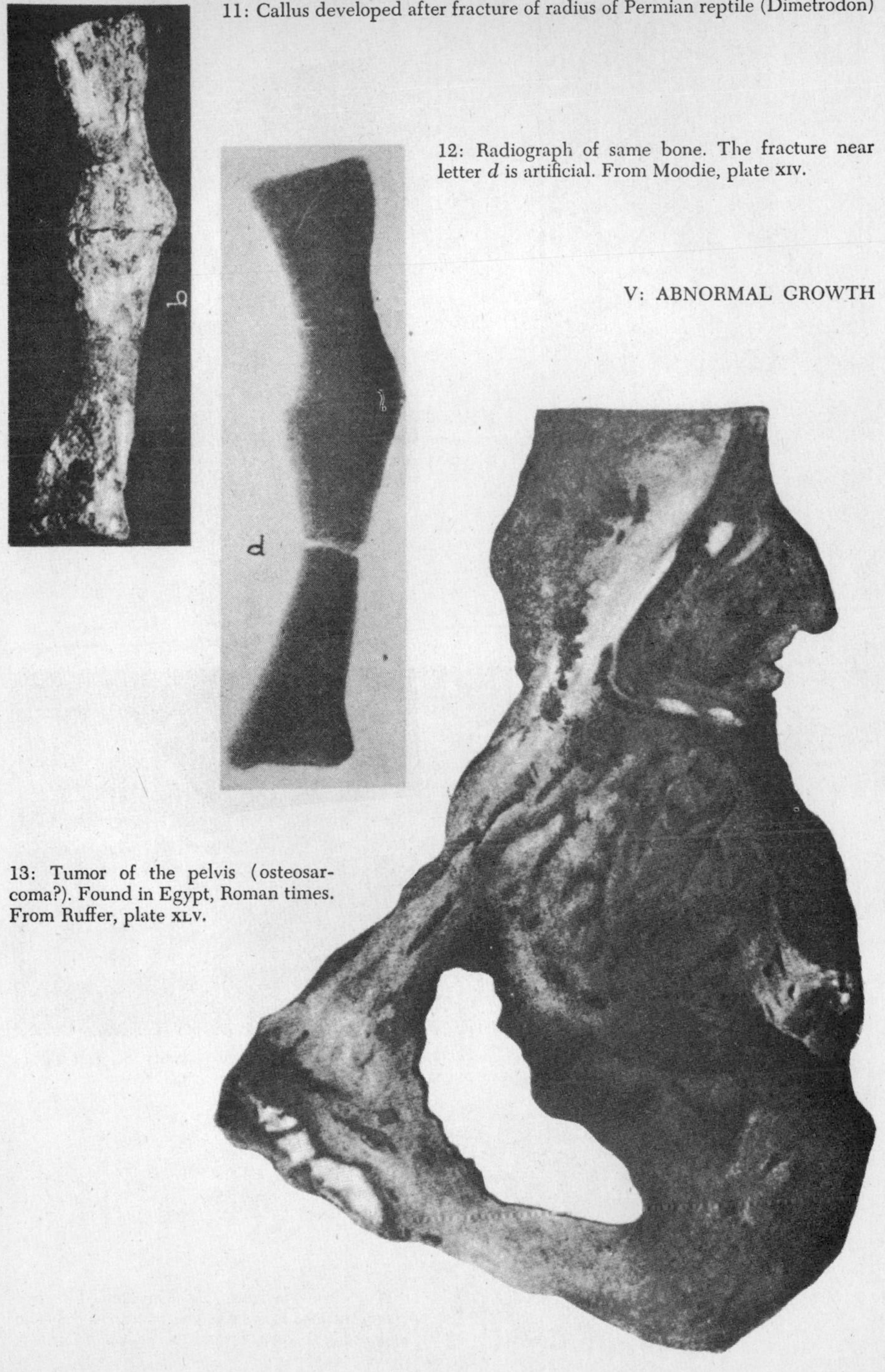

11: Callus developed after fracture of radius of Permian reptile (Dimetrodon)

12: Radiograph of same bone. The fracture near letter *d* is artificial. From Moodie, plate XIV.

V: ABNORMAL GROWTH

13: Tumor of the pelvis (osteosarcoma?). Found in Egypt, Roman times. From Ruffer, plate XLV.

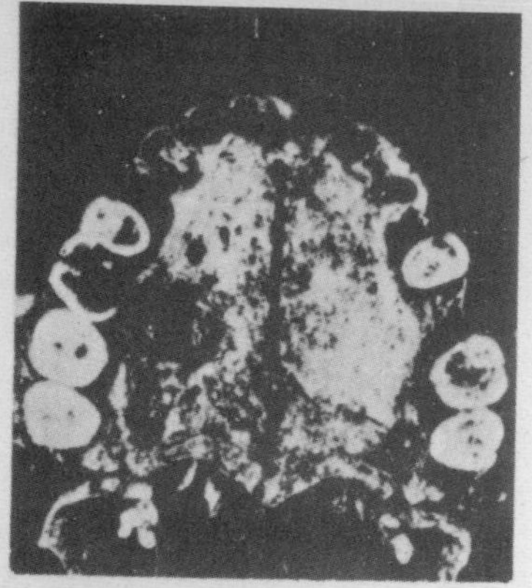

14: Coptic skull. Caries of first right molar, abscess that perforated through palate.

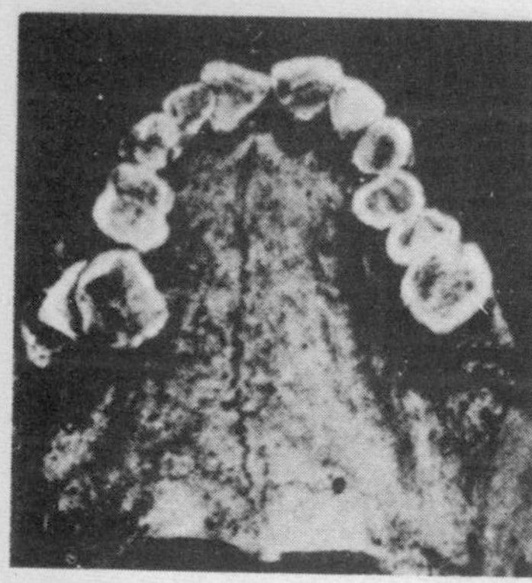

15: Skull of Macedonian period. Attrition of teeth. Accumulation of tartar at first right molar. Traces of suppurative periodontitis.

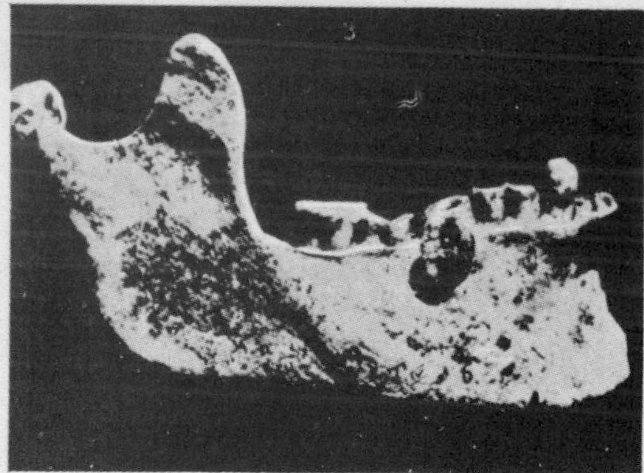

16: Predynastic mandible. Abscess cavity at first right molar. Figs. 14-16 from Ruffer, plate LIX.

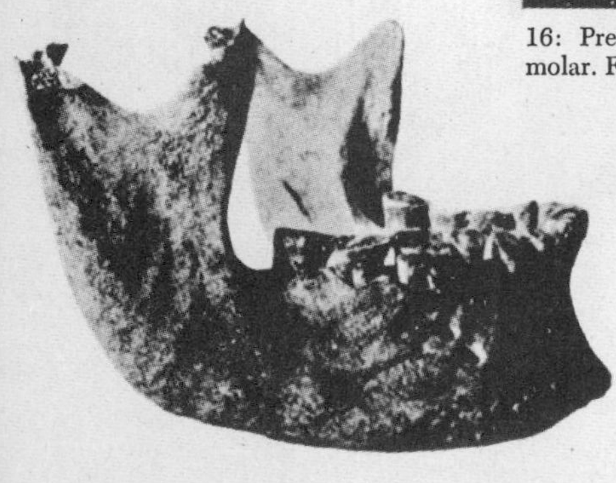

17: Mandible from Old Kingdom. The two perforations may have been made to drain an alveolar abscess. From Moodie, plate LXXV.

VII: ARTERIOSCLEROSIS

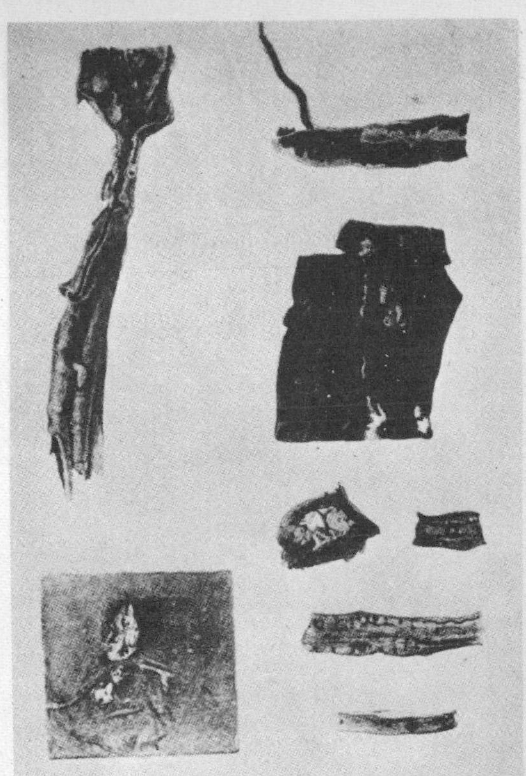

18: Calcified arteries from mummies of XVIIIth to XXIst Dynasties.

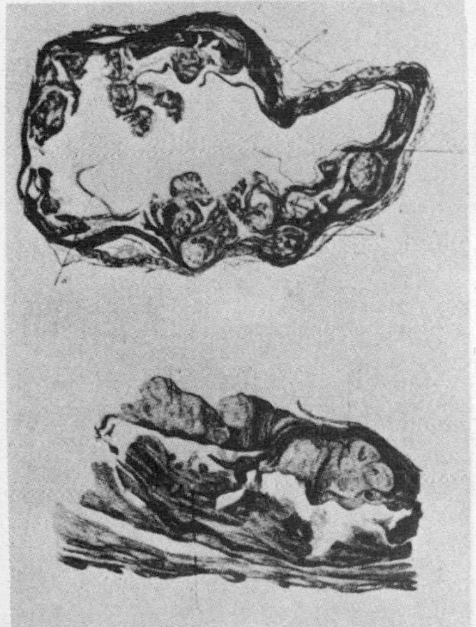

19: Sections through arteries showing calcified patches. From Ruffer, plates III-IV.

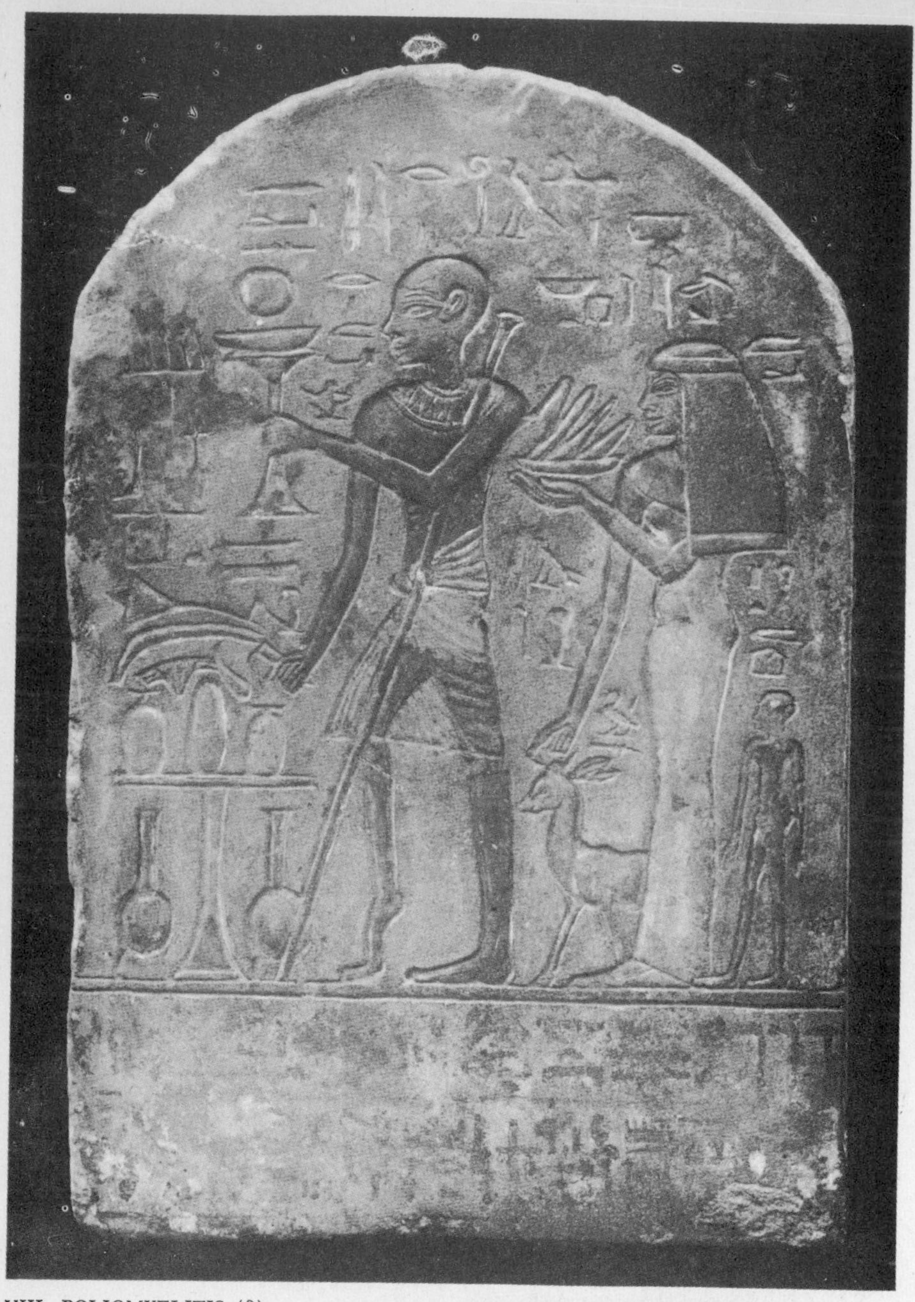

VIII: POLIOMYELITIS (?)

20: Stele of XVIIIth Dynasty in the Carlsberg Glyptothek at Copenhagen. The strongly atrophied right leg with talipes equinus may be the result of poliomyelitis. From *Ciba Zeitschrift*, no. 33, p. 1124.

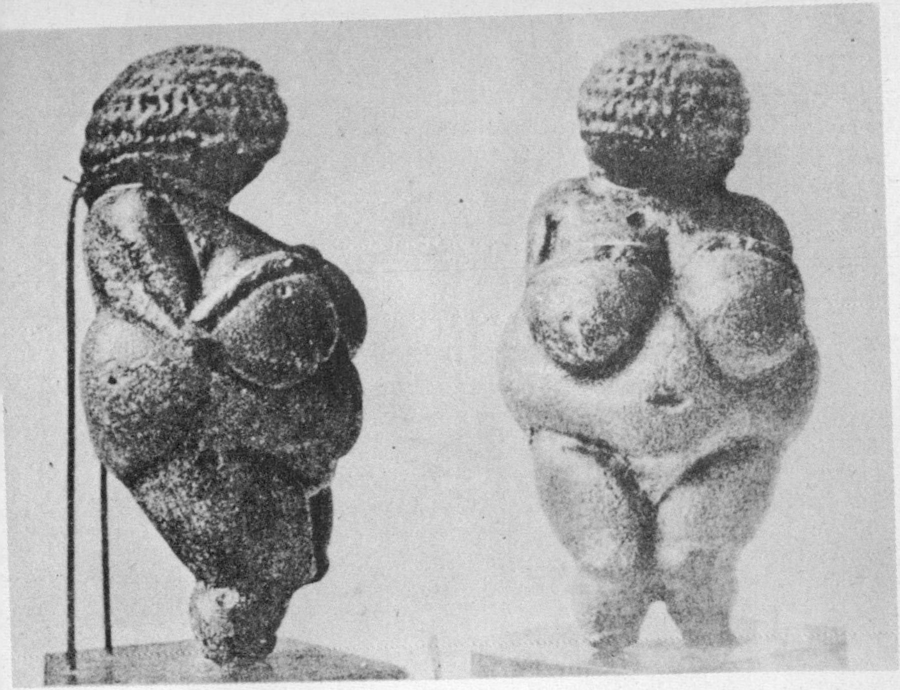

21: The 'Venus of Willendorf' (Lower Austria). Upper Aurignacian limestone statuette. From Kühn, *Malerei der Eiszeit,* Munich, Delphin Verlag, 1922, p. 22.

IX: PALEOLITHIC ART

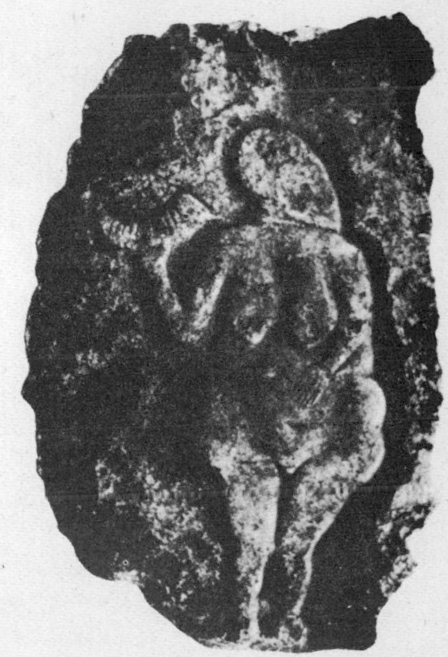

22: The 'Venus of Laussel' (Dordogne) holding a bison's horn. Upper Aurignacian limestone 'false relief.' From *Ciba Zeitschrift,* no. 67, p. 2341.

X: PALEOLITHIC ART

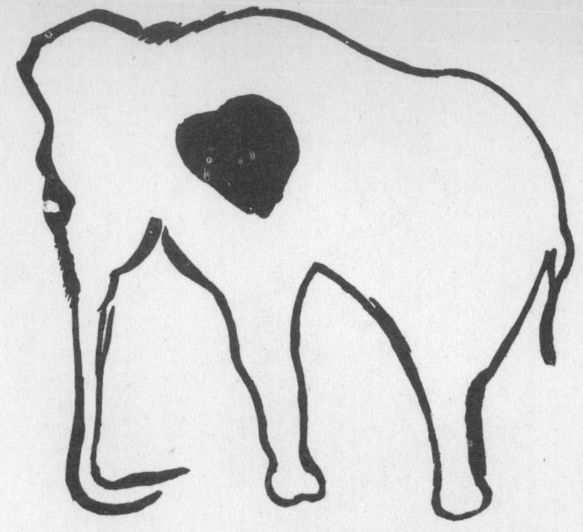

23: Elephant with heart. Paleolithic drawing in a cave at Pindal (Asturias). From Kühn, *Malerei der Eiszeit,* Munich, 1922, p. 42

24: Reindeer stepping over a pregnant woman. Paleolithic carving on reindeer bone. From *L'Anthropologie,* 1895, vol. 6, plate v, fig. 4.

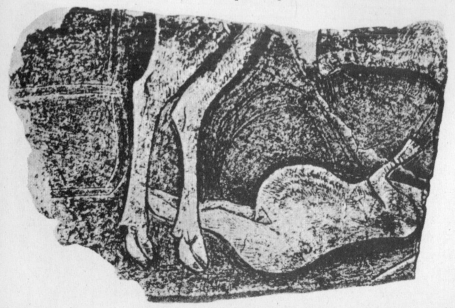

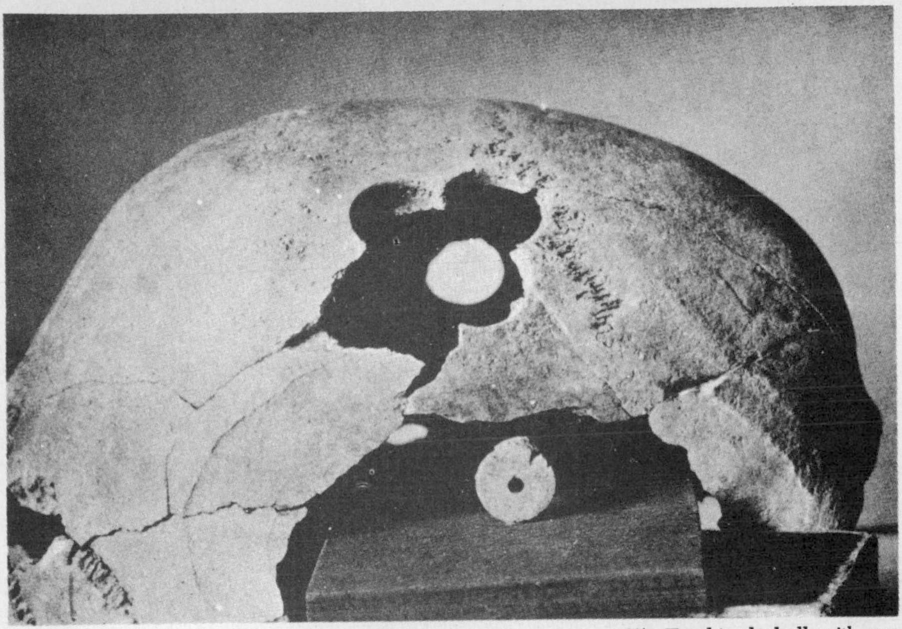

XI: PREHISTORIC TREPHINING

25: Trephined skull with rondelle. From Guntramsdorf (Austria). La Tène period. From *Ciba Zeitschrift*, no. 39, p. 1326.

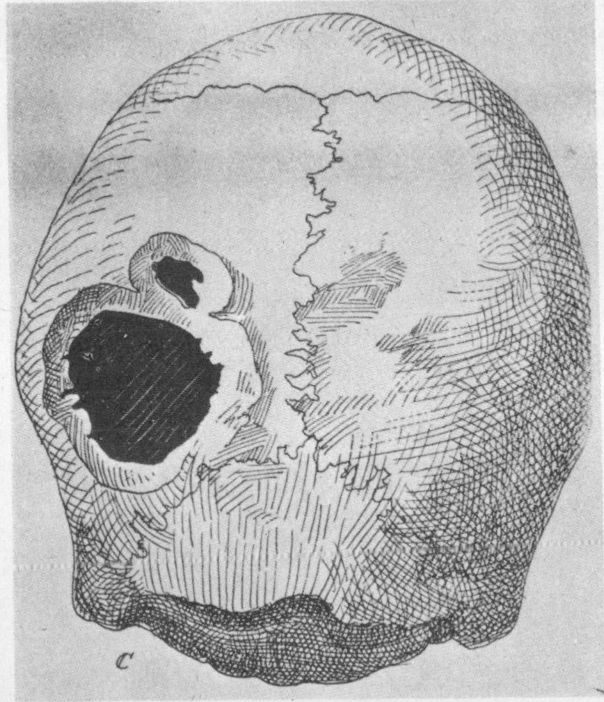

26: Neolithic trephined skull. From a cavern on the Marne (France). From Moodie, *Paleopathology*, pl. LXXII.

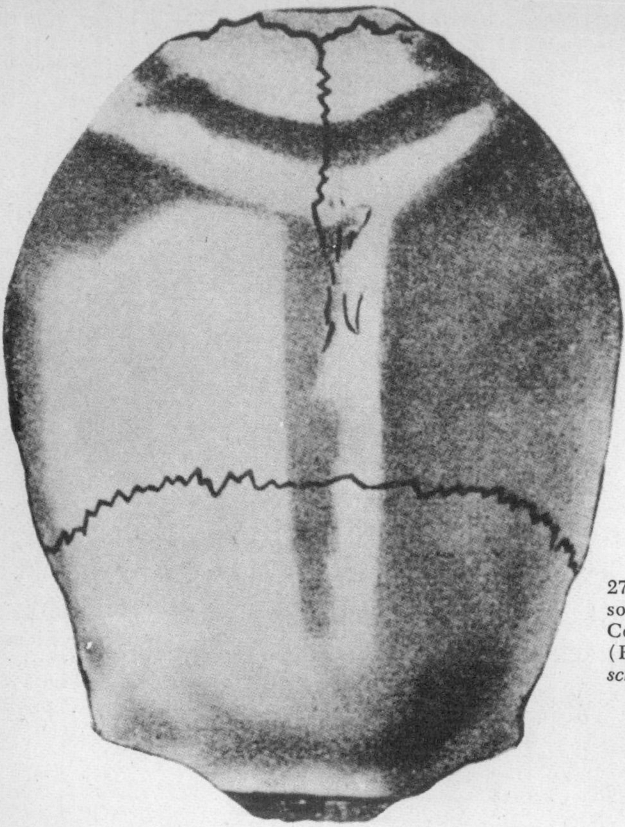

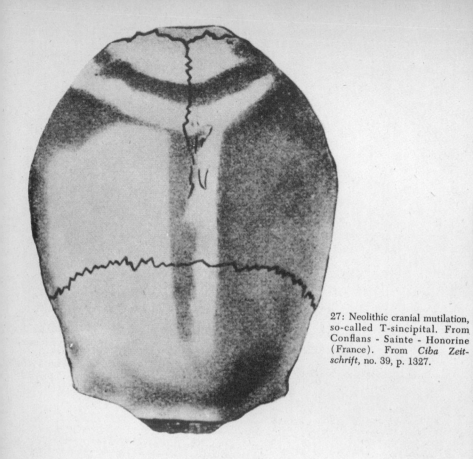

27: Neolithic cranial mutilation, so-called T-sincipital. From Conflans - Sainte - Honorine (France). From *Ciba Zeitschrift,* no. 39, p. 1327.

XII: NEOLITHIC OPERATIONS AND MAGIC

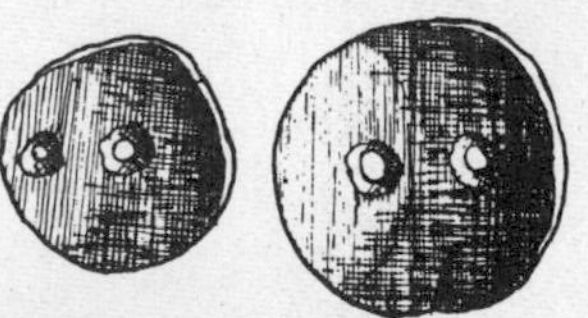

28: Neolithic cranial amulets, or 'rondelles.' Museum of St. Germain. From *Ciba Zeitschrift,* no. 39, p. 1327.

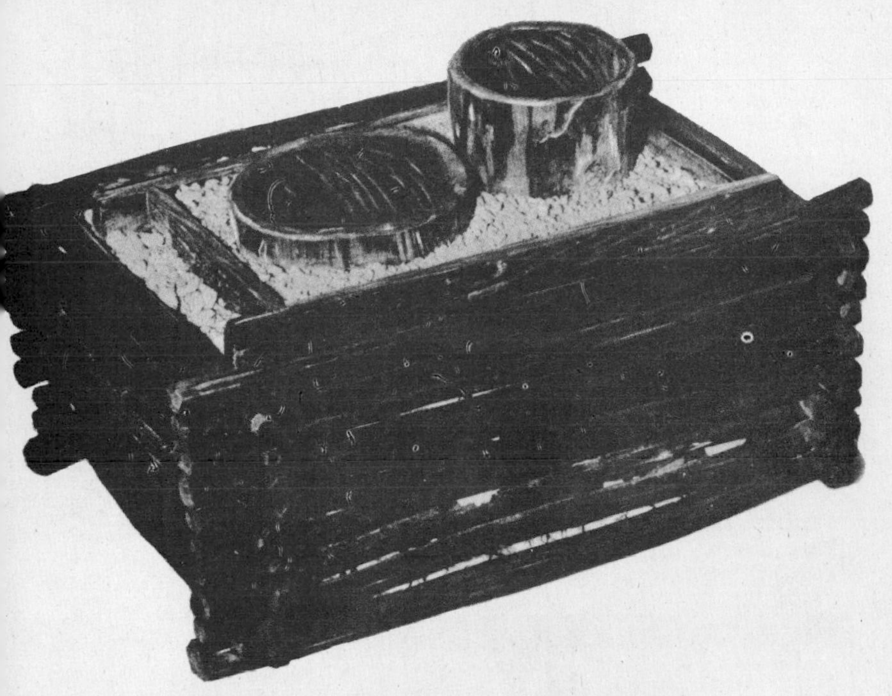

XIII: PREHISTORIC HYDROTHERAPY

29: Bronze Age tubings of the Mauritius spring in St. Moritz (Switzerland). From a reproduction in Schweizerisches Landesmuseum Zürich.

XIV: CAUSATION OF DISEASE

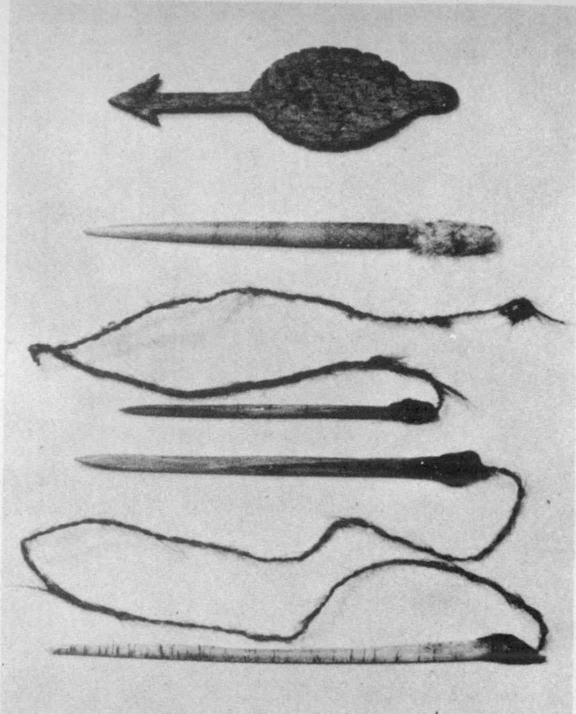

30: Object intrusion. Pointing sticks for magic shot. Australia. Wellcome Historical Medical Museum.

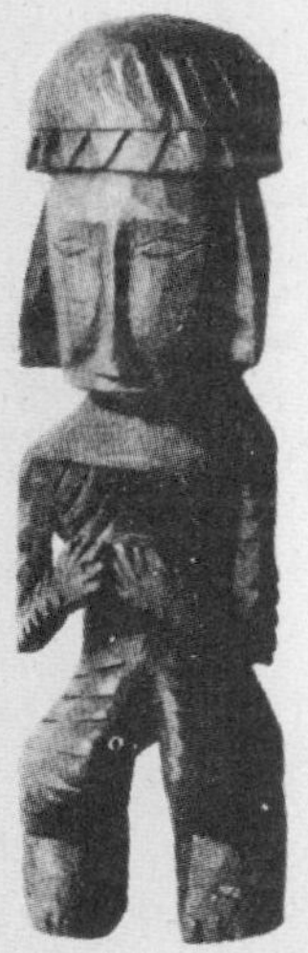

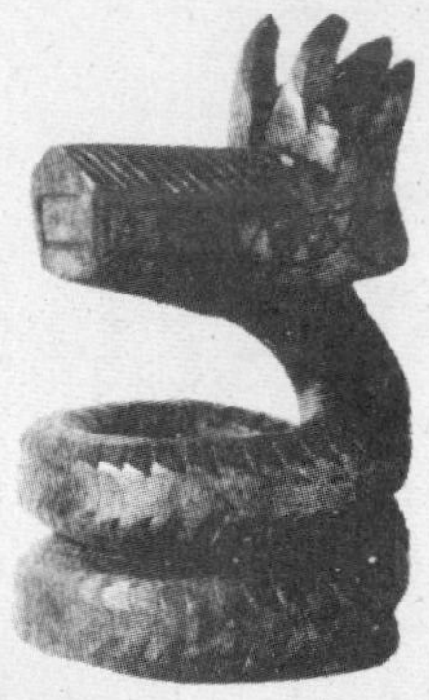

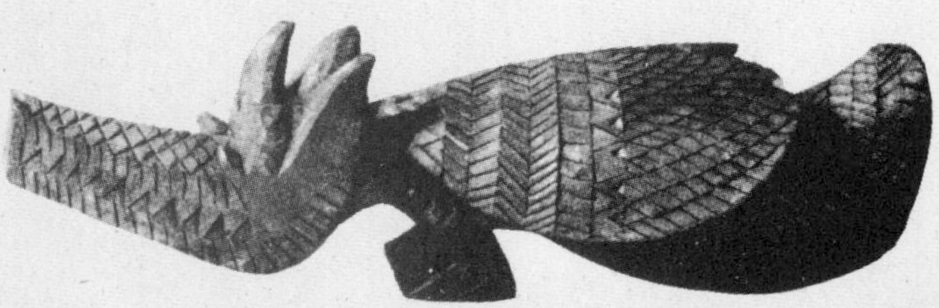

31: Spirit intrusion. Three effigies made of sago pith, representing spirits causing diseases. From Sarawak, Borneo. Wellcome Historical Medical Museum.

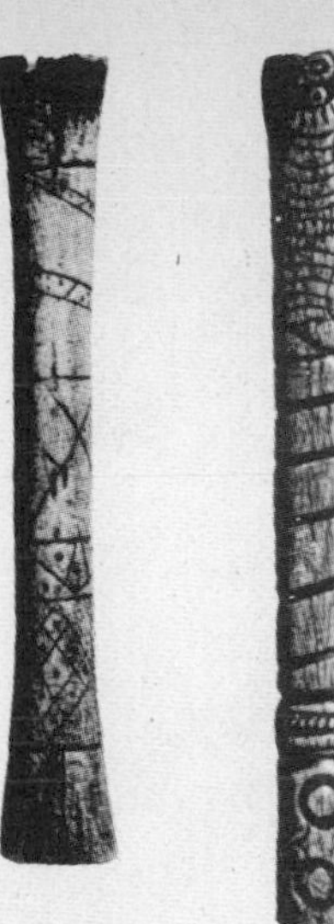

32: Soul abduction. Two soul-catchers, also used for recapturing the soul. North American Indian. Wellcome Historical Medical Museum.

XV: CAUSATION OF DISEASE

33: Sympathetic magic. Nail effigies: vehicles for infliction of disease by human agency. Congo. Wellcome Historical Medical Museum.

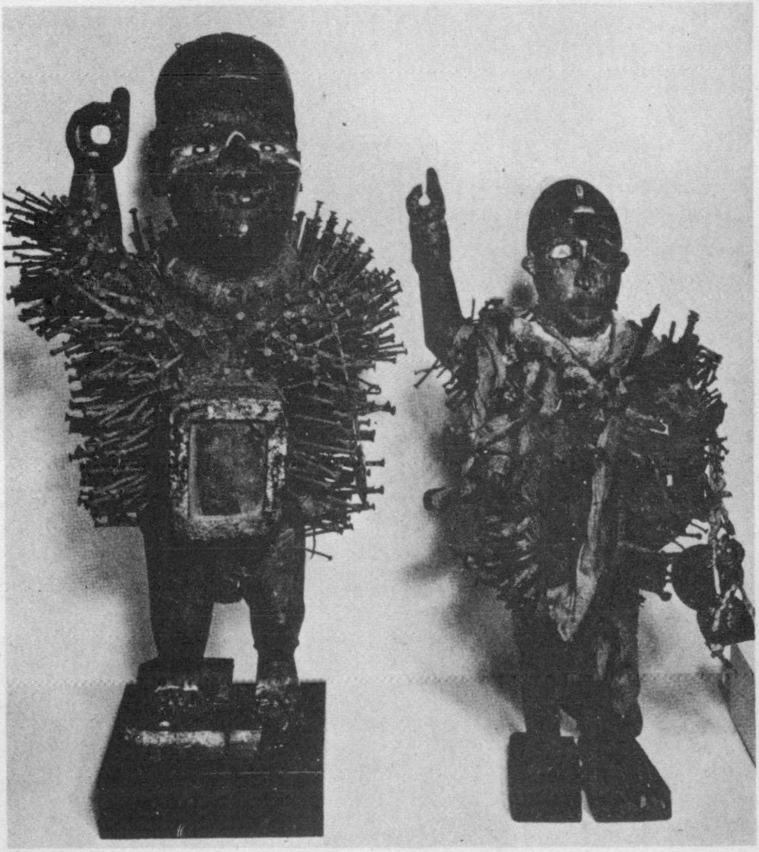

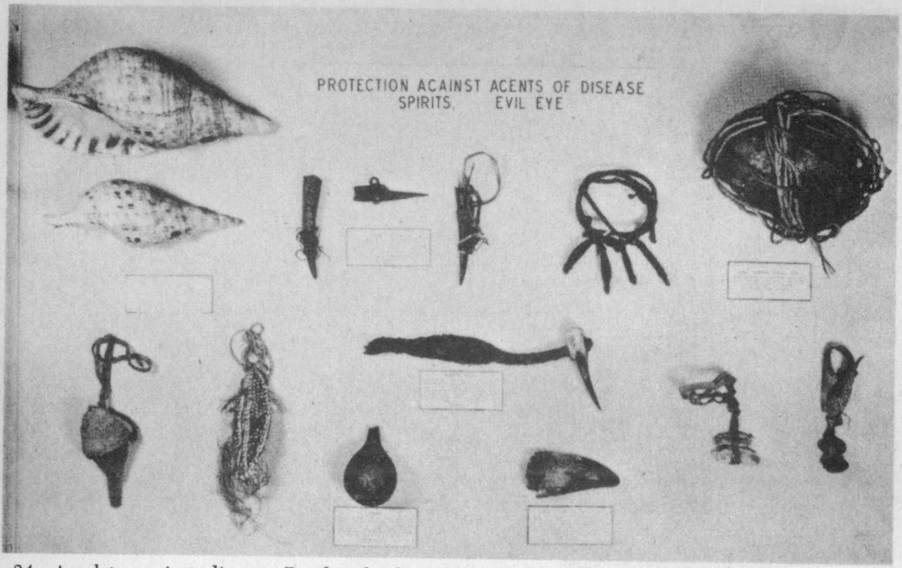

34: Amulets against disease. Pacific islands and Africa. Wellcome Historical Medical Museum.

XVI: PREVENTION OF ILLNESS

35: Amulets and amulet cases. Pacific islands and Africa. Wellcome Historical Medical Museum.

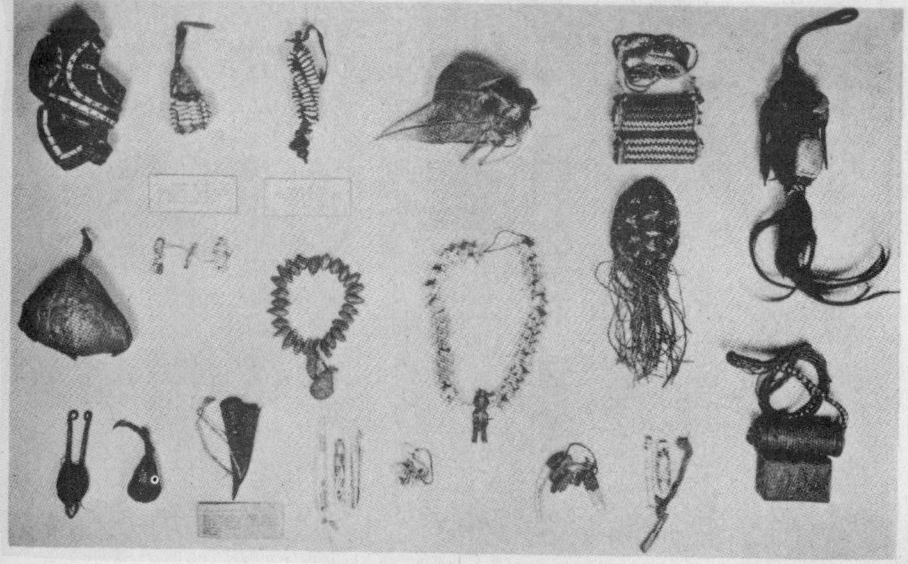

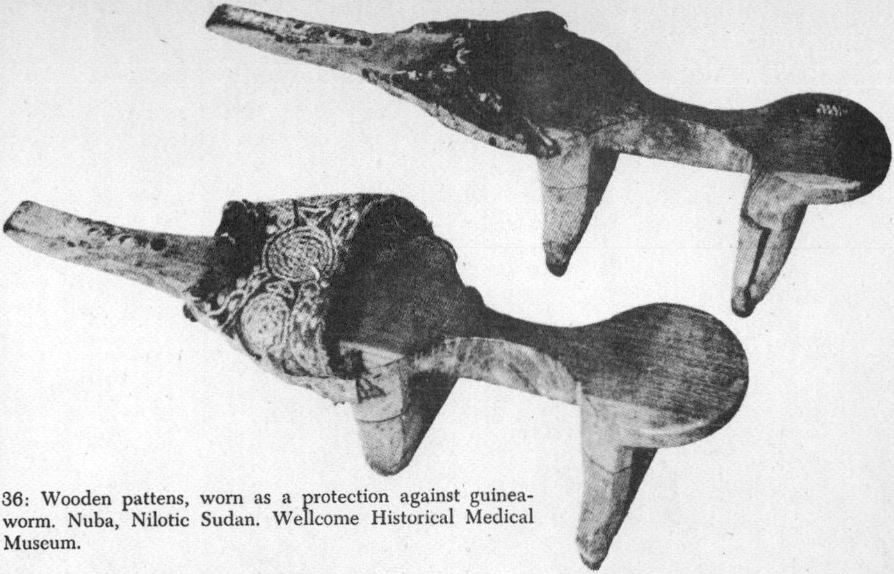

36: Wooden pattens, worn as a protection against guinea-worm. Nuba, Nilotic Sudan. Wellcome Historical Medical Museum.

XVII: PREVENTION OF ILLNESS AND TRANSPORTATION OF SICK

37: Stretcher of the Dacota Indians. After Schoolcraft. From *Ciba Zeitschrift,* no. 10, p. 330.

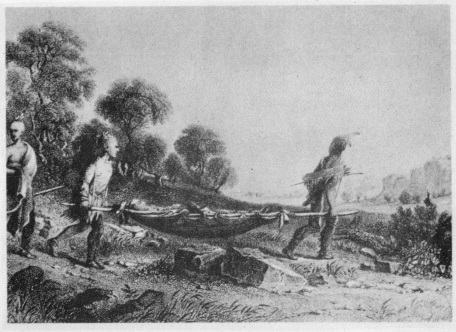

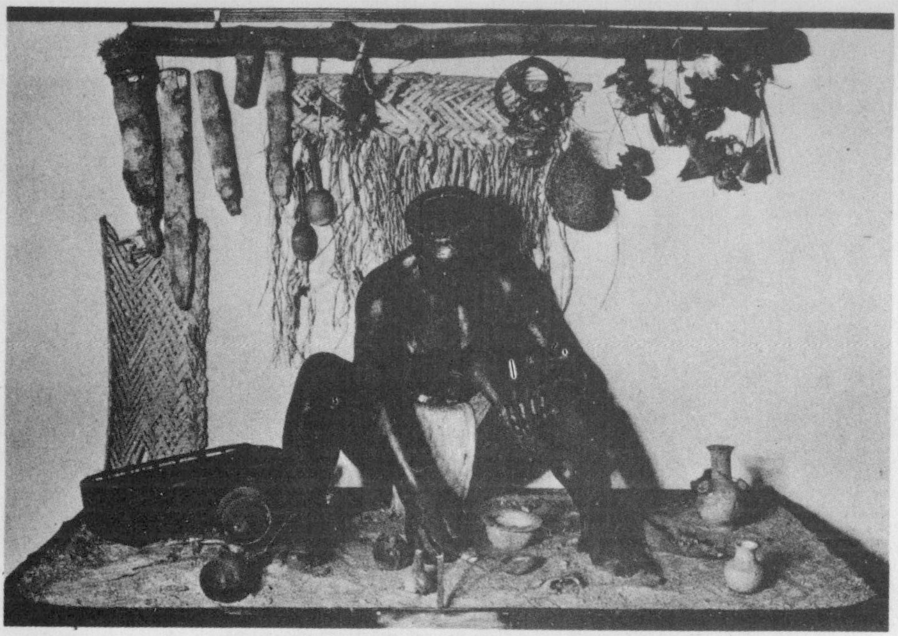

38: Medicine man of a medical Secret Society (*Idiong*), surrounded by his equipment. Ibidio, S. Nigeria. From a plaster cast with authentic equipment in the Wellcome Historical Medical Museum.

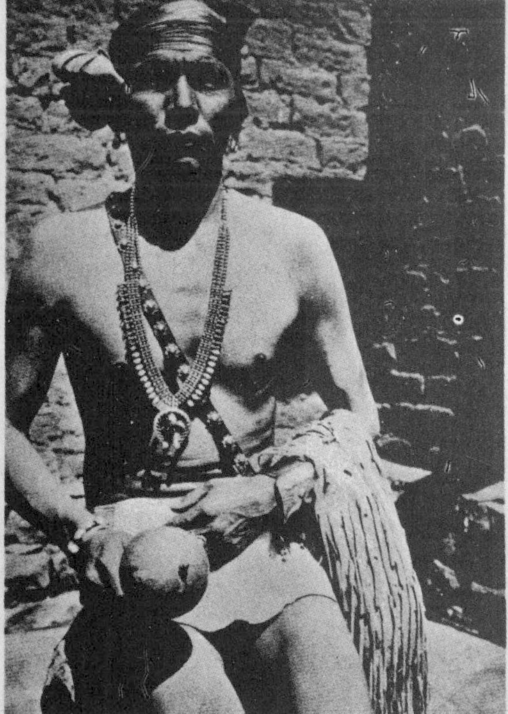

XVIII: THE MEDICINE MAN

39: Medicine man of Navajo Indians. From photograph given to Sir Henry Wellcome by Miss Malvina Hoffman. Wellcome Historical Medical Museum.

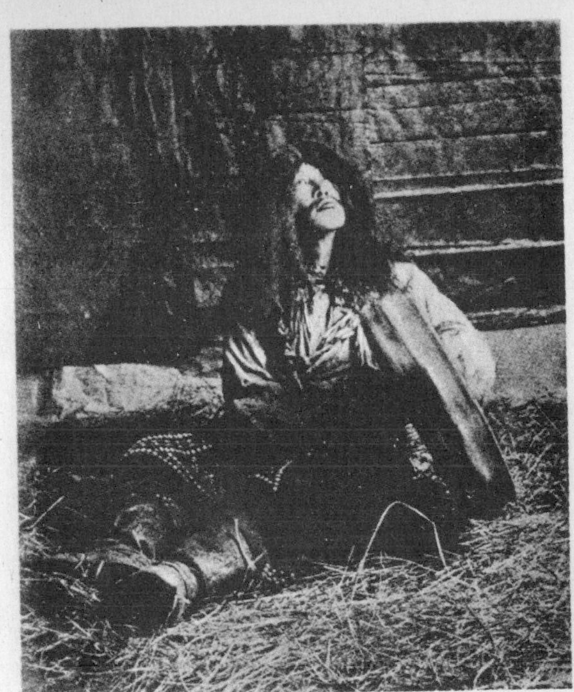

40: A Yakut shaman in the period of preparation. From Nioradze, *Der Schamanismus*, Stuttgart, Strecker und Schröder, 1925, frontispiece.

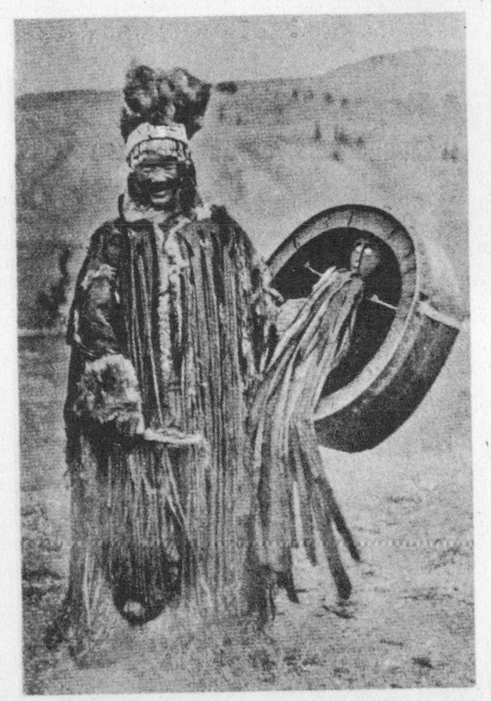

XIX: THE MEDICINE MAN

41: Shaman. Altai region. From Nioradze, *Der Schamanismus*, Stuttgart, 1925, p. 88.

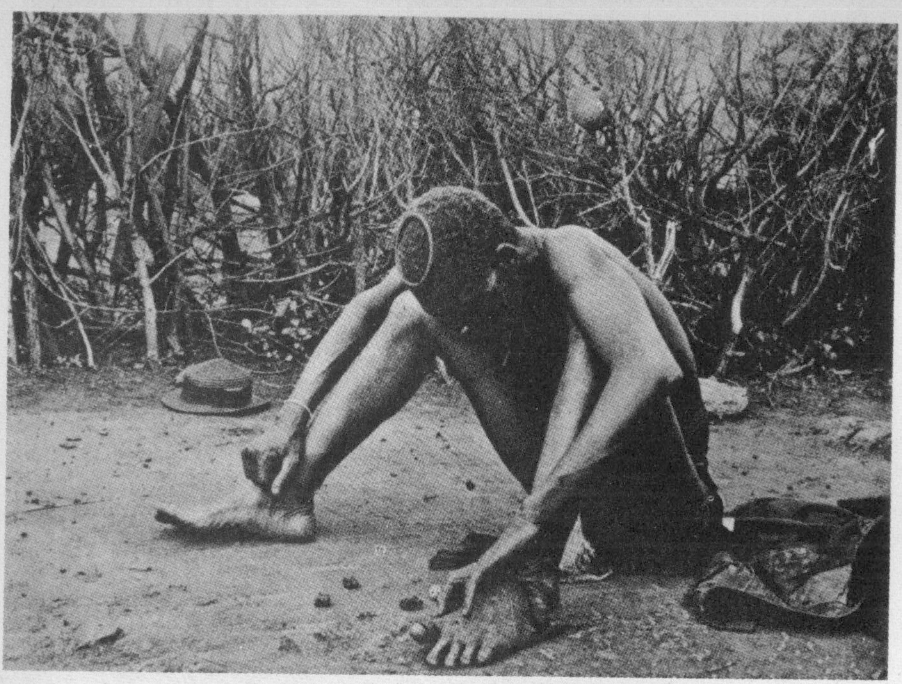

42: Medicine man reading the divining bones for diagnosis of the cause of illness. S. Rhodesia. Photograph in the Wellcome Historical Medical Museum.

XX: DIVINATION

43: Medicine lodge of the Sioux Indians. After Schoolcraft. From Bartels, *Die Medicin der Naturvölker,* Leipzig, Th. Grieben's Verlag, 1893, p. 163.

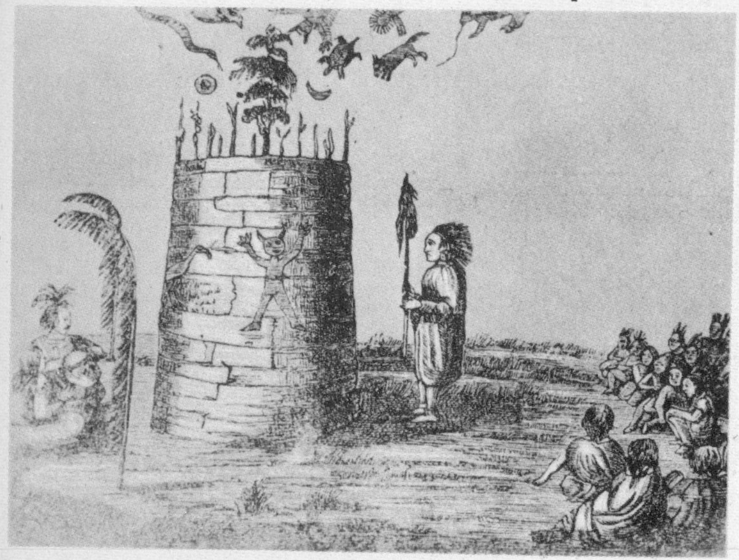

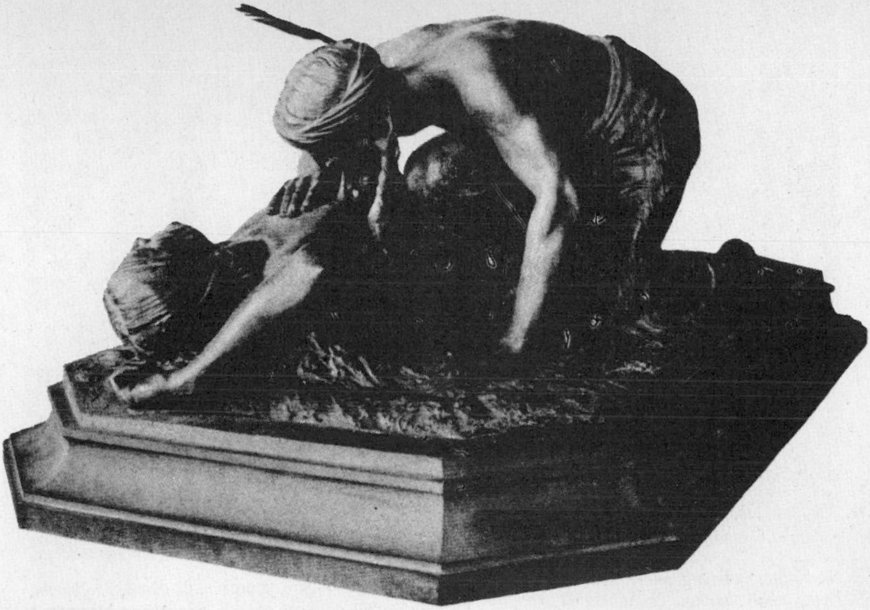

44: Removal of disease by sucking through a bone tube. Ojibway Indians. From sculptured group made for Wellcome Historical Medical Museum by Miss Jane Jackson after pencil drawing by Eric Stone in *Medicine among the North American Indians,* Clio Medica Series.

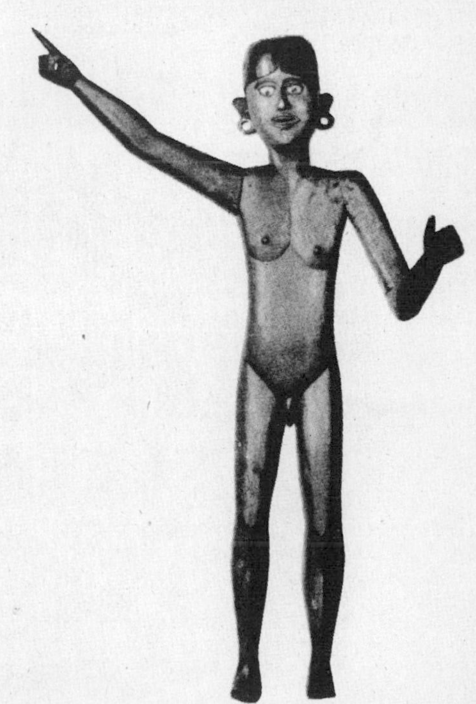

XXI: TREATMENT

45: Anthropomorphic effigy in menacing attitude to frighten away spirits of disease. Nicobar Islands. Wellcome Historical Medical Museum.

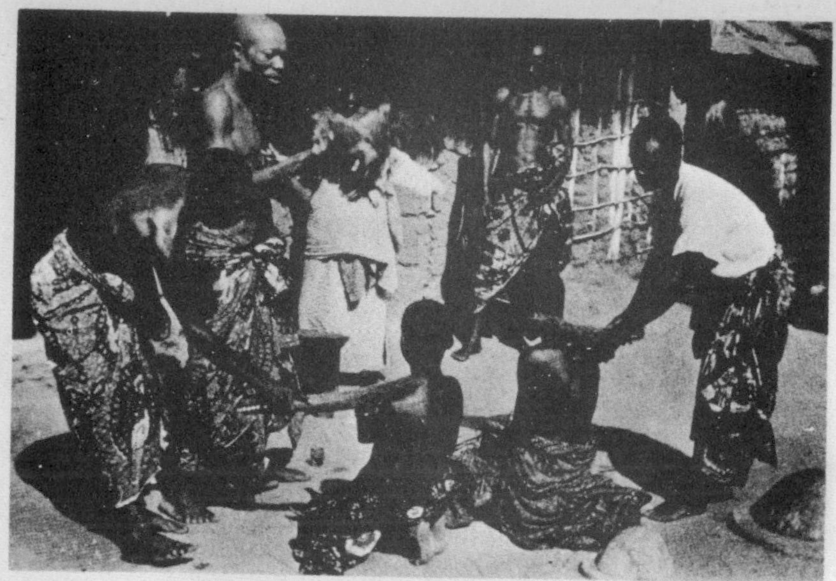

46: Sickness being swept away with small brooms after ritual transference of disease to fowls. Ewe, West Africa. Photo by H. V. Meyerowitz. From a print in the Wellcome Historical Medical Museum.

XXII: TREATMENT

47: Substitution dolls (*Adu*) for transference of disease. Nias Islands. Wellcome Historical Medical Museum.

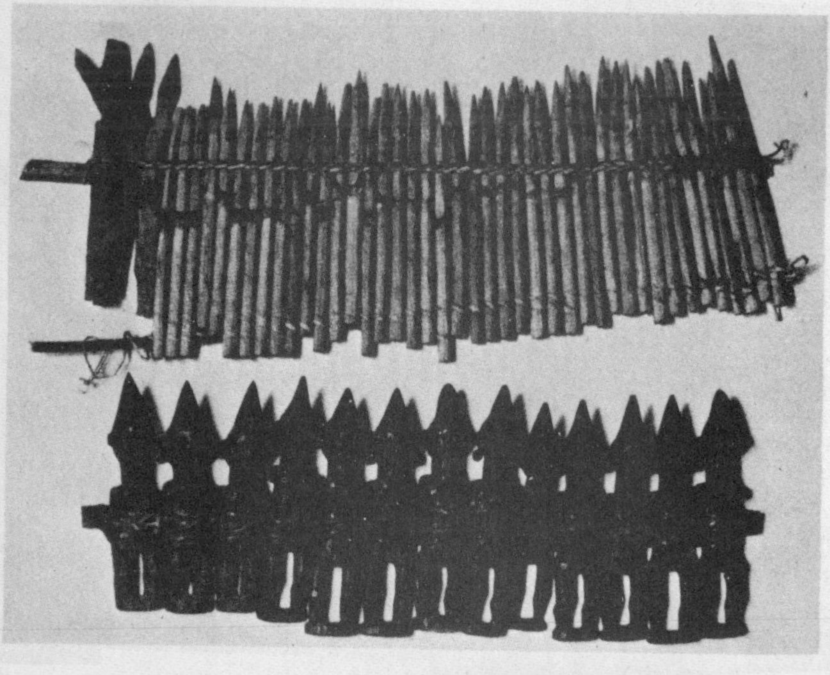

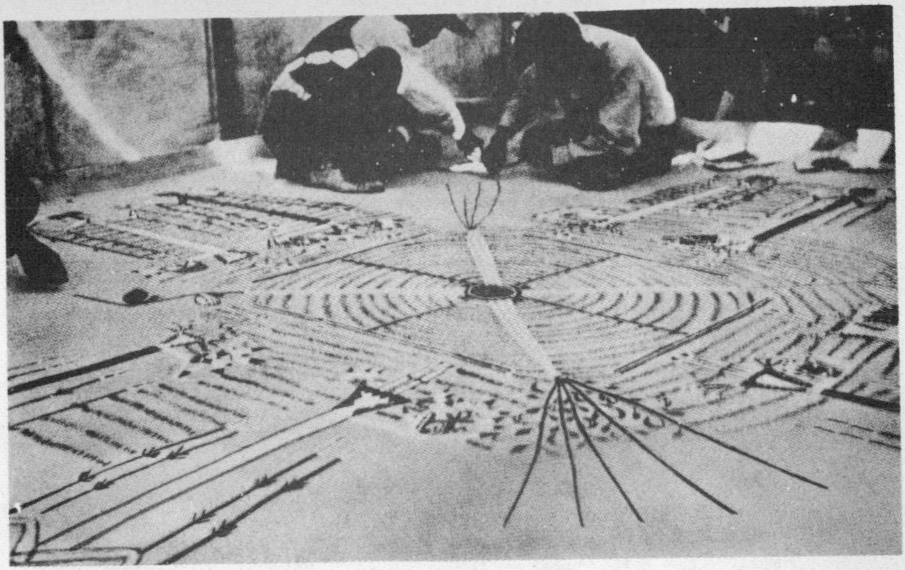

48: Navajo sand-painting. Photo by J. R. Willis, Southwest Post Card Co., Albuquerque, New Mexico.

XXIII: TREATMENT

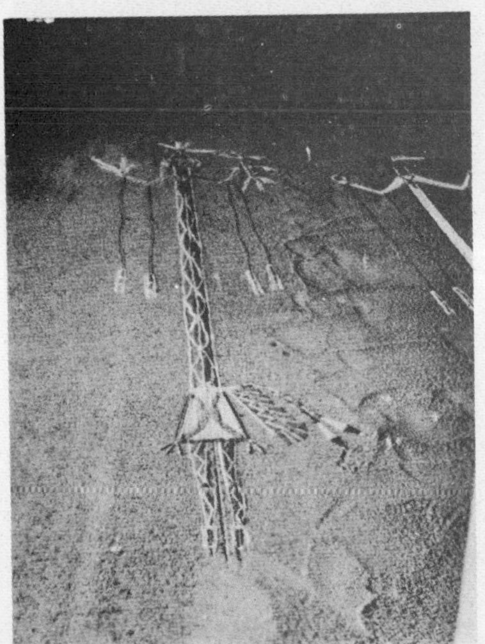

49: Detail of a Navajo sand-painting. Photo by Miss B. M. Blackwood, Pitt Rivers Museum, Oxford.

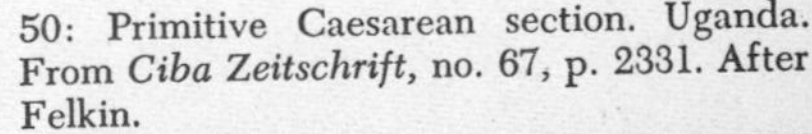

50: Primitive Caesarean section. Uganda. From *Ciba Zeitschrift*, no. 67, p. 2331. After Felkin.

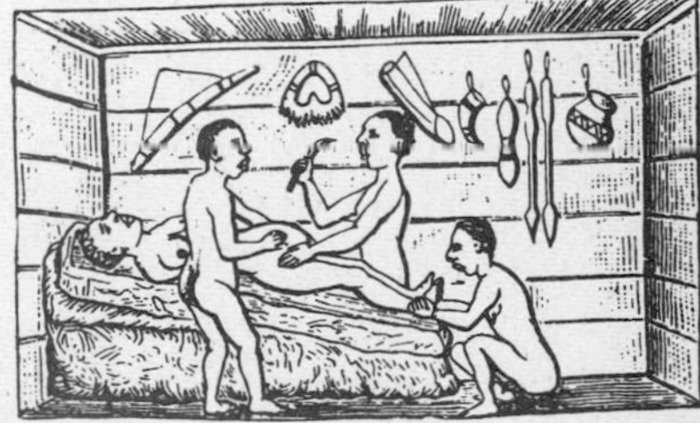

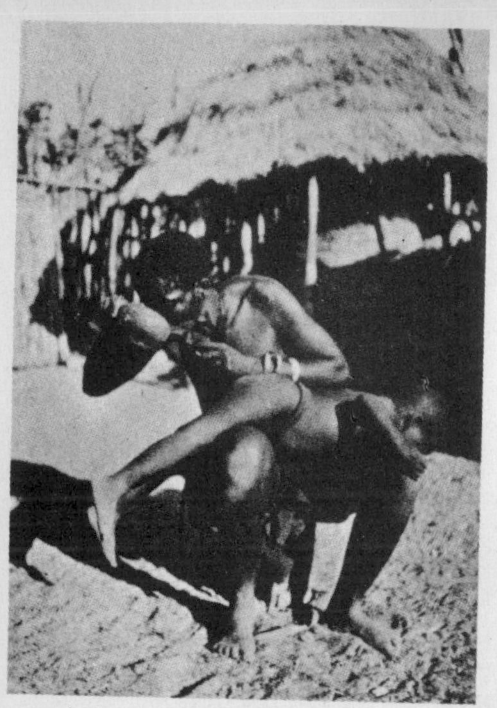

XXIV: TREATMENT

51 and 52: Native mother of the Kwanyama tribe, S. Angola, giving an enema to her baby boy.

Fig. 51: Filling the mouth with liquid.

Fig. 52: Blowing the liquid through a reed into the rectum.

Photograph by Miss A. Powell-Cotton. From a print in the Wellcome Historical Medical Museum.

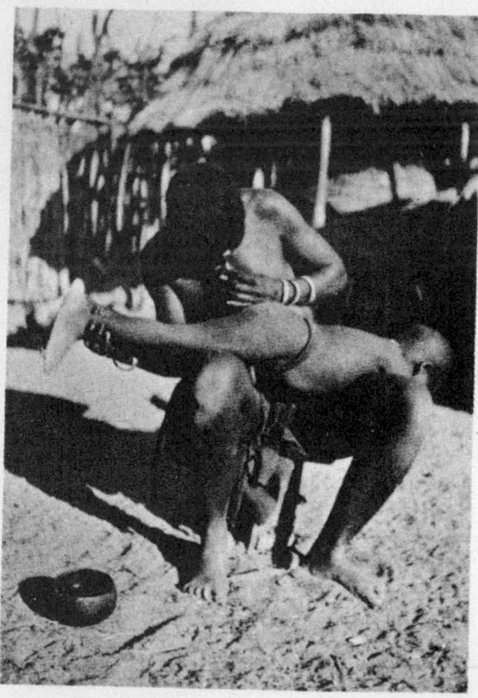

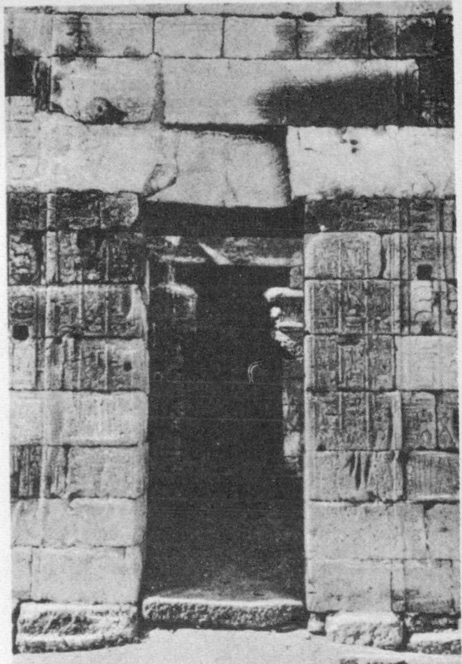

XXV: PREGNANCY AND CHILDBIRTH

53: Entrance to the temple of Amenerdais. Medinet Habu, Thebes. The chapel was for the benefit of childless women and expectant mothers.

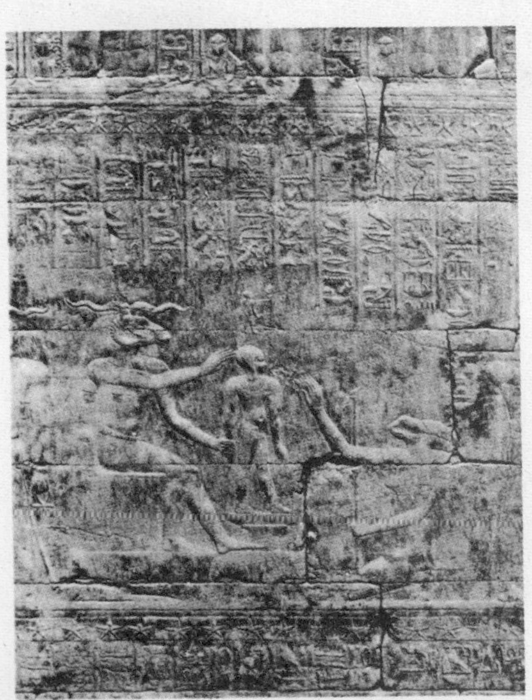

54: Molding of the infant. Birth house of Nektanebis, Temple of Hathor, Dendera. Figs. 53 and 54 from photographs taken by Captain P. Johnston-Saint, in the Wellcome Historical Medical Museum.

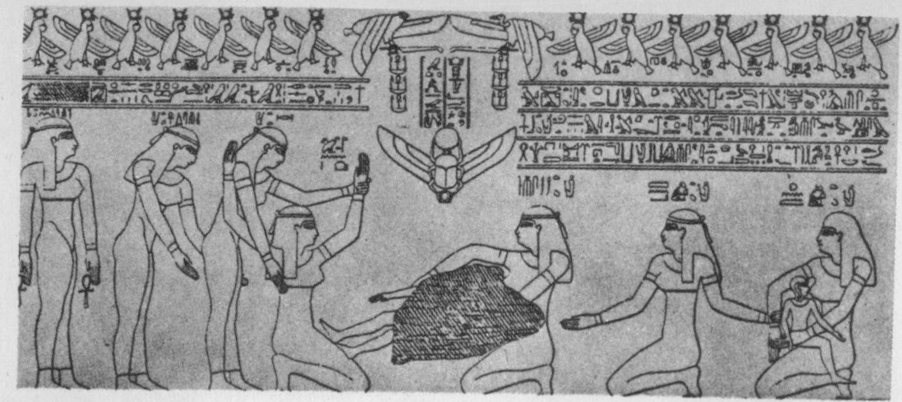

XXVI: CHILDBIRTH

55: The goddess Ritho giving birth to the son of Re. Birth temple at Erment. From Weindler, *Geburts- und Wochenbettsdarstellungen auf altägyptischen Tempelreliefs,* Munich, C. H. Beck, 1915, p. 30. After Lepsius.

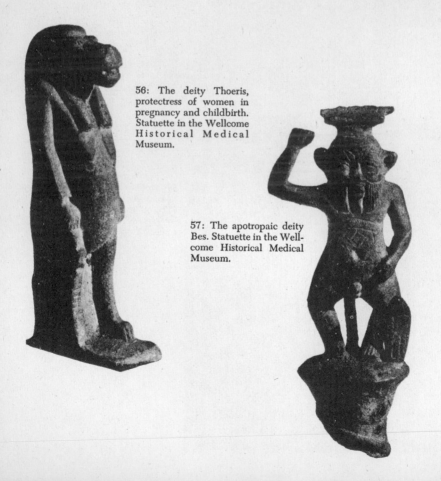

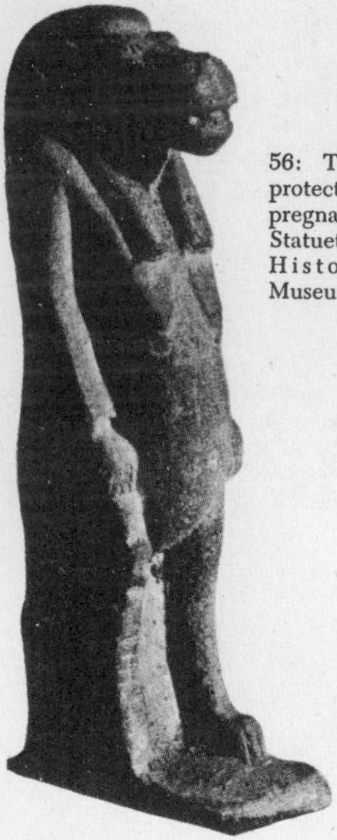

56: The deity Thoeris, protectress of women in pregnancy and childbirth. Statuette in the Wellcome Historical Medical Museum.

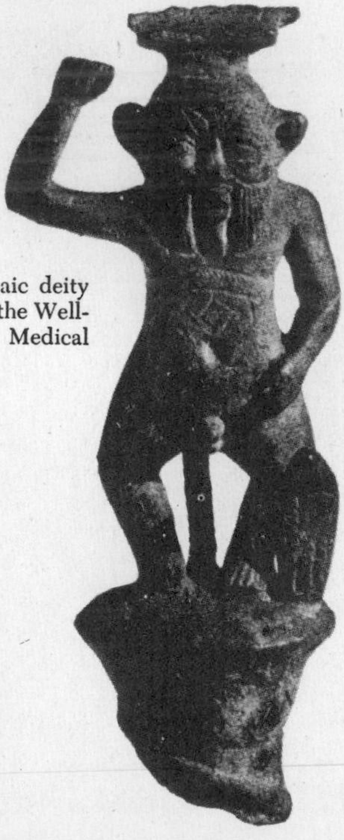

57: The apotropaic deity Bes. Statuette in the Wellcome Historical Medical Museum.

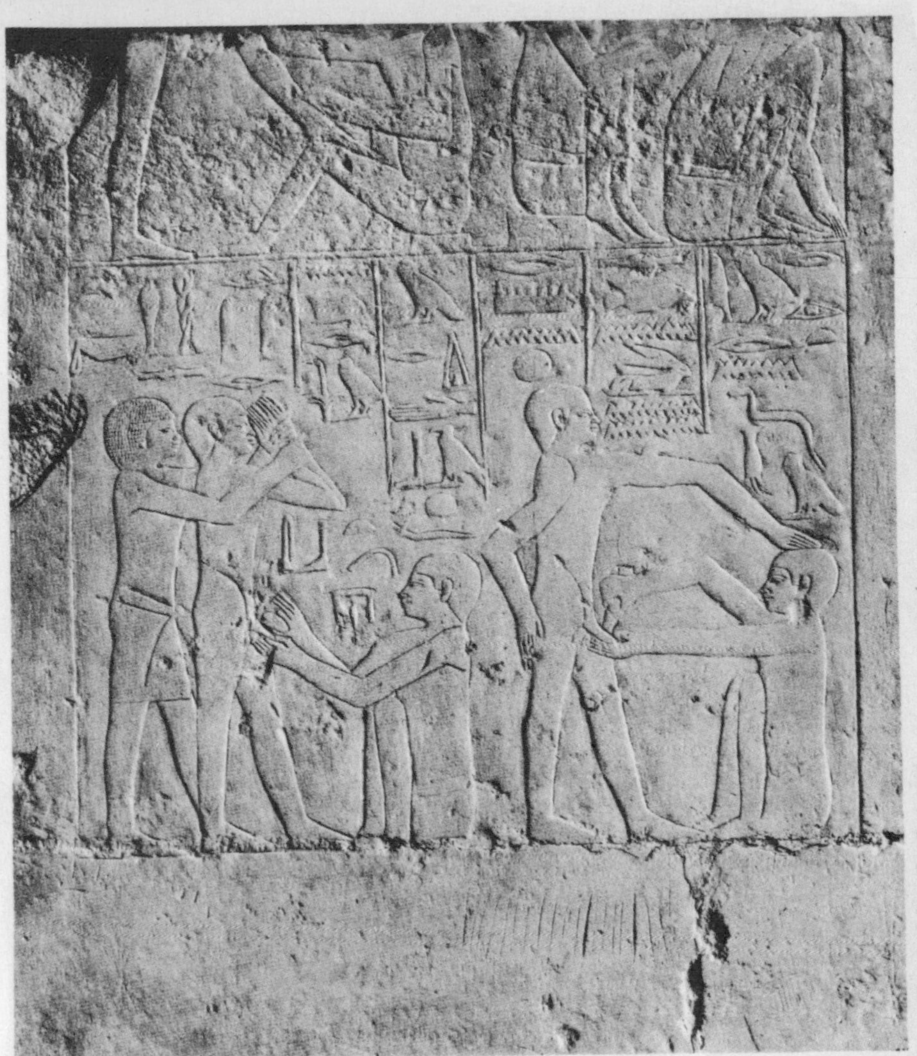

XXVII: CIRCUMCISION

58: Relief showing (lower register) circumcision operation in progress; (upper register) operation on a man's foot (left) and an operation on the back (right). From the necropolis of Sakkara, VIth Dynasty. From a cast in the possession of the Wellcome Historical Medical Museum.

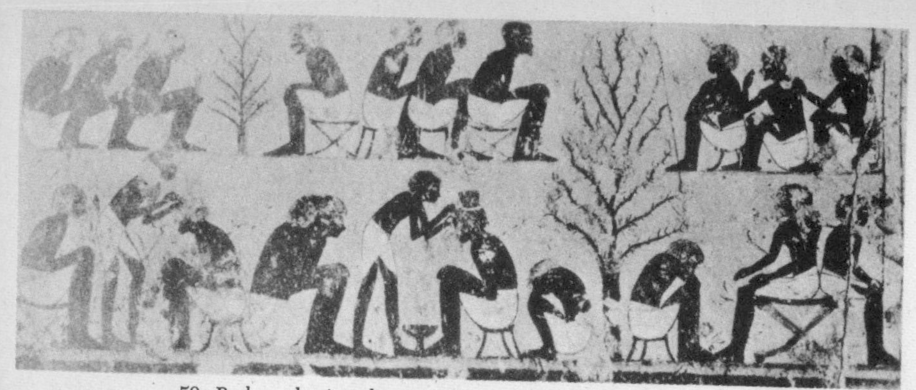

59: Barbers shaving clients in the open air. Wall painting, XVIIIth Dynasty. From Wreszinski, *Atlas zur altägyptischen Kulturgeschichte*, Leipzig, J. C. Hinrichs, 1923, plate 44.

XXVIII: TOILET

60: Woman painting her lips. From Pleyte and Rossi, *Papyrus de Turin*, Leiden, 1869-76, plate 145.

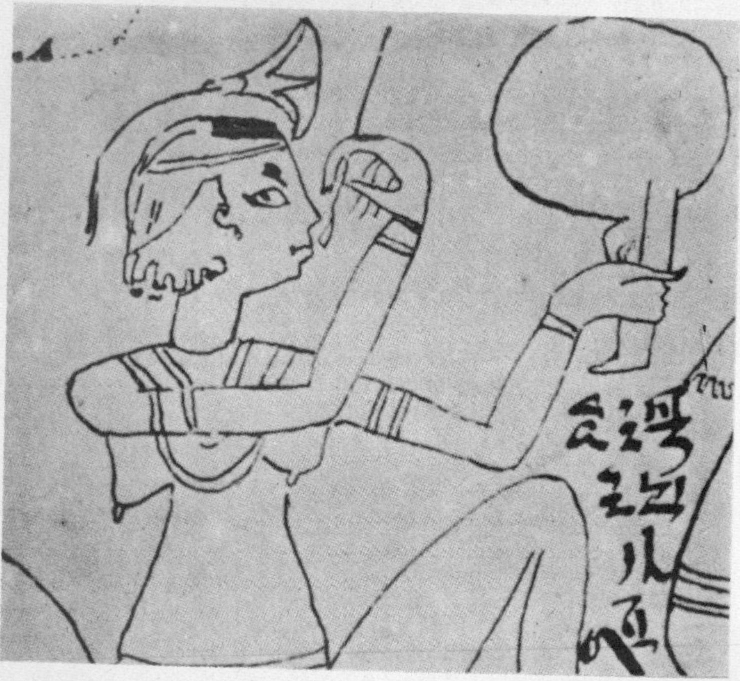

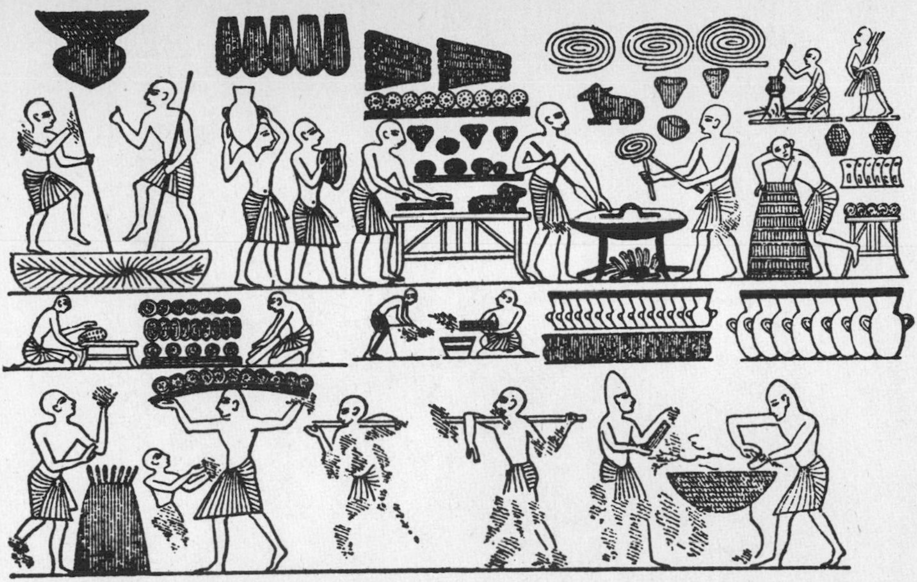

61: Royal bakery and pastry shop. (Right lower corner) brewing of beer. Tomb of Ramses III. From Erman-Ranke, *Aegypten und ägyptisches Leben im Altertum,* Tübingen, Verlag von J. C. B. Mohr (Paul Siebeck), 1923, fig. 71, p. 224.

62: Wine making. Gathering and pressing of grapes. Storing of wine in jars. XVIIIth Dynasty. From Erman-Ranke, fig. 72, p. 227.

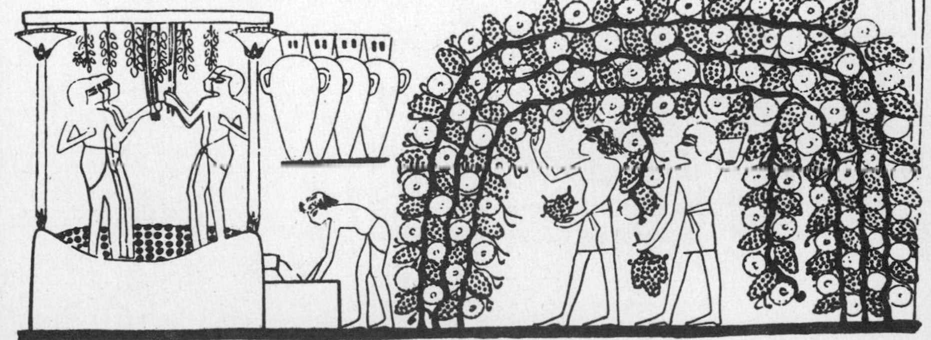

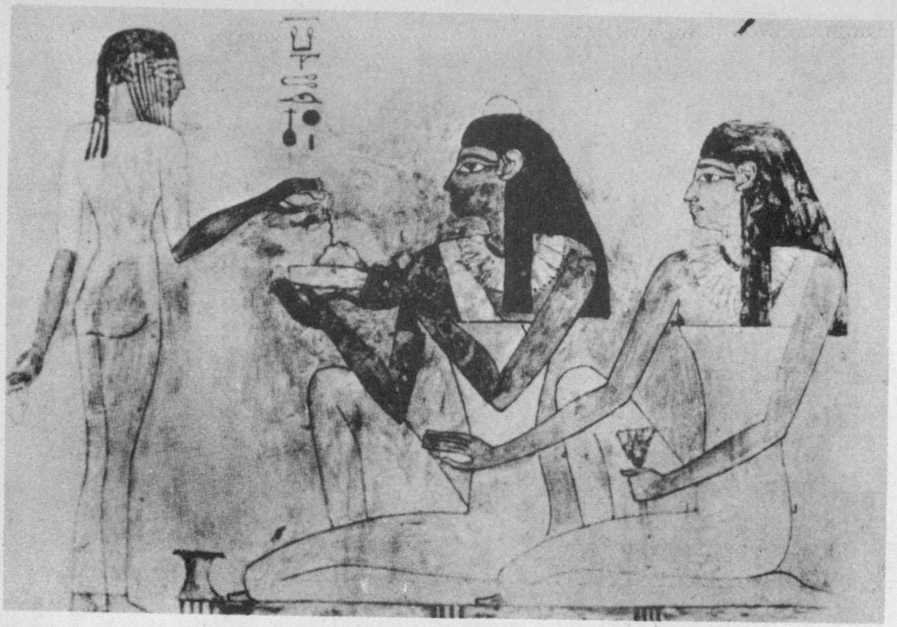

63: Ladies being served with food and drink. Wall painting, fifteenth century B.C. Metropolitan Museum of Art, New York.

XXX: NUTRITION

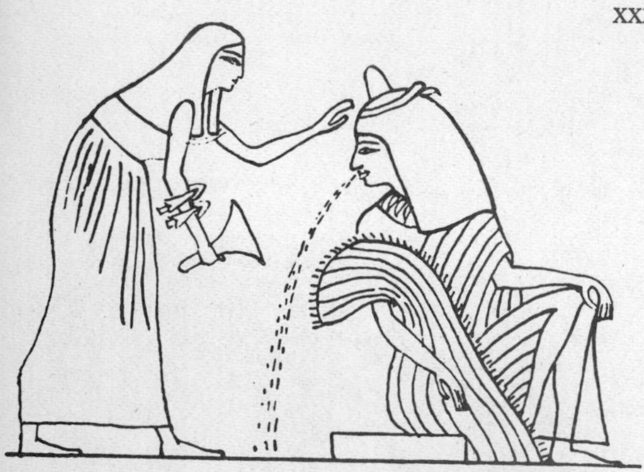

64: Lady at banquet vomiting. New Empire. From Erman-Ranke, fig. 128, p. 288.

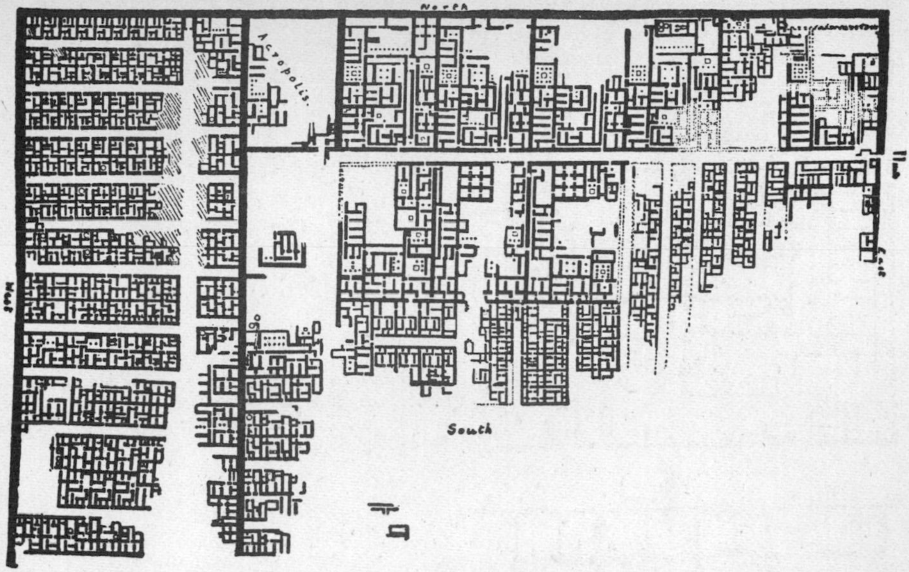

65: Ground plan of the ruins of the town of Kahun built during the XIIth Dynasty. Laborers' quarters in the western section, houses of court and nobility in the much larger eastern section. From Erman-Ranke, fig. 50, p. 198.

XXXI: HOUSING

66: A garden and fish pond. Wall painting in a Theban tomb, XVIIIth Dynasty. From Wreszinski, *Atlas,* plate 92.

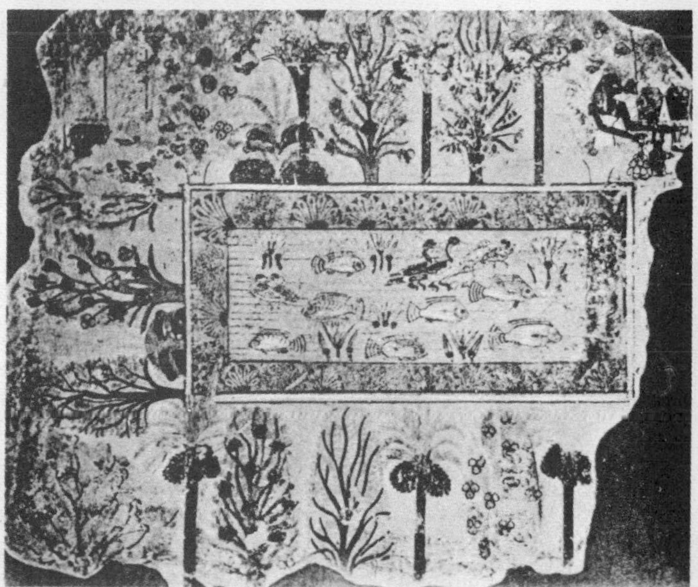

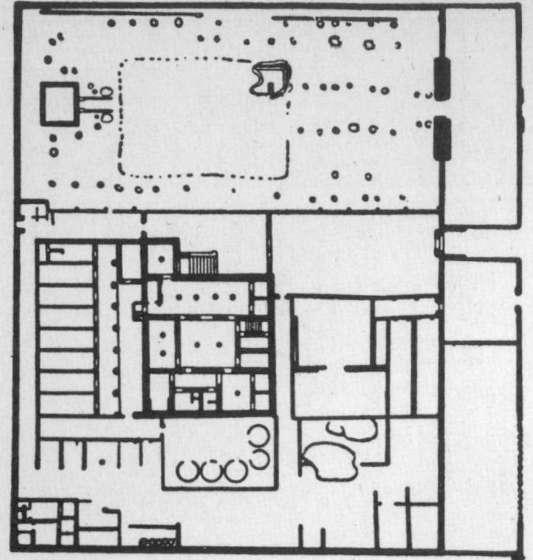

XXXII: HOUSING

67: Plan of a rich man's house in El Amarna, with stables for cattle and sheep, granaries, store rooms, latrines and bath. XVIIIth Dynasty. From Erman-Ranke, fig. 53, p. 202.

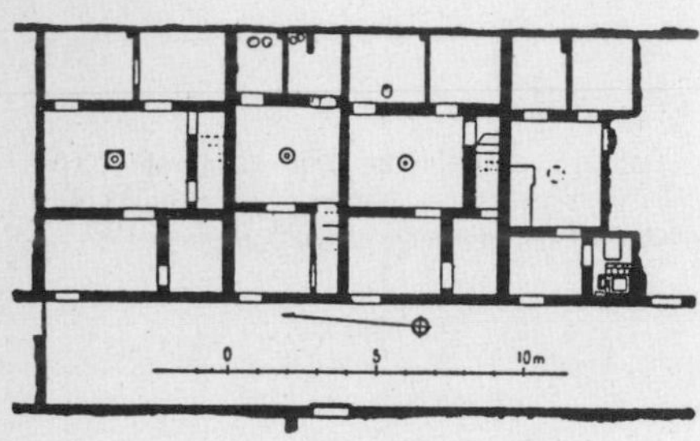

68: Plan of four small houses in El Amarna. Chief room has central pillar; stairs leading to roof. Bathroom in right lower corner. From Erman-Ranke, fig. 52, p. 201.

69, 69a: Remains of a bathroom and a latrine seat. El Amarna. Photograph in the Wellcome Historical Medical Museum.

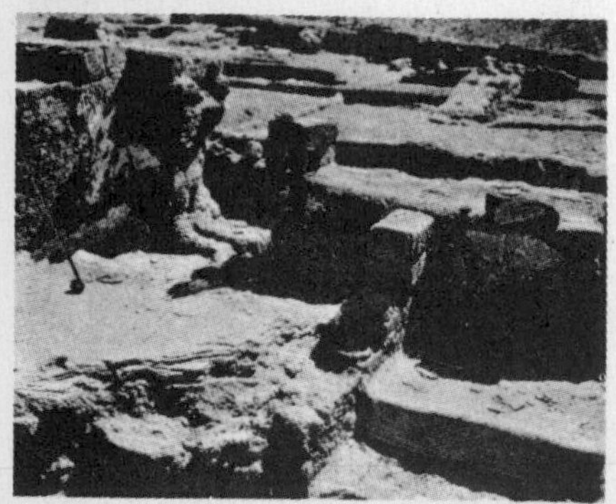

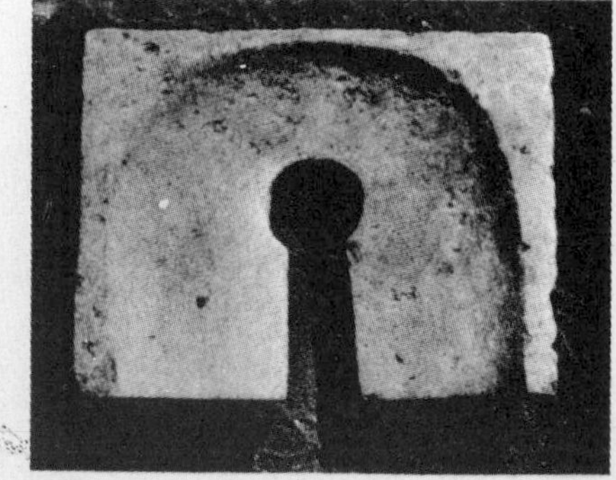

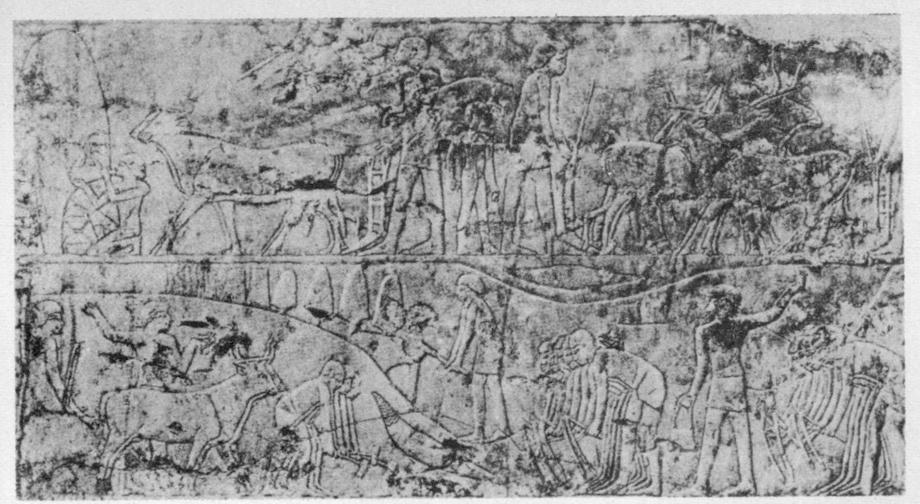

70: Farm labor. Relief from tomb of Khaemhet. XVIIIth Dynasty. From Wreszinski, *Atlas,* plate 9.

XXXIII: LABOR

71: Leather worker and shoemaker. Relief from tomb of Ebe. XVIIIth Dynasty. From Wreszinski *Atlas,* plate 133.

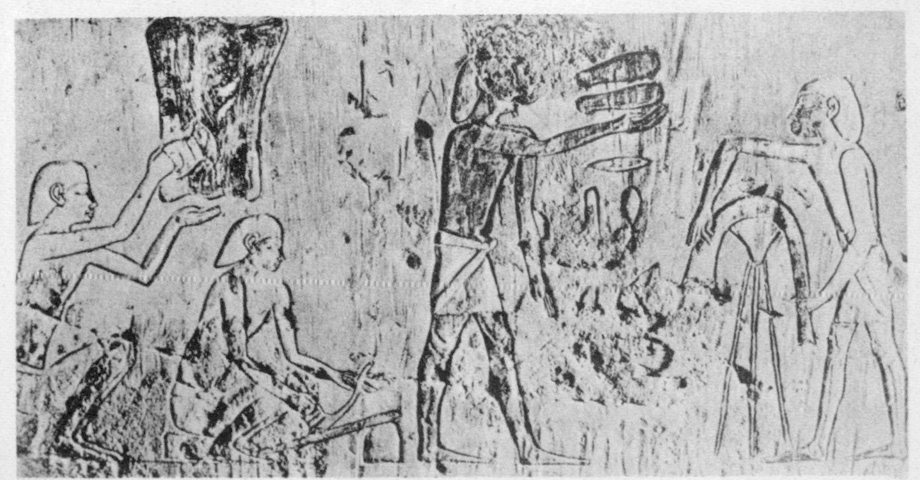

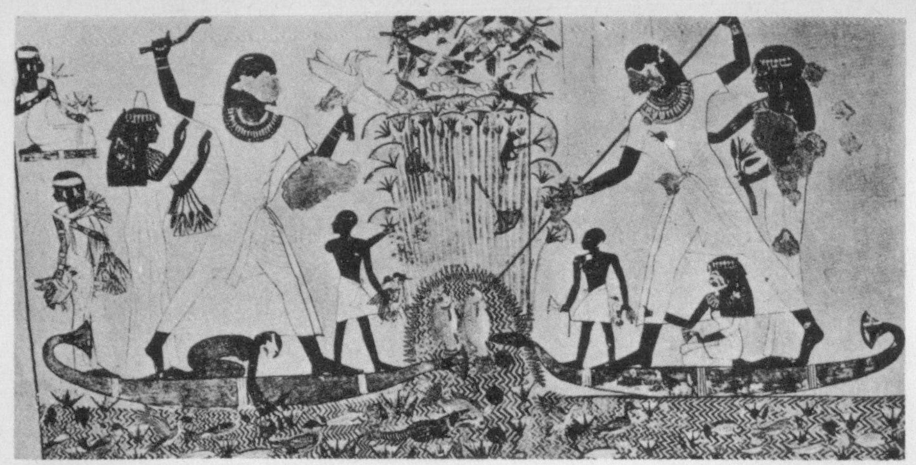

72: Hunting and fishing. Wall painting. XVIIIth Dynasty. From Wreszinski, *Atlas,* plate 2.

XXXIV: REST AND RECREATION

73: Game played on a board. Wall painting. XIX-XXth Dynasty. From Wreszinski, *Atlas,* plate 49.

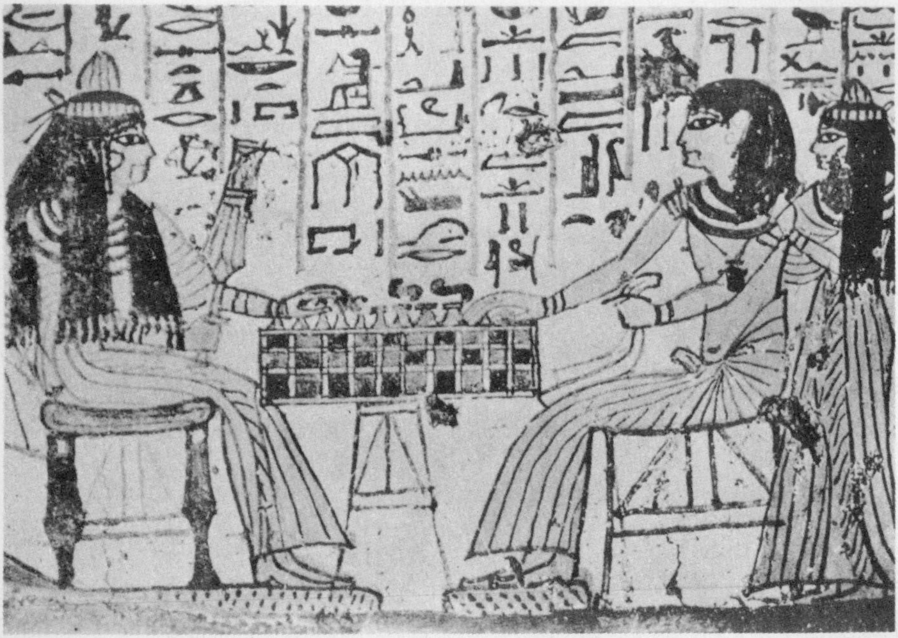

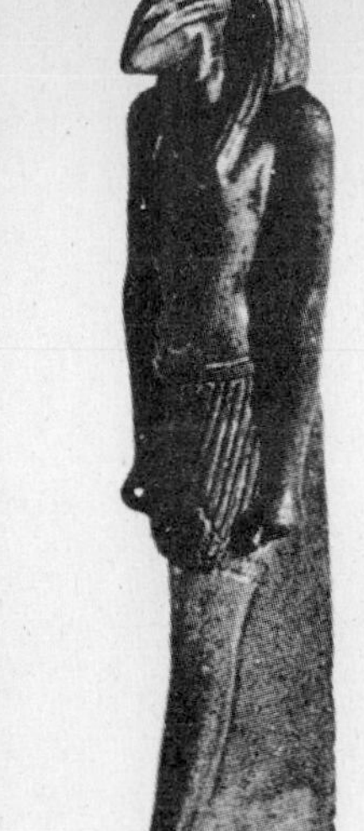
74: Thoth.

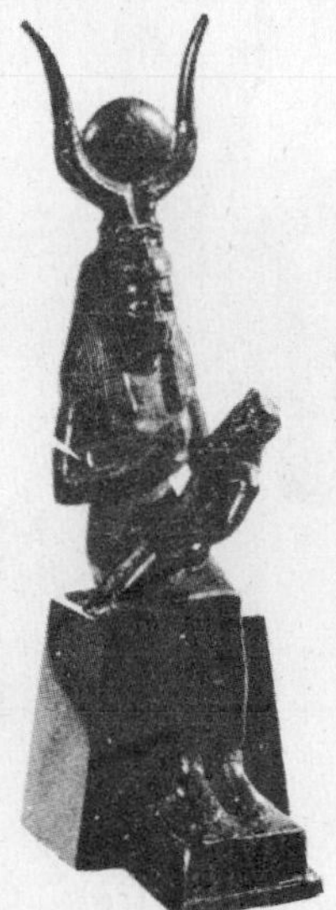
75: Isis, with Horus the child.

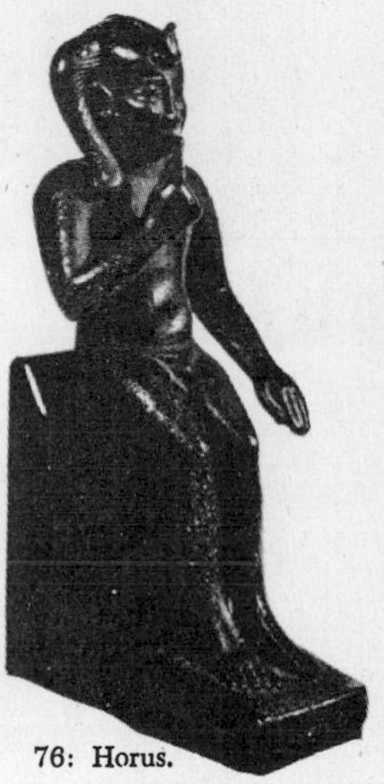
76: Horus.

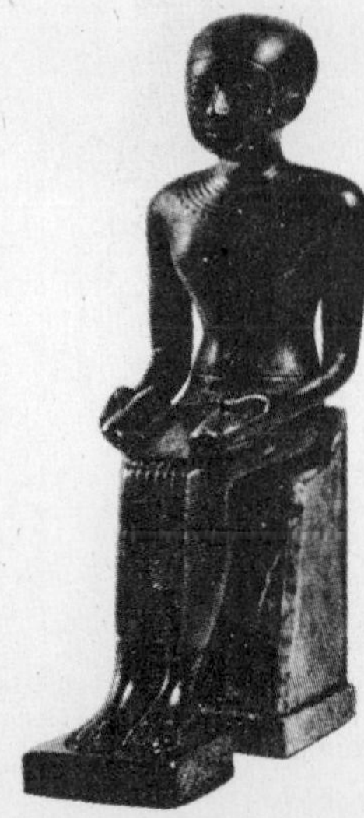
77: Imhotep.

All these illustrations after statuettes in the possession of the Wellcome Historical Medical Museum.

XXXVI: HEALING DEITIES

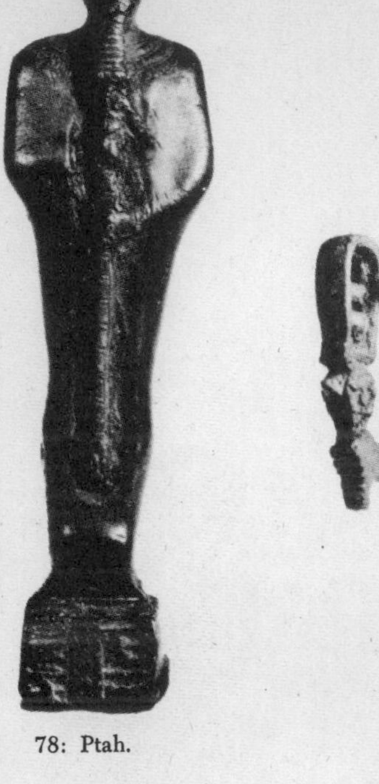

78: Ptah.

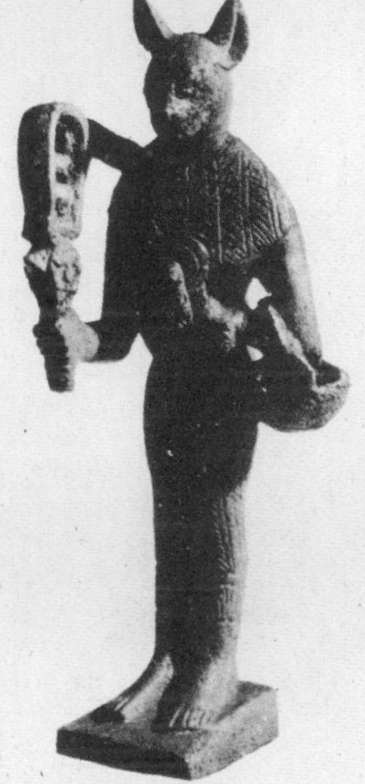

79: Ubastet.

80: Neith.

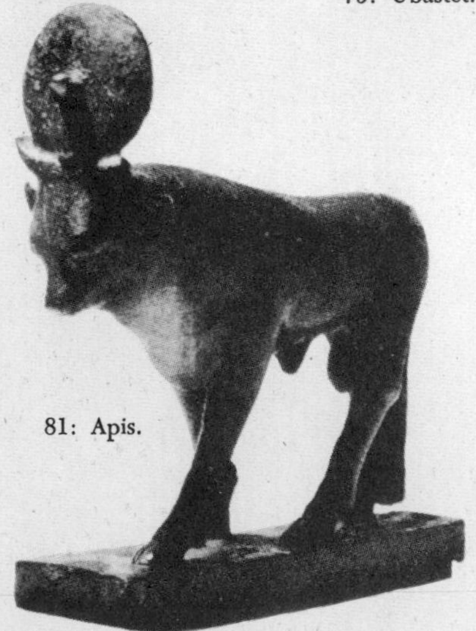

81: Apis.

All these illustrations after statuettes in the possession of the Wellcome Historical Medical Museum.

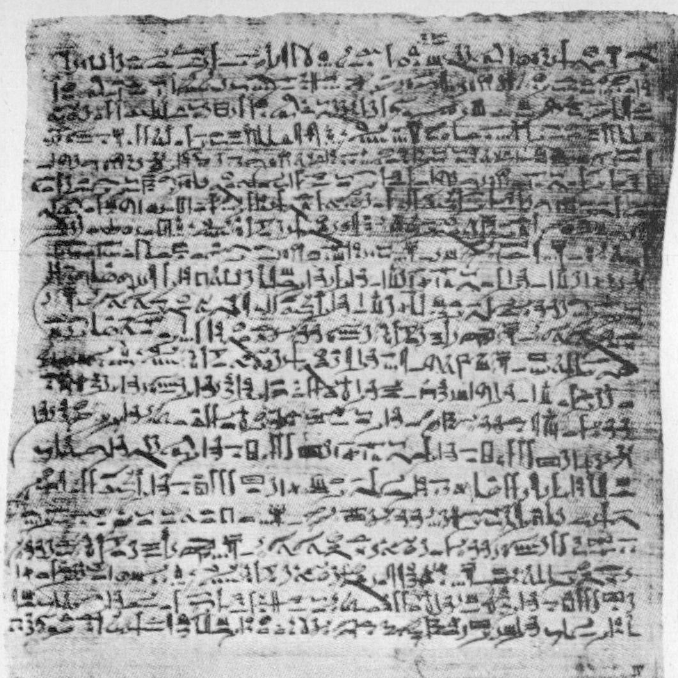

XXXVII: MEDICAL LITERATURE

82: Papyrus Edwin Smith, column 5. From Breasted, *The Edwin Smith Surgical Papyrus,* Chicago, 1930, plate v.

83: Papyrus Ebers, column 40. From Georg Ebers, *Papyrus Ebers,* plate XL.

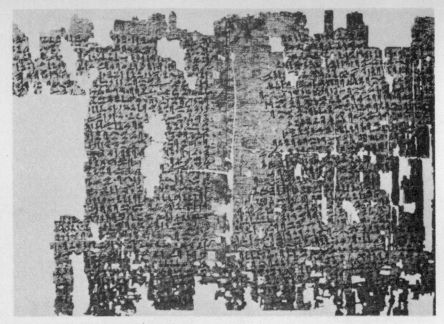

84: Gynaecological Papyrus of Kahun, pp. 1 and 2. From *The Petrie Papyri. Hieratic papyri from Kahun and Gurob.* Edited by F. L. Griffith, London, 1898.

XXXVIII: MEDICAL LITERATURE

85: London Medical Papyrus, p. 14. From Wreszinski, *Der Londoner medizinische Papyrus und der Papyrus Hearst,* Leipzig, 1912.

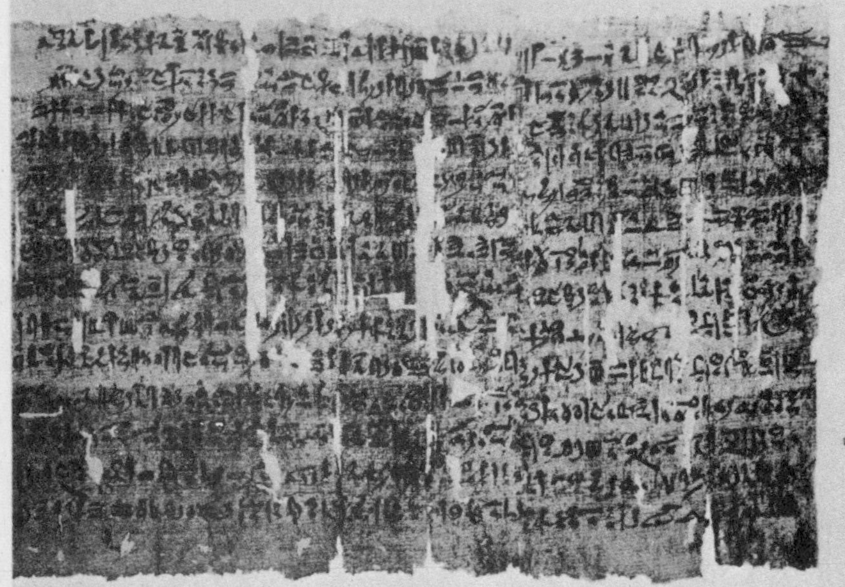

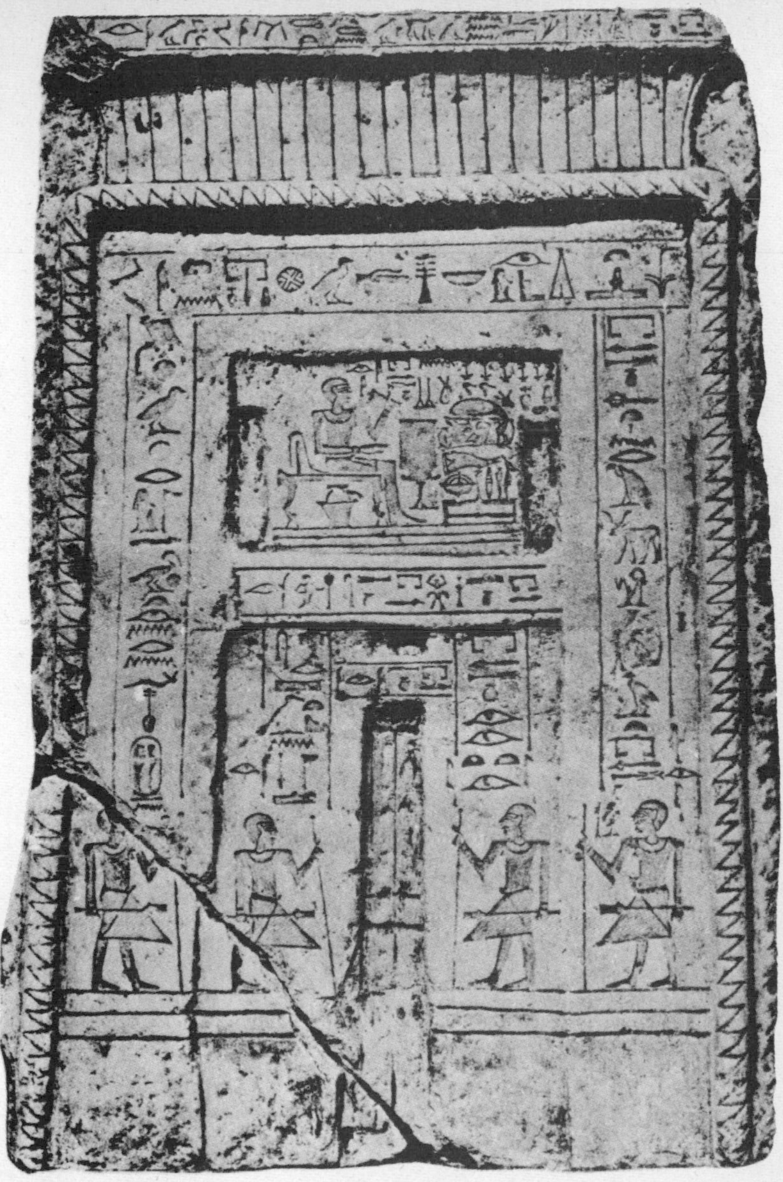

XXXIX: PHYSICIANS

86: Stele of court physician Irj, represented four times standing and once sitting in front of a table with sacrificial food. End of Old Kingdom. From Junker, 'Der Hofarzt Irj,' *Zschr. ägypt. Sprache*, 1928, vol. 63, plate II.

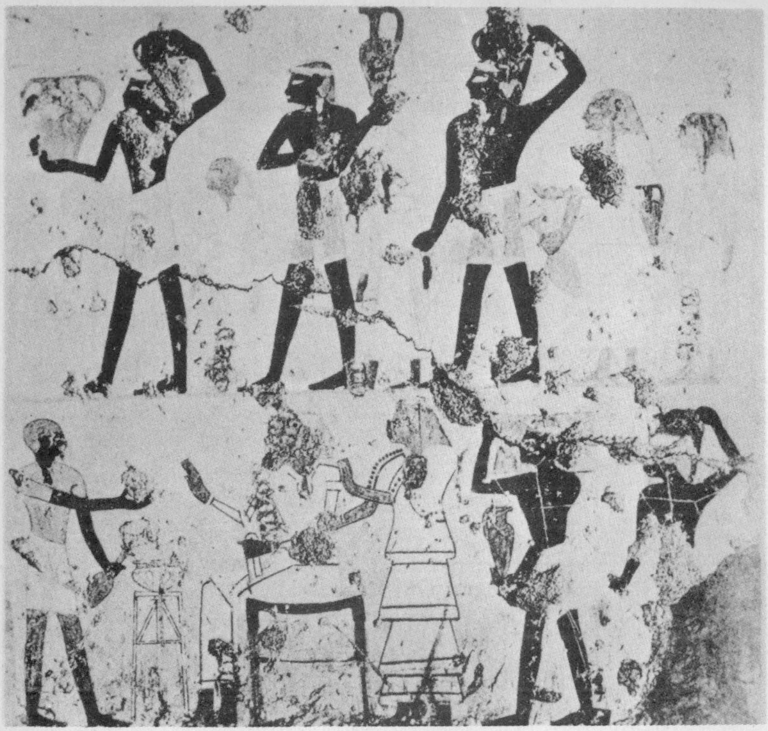

87: Syrian prince (seated) consulting the Egyptian physician Nebamon. The physician is in the left lower corner holding a bottle and handing a potion to his patient. Wall painting. XVIIIth Dynasty. From Wreszinski, *Atlas*, plate 115.

XL: PHYSICIANS

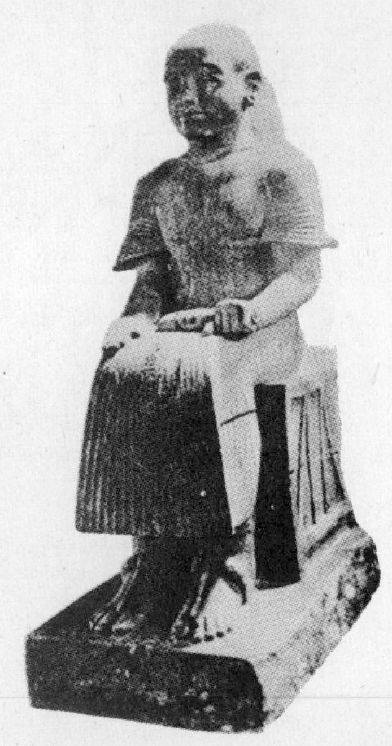

88: Statue of physician Iwti (XIXth Dynasty ?). Leiden, Rijksmuseum. From Fonahn, 'Der altägyptische Arzt Iwti,' *Arch. Gesch. Med.*, 1909, vol. 2, plate VI.

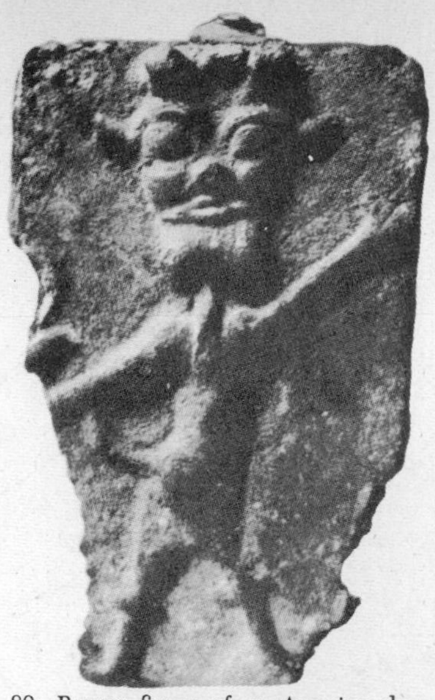

89: Bronze figure of an Assyrian demon. British Museum. From *Ciba Zeitschrift,* no. 25, p. 861.

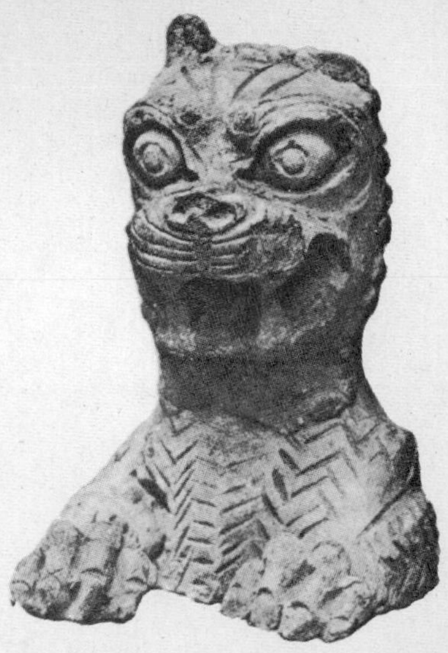

90: Bronze figure of an Assyrian demon. British Museum.

XLI: CAUSATION OF DISEASE

91: The demon Pazuzu. Assyrian bronze. Louvre. From *Ciba Zeitschrift,* no. 25, p. 864.

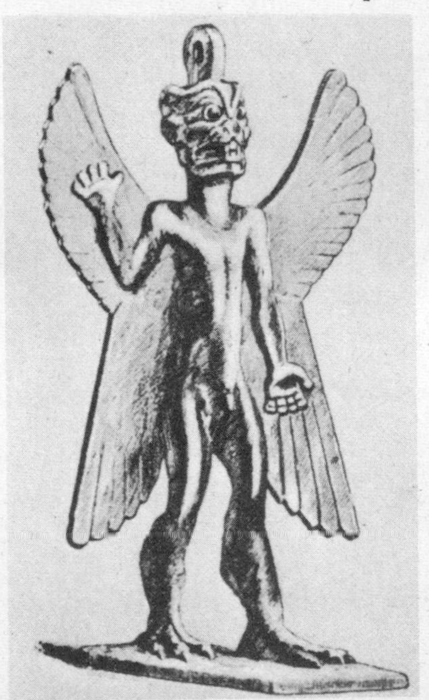

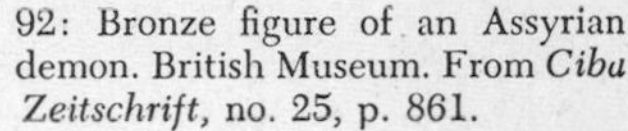

92: Bronze figure of an Assyrian demon. British Museum. From *Ciba Zeitschrift,* no. 25, p. 861.

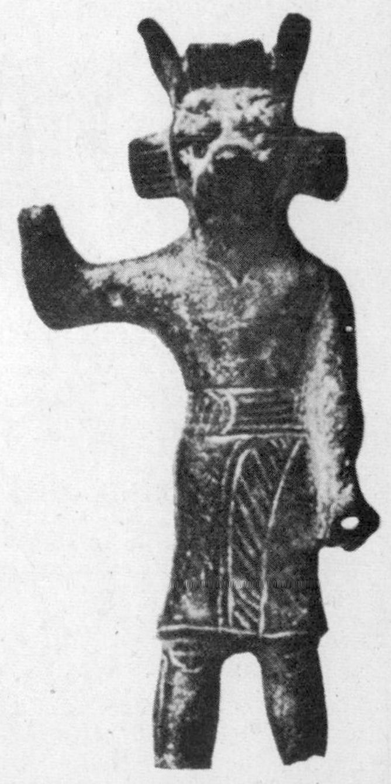

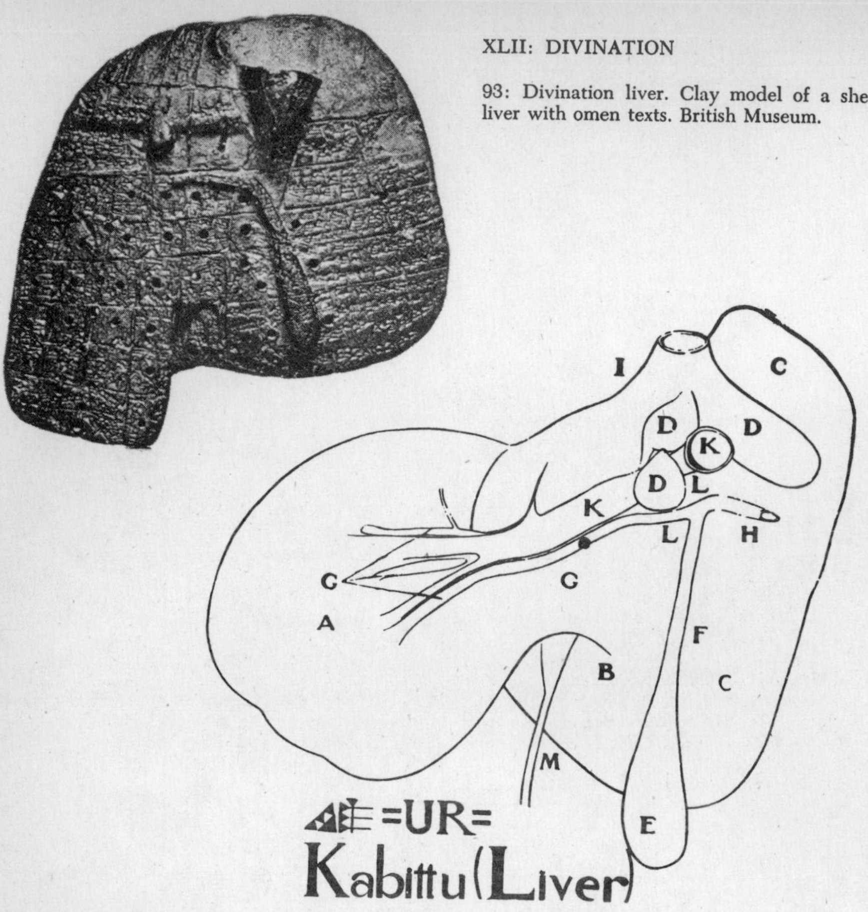

93: Divination liver. Clay model of a sheep's liver with omen texts. British Museum.

94: Drawing of a sheep's liver with Latin and Babylonian-Assyrian designation of parts. After Jastrow. From *Proc. Roy. Soc. Med.*, Sect. Hist. Med., 1914, vol. 7, p. 121.

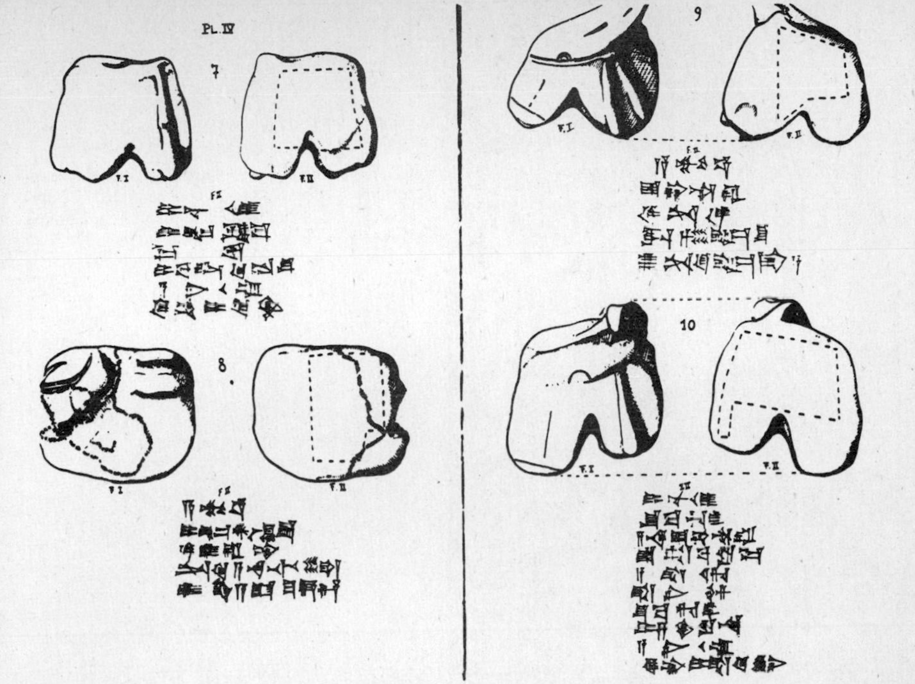

95: Clay models of liver from Mari (Tell-Hariri). After Rutten. From *Rev.Assyr.*, 1938, vol. 35, plates IV-V.

XLIII: DIVINATION

96: Etruscan bronze model of a liver from Piacenza. From Contenau, *La Divination chez les Assyriens et les Babyloniens*, Paris, Payot, 1940, fig. 10, p. 279.

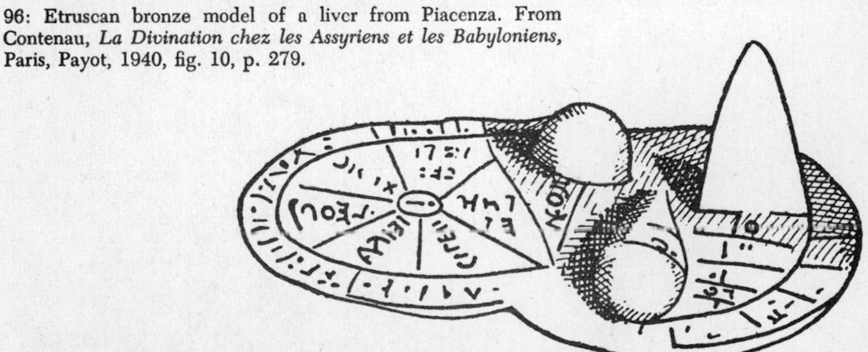

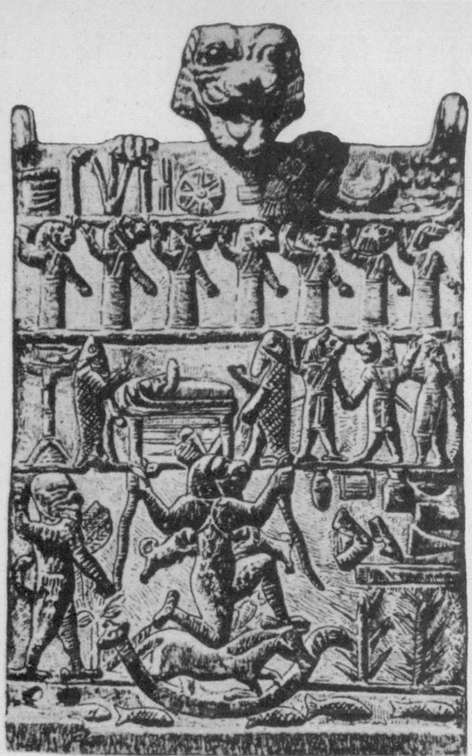

XLIV: TREATMENT

97: Assyrian bronze plaquette probably representing the cosmos (Heaven and Underworld) and in the middle an exorcism. Louvre.

98: Verso of the same plaquette representing a winged deity. From *Ciba Zeitschrift,* no. 25, pp. 862 and 863.

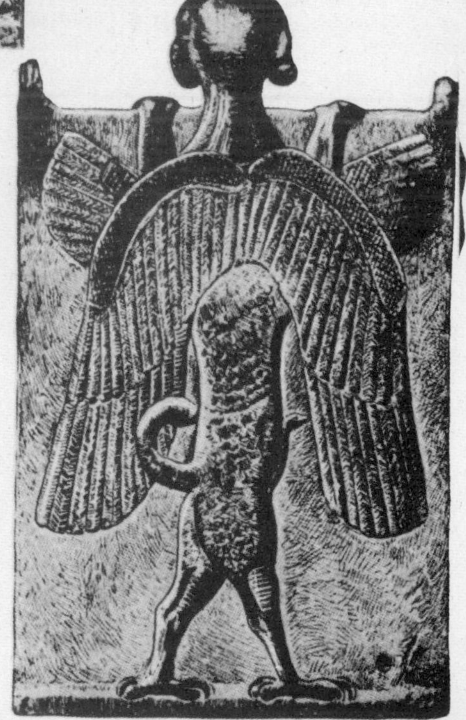

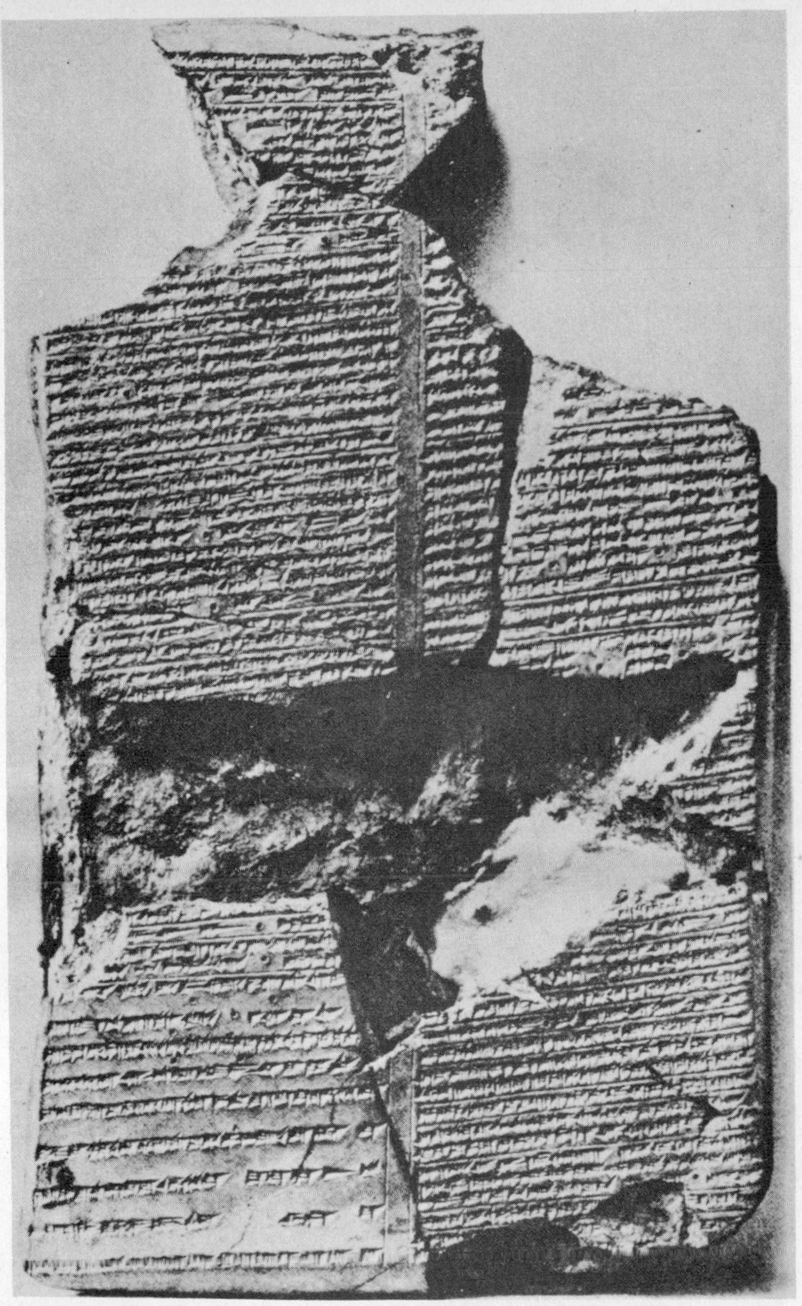

XLV: MEDICAL LITERATURE

99: Cuneiform tablet with medical text. British Museum, K 191. From *Ciba Zeitschrift*, no. 25, p. 852.

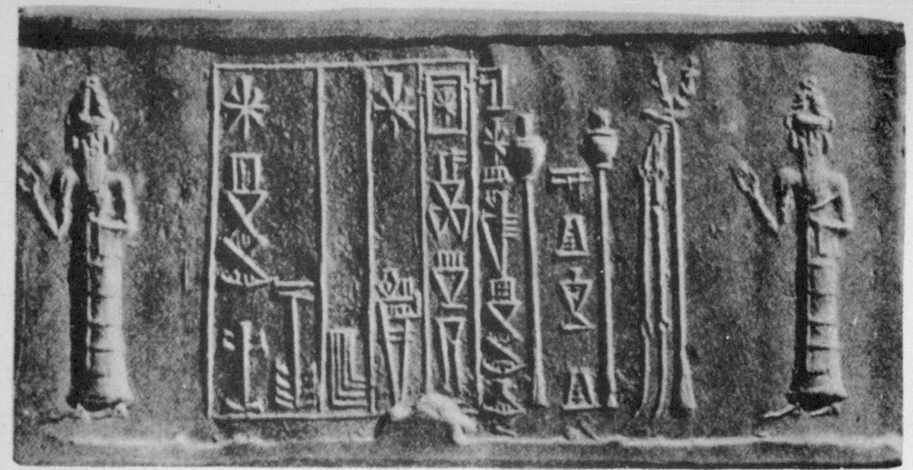

100: Cylinder seal of the physician Ur-Lugal-edinna. Louvre. From Contenau, *La Médecine en Assyrie et en Babylonie,* Paris, Maloine, 1938, fig. 24, p. 41.

XLVI: PHYSICIAN

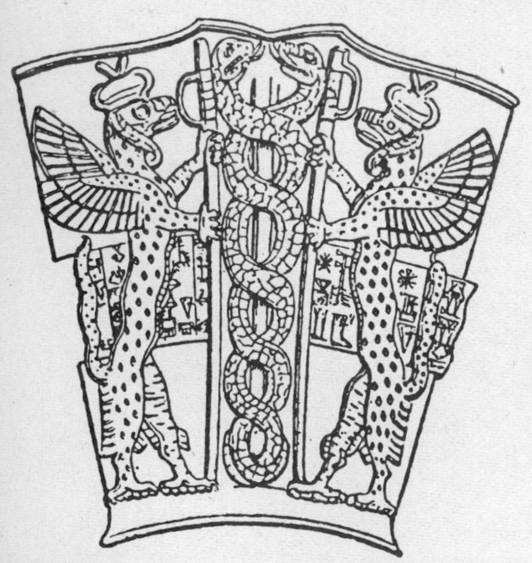

101: Emblem of the god Ningizzida. From Meissner, *Die babylonisch-assyrische Literatur,* Potsdam, Athenaion, 1927, fig. 85, p. 77.

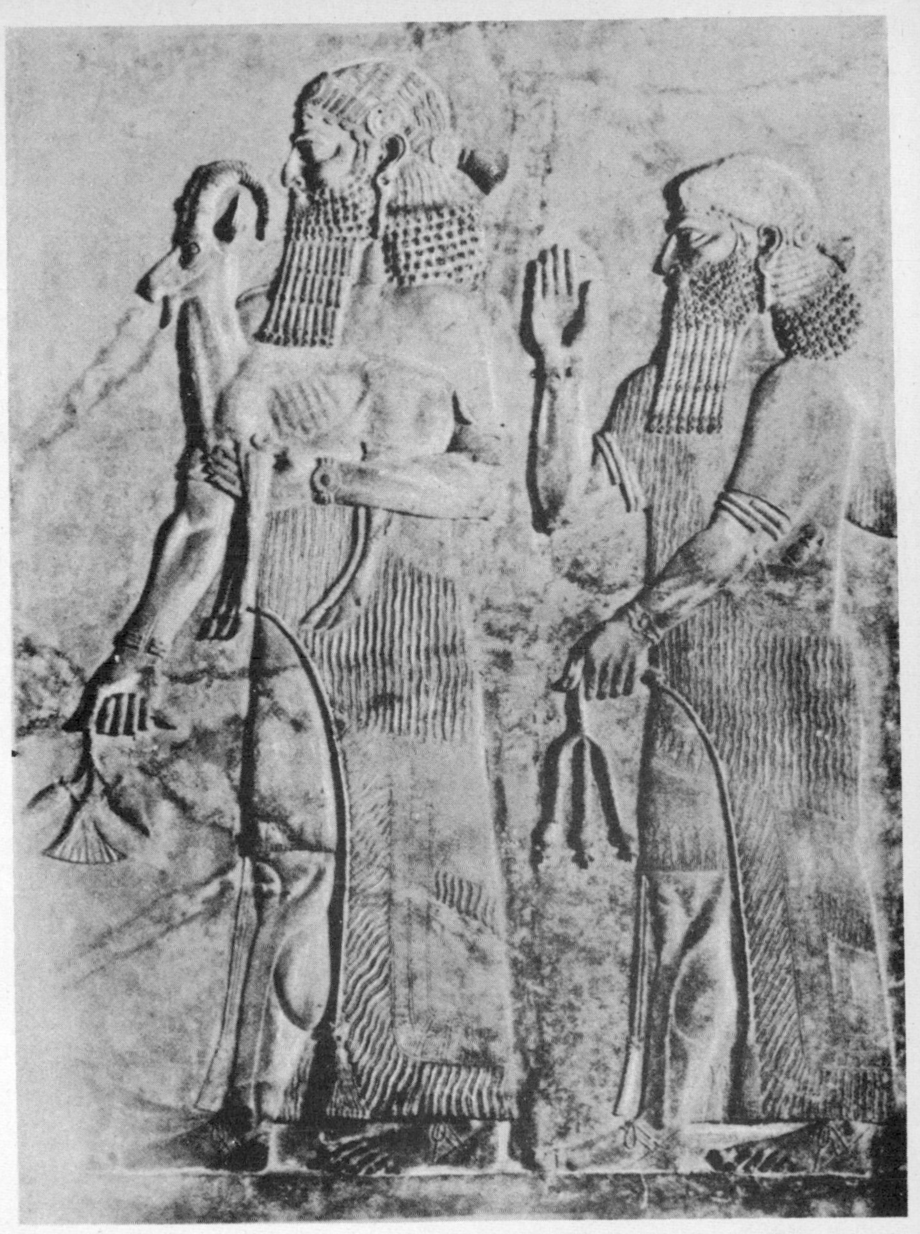

XLVII: DRUGS

102: Two priests one of whom carries a gazelle and the other a poppy. Louvre. From Contenau, *La Divination chez les Assyriens et les Babyloniens,* Paris, Payot, 1940, plate III.

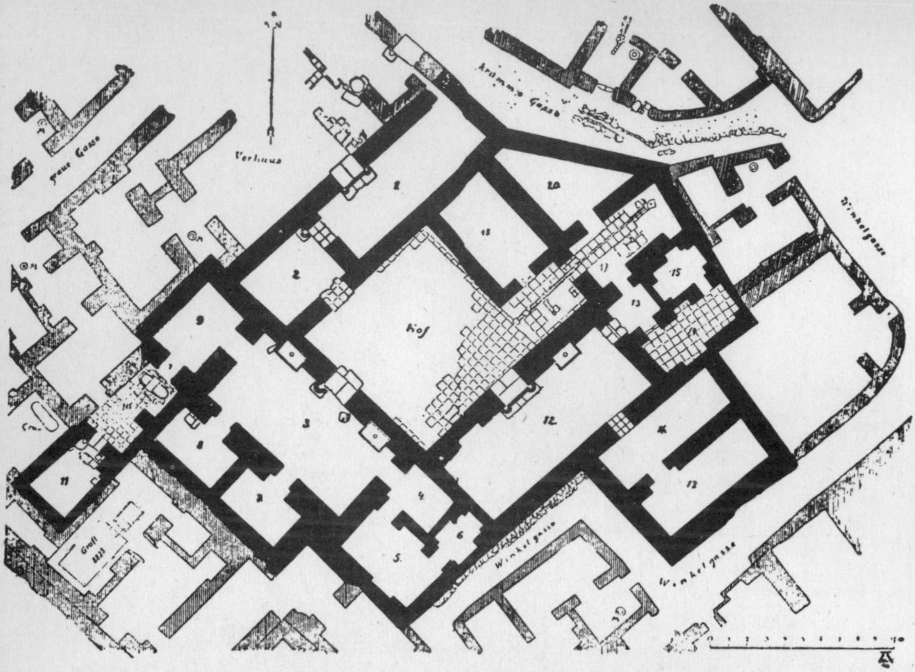

103: Plan of an Assyrian house in Ashur. From Hunger and Lamer, *Altorientalische Kultur im Bilde*, Leipzig, Quelle und Meyer, 1923, fig. 142. p. 75.

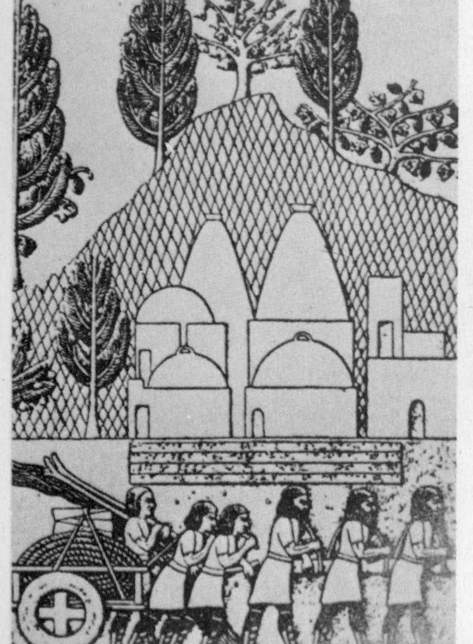

XLVIII: HOUSING

104: Profile of Assyrian houses. From Contenau, *La Civilisation d'Assur et de Babylonie*, Paris, Payot, 1937, fig. 24, p. 147.

*

1. Beginnings, Principles and Patterns

For hundreds of thousands of years man lived like a beast in the forest, covered with hair, grubbing for food, sleeping in trees and later in caves.[1] Thousands of generations were born, lived in animal fashion, and died before man's brain developed more gray substance than other animals possessed, and he began to use stones as tools with which he could struggle more effectively against the hostile forces of nature. They were simple enough, these early tools: flint, round so that it filled a man's fist, could be used as a hammer or as an axe when it was sharp and pointed on one side. These were the eoliths, stones that mark the dawn of human civilization.

Centuries and millennia passed and man gradually learned to make improved tools, to make drills, knives, scrapers, spearheads of flint; and of bone he made harpoons, javelin points, awls, and needles. He learned to use the fur of animals to protect himself against the cold and, greatest of all discoveries, he learned the use of fire. Man of the Old Stone Age [2] was a hunter who lived in caves on the walls of which he sometimes painted in black and bright ochre the animals that were the object of his hunting: the reindeer, the boar, the bison, the horse, and the mammoth. On reindeer antlers and mammoth tusks he carved animals, and he made statuettes in ivory, limestone, or soapstone representing women, sometimes realistically, sometimes with great emphasis on the sex organs and secondary sex characteristics.[3] The dead were buried in a sleeping position, painted with ochre and decorated with necklaces or crowns of shells, with various implements placed beside them.

We know that paleolithic man suffered from diseases and that he was all too familiar with the pains and disabilities caused by arthritis. We should like to know whether he reacted against them and, if so, in what way. We should like to know whether he made any conscious efforts to maintain his health and to prevent illness apart from such elementary measures as seeking shelter, keeping sufficiently warm, and satisfying his appetite. If we set the beginning of the upper paleolithic at about 30,000 B.C. and could answer the questions just raised, we should be able to witness the very dawn of medicine.

There can be no doubt that the Cro-Magnon race, which took the place of the Neanderthal man in Western Europe and initiated the Aurignacian period, was an intelligent race of skilful men and keen observers. Their cave paintings are a vivid testimony not only to their artistic skill but to their great power of observation. On one such painting in the cavern of Pindal the Aurignacian artist drew in red ochre the outlines of a mammoth, and in the center of it he placed a dark spot that may well be the heart: the organ that must have attracted the attention of man from the earliest times because he found it beating as long as there was life, because he soon must have discovered that the best way to kill an animal was to hit it through the heart, and perhaps also because he felt his own heart hammering in the breast when fear seized him. If the dark spot of the mammoth of Pindal actually represents the heart, we may well consider this the earliest anatomical picture.

Burial customs indicate that paleolithic man probably had religious beliefs. Leading a life of hardship, surrounded by the hostile forces of a nature that he could not understand, he came to believe in a life after death. The red color of ochre was symbolic of the life-giving blood, the shells, of the woman's vulva through which life was born; and implements were given the dead in the grave so that he would not be deprived of them in the hereafter. The statuettes of women, with large breasts, vulva, and buttocks and with no face or limbs, mere bundles of sex, may well be idols, representing a Great Mother.[8a]

A carving showing a reindeer stepping over a woman in childbirth has been interpreted as talisman picturing a magic rite. Max

Höfler quoted parallels from ancient mythology to prove that the idea was that strength would be imparted by the strong animal to the weak woman through the magical act of its stepping over her.[4]

But we have no evidence whatsoever of any paleolithic medicine. Disappointed we turn to the next period in the history of mankind, the New Stone Age, which in Europe set in between 7000 and 10,000 years ago.[5]

The transition from the paleolithic to the neolithic period, from a food-gathering to a food-producing economy, marks perhaps the greatest step in the history of civilization. It is still controversial whether this development took place slowly and gradually or whether it was initiated or at least accelerated by the invasion of foreign tribes from the East. The stone was polished now and tools were articulated. With improved tools man became independent of the cave. He could clear the forest, fell trees that served as building materials for huts, which, built closely together, formed a village that was frequently protected by a wall. Still better protection was sought by building the huts on piles in the lakes.[6] A tree hollowed out was a boat. Some of the greatest inventions were made at that stage. Whoever found that the wild bull could be changed into the docile ox by castration certainly made a great contribution to civilization.[7]

The land was plowed and grain was grown which could be stored, so life became more secure. The wild horse was domesticated. Cattle, sheep, goats, pigs were bred; they provided meat and milk for food, hides for clothing, fibers for textiles.

The domestic arts and crafts developed. The basket made of willow shoots and the animal-skin bag were the chief containers for solid and liquid substances.[8] Whoever had the idea of coating the inside of a basket with clay invented pottery. Every house had its loom and flax was used to make ropes, nets, mats, and clothing. It is very likely that sheep's wool was used at that early time also. And while the great art of the Aurignacian period had long been lost, people now satisfied their artistic needs by decorating the objects of everyday life. Pottery was ornamented with designs reminiscent of its basket origin; and textiles were sometimes embroidered.

With developing civilization social life became more complex.

Paleolithic man, gathering the fruits of the forest and hunting wild animals, was not tied to the soil. He went wherever the hunting grounds seemed promising. He owned little: the woman who slept with him and bore him children, the fur that kept him warm, a few stone implements. Social organization was probably limited to the family or to small groups of families who shared a cave for a while.

Conditions changed when man became a producer, a farmer, tilling the soil, breeding animals, living in villages. Families joined to form larger social groups, living and working together, following definite sets of rules. Women played an increasingly important part in the life of the group, doing farm work and attending to the home industries, while the men took care of the animals, were hunters and fishermen, traders, and also warriors. It is quite possible that matriarchy was the rule where agriculture was the predominant occupation, while patriarchy was found rather among cattle breeders. Ownership of the means of production gave power.

Hundreds of megaliths, stone monuments, have been preserved in Western Europe from neolithic times: menhirs or simple stone pillars, cromlechs or stone circles, dolmens or stone chambers, tombs erected for the dead, monuments of a cult the character of which remains dark.

Developing civilization must have affected the incidence of illness among prehistoric populations. Many hazards were reduced; the supply of food was more secure and the protection against cold and enemies was better. On the other hand it is quite possible that the natural resistance of man was reduced largely because of an increased dependence on the products of civilization. At any rate we know from paleopathological studies that neolithic man suffered from a great variety of diseases. And again we should like to know how he reacted against them.

The lake-dwellers cultivated or gathered over two hundred different plants,[9] among which are not a few that possess medicinal qualities.[10] We have no way of ascertaining that any one of them was used as a drug in the treatment of disease, but it is quite possible that some of them were actually used for such a purpose.

It is also possible that neolithic man treated diseases with the waters of mineral springs, drinking them or bathing in them.

Through their temperature, smell, flavor, the way they came out of the soil as geysers or bubbling with carbon dioxide, they must have attracted the attention of man at an early period. Archaeological findings in St. Moritz, in the Swiss Grisons, have revealed that the highly mineralized ferruginous spring that occurs there was used in the Bronze Age, if not earlier. Two heavy wooden pipes with a diameter of over three feet were found, at the bottom of one of which were two bronze swords. Remnants of a third wooden pipe near by point to a still earlier use of the spring. It is not likely that people would have taken so much trouble if the water had not been needed for some special purpose. Drinking water was available in unlimited quantities from the lake and from numerous ordinary springs. Hence it is very probable that the water was used for the treatment of ailments, as it still is today.[11]

Neolithic man was a skilful craftsman, and we should not be astonished if he had applied his skill to surgical operations. There is evidence that attempts were made to remove arrows from the body, sometimes successfully, sometimes not.[12] Skulls have been found on which large fracture wounds had healed remarkably well,[13] and it seems probable that some treatment was applied to them if nothing else but compression to stop the hemorrhage. Karl Jäger, who made a study of prehistoric bones, stated that 53.8 per cent of fractured extremity bones had healed with such excellent results that one had to assume that prehistoric man was skilful in the treatment of fractures.[14] His statement was generally accepted by medical historians and was repeated frequently,[15] but it was overlooked that his assumption was based on the examination of only thirteen fractured bones. As we mentioned before, well-healed fractures are frequently found also among wild animals.[16] The earliest splints that have come to light came from an Egyptian tomb of the Vth Dynasty.[17]

This does not mean that prehistoric man could not have been familiar with the method of splinting fractures. I, for one, am convinced that this, like so many other treatments, particularly those of a technical nature, was invented spontaneously in various parts of the world. We can well imagine the process. A man went hunting, slipped over a wet rock, broke a leg, crawled back to the hut or was carried by his mates. Once in the hut he was placed near the fire, remained lying for weeks suffering pain at the slightest motion until the fracture was at last healed. But when he got up he found himself a cripple, limping forever because the leg had become inches shorter than it had been before. This must have happened many times for thousands of years until somebody, a man of genius, one of those early inventors, had the bright idea to stretch the broken leg to its normal length. He did it while the patient howled in pain. Then he found that the stretched leg would not remain in the desired position but somehow had to be kept stretched. He looked around, saw a piece of board, or a piece of bark, attached it to the leg and the now splinted fracture healed without shortening.

We have no evidence that this actually happened as early as the neolithic period, but we have plenty of evidence for another much more daring operation, the trepanation of the skull. The first trephined neolithic skull was found in France as early as 1685, and another was found in 1816, but at that time it was assumed that the hole in the wall of the cranium was traumatic, the result of a wound.[18] The problem was approached from a different angle when the French anthropologist Prunières demonstrated in 1873 at the annual convention of the French Association for the Advancement of Science, in Lyon, an oval piece of bone cut from a parietal bone that he had found in a skull in a dolmen of the Lozère. He considered this 'rondelle' to have been an amulet.[19] In the following years new excavations and the systematic exploration of museum specimens revealed a great many trephined skulls and a great many rondelles, round or oval pieces of bone cut out of skulls. The French surgeon and anthropologist, Paul Broca, took up the study of prehistoric trephining with great eagerness and published a series of monographs on the subject.[20] It so happened that just at that time trepanation, which had been widely practiced in surgery in the case of fractures from the days of Hippocrates on to the early nineteenth century and which had then been almost abandoned, was being reintroduced, so that the attention of anthropologists and surgeons was focused on this operation; it is no wonder that this coincidence of interests gave rise to wild speculations.[21]

Prehistoric trephined skulls were found in France first of all, where over two hundred have been excavated so far. But France is by no means the only country that has yielded such material. Similar skulls have been found in the Western Mediterranean basin, in Spain, Portugal, Algiers, and Italy; in Great Britain,[21a] in Switzerland, Germany, Bohemia, Austria; north of France, in Belgium, Denmark, Sweden, and as far as Poland and Russia.[22]

Primitive trephining, moreover, was practiced in America, primarily in Peru [23] and Mexico,[24] but also in North America as far as Canada and in South America as far as Argentina.[25] The operation is still performed by lay practitioners in the Balkans, among the Cabyls of the Atlas, and in a number of primitive tribes of the South Pacific.[26]

When the first trephined neolithic skulls were found in France it seemed almost incredible that man at that early time should have dared to undertake such a dangerous operation that could easily be fatal. And how could it be done with the primitive instruments that were man's only tools? Experiments performed on cadavers showed, however, that it was not only possible but relatively easy to trephine a skull with a sharp flint. It could be done either by scratching the bone, or by making a circular incision that was gradually deepened, or finally by drilling a series of small holes arranged in a circle and then cutting the bridges between them.[27] All three methods must have been used at times, as the edges of trepanation holes show. These edges also tell us that individuals survived these operations in many cases, because bony scars had been formed. The operation was usually practiced on the parietal bone, sometimes on the frontal and occipital bones. The operator apparently knew that cutting through the sagittal suture would inevitably lead to fatal hemorrhage. Some perforations are small, others very large, and multiple perforations have been found, particularly in American material.

Why did prehistoric man perform such operations? It is impossible to answer the question with any degree of certainty, and all we can do is speculate on the subject. For over two thousand years surgeons trephined skulls in the Western World chiefly in the case of fractures, to relieve compression of the brain and to create an opening through which splinters could be removed and blood and other matters could be drained. The neolithic skulls with very few exceptions [28] do not show any sign of fracture, so that trephining must have been practiced for some other reason.

But then, ancient and medieval surgeons trephined skulls also in the treatment of epilepsy and similar convulsive diseases, and some still did it in the seventeenth century, 'that the evil air may breathe out.' [29] Primitives today open the skull of people suffering from severe chronic headaches and similar symptoms.[30] Could it be that neolithic man did it for the same, that is for medical, reasons? It is possible, and yet the problem is infinitely more complex than it looks at first sight, because trepanation was practiced not only on living individuals but also on the dead, and the round pieces of bone that were obtained in such a way, the 'rondelles,' were carefully preserved. Many were found to be perforated, which means that they were worn as necklaces. When an individual who had been successfully trephined died, rondelles or other fragments were cut out of his skull in such a way that they would include part of the edge of the original perforation. It seems highly probable that these rondelles were used as amulets.

All these practices point to magic or religious beliefs. Hence Broca in the beginning of his studies strongly denied the possibility of any surgical purpose, and considered the operation an initiation rite comparable to the tonsure of the priest. Later when trephined skulls were excavated in increasing numbers and it was found that the operation was performed on men and women indiscriminately, he changed his views and assumed that the purpose of the operation was to liberate epileptics, demoniacs, people afflicted with any forms of convulsion, from evil spirits. The fact that individuals survived the operation gave them a character of sanctity, so that after their death the bones of their skulls became relics, pieces of which were used as amulets protecting against convulsive diseases.[31]

Broca permitted his imagination to carry him rather far, but it is likely that the explanation of prehistoric trephining is to be sought along some such line in a combination of medical, magical, and religious views and practices. We must be aware, however, that there can be no certainty in the matter and that we can do no more than guess on the basis of analogy with conditions in totally different civilizations. This also applies to the interpretation of another neolithic mutilation, the so-called Sincipital T.

In 1895, L. Manouvrier described a strange mutilation found on a number of female skulls from ossuaries of the Seine-et-Oise, northeast of Paris.[32] It consisted of a T-shaped scar beginning on the frontal bone, running all along the sagittal suture, and branching into two parts along the posterior edge of the parietal bones. While the T-shape was the rule, a few skulls were found with straight-line or oval cicatrices. The scars may have been caused by deep incisions through the scalp or possibly by cauterization.

We have no way of ascertaining the reason for which this obviously painful operation was performed, whether it was for therapeutic, magical, religious, or cosmetic ends, or possibly as a punishment. The scalp was cauterized by Arabic physicians in the treatment of epilepsy, melancholy, and other nervous diseases.[33] Oval scars similar to one described by Manouvrier were found on skulls of the Guanches, early inhabitants of the Canary Islands, who 'made large scarifications with their stone knives on the skin of the part affected, and then cauterized the wound with roots of Malacca cane dipped in boiling grease; preference being given to the use of goat's grease.' [34] Deep scarifications of the forehead were practiced by Alexandrian surgeons in the treatment of eye diseases.[35]

These are all interesting analogies, and, while it is possible that neolithic man did perform these T-shaped cuts for similar reasons, we cannot do more than speculate about it.

Interesting as these prehistoric remains are as early testimonies of the awakening of man's mind, they give us very little information about man's attempts to protect and restore his health; nor is this to be expected from a civilization that flourished thousands of years ago and had no script and therefore no written literature. All we may expect, having only direct sources, is a few indications chiefly about the material side of man's life: the food he ate, the dwellings he used as shelter, the objects of his everyday life, his tools, and weapons. We are informed about his craftsmanship and artistic skill, but when it comes to ascertaining his mode of production and distribution, his social organization, his religion and medicine, all we can do is speculate, drawing analogies from our knowledge of early civilizations that possessed a written literature and from the study of contemporary primitive tribes.

I think there can be no objection to such speculation so long as it is done cautiously and we remain aware of its hypothetical character. The problem of the origins and beginnings of medicine is an extremely interesting one and we should at least make an attempt to form a view on the subject.

Man is a mammal and like other animals, he is equipped with instincts that drive him to commit actions tending to preserve the individual, to propagate his kind, and to omit actions inimical to such a purpose. The newborn babe needs no instruction to suck the mother's breast. All animals seek the food that their organism requires and so did man at all times. We may readily assume that his instincts were the purer the less developed his civilization was, that is, the less his actions were the result of reflexes conditioned by a more complicated social environment. It can only be attributed to instinctive behavior that man all over the world, under the most different geographic conditions, invariably found a balanced diet,[36] one best adapted to the climate.

When illness has taken hold of the animal organism, instincts manifest themselves in a special way. The body craves what it needs to overcome the lesion and restore health. The dog taken by a fever seeks rest in a quiet corner, but is found eating herbs when his stomach is upset. Nobody taught him what herbs to eat, but he will instinctively seek those that make him vomit or improve his condition in some other way.

And just as man in health sought and instinctively found the animal parts, plants, and minerals that his organism required for sustenance, so man in illness craved and instinctively found other plants, animal parts, or minerals that his body needed to overcome illness, or he ate foodstuffs in different combination or quantity. There is no sharp borderline between food and drug. Figs are food, but eaten in large quantities they act as a purgative. Citrus fruits are food to the healthy individual and a specific remedy to one suffering from scurvy.

If we accept the theory according to which man found his food by instinct—and I do not see what other explanation there could be—then we must also assume that he found drugs instinctively. Only this can explain the fact that almost all primitive people possess a—sometimes considerable—druglore,[37] which we shall have to discuss in greater detail later on. Instinct is apparent in these matters even in our sophisticated present civilization. Even today pregnant women can be seen eating whitewash from the wall because their organism is in need of calcium, and every physician or nurse knows of patients craving for just what their condition requires: pickles when they need acid, or a cup of coffee that will provide the amount of caffeine needed to stimulate a slackening circulation.

There is no doubt in my mind that dietetic and pharmacological therapy were born of instinct. Later, of course, with developing civilization man was conscious of his knowledge of foods and drugs; he extended it and passed it on from father to son or rather from mother to daughter, because it was the women who prepared the food and therefore also knew best how to prepare a healing potion.

Instinct was the source from which other methods of treatment sprang, such as physical therapy.[38] An individual hurts his leg and spontaneously, without thinking, he rubs it. This rubbing, developed into a system, became massage. Another individual suffers from lumbago, crawls to the fire, and once he feels the heat his pain becomes more tolerable. From such simple instinctive reactions, the many methods may have developed for the application of heat—and in other cases, of cold—in the form of water, steam, sand, or the poultice. The water buffalo and other cattle seek the water not only because it is cooler than the air but to keep insects and parasites off. Other animals roll themselves in mud so as to be covered by a protective layer. The cat buries its feces carefully and licks itself constantly to keep clean and free from parasites; and it is most amusing to watch the antics of a wild rabbit making its morning toilet. In this endeavor to ward off parasites, animals even help one another. Man too must have struggled against parasites, must instinctively have tried to keep clean, washing his body, bathing in rivers and lakes. The fight against parasites is one root of hygiene.

Surgery also is an old method of treatment that originated in instinctive actions. A thorn that entered the skin was removed by early man just as it is by animals, and so were other foreign bodies as long as they were accessible. An animal licks its wounds and man may well have done it also. He may have stopped a hemorrhage through compression just as he must have practiced bleeding at an early stage. Scratching became scarification and sucking became cupping. Bleeding as a method of treatment was so universal that it also must be derived from instinctive actions, although early observations probably contributed to a rapid development of the method: the fact that individuals suffering from fever diseases suddenly felt relieved when they had a spontaneous hemorrhage, bleeding from the nose or when menstruation set in.

Surgeons like to claim that their art is the earliest form of medical treatment.[39] They point out that there can be no doubt that man suffered injuries at all times, while it is uncertain when he first suffered from internal diseases; and they further maintain that the woman who first cut an umbilical cord performed a surgical operation. I think that such controversies are extremely futile, since they are not based on evidence but on speculation only. If the cutting of an umbilical cord is considered a surgical operation, then we must admit that there was surgery among animals also. And one could present just as good arguments for the greater antiquity of dietetic and possibly pharmacological therapy, stressing the fact that man at all times ate food and that the instinctive regulation of the intake of food according to the conditions of the organism was a form of treatment. But, as I just said, there is no point in engaging in discussions that cannot be more than a parlor game.

We mentioned that the fight against parasites was one root of hygiene. Another is probably to be sought in the fact that the sex urge drives individuals to seek healthy mates. We may therefore assume that young men and women at an early stage strove to maintain their health by cultivating their body in order to be attractive to the other sex.

We must also remember that the animal organism possesses in pain a marvelous alarm mechanism, which undoubtedly played a part in the beginnings of medicine. Pain makes us conscious of our body and signalizes that something that belongs to us is threatened.[40] Without pain, we should injure ourselves constantly, burning our fingers, biting our lips, chewing our cheeks. As a matter of fact, experiments have revealed that rats bite off their extremities as soon as they are anesthetized. When I feel a pain I suffer, and I instinctively act so as to relieve it. We can well imagine that early man suffering an acute pain in the stomach felt impelled to act, pressed his epigastrium with both hands, applied heat or cold, drank water or some decoction until he felt relieved. Pain, in other words, released a series of instinctive actions, some of which were more effective than others. With developing civilization man learned to differentiate between treatments, became aware of them, remembered them, and passed them on. Thus a certain body of empirical medical lore—house remedies we should call them—was acquired and became the common knowledge of the group.

Instinctive self-help came first, but mutual aid can also be assumed for an early stage, since it is common among animals. While I am writing these lines two squirrels are on my window sill cheerfully delousing each other. It is winter, not the mating season, and their action is not a mere gesture of courtship. That paleolithic men helped one another is evidenced by his burial customs.

Now we know a little more about the beginnings of medicine but still very little. It seems quite obvious that Magdalenian man, who created the cave paintings, and even to a greater degree neolithic man, who wore rondelles on a string around his neck, must have had some thoughts about the course and nature of disease, views that must have determined some of their actions, just as they must have had thoughts about the cause and nature of lightning, thunder, floods, and other natural phenomena that threatened life. Whenever people invented the script and wrote down their old traditions, we find a highly developed mythology explaining the phenomena of nature, including disease. The explanations have a religious or magical character and are so similar in all ancient civilizations that it would be difficult to interpret this similarity as the result of diffusion alone. It seems instead that man, having reached a certain stage of civilization, faced with the same phenomena, lightning, thunder, disease, et cetera, came spontaneously to similar explanations, particularly since the conceivable number of explanations is limited.[41] There can be no doubt that these views are infinitely older than the oldest written records, and we may assume that the earliest medical theories that sprang up spontaneously thousands of years ago in various sections of the globe had such a religious magical character.

The old civilizations are gone and the written records they left behind are not numerous. But then we find magic religious theories of disease today also, namely, among primitive peoples, and we naturally feel tempted to fill in gaps in our knowledge of the past from the study of contemporary primitive tribes. The question is whether this is feasible and justifiable.

There are today scattered over the world a quite considerable number of social units, tribes[42] commonly designated as primitive because they have no script and because their technology is very simple compared with ours. The Greeks knew such peoples and called them barbarians. To the explorers of the Renaissance they were savages and to Jean-Jacques Rousseau and his followers they were noble savages, people who lived the life of nature, unspoiled by civilization. The French spoke of *naturels;* the Germans still designate them as *Naturvölker,* peoples whose life is highly dependent on nature, while the *Kulturvölker,* the civilized people, have mastered nature through their technology.[43]

Under the influence of the theory of evolution anthropologists and sociologists in the nineteenth century assumed that the various types of human culture represented evolutionary stages in a development from simple to more complex forms.[44] Indeed it was easily apparent that the Egyptians, the Babylonians, and others had all gone through a scriptless period, had all had a simple technology in the beginning. The similarity of cultural forms was striking, and even in young civilizations—even today among us—magic and religious beliefs are found that are almost identical with those of primitive people; since they cannot be explained by diffusion it is usually assumed they are survivals of early beliefs.

In such a light, the primitives appeared as people that represented the first stage in the evolution of human civilization, people who for racial or other reasons had been arrested in their development, unable to evolve to the next stages. By watching them we were watching the dawn of civilization, and by studying their medicine we were studying the beginnings of man's reaction to disease.

This was an extremely attractive theory which actually stimulated a great many valuable investigations. Today, however, we know that the problem is not quite so simple. The primitives are very different from one another. They have not been entirely static during the centuries and millennia but have had a history also. This is particularly clear in the case of many African tribes that possess a rich oral literature in which the events of centuries are recorded.[45] Some primitives of today once had a higher civilization and have degenerated. We also know that the development of culture in various parts of the world did not always follow the same lines, pass through the same stages, from stone to bronze and iron, from basketry to pottery, from matriarchy to patriarchy, and so on. It is impossible, therefore, to accept the evolutionary theory of culture integrally and in the simplified form in which it was presented.[46] And it is impossible to identify without further ado the medicine of today's primitives with prehistoric medicine.

I think, however, that it would be a great mistake to eliminate the concept of evolution altogether from the history of civilization, particularly in such a field as the history of medicine. All ancient civilizations have developed according to a certain pattern, which is very much the same if we conceive it broadly enough and do not let our vision be dimmed by details. They all started from primitive beginnings; developed their own forms, technical, economic, social, religious, artistic; had a period of flowering when the creative forces were at their height; lingered on for a number of centuries in full possession of their faculties and achievements until the forms became rigid, disintegrated, and a new people took over. The parallelism in the development of ancient civilizations is undeniable, and the analogies are so numerous that they cannot be overlooked; and they are not only on the surface.[47]

In art there is a development, although not necessarily a progressive one. There is a definite development from Bach to Haydn and Mozart, to Beethoven, Brahms, and Schönberg. Every composer usually starts out with the means of his predecessors. But we could not say that Brahms is superior to Bach, or Schönberg to Beethoven; they are different. In technology, however, and this includes the technological side of medicine, there is an evolution, a progressive development. Our present chemotheraphy of infectious diseases is not only different from the treatment of the same diseases by Sydenham or by Hippocrates but is superior, because it cures more people. Medicine is a craft the effectiveness of which can be measured and therefore expressed in figures. The general death rate of a group, its infantile mortality rate, and average life expectancy are indices that show not only whether its standard of living is high or low but also whether its medicine and health services are advanced or backward. The two usually go together.

Hence, in medicine, we certainly can distinguish between primitive and advanced conditions; and this book will show how experience and knowledge accumulated in the course of time, how theories succeeded one another, each one lifting the veil a little higher. There can be no doubt that the beginnings of medicine were primitive everywhere and that conditions were probably similar in many ways to those we find among some of today's primitive peoples.

The study of primitive medicine is extremely interesting and is important for various reasons. One, we just mentioned, namely, that it throws light on early conditions that prevailed in ancient civilizations. Another reason is that it reveals certain psychological mechanisms, certain beliefs and practices that are also found among civilized peoples today, either as part of what is commonly called folk-medicine or as superstitions that are sometimes widespread even among the educated classes.[48] We shall have many opportunities to point to such survivals.

And, finally, we must be aware that the study of primitive medicine, of primitive culture at large, has practical significance also. Most primitives are colonial people or have the status of such within a nation; they must be administered. Although their health was neglected for a long time, it has at last been found that no labor may be expected from sick natives and that it is to the white man's advantage to provide modern health services for them.[49] Just as the colonial administrator cannot fulfil his task unless he is thoroughly versed in anthropology, in the same way the colonial doctor will soon find that he has much better results and a much better contact with his native patients if he is familiar with their tribal medicine and is able to translate his prescriptions into terms and concepts that they may understand.[50]

A brief discussion of primitive medicine presents considerable difficulties because there is a great diversity of primitive cultures and therefore of medicines also. Culture, whether primitive or not, always has a certain configuration that forms a pattern.[51] Medicine of a primitive tribe fits into that pattern, is one expression of it, and cannot be fully understood if it is studied separately. The tendency among anthropologists, therefore, is to describe not the parts—economy, law, religion, medicine, et cetera—but the whole, the pattern, and the parts within it.[52]

This certainly is a correct approach, one that is not peculiar to anthropology but applies to the history of civilization at large. Hippocratic medicine is also part of a cultural pattern and must be studied within that framework. There can be no doubt, however, that primitive medicine, as it appears within the various culture patterns, consists of a relatively small number of elements, which are very much the same in all primitive cultures and vary only in their combination. These elements are very different, however, from those that constitute the scientific systems of medicine of later ages. They determine the color and character of primitive medicine; and while the anthropologist who studies the culture of primitive tribes is interested primarily in the combinations of these elements, we here who study the various approaches to the problems of medicine are interested in the elements themselves. In the following pages we shall discuss them briefly, and in doing so we are fully aware that we are not picturing the medicine of a given tribe or tribes but that we are searching for common elements, that we are abstracting and generalizing.

NOTES

1. About early man, see M. Boule, *Les Hommes fossiles*, 2nd ed., Paris, 1923; E. Werth, *Der fossile Mensch*, Berlin, 1921; Arthur Keith, *New Discoveries*

Relating to the Antiquity of Man, London, 1931; Raymond W. Murray, *Man's Unknown Ancestors*, Milwaukee, 1943.

2. See J. Déchelette, *Manuel d'archéologie préhistorique, celtique et gallo-romaine.* I. *Archéologie préhistorique*, Paris, 1924; G. G. MacCurdy, *Human Origins, a Manual of Prehistory*, New York and London, 1924, 2 vols.; Henry Fairfield Osborn, *Men of the Old Stone Age*, 3rd ed., New York, 1934; R. R. Schmidt, *Die diluviale Vorzeit Deutschlands*, Stuttgart, 1912; E. Dennert, *Das geistige Erwachen des Urmenschen*, Weimar, 1929; *Reallexikon der Vorgeschichte*, ed. by Max Ebert, Berlin, 1924-9, 14 vols.
3. The literature on paleolithic art is very extensive and can be found in the manuals of archaeology. Basic are the publications of E. Cartailhac, l'Abbé E. Breuil, L. Capitan, and others, *Peintures et gravures murales des cavernes paléolithiques*, published under the auspices of the Prince of Monaco from 1906 on. See also S. Reinach, *Répertoire de l'art quaternaire*, Paris, 1913. Some recent publications with very good illustrations are Herbert Kühn, *Die Malerei der Eiszeit*, Munich, 1922, and Max Raphael, *Prehistoric Cave Paintings*, New York, 1945. See also monographs in general histories of art such as Eckart von Sydow, 'Die Kunst der Naturvölker und der Vorzeit,' *Propyläen Kunstgeschichte*, vol. I, Berlin, 1923.

3a. About these statuettes see Hančar, *Prähist. Zschr.*, 1939-40, 30-31:85-156.

4. M. Höfler, 'Ein alter Heilritus,' *Arch. Gesch. Med.*, 1914, 7:390-95.
5. John M. Tyler, *The New Stone Age in Northern Europe*, New York, 1921.
6. J. Heierli, *Urgeschichte der Schweiz*, Zurich, 1901; A. Schenk, *La Suisse préhistorique*, Lausanne, 1912. The lake dwellings of central Europe first appeared in the neolithic and were continued during the Bronze Age.
7. V. Hehn (*Kulturpflanzen und Haustiere in ihrem Übergang aus Asien nach Griechenland und Italien sowie in das übrige Europa*, Berlin, 1870, 8th ed. by O. Schrader, Berlin, 1911) thought that it was done in connection with certain religious views.
8. The bag of goat skin is still the chief container for water and other liquids all over the Orient.
9. Oswald Heer, *Die Pflanzen der Pfahlbauten*, 68. *Neujahrsbl. Naturforsch. Ges. Zurich*, 1865; E. Neuweiler, *Die prähistorischen Pflanzenreste Mitteleuropas mit besonderer Berücksichtigung der schweizerischen Funde*, Zurich, 1905; H. Brockmann-Jerosch, 'Vergessene Nutzpflanzen,' *Wissen und Leben*, vol. 7, 1914, 'Älteste Kultur- und Nutzpflanzen,' *Vierteljahrsschr., Naturforsch. Ges. Zurich*, vol. 62, 1917.
10. Such as e.g. *Papaver somniferum L., Sambucus ebulus L., Fumaria officinalis L., Verbena officinalis L., Saponaria officinalis, Menyanthes trifoliata L.*, and others listed in E. Neuweiler, 'Die Pflanzenwelt in der jüngeren Stein- und Bronzezeit der Schweiz,' *Mitt. Antiqu. Ges. Zürich*, 1924, 29 (4):253ff.
11. Replicas of these pipes are in the National Museum at Zurich and at the Engadine Museum at St. Moritz.
12. See A. F. Le Double, *La Médecine et la chirurgie dans les temps préhistoriques et protohistoriques*, Paris, 1911 (a pamphlet of 38 pages).
13. Karl Jäger, *Beiträge zur frühzeitlichen Chirurgie*, Wiesbaden, 1907 (with an atlas of 13 plates), p. 115: Schädelfrakturen.

14. Loc. cit. p. 17. It must be said, however, that Jäger himself did not attribute much importance to these figures and that he was aware that his material was too small to permit far-reaching conclusions.
15. So by Karl Sudhoff who stated explicitly that fractures must have been splinted at that time, *Kurzes Handbuch der Geschichte der Medizin*, Berlin, 1922, p. 8.
16. Adolph H. Schultz, *Bull. Hist. Med.*, 1939, 7:571-82.
17. G. E. Smith, 'The Most Ancient Splints,' *Brit. Med. J.*, 1908, 1:732.
18. Déchelette, loc. cit. p. 475.
19. *Ass. franç. avancem. sciences*, Congrès Lyon, 1873, p. 704.
20. The chief publication of Paul Broca on the subject is 'Sur la Trépanation du crâne et les amulettes craniennes à l'époque néolithique,' *Congrès internat. anthrop. et arch. préhist. VIIIe session*, Budapest, 1876, pp. 101-96; reprinted in *Rev. Anthrop.*, 1877, p. 142ff. and as a separate pamphlet, Paris, E. Leroux, 1877. Broca's other numerous papers on the subject are listed in E. Guiard, *La Trépanation cranienne chez les néolithiques et chez les primitifs modernes*, Paris, 1930, p. 111f.; see also V. Busacchi, 'La trepanazione del cranio nei popoli preistorici (neolitici e precolombiani) e nei primitivi moderni,' *Atti. Mem. Accad. Storia Arte Sanit.*, 1935, vol. 34, no. 2 and 3.
21. Lucas-Championnière, *Les Origines de la trépanation décompressive. Trépanation néolithique, trépanation pré-Colombienne, trépanation des Kabyles, trépanation traditionelle*, Paris, 1912.
21a. T. Wilson Parry, 'The Prehistoric Trephined Skulls of Great Britain together with a Detailed Description of the Operation Probably Performed in Each Case,' *Proc. R. Soc. Med.*, Sect. Hist. Med., 1921, 14:27-42.
22. E. Guiard, loc. cit. note 21, p. 101.
23. M. A. Muniz and W. J. McGee, 'Primitive Trephining in Peru,' 16th *Ann. Rep. Bur. Amer. Ethnol.*, Washington, 1897.
24. C. Lumholtz and A. Hrdlička, 'Trephining in Mexico,' *Am. Anthrop.*, 1897, 10:389-96.
25. H. L. Shapiro, 'Primitive Surgery, First Evidence of Trephining in the Southwest,' *Nat. Hist.*, 1927, 27:266-9; E. F. Greenman, 'A Report on Michigan Archaeology,' *Am. Anthrop.*, 1926, 28:312-13; H. I. Smith, 'Trephined Aboriginal Skulls from British Columbia and Washington,' *Am. J. Phys. Anthrop.*, 1924, 7:447-52.
26. O. von Hovorka and A. Kronfeld, *Vergleichende Volksmedizin*, Stuttgart, 1909, vol. II, p. 444ff.; Guiart, loc. cit. p. 58ff.
27. Lucas-Championnière, loc. cit. p. 75ff.; Guiart, loc. cit. p. 80ff.
28. Carrière and Reboul, 'Un Cas de trépanation préhistorique faite pendant la vie et suivie de guérison opératoire observée sur un crâne de la grotte sépulcrale de Rousson (Gard),' *Bull. Mém. Soc. Anthrop. Paris*, 1894, p. 351ff.; Petitot, 'La Sépulture dolménique de Mareuil-les-Meaux,' ibid. 1892, p. 344.
29. O. Temkin, *The Falling Sickness*, Baltimore, 1945, p. 224.
30. H. Malbot and R. Verneau, 'Les Chaouïas et la trépanation du crâne dans l'Aurès,' *L'Anthrop.*, 1897, 8:1-18, 174-204.
31. Broca, loc. cit. p. 50ff. of the pamphlet (note 20).

32. L. Manouvrier, 'Le T Sincipital—curieuse mutilation crânienne néolithique,' *Bull. Soc. Anthrop. Paris,* 1895, 4th series, 6:357. Further literature and a good summary of the problem in G. G. MacCurdy, 'Prehistoric Surgery—a Neolithic Survival,' *Amer. Anthrop.,* 1905, N.S. 7:17-23.
33. L. Manouvrier, 'Les Marques sincipitales des crânes néolithiques considérées comme reliant la chirurgie classique ancienne à la chirurgie préhistorique,' *Bull. Mém. Soc. Anthrop. Paris,* 1902, 5th series, 4:494ff.
34. Lehman-Nitsche, 'Notes sur des lésions de crânes des îles Canaries analogues à celles du crâne de Menouville et leur interprétation probable,' *Bull. Mém. Soc. Anthrop. Paris,* 1903, 492ff.; MacCurdy, loc. cit. p. 20.
35. Celsus, vII, 7, 15. See K. Sudhoff, 'Medizin in der Steinzeit,' *Ztschr. f. ärztl. Fortbildung,* 1909, 6:196-200; reprinted in *Skizzen,* Leipzig, 1921, pp. 53ff.
36. K. Hintze, *Geographie und Geschichte der Ernährung,* Leipzig, 1934; V. Ducceschi, 'L'alimentazione umana nelle età preistoriche,' *Mem R. Ist. Veneto Sci. Lett. Arti,* 1936, vol. xxx, no. 1.
37. W. Artelt, 'Studien zur Geschichte der Begriffe "Heilmittel" und "Gift," Urzeit—Homer—Corpus Hippocraticum,' *Stud. Gesch. Med.,* 23, Leipzig, 1937.
38. R. Hofschläger, 'Über den Ursprung der Heilmethoden,' *Naturwiss. Verein zu Krefeld, Festschr. z. Feier d. 50-jährigen Bestehens,* Krefeld, 1908, pp. 135-218; R. Hofschläger, 'Die Entstehung der primitiven Heilmethoden und ihre organische Weiterentwicklung,' *Arch. Gesch. Med.,* 1909, 3:81-103; F. von Oefele, 'Prähistorische Parasitologie nach Tierbeobachtungen,' *Arch. Parasit.,* 1902, 5:117-38.
39. E.g. W. von Brunn, *Kurze Geschichte der Chirurgie,* Berlin, 1928, p. 1.
40. See the study of V. von Weizsäcker, 'Die Schmerzen. Stücke einer medizinischen Anthropologie,' *Die Kreatur,* 1926-7, 1:315-35.
41. Bastian's *Elementargedanke* has been strongly opposed by the 'diffusionists,' who assumed that civilization was spread over the world from one focus or a few single foci. The psychological school, however, from W. Wundt to the various brands of psychoanalysts maintains that man's basic mental mechanisms have always been the same. A. Bastian, *Der Menschheitsgedanke durch Raum und Zeit,* Berlin, 1901, 2 vols.; W. Wundt, *Völkerpsychologie,* Leipzig, 1900-1920, 10 vols.; S. Freud, *Totem und Tabu, Einige Übereinstimmungen im Seelenleben der Wilden und der Neurotiker,* Leipzig, 3rd ed., 1922; C. G. Jung, *Wandlungen und Symbole der Libido,* Leipzig and Vienna, 3rd ed., 1938.
42. James G. Leyburn, *Handbook of Ethnography,* New Haven, 1931.
43. The term *Naturvolk* was first used by Herder in 1784 in *Ideen zur Philosophie der Geschichte der Menschheit.*
44. See, e.g. Edward B. Tylor, *Early History of Mankind,* London, 1870; *Primitive Culture,* London, 1871 (6th ed., 1920).
45. See the tales collected by Leo Frobenius, *Atlantis, Volksmärchen und Volksdichtungen Afrikas* (Veröffentlichungen des Forschungsinstituts für Kulturmorphologie), Jena, 1921-8, 12 vols.
46. See the discussion of Franz Boas, *The Mind of Primitive Man,* New York, 1931, pp. 174-96.

47. I once discussed this parallelism as it presents itself in medicine and outlined the various phases through which medicine went in the great civilizations of the past, 'Die historische Betrachtung der Medizin,' *Arch. Gesch. Med.*, 1926, 18:1-19.
48. O. von Hovorka and A. Kronfeld, *Vergleichende Volksmedizin, Eine Darstellung volksmedizinischer Sitten und Gebräuche, Anschauungen und Heilfaktoren, des Aberglaubens und der Zaubermedizin,* Stuttgart, 1908-9, 2 vols.; Georg Buschan, *Über Medizinzauber und Heilkunst im Leben der Völker,* Berlin, 1941.
49. This became particularly clear in South Africa, where the gold mines could not find 300,000 able-bodied younger men among 7½ million natives and had to import labor from the tropical belt.
50. A brilliant study on this subject is Alexander H. Leighton and Dorothea C. Leighton, *The Navaho Door, an Introduction to Navaho Life,* Cambridge, Mass., 1944.
51. Ruth Benedict, *Patterns of Culture,* Boston and New York, 1934.
52. E. H. Ackerknecht exemplified this very graphically in describing culture pattern and medicine of three tribes, the Cheyennes, Dobuans, and Thongas, 'Primitive Medicine and Culture Pattern,' *Bull. Hist. Med.*, 1942, 12:545-74.

*

2. Causation and Nature of Disease

What is disease? What causes it? Practically all primitives know of diseases that require no explanation. They 'come of themselves,'[1] are the obvious consequence of eating or drinking too much, of minor injuries, or similar occurrences. They are not diseases in the strict sense of the word, but minor ailments that do not threaten life, common ailments that are seen every day. The Bantu of South Africa know that food passes through the body and that it may cause discomfort that an emetic or purgative will relieve.[2] They frequently see worms leaving the body with the stools and think that pain is caused when such worms wander through the body. Coughs and colds, fever and rheumatism need no explanation. They come and go, are treated by the patient himself or by family members with what we should call domestic remedies, and little is thought of them. They are a nuisance 'like having debts,' as an old Bantu said to me, and, he added, 'just as unavoidable.'

Similarly the Mano of Liberia do not bother about explaining colds, measles, or toothache. They also know that bees and wasps sting, and are familiar with the results of the bite of snake and scorpion. Even such a disease as yaws in its primary and secondary stages does not call for interpreting. It is so common that the Mano merely says, 'Oh, that is not a sickness, everybody has that.'[3]

In the same way the Zande in the Southern Sudan treats himself in case of a mild ailment. And if he does not know how, there is always an older man around who will recommend a suitable drug.[4] The Fijian considers the frequent colds and coughs from which he suffers—boils, scabies, ringworm, and similar disorders—as 'diseases of the body' due to incidental circumstances. They do not require special attention so long as they take a normal course and respond to the customary treatments. Should this not be the case, then an ailment would immediately become suspicious and would fall into another category.[5] The Apache know of many ailments that are the result of surfeit, want, overexertion, carelessness, or needless daring, of foolishness and old age, ailments that need not be treated ceremonially.[6]

Thus it seems that primitives almost universally distinguish between minor, common, and therefore obvious ailments that they can handle themselves, and serious sickness that is mysterious and cannot be cured unless it has been explained, a process that requires the special knowledge and skill of the medicine man. It may be that such a differentiation is secondary, the result of a later development. If a bee stings me, I experience a painful swelling as a matter of course, but why did the bee sting me and not my neighbor? This may require an explanation. It may be that economic factors played a part, the tendency to simplify life that is found even among primitives today. A ceremonial treatment is complicated and expensive; why have recourse to it for a cold that comes and goes by itself?

Action, however, must be taken in the case of serious illness. Why has an individual been stricken? What is causing his sickness?

Here we must remember that the primitive does not distinguish between medicine, magic, and religion.[7] To him they are one, a set of practices intended to protect him against evil forces and to bring him good luck. He feels threatened by mysterious forces. Spirits inhabit the objects of his environment. The ghosts of the dead are hovering over the village.[8] The transcendental world is real to him, and he partakes in it when he dreams and his soul leaves the body temporarily and has intercourse with the spirits. Dreams are so real to him that he feels responsible for actions committed in dreams.

In order to live safely, primitive man must be on his guard all the time. He must be aware of happenings, even slight ones, and must interpret them. He has a strong interest in causality, and in explaining phenomena he is indifferent to secondary causes and excludes the concept of chance. When three women go together for water to the river, to use an example quoted by Lévy-Bruhl,[9] and the one in the middle is caught by an alligator, it must be explained why she was attacked and not the woman to the left or the one to the right. The most logical explanation is that the two women who escaped bewitched the one who was caught and they will have to face the consequences.

Another point that must be kept in mind is that primitive man is extraordinarily suggestible. This explains his strong response to spells, charms, and other magic devices and the fear he has of breaking taboos. A young Kurnai, in Australia, who committed such an offense by eating a female opossum before he was permitted to do so, fell ill and died in three weeks.[10] Similar cases have been reported from all over the world.

Now, if somebody falls seriously ill there must be a reason for it, and to the primitive mind the most logical assumption is that the individual fell sick because somebody did something to him. This somebody may be a man who harmed the patient through sorcery, in which case we have a magical explanation. Or, this somebody may be a higher power, a spirit or ghost or the deity, in which case we have a religious explanation.

I am well aware that there are no sharp borderlines between magic and religion in primitive culture and that it is often impossible to decide into which category a process falls, so that some anthropologists prefer to use the more general term 'magico-religious.' I think, however, that from our point of view there are certain advantages in distinguishing between the elements of primitive medicine whenever this is feasible, and I believe that the following chapters and volumes will make this evident. In making this distinction, I follow more or less the definition of Rivers, who, by magic, means, 'a group of processes in which man uses rites which depend for their efficacy on his own powers believed to be inherent in, or the attributes of, certain objects and processes which are used in these rites.' Under religion, on the other hand, he comprehends 'a group of processes, the efficacy of which depends on the will of some higher power, some power whose intervention is sought by rites of supplication and propitiation. Religion differs from magic in that it involves the belief in some power in the universe greater than that of man himself.'[11]

How can a man make another individual sick? Here we encounter probably the two oldest and most basic concepts of disease, namely the view that disease is a 'Plus' or a 'Minus,' a 'Too-much' or a 'Not-enough.' Man is sick because there is something in his body that does not belong to it, or he is sick because something has been removed from his organism that is necessary to life. A man makes another individual sick by introducing magically a foreign object into the victim's body, or by removing magically a vital part from it.

The idea of object-intrusion as one of the primary causes of disease is very widespread.[12] It is almost universal on the American continent, is found in northeastern Siberia, southeastern Asia, Australia, and New Zealand, is encountered in Africa in spots, and almost universally in European folklore.

An individual is suddenly stricken with illness and he knows that an object has been shot into his body. This object may be anything from a small pebble, a bit of straw, leather, earth, coal, a piece of quartz, glass, a splinter of wood, a bean, a fishbone, or a shell, to an insect, a worm, or another small animal.[13]

Who made you sick in such a way? A fellow man, a neighbor, a relative, somebody who had a grudge against you and meant to harm you and even to kill you. Either he had the gift of sorcery himself and knew how to cast the spell, or he went to the medicine man, who, being expert in magic, could not only cure people but also bewitch them. In Melanesia the sorcerer used a 'ghost-shooter' to that end.[14] He took a piece of bamboo, filled it with bones of a dead man, leaves, and other ingredients. Then holding his thumb on the open end of the stick, he went in search of the victim. And when he spotted him, he aimed the stick at him, removed the thumb from the opening, and all the evil influence streamed out. The victim, seeing this, felt suddenly stricken, went home, lay down a sick man, and not infrequently died.[15] A somewhat simpler method practiced in the same locality consisted in wrapping the magic objects into a parcel that was placed on the victim's path.[16]

Fejos has given a graphic description of these practices among the Yagua of Peru: [17]

> On the day a shaman intends to practise evil magic he refrains from eating meat and remains in his hammock during the afternoon, with his face turned toward the wall. When night falls he commences to smoke a large cigar and blows the smoke over his whole body until the skin is soft enough for the magic darts to make their exit from his body. He then leaves the house and proceeds toward the dwelling of his intended victim. He always walks and never wears a disguise, such as that of a jaguar or a bird. The shaman is supposed to be able to cover much greater distances than ordinary mortals during the night. Upon arriving at his destination, he silently approaches the doorway of the communal house and pushes aside the screen to locate the hammock of his victim. Once he ascertains where it is, he closes the screen and takes up a position outside the house opposite and close to the hammock. He listens to the person's breathing, then pulls out two, three, or four darts from his body, and with an overhand motion 'throws' them in the direction of the breathing sound. The darts pass through the palm screen wall without difficulty, and enter the body of the victim, who does not wake 'because it does not hurt then but only later.' The darts which are now lodged in the unfortunate individual will rot away, and he will die, sometimes within a single day or night. The time required for the evil spell to take effect varies, however, with the shaman's strength and ability to make the darts effective.

It was particularly diseases with acute pains that were attributed to such a cause. rheumatic disorders, lumbago, sciatica, stitches, pleurisy. Lumbago is still popularly called *Hexenschuss* in German, 'shot of the witch.' It was due to the 'shot of the elf' in Wales.[18] Elfs are elemental spirits, and among primitives also the view is found that foreign objects may be shot into the victim's body not only by fellow men using sorcery but also by spiritual beings, by the deity,[19] a view that is not infrequent in higher civilizations. The arrows of the Almighty were within Job and their poison drank up his spirit.[20] Apollo punished the people with pestilence by shooting his darts at them.[21]

Another point that must be mentioned in this connection is that to some primitive peoples it is not so much the object that causes sickness as rather the spiritual essence contained in the object, so that the real cause of the disease would be intrusion by a spirit.[22] This may well be the case, and it merely confirms that there are no sharp borderlines in primitive medicine. Still, there is a difference between pure spirit intrusion or possession by a demon and the presence of a spirit bound to an object.

Tylor in 1870 expressed the view that the concept of disease caused by object intrusion had a single origin and spread by diffusion.[23] Clements in 1932 elaborated this thesis considerably, ascribing the origin of the concept to the Old World paleolithic, whence it would have spread through Asia, where it would have been lost later in most places. And, finally, it would have been brought to America with the migrants who crossed the Bering Strait toward the end of the Pleistocene.[24]

It is needless to say that such a theory is highly speculative. The large gaps in Asia are not too easy to explain and the very fact of the wide distribution of the concept raises a suspicion of plural origin, particularly since there is a certain relation between this concept and that of parasitism. I would not use the idea of the toothworm as an argument for the single origin.[25] Worms are the obvious parasites, and while man could not know how they entered the body, it was apparent how they left it. Once it was assumed that worms cause pain by attacking various parts of the organism, it seemed likely that they would also cause the most violent pain, the toothache.

Whatever the origin of the concept of object intrusion may have been, there can be no doubt that it is very old. And so must also have been the other basic concept according to which disease was caused by the loss of something essential to life, by the loss of what we call the soul, or of the organ considered the seat of the soul.

The belief in a soul seems to be universal among primitives, in a double of man, an ethereal image, finer in texture than the body, an essence that leaves the body in sleep, coma, and death.[26] A man dies; his body rots, is buried, or burned, but we see him exactly as he was, can talk to him, namely in dreams. And so, the primitive concludes, something that was part of him is still alive although the body died. We sleep, we know, since everybody can testify that we have been lying on the floor of the hut or in the hammock all night, and yet we have been far away, have met people, have talked to them, have had adventures. As long as body and soul are together as they should be, man is normal and in good health, but he becomes sick if the soul leaves him, is abducted, and he dies if the soul does not return.

The soul resides in the body at large or is localized in certain parts, in the kidney fat, according to Australian tribes,[27] or fat of the omentum,[28] in the heart, as the Tukano of the northwest Amazon River believe,[29] in the liver,[30] or gall bladder.[31] Whoever abducts these organs takes the soul away with them.

How can the soul be removed in order to make an individual sick? In different ways. On the Hervey Islands, in Australia, the medicine man constructs a magic device, a soul trap consisting of a rope of coconut fiber, ten feet long, with loops. It is hung on a tree in the victim's path. He comes, sees the noose, knows what it means; his soul is caught and he will die unless help is given him.[32] Or the soul has left the body while I am dreaming; it is wandering around and has lost its way, does not find its way back. Or it has met with an accident, has been caught by the ghosts of virgins, as the Annamites think. They lure mortal man with strange laughter, and if he answers their call he loses his soul and becomes raving mad.[33] A sudden fright may cause the loss of the soul; [34] or among the Ammassalik-Eskimos of East Greenland, it is believed that a child may lose his soul when he falls down.[35] Young children are more susceptible to soul loss than adults. The soul leaves them and returns to them through the fontanel.[36] On the Island of Nias in Indonesia, it is believed that a man's shadow is endowed with soul, and by taking the shadow away the soul is affected.[37] In the folklore of a number of people, the view is encountered that sneezing indicates that the soul has left the body or, more frequently, that it has returned to it. At any rate, it provides an opportunity for wishing the individual health and good luck.[38]

If the soul can be persuaded or forced to return to the body it left, the patient will recover. But if the captured soul has been buried, as the Cherokee believe,[39] or worse, if it has been devoured by cannibal spirits, such as are known to Siberian tribes,[40] the case is hopeless and the patient will die.

The magic shot explains acute painful diseases that befall an individual suddenly, while the loss of the soul is responsible for diseases that make one unconscious, or for chronic diseases in the course of which the patient withers away. But here as everywhere in primitive medicine there are no sharp borderlines.

The belief in loss of the soul as a cause of disease is widespread.[41] Its chief center seems to be Siberia, where it is the foremost theory of disease. But it is also generally found in Indonesia, Papuo-Melanesia, northwestern America, and in spots on every continent. Clements believes that the theory originated in the upper paleolithic. It is highly probable that man at that time had developed the concept of a soul, but whether he connected it with disease or not at that early stage again remains guesswork.

So far we have seen that an individual, skilled in magic, can cause sickness in a fellow man by introducing a foreign object into his body or by removing his soul. But there are other methods of magic for inducing sickness and death, the methods of sympathetic magic.

Since J. G. Frazer's investigations,[42] one usually distinguishes between imitative or mimetic [43] and contagious magic. They are both methods of sympathetic magic in that in both cases the harm is not done to the victim directly but to something that is part of him, and he then suffers by sympathy. In imitative magic the sorcerer makes an effigy of the victim, drawing his image or making a puppet. In doing this he conjures the victim, and now having a hold over him he pierces the image with pins; burns, buries, or damages it in some other way; and the distant victim falls sick and possibly dies.

The rituals vary but the basic idea is always the same. On the Aru Islands in Indonesia, a picture is made of resin, which is thrown into the sea while imprecations are being pronounced. In Victoria the sorcerer makes a wooden model of the part of the body that is to be hit. It is then hung near the fire, incantations are sung, and the far-away victim suddenly feels an intense pain in that part. In the Babar Archipelago, in Indonesia, an effigy is made from a koli-leaf. The sorcerer then cuts off its head, puts what is left with wax into an egg, and burns the whole.[44] The Lerons of Borneo leave the victim's wooden image in the jungle; it decays gradually and while it does so the patient withers and dies. On Jervis Island, north of Queensland, human effigies of stone and wood can be bought ready made. All one has to do is give them the name of the victim and perform the magic manipulations on them. Examples could be multiplied indefinitely because imitative magic is universal and, one may add, timeless. Today still, photographs are stuck with pins vengefully, or they are torn or burned with a desire to harm, and not only among primitives.

This belief also explains the reluctance of many primitives to being photographed or painted, a difficulty that every worker in the field has experienced.[45] The few examples we gave also show that the magic action of harming an effigy is frequently combined with incantations, or the magic power of the word.[46] They furthermore show that an individual's name is also part of his person, and a not unimportant one. If you know the name, the full name that identifies him, you can write it on a leaf, or on a piece of bark or paper, which can then be destroyed.

Imitative magic acts on a man's effigy, his name, and possibly his shadow, which is an image also; while contagious magic deals with products of the victim's body, such as hair clippings, nail parings, a tooth, excrements, spittle, or objects that touched him, bits of his clothes, his food or dwelling, and even his footprint. If you can get hold of such a part, you have power over the whole, because the harm you inflict on the part will affect the whole by magical contagion. The Kai of New Guinea have an explanation for it. They believe that soul substance permeates not only the whole body but everything that is in touch with it. Hence, if you have hair clippings of an individual, or his loincloth, you can act on his soul.[47] There is frequently a similarity in the rite performed and the desired effect. Thus in Victoria it is believed that burning of hair clippings causes fever, while on Serang, burning of hair with some of the victim's food produces a violent headache, and burning of excrements, dysentery.[48] In Australia sharp stones placed in an individual's footprints are expected to induce lameness.

Frazer pointed out that contagious magic had one advantage in that it forced those who held such beliefs to be clean, to bury their feces, their spittle and other secretions, their refuse and rubbish so that the enemy would not be able to find them.[49]

There is one more form of magic that must be mentioned in this connection although it is not common among primitives today. It is localized primarily in Mediterranean countries and the Near East, where it occurred in remote antiquity and is still a generally accepted belief among the people. I mean the magic power of the evil eye.[50]

The notion is that some individuals have the faculty to cast a spell on others by glancing at them, catching their eyes. Some do it involuntarily, because they are cursed with this evil power that they cannot but exert on whoever happens to cross their path. Some of them are very ugly, others, on the contrary, very beautiful people. There are, on the other hand, individuals who use this power knowingly. They are filled with envy, with jealousy, with the desire to possess something or somebody. This intense desire is expressed in the eye, which emanates a radiance that hits the victim like a curse.[51] Whoever falls under the spell, under the glance that 'fascinates,' must expect misfortune; something will go wrong and he is lucky if he only loses money. More often he will have an accident or will become sick and may even die. Children and young animals are more exposed and more defenseless than adults and, therefore, need added protection.

It is a strange belief which has persisted through the centuries and millennia with incredible tenacity. Whoever has lived in Mediterranean countries has encountered people who were supposed to have the evil eye, and free from superstitions as he had thought himself to be, he could not help but feel ill at ease. And in those countries everybody knows of people who have been victims of the evil eye.

We mentioned before repeatedly that there is no sharp borderline in primitive culture between magic and religion. As a matter of fact, magic, religion, and medicine are one to the primitive mind. A man may cause illness by sending through magic not a stone but a demon into the victim's body, and on the other hand a deity may punish a man with illness by introducing a foreign object into him or abducting his soul. If we differentiate between various concepts of disease, we do it for the sake of simplicity, in order to have a clearer view of the constituent elements of these beliefs and practices, but we know that these elements occur in a great variety of combinations.

The belief in spirits that reside in animate and inanimate objects of man's environment, in the elements of nature, spirits that interfere in man's life for good or evil and therefore may cause disease, is extremely widespread, in fact almost universal. In Indonesia, action of spiritual or divine beings is considered the chief cause of illness,[52] and this is true of Polynesia, where religion permeates all aspects of life.[53] The Cherokees, in America, know many spirits [54] that are neither good nor evil, but when these are offended, when they feel provoked by man, they hit back and cause sickness. Thus the spirit of fire is resentful when a person throws the offal of anything he has chewed into the fire, and the result is a toothache. Urinating on the ashes leads to an 'itching of the privates which causes the patient to scratch the parts affected thus producing painful sores.' [55] The spirit of the moon causes blindness.[56] And the river 'sends disease to those who insult it by such actions as throwing rubbish into it, by urinating into it, etc. As a vengeance for the latter act, it causes a disease from a description of the symptoms of which it appears that enuresis is meant.' [57]

Spirits may cause sickness in many ways, not only by entering the victim's body. They attack and strike man.[58] The Sakai of the Malay Peninsula believe that the spirits lie in wait until the victim passes, then hit his shadow with clubs.[59] According to Central Australians, the spirits use a pointing-stick that is hooked at one end. 'This is projected into the body of the victim, and every now and then the spirit gives a malicious tug at the hair string which is attached to the hook, so as to increase the victim's pain.'[60] Indeed, there are many forms of pain that would suggest such a method of torture.

A very common form of disease causation by spirits, particularly in the Old World, is the so-called spirit intrusion. The spirit enters the patient's body, thus causing sickness. The spirit is the disease and the patient is cured when the disease, i.e. the spirit, has been driven out. The Mosquito Indians of Nicaragua believe that the spirit resides not in the body as a whole but in the sick organ.[61]

Clements makes a sharp distinction between spirit intrusion and possession, and I think with very valid arguments.[62] A stomach ache may be caused by a spirit who does not make himself known. If he is found out, it is through the medicine man's diagnosis. In the case of possession, the spirit is vocal; he speaks through the victim. Mental and nervous diseases are explained in such a way, delirium, hysteria, epilepsy, and others. The victim of possession, moreover, need not necessarily be a sick man; he may be considered a holy man, one who is in close touch with the transcendental world, a prophet.

The concept of spirit intrusion as a cause of disease is widespread, but it seems to be missing in Australia and Tasmania, among the Negritos of the Malay Peninsula, and the Pygmies of the Philippines, all tribes of very low cultural development. It does occur among the American Indians but by no means universally.[63]

All spirits may cause illness when they are provoked, but many tribes differentiate between good and evil spirits, and among the latter they know of specialists whose function it is to cause diseases. Thus smallpox is considered an evil spirit by the Dyak of Borneo[64] and by the Yoruba of West Africa, where the demon comes with an assistant who wrings the neck of the sick.[65] The Singhalese are famous for the twenty-four types of demons they distinguish, with specialists for every disease.[66]

Spirits of a special kind who are also instrumental in causing sickness are the ghosts of the dead, particularly of those who have died recently. To most primitive peoples the world of the dead is a very real one. The spirits of the ancestors are never far away; they take an active part in one's life, bring good luck and bad; one sees them and talks to them in dreams.[67] People are afraid of the dead. When the soul leaves the body, it is not yet reconciled to its fate and may wish to come back to life by entering into some other body, into that of a relative, thus causing illness. This fear is reflected even today in burial customs that tend to make it difficult for the dead to return and to recognize his relatives. The opening of the house through which the corpse was taken out is walled up; the traces of the funeral procession are erased and the mourners make themselves unrecognizable by all wearing clothes of the same color, one that they usually do not wear.[68]

Particularly feared are the ghosts of people who died without having fulfilled their mission on earth, young children, brides, women in childbirth or childbed. They more than any other dead must be eager to return to life or, feeling lonely, they may wish to kill some who were close to them so as to enjoy their company in the world of the spirits.[69]

The ancestral spirits, however, may also send sickness as punishment for a break of taboo, just as other spirits or the divinity may punish man in such a way for the breaking of a taboo or the failure to follow certain observances.[70] This concept of disease is obviously deeply rooted in Polynesia, where the concept of taboo is highly developed. It is found on the American hemisphere among many Indian tribes, and while it occurs among some of the most primitive peoples, such as the South Australians, the Pygmies of the Philippines, and those of the Malay Peninsula,[71] we shall see later in this volume that the concept of disease as a punishment for sin played a dominating part in the Semitic civilizations of the ancient Orient.

Some taboos are very old. They have been observed in a tribe since time immemorial and have determined social relationships. Such are the food taboos. The killing and eating of a totem animal is an infraction of a taboo that is invariably punished. Among the Mano of West Africa cannibalism was common in the past, but it was taboo to eat a member of the family or clan. The same prohibition applied to totem animals that were considered 'brothers.'[72] Among the Bantu, all animals killed by lightning are taboo, and women may not eat the meat of an animal that has aborted or died in calving lest she suffer the same fate.[73]

Old are also the taboos that govern sex relations. The prohibition against having intercourse with a menstruating or pregnant woman or one in childbed is extremely widespread. If a Mano infant cries much, this is due to the fact that the parents had intercourse while the mother was pregnant with him.[74] The idea that a man suffers not only for his own sins but also for those of his ancestors is not unknown in primitive society,[75] just as the concept of an 'uncleanness' that affects the fellow man in some way is also encountered. Zulus who have just had sexual intercourse, menstruating women, and mourners are not permitted to go close to a sick man or one wounded, because their presence would retard the process of healing.[76]

Taboos not only are old tribal prohibitions sanctified by tradition but may have been set by an individual for a special purpose. Thus in Melanesia the owner of fruit trees, coconut palms, of betel vines may wish to protect himself against theft of the fruit, and he, or whoever knows the rites, will impose a taboo on these trees 'in the name and under the sanction of the ghosts of the dead.'[77] Whoever steals fruit from the trees so protected does not commit a crime but a sin, a sacrilege, and is punished not by his fellow men but by the spirits that he has offended. He falls sick and can be cured only if the ghosts, after having been placated by a gift to the man who imposed the taboo and now intervenes for the sinner, are willing to remove the penalty.

All taboos are in the name and under the sanction of a fetish, spirit, ghost, or the deity, and it is he who punishes the violator. And sickness is the most frequent form of punishment.

It may very well happen that an individual breaks a taboo unintentionally. He may not even know that he committed such an offense. But he is sick and it is the medicine man's task to find out what has caused the disease. He will press the patient with questions, and if breach of taboo is the cause, confession is the first step toward recovery.

These are, briefly discussed and in a somewhat simplified way, the major elements of the primitive concept of disease. Some have a decidedly magical, others a definitely religious character, but it must be repeated once more that there are no sharp borderlines and that in the mind of primitive man, magic, religion, and medicine constitute an inseparable whole.

NOTES

1. W. H. R. Rivers, *Medicine, Magic, and Religion,* London, 1924, p. 40ff.
2. A. Winifred Hoernlé, 'Magic and Medicine,' *The Bantu-Speaking Tribes of South Africa,* edited by I. Schapera, London, 1937, p. 227.
3. George Way Harley, *Native African Medicine, with Special Reference to Its Practice in the Mano Tribe of Liberia,* Cambridge, Mass., 1941, p. 21.
4. E. E. Evans-Pritchard, *Witchcraft, Oracles and Magic among the Azande,* Oxford, 1937, p. 488.
5. Dorothy M. Spencer, 'Disease, Religion and Society in the Fiji Islands,' *Monographs of the American Ethnological Society,* New York, 1941, p. 20.
6. Morris Edward Opler, *An Apache Life-Way, the Economic, Social, and Religious Institutions of the Chiricahua Indians,* Chicago, 1941, p. 216.
7. Rivers, op. cit. p. 4.
8. See L. Lévy-Bruhl, *La Mentalité Primitive,* Paris, 1922.
9. Ibid. p. 35.
10. A. W. Nieuwenhuis, 'Die Anfänge der Medizin unter den niedrigst entwickelten Völkern und ihre psychologische Bedeutung,' *Janus,* 1924, 28:97.
11. Rivers, p. 4.
12. Forrest E. Clements, *Primitive Concepts of Disease,* University of California Publications in American Archaeology and Ethnology, 1932, 32 (2):185-252, an important publication, with 4 maps.
13. Max Bartels, *Die Medicin der Naturvölker, ethnologische Beiträge zur Urgeschichte der Medicin,* Leipzig, 1893, p. 21ff.
14. Rivers, p. 13.
15. R. H. Codrington, *The Melanesians,* London, 1891, p. 205.
16. Rivers, p. 14.
17. Pál Fejos, *Ethnography of the Yagua,* Viking Fund Publications in Anthropology, No. 1, New York, 1943, p. 92.
18. Dan McKenzie, *The Infancy of Medicine, an Enquiry into the Influence of Folk-lore upon the Evolution of Scientific Medicine,* London, 1927, p. 56; Bartels, loc. cit. p. 26.
19. Rivers, p. 13.
20. Job, 6:4.
21. Ilias, 1:43-53; *see also* H. E. Sigerist, 'Sebastian-Apollo,' *Arch. Gesch. Med.,* 1927, 19:301-17.
22. Clements, p. 188.

23. E. B. Tylor, *Early History of Mankind*, London, 1870, p. 281.
24. Clements, op. cit. p. 209ff.
25. Ibid. p. 212.
26. Ibid. p. 229f.; McKenzie, p. 63; Paul Radin, *Primitive Religion, Its Nature and Origin*, New York, 1937, p. 268ff. Many primitives believe in a plurality of souls.
27. Bartels, p. 37; Lévy-Bruhl, p. 151.
28. Rivers, p. 15.
29. Clements, p. 228.
30. Ibid. p. 234.
31. According to the Great Lakes Ojibway; Clements, p. 234.
32. Bartels, p. 38, after C. W. Pleyte, 'Zwei neue Gegenstände von den Hervey-Inseln,' *Zeitschr. f. Ethnol.*, 1887, 19:30.
33. Bartels, p. 38.
34. Clements, p. 234.
35. A. W. Nieuwenhuis, 'Die Ammassalik-Eskimo von Ost-Grönland,' *Janus*, 1925, 29:40.
36. Clements, p. 233.
37. J. P. Kleiweg de Zwaan, *Die Heilkunde der Niasser*, Haag, 1913, p. 48; McKenzie, p. 64; Bartels, p. 39.
38. Leo Kanner, 'Superstitions Connected with Sneezing,' *Medical Life*, 1931, 38:549-75.
39. James Mooney, '*The Swimmer Manuscript, Cherokee Sacred Formulas and Medicinal Prescriptions, Revised, Completed and Edited by Frans M. Olbrechts*,' Smithsonian Institution, Bureau of American Ethnology, Bulletin 99, Washington, 1932, p. 16.
40. Rivers, p. 66; Clements, p. 234.
41. Clements, p. 225ff., map 4, p. 227.
42. Sir James George Frazer, *The Magic Art and the Evolution of Kings*, London, 1917, vol. 1, p. 52ff.
43. Also called homoeopathic magic, a term which I prefer to avoid since in the history of medicine homoeopathy is a definite pharmacological theory.
44. These examples are from Bartels, p. 35, the following ones from Frazer, loc. cit. p. 59.
45. In South Africa I overcame it by bribing the natives with lollipops. They are so keen on sugar that there is nothing they would not do for it.
46. Rivers also points this out, p. 21.
47. See Rivers' lengthy example, p. 19ff.
48. The two examples from McKenzie, p. 55, the next from p. 50.
49. Frazer, vol. I, p. 175.
50. There is much literature on the evil eye. Some of the most important is: W. W. Story, *Castle of St. Angelo and the Evil Eye*, London, 1877; F. T. Elworthy, *The Evil Eye*, London, 1895; idem, article in James Hastings, *Encyclopædia of Religion and Ethics*, New York, 1912, 5:608-15; S. Seligman, *Die Zauberkraft des Auges und das Berufen*, Hamburg, 1922; A. Castiglioni, *Incantesimo e magia*, Milan, 1934 (*Adventures of the Mind*, New York, 1946).
51. See the very convincing psychological analysis of McKenzie, p. 256f.

52. Rivers, p. 66.
53. Ibid. p. 94.
54. *The Swimmer Manuscript*, loc. cit. p. 43ff.
55. Ibid. p. 21.
56. Ibid. p. 22.
57. Ibid. p. 23.
58. Bartels, p. 12; Clements, p. 188.
59. W. G. Sumner, A. G. Keller, and M. R. Davie, *The Science of Society*, New Haven and London, 1927, vol. 4, p. 785 (hereafter cited as Sumner).
60. F. J. Gillen, *Magic among the Natives of Central Australia*, see Sumner, 4:782.
61. Bartels, p. 12.
62. Clements, p. 188ff.; see also p. 219ff. and map 3, p. 217.
63. See Clements' map, p. 217.
64. Sumner, p. 785.
65. Ibid. p. 782.
66. Bartels, p. 12.
67. Lévy-Bruhl, p. 51ff.
68. Sumner, 2:863ff.
69. Bartels, p. 18.
70. Rivers, p. 73.
71. See Clements, pp. 187, 204-9, and map 1, p. 203.
72. Harley, p. 34.
73. Shapera, *The Bantu-Speaking Tribes of South Africa*, p. 133f.
74. Harley, p. 35.
75. Spencer, p. 28.
76. Shapera, op. cit. p. 108.
77. See Rivers' very graphic example from the island of Eddystone, one of the western islands of the British Solomons, pp. 32-7.

*

3. Prevention

As we have seen, primitive man feels surrounded by an infinity of hostile forces. The magic of his fellow men, the wrath of the spirits, and of the ghosts of the dead are a constant menace. Some primitive peoples are haunted by the idea of sickness and death, and a large part of their activities is devoted to warding off evil influences.[1]

How can an individual in the midst of so many dangers that threaten him hope to maintain his health and lead a normal and happy life?

We must remember that the logic of primitive man is different from ours. The fact that he is inclined to neglect secondary causes, that he does not readily admit that something may happen by accident, and the fact that he firmly believes in magic and in the omnipresence of spirits obviously lead him to different conclusions than we should reach. And yet he is perfectly logical within his own sphere, and we realize it as soon as we accept his premises. The medical field is an excellent example of this because all actions taken are the logical result of the concepts held of disease. This applies to the treatment as well as to the prevention of illness.

Thus in Polynesia and wherever we encounter the concept that disease is a sanction for the breaking of a taboo, the individual wherever he goes will be extremely cautious, looking out for taboo signs. If in Eddystone Island he sees next to a tree the sign of the *Kenjo*, several plants with four leaves or four shoots placed in a forked stick; or the sign of *Kirengge*, which in addition to the plants includes a stone, a coral, and a certain butterfly,[2] then he knows that these are taboo signs that protect the trees and their fruit, and he will be very careful not to touch them.

Since disease comes from the ghosts of the dead, innumerable methods of protection against them have been devised. The notion that the corpse is unclean, so strongly expressed in the Old Testament, the idea that some evil force comes from it, is very widespread, and it is not unusual that the dying or dead man is simply abandoned, that the hut is destroyed in which he died, or that he is carried outside the hut for the final agony.[3] We mentioned before that the purpose of many funeral rites was to make the mourners unrecognizable to the dead and to make it difficult for him to find his way back.

These negative measures, however, that merely tend to keep the dead away are not sufficient. The ghosts cannot be banished permanently; they are ever present and must be propitiated. Offerings of food, of betel or tobacco, whatever they liked while they were alive, are brought to them. Songs and dances are performed to please them and the more is done the more important the deceased man was, because the ghost of a chief or a medicine man can do infinitely greater harm than that of a poor man, of a slave, or of a woman.[4] The important dead will bring evil happenings, sickness, crop failures, wars, unless they be kept placated and satisfied. This may require that the individuals responsible for their death be found out and punished.[5]

The Bantu of Africa live in constant communion with their ancestral spirits. Whenever an animal is slaughtered or beer is brewed, a special offering is brought to them as a matter of routine; and they may expect special sacrifices when unusual events occur in the family, the birth, or initiation of a child, a marriage, the happy return of a warrior, or a death.[6] The cult of the ancestors is a strong, policing force in a tribe because they are close to their descendants, carefully watch their actions, meting out rewards and punishments; and if an individual wants to avoid sickness and other mishaps, he must abide by the many rules of conduct of his social group so as to win the support and avoid the wrath of the ancestral ghosts.

All this obviously also applies to other than the ancestral spirits, to the many forces that surround man and interfere in his life, for good or evil, but more often for evil. They too must be placated and propitiated if one wishes to avoid sickness.

Illness believed to be caused by magic must be prevented by counter-magic, and wherever the magic concept of disease prevails a great variety of protective measures have been devised and a great many objects with magic properties are found to be used for such a purpose. Here we must distinguish between fetish, amulet, and talisman, although the borderlines are by no means sharp and it is sometimes difficult to decide into which category a specimen falls. A *fetish* is an object that is the seat of magic power. It may be the abode of a spirit or may have been charged by the medicine man with the mystic power, mana, or manitou, or whatever it may have been called. It may be an object of worship, in the sense in which President de Brosses in the eighteenth century described fetishism as an early form of religion.[7] The owner of a fetish expects it to act according to his intentions. Among the Mano of

Liberia, 'if such a fetish seems slow in performing its duty the owner will take one grain of melegueta pepper, chew it up with a piece of white kola, spit it onto the fetish held in both hands, and say, "Are you really medicine? What can you do?" Then the fetish will be vexed and anxious to show what it can do. It will obey the owner's request.'[8] The fetish may be used for good or evil. Buried under the entrance of a hut it may cast an evil spell on whoever steps over it, or it may protect against magic. The African fetish often has the form of a man or animal, while with the American Indians the chief form of fetish is represented by the medicine bundle, a sacred bundle that contains various objects collected by a youth under divine inspiration and guidance.[9]

Harley gives a graphic description of the various methods used by the Mano as preventives against witchcraft.[10] Two vines twisted together constituted a barrier that no enemy could cross. The blacksmith dedicating a new shop consecrated his iron tools by sacrificing a chicken and performing magic rites intended to prevent individuals, men and women, endowed with *wi*[11] or witchcraft from entering the shop. Blood was rubbed on the irons. All iron was supposed to have magic properties since it was made in sacred fire.

The Mano also had secret societies, the purpose of which was to protect the members against witchcraft. Thus the members of the Yufa Society received a kind of fetish in a leather pouch supposed 'to have power to change itself into a man and catch a witch by beating him in the night while on a journey,'[12] and the members of the Sukba Society combined witch smelling with fire jumping and had a powerful fetish, a horn of medicine.

Amulets are also objects that possess magic properties but their action is directed to one purpose, namely, to ward off evil, to catch and neutralize black or evil magic directed toward the owner of the amulet. Thus amulets are one of the chief means of preventive medicine where the concept is held that disease is the result of witchcraft. The use of amulets is by no means limited to primitive society; we find it everywhere at all times, and even today in our 'enlightened' Western societies there is hardly an individual who does not consciously or unconsciously wear some kind of amulet. In times of stress and strain, of war and epidemics when life is particularly endangered, the tendency to have recourse to magical means of protection is very prominent even today.

There is an infinite variety of amulets. Every object after all may assume apotropaic, or warding-off, qualities if it has been 'consecrated' by somebody who has the power to do it. We may, however, distinguish between certain groups of amulets.[13] One consists of sharp and cutting objects, teeth of animals, claws of eagle or bear, small knives, all objects that have the faculty to cause wounds. It seems as if they emanated this quality and thus were able to meet and destroy the evil magic. Another extremely widespread group of amulets is represented by reproductions of the genitalia, male and female, phallus and cowrie shell. It is probably their life-bearing property that gives them their protective power. In Mediterranean countries, the most popular gesture to ward off the influence of the evil eye is the *fica,* whereby the thumb is pushed through index and middle finger, an obscene gesture that has been practiced for several thousand years. Hand and comb, the instruments used to remove vermin, are frequently found as amulets. Others are reproductions of foot, leg, heart, or eye of animals, snake, and scarab. The diamond and other precious stones are powerful amulets. Their glittering attracts the evil eye, holds it, and neutralizes its effect. All jewelry had magic significance once; it is ornament today but in its style it still frequently reflects its origins. We shall see in the next volume of this book that antiquity produced a considerable literature on the magic virtues of stones. There is hardly anything under the sun that could not under proper conditions assume the qualities of an amulet, whether it be feathers of a buzzard or the scent bag of a skunk that the Cherokees use for such a purpose.[14] More complex amulets that combine objects and the magic power of the written word are found frequently in Egypt and other higher civilizations.

Not only man is threatened by sorcery but also man's most treasured possession, his domestic animals. If the horse suddenly limps, the camel dies without apparent reason, the cow succumbs to the pains of labor, or the goat gets lost in the mountains, the most logical explanation is that an evil spell has been cast on it or that it has been the victim of spirits. Animals too are affected by the evil eye. They too, therefore, require protection against magic. The clear-sounding bells of the goats and the bass of the large cowbells so characteristic of the Alps serve not only to locate an animal gone astray but are, first of all, intended to drive evil spirits away. Horses, mules, and donkeys, particularly in Mediterranean regions, are covered with amulets, shining brass discs, half-moons, and stars.

Like the amulet, the *talisman* is also an object that possesses magic properties, but it acts in a different way. While the amulet wards off evil magic, the talisman brings good luck. The clover with four leaves and the horseshoe are examples of talismans still popular today. An animated talisman, a person or animal that brings good luck, is a *mascot.*

So far we have discussed religious and magical means of preventing sickness. Their choice was determined by the prevailing concept of disease. We know, however, that certain conditions that we consider pathological, the minor ailments of everyday life, are taken for granted by the primitives, are accepted without explanation, and treated with domestic remedies. Similarly we find that primitives practice a certain hygiene that is perfectly rational in our sense of the word and that they do not in any way connect with medicine.

African natives are on the whole very clean. Among the Mano of Liberia the men have a hot bath every day at sunset and the women go to the river where they wash their skin and the clothing of the family.[15] Whoever has traveled in Africa has seen natives cleaning their teeth endlessly with a stick used as a toothbrush. Hygiene and cosmetics frequently overlap. Another very common sight is that of a woman delousing the children's hair, or that of her husband. Huts are usually clean and tidy. In South Africa it is striking to see how clean and well kept the huts in native locations are, while housing developments for the mixed or so-called Cape colored population are run down in no time.

Primitives know how to prepare their food. In many places they learned to bake bread from a great variety of cereals. Some dishes of the American Indians are delicious, such as a fish wrapped in fragrant wet seaweed and cooked in hot ashes. In all colonies the conquerors took over from the natives foods and dishes, which from the colonies often reached the homeland. Sometimes their cultivation became almost universal, as was the case with the potato, the tomato, and maize that came from America. Plants that are now favorite fruits and vegetables in America, such as alligator pear, kidney and lima bean, squash, sweet potato, oca, peanut, pineapple, and others in addition to those mentioned before, were cultivated by the Indians prior to the discovery of the New World.[16]

Primitives also knew how to preserve food. In the North, meat and fish could be kept frozen. In other climates they were dried. The Indian pemmican is a well-known example of a preserved food. The dried meat of buffalo, or in other regions of deer and moose, were pounded with stone hammers, packed tightly in bags, and sealed off with melted fat. There was another variety, with vitamins added in the form of ground wild cherries, the berry pemmican. This provided a compact food of high nutritional value that could be carried on expeditions.[17]

Under the most different climates primitives devised a balanced diet.[18] If they had not, they would soon have died out. The great deal of malnutrition among them today is the result of prevailing social and economic conditions, the consequence of colonial exploitation. As long as the Bantu were in possession of their homeland, they had a balanced diet consisting chiefly of milk, mealy meal (ground African corn), and indigenous herbs. Once the white man took their land away and they were reduced to living on small overstocked farms, the cows had not enough milk, the land produced not enough corn, and the people in contact with the white man forgot the use of herbs. A similar process took place in many colonies.

Primitives often use certain preventive and protective measures just as they use house remedies without thinking of medicine. Thus according to Harley,[19] the Mano smear red palm oil and the leaf of a plant, *Alchornea cordifolia,* on feet and ankles to prevent ground itch or hookworm. Another plant is taken to prevent diarrhea after having eaten new rice. When a child is weaned and is given the first solid food, leaves of certain plants are added. The mother in doing this has no particular thoughts about it. She does so because it is commonly done and because mothers know that if it were not done the child might vomit.

Here as in all other aspects of primitive medicine we cannot separate religious, magical, and empirico-rational elements. If a primitive does not urinate or throw rubbish into the river from which he takes his drinking water, this looks to us like a very rational hygienic measure, yet we know that he abstains from such an action so as not to offend the spirit of the river. And if he buries his feces, he does it not for hygienic reasons but because he is afraid of contagious magic.

Sickness that strikes the individual is bad enough, but worse are epidemics that visit and decimate entire tribes. The severity of the menace drives people, civilized or primitive, to act, and for thousands of years, until the scientific era, the main reactions to epidemics have been much the same. The first impulse is to flee from the infested locality. The Kubu who live in the forests of South Sumatra, one of the most primitive tribes in existence, know of no other reaction than flight.[20] When smallpox or some other epidemic reaches them, they move on, deeper into the forest, and simply abandon their sick, who thus are dead socially before physical death has overcome them. Nomad or semi-nomad tribes obviously find it easier than sedentary tribes to flee before an epidemic. The Navahos do not hesitate to abandon their hogans, while the Hopis remain in their pueblos and die in large numbers.[21]

It was probably easier for primitive and early civilizations to develop a clear concept of the contagiousness of disease than it was for later civilizations, for the good reason that among primitives and in early antiquity we usually find an outspoken magico-religious concept of contagion. If soul substance was contained in every object that an individual touched, he could be hit by magic through any such object, as we discussed before. On the other hand, if evil was in an individual it could be spread not only through direct contact but also through the objects that he had touched. Not only the dead were dangerous, but their clothing and other possessions were too, and the same was true of the sick, or of certain sick people at least.[22]

Flight is one protective measure, but it does not always help. An epidemic may travel as fast as human beings do. Another method of prevention, therefore, is directed against the cause, and for thousands of years, and today still among primitives, epidemics were attributed to the wrath of the deities. Since such a disease is a collective one, the measures of appeasement had to be collective also.

With the Cherokee, as soon as there were rumors of an epidemic breaking loose—when it was known that a nearby settlement was affected or when there was a case of illness which was pronounced by the old people, who had witnessed previous epidemics, to be a case of the disease in question—one of the most reputed medicine men announced his intention to hold a medicine dance to safeguard the people against the coming evil. The whole community turned out at the scheduled time; the medicine dance was danced, the medicine 'against all diseases' was prepared by the medicine men and drunk by the people.[23]

Similarly, the Apache tried to stave off epidemics by performing the masked-dancer rite. 'When I hear of disease coming,' a Mount Spirit medicine man said, 'I paint them and tell them to chase the disease away with the sticks.'[24] 'When sickness is around, the masked dancers and the clown are made on a hill and then come to the people below, making fires on the way down. In this way they keep sickness away.'[25]

The epidemic of influenza of 1918-19 was an event against which primitives mobilized all their resources[26] with as little result as we had with scientific medicine.

Of all epidemic diseases, one of the most dreaded was undoubtedly smallpox. We know little about its early history,[27] but it seems that it might have originated in Africa, from where it spread to Asia and Europe. At any rate it was unknown in America before the Conquest, and when the Spaniards brought the disease the Indians were almost wiped out.[28] The same happened whenever European colonists came in contact with a population that had never experienced smallpox.

It is interesting to find that primitives possessed a method that protects effectively against this disease, the preventive inoculation of smallpox, the precursor of Jenner's vaccination.[29] It obviously is impossible to tell where exactly and at what time it was discovered, whether the discovery was made once and spread through diffusion, or whether it was made repeatedly in various parts of the globe. The knowledge that no individual ever suffered from the disease twice must have been universal, and a pock-marked face was a visible sign of immunity. Still, from such observation to the actual inoculation of the disease there was a long way to go.[30]

Whatever the origin of variolation may have been, there can be no doubt that it was practiced in the seventeenth century in Africa and Asia and that there was a beginning of it in European folk-medicine. As early as 1716 Cotton Mather, a preacher in Boston, wrote that he had heard from one of his Negro slaves that the inoculation of smallpox was often practiced in Africa.[31] It is still practiced today by the Ashanti and Mano on the West coast, the Somali in the East, and numerous central African tribes.[32] It was practiced so successfully in North Africa that a French army physician recommended its use whenever vaccine was not available.[33]

As far as Asia is concerned, our starting point is the fact that inoculation was known in Constantinople in the early eighteenth century, where it was practiced by Greeks from Thessaly. A Greek physician in Constantinople, Emmanuel Timoni, was the first to draw attention to the subject.[34] Whence did the knowledge of inoculation come to Turkey and Greece if not from Asia? And, indeed, as soon as Western physicians were familiar with variolation, they found it practiced in wide sections of Asia, throughout the Russian empire, in India and China.[35]

Methods varied. In Africa a light incision was made, to which serum from the pustule of a patient was applied. In Central Asia scabs were ground with water, were kept for about a week, and the virus thus attenuated was then inoculated with pins. In China, pulverized scabs were blown into the nose, and in Central Europe in the seventeenth century, 'Pockenkaufen,' the purchase of pocks, was a folk-medical custom. Children were sent to the smallpox hospital where for a few pennies they bought scabs with which they were made sick.[36]

Methods varied but the basic idea was the same. It was to make individuals, particularly children, immune against a much dreaded disease by inoculating them with the virus of this very disease, but in such a way that they would have it only in a mild form. It is a bold idea, comparable only to the immunization against snake venom as practiced by African tribes.[37]

NOTES

1. See E. H. Ackerknecht, 'Primitive Medicine,' *Transact. New York Acad. Science,* 1945, II, 8:26-37.
2. Rivers, *Medicine, Magic, and Religion,* London, 1924, p. 33.
3. Numerous examples in Sumner, *The Science of Society,* New Haven and London, 1927, 2:851.
4. Lévy-Bruhl, *La Mentalité primitive,* Paris, 1922, p. 64.
5. Ibid. p. 65.
6. Schapera, *The Bantu-Speaking Tribes of South Africa,* London, 1937, p. 254f.
7. C. de Brosses, *Du Culte des dieux fétiches ou parallèle de l'ancienne religion de l'Egypte avec la religion actuelle de Nigritie,* Paris, 1760. About fetishism see E. B. Tylor, *Primitive Culture,* London, 1920, p. 145ff. Sumner 2: 979ff.; W. Born, 'Fetish, Amulet and Talisman,' *Ciba Symposia,* 1945, 7:102-32.
8. Harley, *Native African Medicine* . . . Cambridge, Mass., 1941.
9. Born, loc. cit. p. 106ff.; M. R. Harrington, *Sacred Bundles of the Sac and Fox Indians,* Philadelphia, 1914.
10. Harley, pp. 172-6.
11. According to Harley (p. 23), '"Wi" may be defined as a special kind of *mana* which a person may have without knowing it, and which gives him power over others to cause sickness and death, though the term is used also in a general sense to indicate any kind of witch substance.'
12. Ibid. p. 174.
13. About amulets see Elizabeth Villiers, *Amulette und Talismane und andere geheime Dinge,* bearbeitet und erweitert von A. M. Pachinger, Munich, 1927; S. Seligmann, *Die magischen Heil- und Schutzmittel aus der unbelebten Natur, mit besonderer Berücksichtigung der Mittel gegen den bösen Blick,* Stuttgart, 1927; M. Kronfeld, *Zauberpflanzen und Amulette,* Wien, 1898.
14. James Mooney, *The Swimmer Manuscript* . . . Smithsonian Inst., Bur. Amer. Ethnol., Bull. 99, Washington, 1932, p. 76.
15. Harley, p. 74.
16. A list of such plants is given in Clark Wissler, *The American Indian,* New York and London, 2nd ed., 1922, p. 15; see also G. F. Carter, 'Origins of American Indian Agriculture,' *Am. Anthrop.,* 1946, 48:1-21.
17. Wissler, p. 7.
18. Carl Seyffert, 'Einige Beobachtungen und Bemerkungen über die Ernährung der Naturvölker,' *Zschr. Ethnol.,* 1931, 63:53-85; also C. B. Davenport, 'The Dietaries of Primitive Peoples,' *Am. Anthrop.,* 1945, 47:60-82.

19. Harley, p. 73f.
20. On account of their extremely primitive status the Kubu have been studied carefully by Dutch and German ethnologists. See G. J. van Dongen, 'De Koeboes der Ridanrivier,' *Tijdschr. voor het Binnenlandsch Bestuur,* 1906, vol. 30; B. Hagen, *Die Orang Kubu auf Sumatra,* Frankfurt a. M., 1908; W. Volz, *Im Dämmer des Rimba,* Breslau, 1921; A. W. Nieuwenhuis, *Janus,* 1924, 28:42-60.
21. Dane Coolidge and Mary Roberts Coolidge, *The Navajo Indians,* Boston, 1930, p. 15.
22. See our discussion of sympathetic magic in the preceding chapter.
23. *The Swimmer Manuscript,* p. 75.
24. M. E. Opler, *An Apache Life-Way,* Chicago, 1941, p. 276.
25. Ibid. p. 276.
26. Ibid. p. 277f., where a graphic description is given of how influenza came to the Chiricahua Indians and how they reacted against it. Among other precautions they were exhorted 'not to say anything bad about this sickness. Don't mention it, or it will come back.' At that time the masked-dancer rites were also performed to keep away sleeping sickness.
27. P. Kübler, *Geschichte der Pocken und der Impfung,* Berlin, 1901.
28. G. Sticker, 'Krankheiten in Mittelamerika zur Zeit des Columbus,' *Janus,* 1924, 28:232-301.
29. Non-medical writers are inclined to confuse vaccination and variolation. *Vaccination,* as the name indicates, is the inoculation of cowpox, a disease of cows, which, however, is transmissible to humans and protects them against smallpox. In *variolation,* on the other hand, the virus of the human disease smallpox is inoculated directly, usually after having undergone manipulations that attenuate it.
30. About the history of the inoculation of smallpox or variolation, see A. C. Klebs, 'The Historical Evolution of Variolation,' *Johns Hopkins Hosp. Bull.,* 1913, 24:69-83, of which reprints were issued with a bibliography of 600 items; also, A. C. Klebs, *Die Variolation im achtzehnten Jahrhundert. Ein historischer Beitrag zur Immunitätsforschung,* Giessen, 1914. I strongly feel that a re-examination of the sources on Africa and Asia is needed, and further research may well produce new evidence.
31. G. L. Kittredge, 'Some Lost Works of Cotton Mather,' *Proc. Mass. Hist. Soc.,* 1912, 45:418-79. The crucial passage (p. 422) reads: 'Many months before I mett with any Intimations of treating ye *Small-Pox,* with ye Method of Inoculation, any where in *Europe;* I had from a Servant of my own, an Account of its being practised in *Africa.* Enquiring of my Negro-man *Onesimus,* who is a pretty Intelligent Fellow, Whether he ever had ye *Small-Pox;* he answered, both, *Yes* and, *No;* and then told me, that he had undergone an Operation, which had given him something of ye *Small-Pox,* and would forever praeserve him from it; adding, That it was often used among ye *Guramantese,* and whoever had ye Courage to use it, was forever free from ye fear of the Contagion. He described ye Operation to me, and shew'd me in his Arm ye Scar, which it had left upon him; and his Description of it, made it the same, that afterwards I found related unto you by your *Timonius.*'

32. H. Gros, 'La Variolisation,' *Janus*, 1902, 7:169-74.
33. Ibid. p. 174.
34. In a letter presented to the Royal Society by John Woodward with the title: 'An Account, or History, of the Procuring the Small-Pox by Incision, or Inoculation; as it has for some time been practised at Constantinople. Being the Extract of a Letter from Emanuel Timonius . . . dated . . . December 1713,' *Phil. Trans.*, 1714, No. 339, art. v.
35. The literature is listed in the two publications of Klebs, whose important collection of books on variolation is now in the Historical Library of the Yale University Medical Library.
36. I think it would be worth while to examine the possibility of variolation having been an Arabic invention, which had been spread to the East and West with the Arabic conquest and was practiced particularly in the slave trade.
37. E.g. Harley, p. 213ff.

*

4. The Sick Man

An individual's vigilance has broken down. He has transgressed a taboo, offended a spirit, or fallen a victim to a fellow man's magic. He may have committed a sin quite unintentionally, just as we may happen to drive through a red traffic light. Or he may have insulted a ghost or a neighbor in a dream, an offense for which he must accept responsibility. Constant watchfulness and skill are required to steer a safe course through the reefs of everyday life, to comply with the many religious and social rules, to avoid breaking prohibitions, and to be prepared to ward off magic by counter-magic.

But even the most careful individual will stumble at times or will become the innocent victim of evil powers. As a result, calamities of various kinds will visit him. His cattle may die, his boat may be wrecked, his hut with all his property may burn down, or he himself may have an accident or may become sick.

What happens in primitive societies when an individual has fallen ill? Nothing, as a rule, in the case of minor ailments. They are not considered diseases and do not give the sick man a special position in society. They are treated with domestic remedies and disappear, as they came, without requiring an explanation and without preventing the patient from sharing in the life of the group.

Things are different in the case of a serious illness, when pneumonia, smallpox, typhoid fever, or any such disease has taken hold of a man, or when he has suffered an accident, has broken a leg, or had his skull cracked. Such an occurrence invariably and, I may add, in all civilizations gives the sick man a special position in society, one which is determined primarily by two factors, the physical condition in which the patient finds himself and the attitude of a given society toward the phenomenon, disease—its valuation of health and disease.

This sick man is weak and helpless, like a child or an old man. He cannot move, cannot attend to his accustomed occupations, cannot fulfil what is normally expected of him. The rhythm of his life is different from that of those in good health. Disease isolates, always and everywhere. Being helpless, the sick, like the aged, are dependent on others, and because the physical condition of the two groups is very similar we often find that the attitude toward them is the same.[1]

The sick, the crippled, and the aged are a burden on society because they are unable to contribute their share of labor to the common welfare. Two basic attitudes toward them are observed among primitive peoples. Some accept the burden, treat them kindly, feed them, attend to them, honor the aged, and are prepared to bring any sacrifice to have the sick treated by the medicine man and if possible cured. Others, however, get rid of the handicapped, kill them, and sometimes eat them. This would appear to be a simple classification, and it looks as though we had two groups of peoples, the one savage and the other more civilized. Actually conditions are much more complicated, as we shall see in a moment.

The view that man was savage first, then became civilized, and that good treatment of the sick and aged is a criterion of higher civilization is contradicted by the facts, so far as primitive societies are concerned. Indeed, we find quite generally that food-gathering, fishing and hunting, communities are inclined to treat their handicapped members well. Where life is hard and the food supply uncertain, the sharing of food becomes a necessity. The Australians of New South Wales take care of the sick and aged for a long time. Among the tribes of Central Australia it happens that a sick old man is given blood of a young man to drink. In New Britain, in Melanesia, when the parents of a married woman are sick, the young couple leaves its hut, moves to the parents-in-law, and attends them as long as is needed. The Kurnai, of Victoria, carry the sick and infirm when the tribe moves.[2]

Even among such peoples, however, the sick and infirm may be sacrificed in special circumstances: when the food or water gives out, when the tribe is starting out on a long migration, or in case of epidemics when the fear of the sick is such that he may be abandoned, as we found with the Kubu.

Such an attitude, however, is different from the habitual destruction of the sick and weak that is encountered sometimes, particularly among agricultural and pastoral tribes where the social organization and property relations are more complex and the sharing of food is not obvious. But conditions are complicated here too, because the motivations vary a great deal. Economy is undoubtedly the chief cause for the elimination of the sick and infirm. They are socially useless and there is no point in preserving them. In New Caledonia the hopelessly sick are left to themselves or killed with a blow on the head.[3] Among the Záparos of Ecuador a family council is convened and, if it comes to the conclusion that the sick man is a useless member of the group and a burden to the family, he is strangled to death.[4] Before the sick lose too much flesh, the cannibal Bobos of the Western Sudan kill them and eat them. Tautain reports the experience of a man who, while he went on a business trip, left his wife with a Bobo friend. When he returned, he found his wife gone and was handed over 60,000 cowries instead. The friend explained that as the woman had suddenly fallen ill and had been losing weight rapidly, in order to protect the husband's interests, he had killed her in time and had sold her on the market.[5] Many tribes differentiate between young and old, and between rich and poor. While an old patient may be killed without much ado, the sick young man will be spared because his chances of recovery are better. Similarly, a patient of high rank may be treated with greatest care in a group that does not hesitate to kill the sick poor.[6]

Another motive for the destruction of the sick is fear, fear of evil spirits and evil magic, and fear of contagion. An individual who is possessed by a spirit is considered dangerous by some because the spirit may escape and enter another's body. This is why mental patients are buried alive, or killed in some other way on various islands of the Fiji and New Hebrides and also in parts of Africa. By burying the sick, the spirit is destroyed with him. This attitude contrasts with that of some American Indian tribes who treat the insane well, looking upon them with reverence as the carriers of transcendental forces.[7] Not only witches are dangerous but in some cases also the victims of witchcraft. If among the Bangala of the Belgian Congo an individual becomes very lean and has a strange gleam in his eyes, he is put to death to destroy the magic in him.[8] Danger threatens from the dead, and it may therefore be wise to carry the dying man far away from the habitations and bury him alive.

The fear of epidemic diseases and the fact that their contagiousness was well known to many primitive peoples have been mentioned before, and we saw that the chief and most elementary reaction was flight. Some peoples were more aggressive. They did not abandon the sick but killed them in an attempt to destroy the disease with them. Thus the Indians of the Gran Chaco, when an epidemic broke out, set fire to the patients' huts and together with the hut burned the sick and the disease. Similarly the Indians of Ecuador buried alive or, at any rate, killed the first individuals who showed symptoms of a contagious disease.[9]

The sick and crippled and the aged are killed in some tribes as a result of totally different motives, namely respect and compassion, strange as this may seem.[10] The killing becomes what we should call a mercy killing. The sick and infirm are relieved of suffering and misery. They often ask it as a favor. On the Island of Vao, in Melanesia, infirms and invalids entreat their relatives to kill them. The families do it reluctantly, prepare a last meal, and then follow the invalid's desire and strangle or bury him.[11] Even the eating of a family member who has thus been killed may be considered a sign of filial respect. He is absorbed by the family, body and soul. This is an act of cannibalism that has a definite magic religious meaning and is not due to gluttony.[12]

It also happens not infrequently that the sick and infirm commit suicide. This has been reported of a number of tribes, Polynesians, Siberian tribes, Eskimos, some African and other peoples.[13]

The attitude toward the handicapped may vary within one and the same tribe according to the nature of the handicap. Thus the Bayaka in the Congo respect the blind but deride the deaf.

The sick man in primitive society is the victim of transcendental forces, the innocent victim sometimes, but more often he suffers because he or a member of his family has committed an offense. Disease thus is a social sanction, and in many tribes it is the most important social sanction they know. Where such a view prevails, disease plays an extremely important part in society, and the task of medicine is very much broader than the one it has to face with us. Ackerknecht justly pointed out that the primitive healers, in addition to their medical functions, had to assume parts played in civilized societies by judges, priests, soldiers, and policemen.[14]

Patients at all times had, and still have, a strong desire to understand the meaning of their being sick. Why do I suffer? Why am I sick? Why am I plagued with a gastric ulcer that poisons the joy of eating? Why have I developed a cancer that will kill me? What have I done to deserve such a fate? These are questions the physician today may hear all the time and if he answers by pointing out the importance of heredity, human constitution, environment, working conditions, mode of living, and similar factors, he will hardly satisfy his patient's curiosity and need for causality. Why should I be sick while my neighbor who lives exactly as I do is enjoying the best of health? The moral interpretation of disease, its integration into the pattern of an individual's life, seems to satisfy a primitive atavistic need that is still alive in our societies. In the case of venereal diseases the interpretation seems obvious. An individual is sick as a punishment for having sinned, for having committed an offense against the code of bourgeois morality. And it seems the more meaningful because he is stricken in the organ with which he has sinned. As modern physicians, we fight such an attitude and brand it a primitive survival. We refuse to accept disease as a social sanction because we are determined to wipe out disease and because we think that a modern society has other sanctions available.

Conditions are different in primitive societies where disease is well understood as the logical consequence of the patient's—or his family's—behavior. The fact, however, that disease is a sanction and makes an individual's guilt apparent to all gives the patient a special position in society, one that is burdened with a certain odium. The patient, moreover, is a man who on account of his condition is in more intimate contact with the world of the spirits than other people. His soul may have been abducted and on its wanderings has intercourse with the spirits, is lured by them or fights with them. Or the patient is possessed by a demon who now resides in him and talks through his mouth. All this accentuates the special position that the sick man holds in society, makes him an object of awe, a *res sacra.*

In a number of tribes, and particularly among American Indians, it is believed that a man who was seriously sick and recovered will never again be the same as he was before his illness. The fact that he was in close touch with the transcendental world gives him a special position once and for all, and the fact that he was attacked by evil forces but did not succumb to them shows that he has some power over them. As a result, former patients would enroll in medicine societies. The members were not necessarily medicine men, not full-fledged healers, but rather assistants to such. Some societies were specialized for the treatment of one ailment or one group of diseases. Thus among the Seneca, one of the Iroquois tribes, the 'Little Water Company' possessed a remedy that cured wounds. The members of the Society met four times a year in secret convention and performed rites intended to preserve the power of their medicine.[15] In this, as in the case of other societies, a legend related the origin of the company, which in the words of Corlett ran as follows: [16]

Once upon a time there was a fine young chief who not only was popular with his people, but was also a great hunter who always observed the necessary proprieties when killing animals. For this reason, when the young chief was sorely wounded and left for dead on the field of battle, his friends the animals (for they are the great medicine people) gathered around him. After a council they agreed that a wonderful medicine should be made to cure their friend. All of the good animals helped in one way or another to brew this potion, some even giving up their lives that their friend might live. As the young chief regained consciousness he not only recognized his friends but also understood the charm song which the animals were singing, and this song they taught him as well as the dance that went with it. But the young chief could not be told the various ingredients of the medicine, for he was married, and the secret could be given only to a virgin youth. Some time after this, when the chief had returned to his people, an occasion for another war party arose. Before the conflict, the group heard a mysterious voice singing and the chief recognized this as the medicine song of the animals who had saved him. So he sent a number of youths to find the singer and learn the secret of the medicine. They located the mysterious voice as coming from a magic corn stalk whose roots spread in the four directions. After a ceremony the youths were given the composition of the medicine and taught the song which makes the medicine strong and preserves it. This medicine was used after the raid was over, and was found to cure all wounds.

Medicine societies are particularly popular among the Pueblo Indians, the Hopi, the Zuñi, and the Acoma. The latter have four large societies, the Fire, the Flint, the Thundercloud, and the Kabina.[17] Most of the members are patients who have been cured through the services of one of the societies. We shall say more about them when we discuss the treatment of disease, but we should mention here that Pueblo Indians also have societies for other than medicinal purposes. Thus the Hopi are well known for their snake dance, a rite intended to purify the village and to bring rain for the crops. It is performed by a society that is supposed to possess a remedy that makes its members immune from the bite of the rattlesnake.

Basically different from these American medicine societies are the numerous secret societies of Africa. They are primarily associations for the practice of black magic and have, therefore, been outlawed by most colonial powers.[18] They are not associations of former patients and are open to men and sometimes women who apply for initiation. The closest parallel to a certain type of American society is probably an association such as the *Bo Kona,* a Mano Society for the treatment of snakebite.[19]

Although the sick man, as we saw, is sometimes abandoned and killed, there can be no doubt that he is given much attention and is treated kindly among a great many primitive peoples. Cheyenne women are willing to sacrifice a finger for the recovery of a sick family member,[20] and mutual aid is a generally accepted duty among the Cherokees. If the head of a family is sick at the time of plowing, sowing, or harvesting, or the family is in need of firewood, the members of the community help out spontaneously and cheerfully perform the sick man's work without compensation, just as they help to rebuild a tribesman's hut if it has been destroyed by fire.[21]

NOTES

1. The two chief studies on the subject are: John Koty, 'Die Behandlung der Alten und Kranken bei den Naturvölkern,' *Forschungen zur Völkerpsychologie und Soziologie,* vol. XIII, Stuttgart, 1934; Leo W. Simmons, *The Role of the Aged in Primitive Society,* New Haven, 1945. See also Lévy-Bruhl, *La Mentalité primitive,* Paris, 1922, pp. 332ff.
2. These examples from Koty, pp. 21-5.
3. The literature on New Caledonia is in Koty, p. 37.
4. A. Simson, 'Notes on the Záparos,' *J. Anthrop. Inst. Great Brit. Ireland,* 1878, 7:507.
5. Dr. Tautain, 'Quelques Renseignements sur les Bobo,' *Rev. Ethnol.,* 1887, 6:230-31.
6. Examples in Koty, p. 345.
7. Ibid. pp. 36, 38, 345f.
8. Ibid. p. 337, from A. Chapaux, *Congo,* Bruxelles, 1894, p. 536.
9. The literature in Koty, p. 289.
10. Ibid. p. 314ff.
11. F. Speiser, *Südsee, Urwald, Kannibalen,* Leipzig, 1913, p. 71.
12. J. Hastings, *Encyclopædia of Religion and Ethics,* New York, 1913, 3:200.
13. About suicide of the aged see Simmons, loc. cit. pp. 229-30; J. Wisse, *Selbstmord und Todesfurcht bei den Naturvölkern,* Zutphen, 1933.
14. E. H. Ackerknecht, 'Primitive Medicine,' *Trans. New York Acad. Sci.,* 1945, II, 8:26-37.
15. A. C. Parker, 'Secret Medicine Societies of the Seneca,' *Amer. Anthropol.,* 1909, N.S. 11:161-85.
16. W. T. Corlett, *The Medicine-Man of the American Indian and His Cultural*

Background, Springfield and Baltimore, 1935, p. 137f. By permission of Charles C Thomas.

17. Ibid. p. 151ff. *Kabina* is a term for which there is no equivalent in English.
18. K. J. Beatly, *Human Leopards,* London, 1915; Harley, *Native African Medicine* . . . Cambridge, Mass., 1941, p. 139ff.; Evans Pritchard, *Witchcraft, Oracles and Magic among the Azande,* Oxford, 1937, p. 511ff.
19. Harley, p. 105ff.
20. E. H. Ackerknecht, 'Primitive Medicine and Culture Pattern,' *Bull. Hist. Med.,* 1942, 12:555.
21. J. Mooney, *The Swimmer Manuscript* . . . Smithsonian Inst., Bur. Am. Ethnol., Bull. 99, Washington, 1932, p. 80f.

*

5. The Medicine Man

The medicine man holds in primitive society an infinitely more important position than the physician does in a modern community. The medicine man is concerned not only with the people's health but with their entire welfare, ranging from crops to victory in war. It is his function to avert evil that may threaten the individual or tribe in any form, to propitiate the spirits for the benefit of his people, and also to destroy the enemy. He is, therefore, priest, sorcerer, and physician in one. He is, moreover, very often the chief of the tribe, the king who rules over the people. And in addition he frequently is the bard of the group, who knows the stories and songs that tell of the origin of the world and of the deeds of the tribe and its heroes in a far remote age. He thus fulfils another function, one that is very important in a scriptless society.

It is an insult to the medicine man to call him the ancestor of the modern physician. He is that, to be sure, but he is much more, namely the ancestor of most of our professions. We connect him with healing first of all, partly because healing actually is one of his main tasks and also on account of the name 'medicine man,' which is not a good term. Indeed since civilized societies do not have any corresponding universal profession, we have no term available to designate this complex personage, at least not one that could be applied with good reason to all primitive peoples.

When we speak of 'medicine man' we use a term derived from American Indian languages but one that is very misleading because the concept that is translated by 'medicine,' for lack of a better word, is infinitely broader, one that embraces the totality of the transcendental forces. Many ethnologists, therefore, prefer to use the term *shaman.* We shall see later, however, that the Siberian shaman is a medicine man of a very special kind, and hence it is not appropriate to use this term in connection with Australian or American Indian tribes.

Since the English language is rich in terms that designate healers, English and American anthropologists have suggested using such words as seer or leech. Thus Loeb wishes to distinguish between shaman and seer. By shaman he means the inspirational type of medicine man who is voluntarily possessed, through whom the spirit speaks, who exorcises and prophesies. The prototype is the Siberian shaman, of course, but a similar type is found among some other Asiatic tribes, in Africa and Melanesia, on the Fiji Islands and in Polynesia. By seer, on the other hand, he means the non-inspirational type of medicine man who is not possessed but has a guardian spirit that speaks *to* him not *through* him, who does not exorcise and is not a prophet, the medicine man of the American Indians, of Australia, New Guinea, the Negritos.[1]

Rivers frequently uses the term leech. 'When I speak of a leech,' he says,[2] 'I shall mean a member of society whose special function it is to deal with the cure of disease. He may have other functions, such as the formation of rain, the promotion of vegetation, or even the production of disease itself; but in so far as he is dealing with the cure of disease he will be in the nomenclature I shall use, a leech.'

The difficulty with these terms is that they have a strong western medieval flavor, which seems strangely out of place when they are applied to exotic tribes. Leech, moreover, is much too narrow and seer seems a particularly unfortunate designation for the non-inspirational, non-prophetic type, since the word means a prophet, a person who sees visions, one of preternatural insight, especially as regards the future.[3] I prefer, therefore, the use of the traditional term medicine man in its generally accepted broad sense. It is obvious, however, that the medicine men are not the same everywhere. They have something in common, to be sure, because they are members of primitive societies, but otherwise they differ in many respects and the best we can do is to describe the medicine man of certain sample tribes.

We cannot expect to find medicine men in very primitive groups, such as the Kubu of Sumatra whose chief reaction to serious illness is flight. But we do find them among the Australians that are primitive enough, yet more highly developed. A Kurnai told the missionary, A. W. Howitt, how he became a medicine man and we can obtain a clear picture by listening to his tale.[4]

When I was a big boy about getting whiskers I was at Alberton camped with my people. Bunjil-gworan was there and other old men. I had some dreams about my father, and I dreamed three times about the same thing. The first and the second time, he came with his brother and a lot of other old men, and dressed me up with lyre-bird's feathers round my head. The second time they were all rubbed over with *Naial* (red ochre), and had *Bridda-briddas* on. The third time they tied a cord made of whale's sinews round my neck and waist, and swung me by it and carried me through the air over the sea at Corner Inlet, and set me down at *Yiruk*. It was at the front of a big rock like the front of a house. I noticed that there was some thing like an opening in the rock. My father tied something over my eyes and led me inside. I knew this because I heard the rocks make a sound as of knocking behind me. Then he uncovered my eyes, and I found that I was in a place as bright as day, and all the old men were round about. My father showed me a lot of shining bright things, like glass, on the walls, and told me to take some. I took one and held it tight in my hand. When we went out again my father taught me how to make these things go into my legs, and how I could pull them out again. He also taught me how to throw them at people. After that, he and the other old men carried me back to the camp, and put me on the top of a big tree. He said, 'Shout out loud and tell them that you are back.' I did this, and I heard the people in the camp waking up, and the women beginning to beat their rugs for me to come down, because now I was a *Mulla-mullung*. Then I woke up and found that I was lying along the limb of a tree. The old men came out with fire-sticks, and when they reached the tree, I was down, and standing by it with the thing my father had given me in my hand. It was like glass, and we call it *Kiin*. I told the old men all about it, and they said that I was a doctor. From that time I could pull things out of people, and I could throw the *Kiin* like light in the evening at people, saying to it *Blappan* [go!]. I have caught several in that way.

Thus we hear that the young Kurnai was selected and initiated in a dream by the ghost of his father and was given the chief tool of his trade, the piece of quartz with which he caused illness and removed it. The father's ghost was his guardian spirit, talked to him, instructed him, and whatever power he had was due to the ghost.

In addition to the medicine men, the Kurnai had other individuals, the Birrark, also instructed by the ancestral spirits, whose function, however, was not healing but leading the dances and songs, announcing the future, or bringing the ghosts of the dead to the camp.[5] Thus in this very primitive tribe we already encounter a marked specialization.

The Kurnai believed that only the medicine man was able to cause disease, and when a death had been traced to a definite individual, his fate was not enviable. Protected only by a shield or two, he had to fight against the relatives of the deceased. The Arunta, however, the natives of Central Australia, thought that everybody might acquire the power of making a fellow man sick through object intrusion while only the medicine man was able to remove foreign objects, the tiny hooked sticks that were shot magically into the victim's body.

The Arunta medicine man held his power from the ancestral spirits also, but his training and initiation was somewhat more complicated than with the Kurnai.[6] When an individual felt the urge to become a medicine man, he went trembling to the cave that housed the ghosts of the dead. At the entrance he lay down, and while he slept a spirit came and pierced his tongue, his neck, and head with a spear. He was then carried into the cave, to the land of the dead, where the spirits gave him new entrails and introduced magic stones into his body. When he woke up in front of the cave, he felt and behaved strangely at first. For a whole year he was not permitted to practice but was to live in the company of the old medicine men, who instructed him while he was subjected to a number of taboos in regard to food and other things.

The Arunta distinguish three types of medicine man, but these are not specialized groups; the distinction is one of origin. The first two classes are initiated by the ancestral spirits directly and the difference lies merely in the group of spirits that does the initiating. The third class, somewhat less highly esteemed, is trained by the old medicine men without having undergone the initial experience with the spirits. They all have pierced tongues, however, and their functions are very much the same.

The tribes that inhabit the Indonesian island of Nias have medicine men of both sexes and the vocation is frequently, although not necessarily, hereditary.[7] In the northern section of the island a young man who wants to follow his father's profession must wait until he feels ill. Then a medicine man, not his father, will come to see him, treat him, and promise to instruct him. From his father, the candidate learns magic formulas and the handling of the drum; from his other teacher everything else. He assists his teacher and, when the instruction is completed, pays him the equivalent of about eight dollars. It is up to the teacher to decide when his student is ready to practice independently. A banquet is held to celebrate the event. Medicine men are frequently the tribal chiefs or members of chiefs' families. Larger villages often have one male and one female practitioner, while smaller villages may share one.

In other sections of the island a candidate acts as in a frenzy and suddenly disappears into the woods, where he stays in hiding for several days. The villagers assume that he has been abducted by spirits who keep him a captive in a tree. Sacrifices are brought to the spirits to appease them and to induce them to release the captive. Then he comes from the woods dressed in a garment of snakes that are invisible to all except the medicine man, who now assumes the duty to instruct him. He is brought to the burial grounds, to the river, to the top of a mountain, so that he may become acquainted with the spirits of the dead, of the water, and of the mountains.

The Nias people have other healers as well, midwives and the

Dukun, individuals who are familiar with the action of certain drugs and are experienced in massage.

Such healer-herbalists are encountered also among American Indian tribes, the Dakota, Navaho, Apache, Crow, Ojibwa, but here as on Nias the lay healer is a secondary figure who acts only in the case of minor ailments, while serious illness requires the medicine man.[8]

The Indian medicine man has been the object of many studies. His vivid personality attracted the attention of the white men from the date of their first contacts. He was feared when colonists and Indians clashed, but in times of peace he was often helpful to the white man. European doctors were few, and many a sick pioneer in the wilderness was treated kindly and effectively by the Indian medicine man.

Ackerknecht once pointed out correctly that to seventeenth-century Europeans Indian medicine was anything but strange or primitive.[9] This after all, was the time of Molière, and therapy did not consist of very much more than *clysterium donare, postea seignare, ensuita purgare*. Belief in witchcraft and possession by demons had not yet been overcome, and miracle cures in churches were reported frequently. A European peasant and an American Indian had a great deal in common and there was no reason why one of them should have considered the other 'primitive.'

Just as there are great variations in the culture patterns of Indian tribes, the character of their medicine man differs considerably. The profession is open to both sexes but many more men enter it than women, and although no discrimination is made as a rule, it may happen that some ceremonial privileges are denied women. Thus among the Chiricahua Apache a woman medicine man is not permitted to use a sweat lodge nor may she impersonate a Mountain Spirit.[10] Transmission of power by inheritance is exceptional and occurs only in a very few tribes, the Omaha and Hidatsa.[11] With the Blackfoot Indians the medicine man sometimes selects his successor, a bright boy of twelve or thirteen years of age, that he trains for many years, and uses as an assistant until he becomes a full-fledged medicine man himself.[12] The Hopi and Navaho dedicate young boys to the medical clans, and they too undergo a long period of training.[13] Candidates are selected young, particularly in those tribes that have an elaborate and complicated ritual, the mastery of which requires many years of study. In most other tribes the young men or women who decide upon such a career have passed the age of adolescence.

What makes them choose a vocation that brings honor and profits, to be sure, but also hardships and great responsibility? Sometimes it is an extraordinary experience. An Apache woman was struck by lightning but not killed, which was strange enough; when the same woman was attacked and bitten by a mountain lion and escaped, there seemed no doubt that the spirits were calling her.[14] Indeed, it is the powers themselves that select; as an Apache said, 'Perhaps you want to be a shaman of a certain kind, but the power does not speak to you. It seems that, before power wants to work through you, you've got to be just so as in the original time . . . Some hear it; the power speaks to them. Power usually comes in a voice . . . Sometimes it appears to a person in a vision.'[15]

The dream or vision may not come spontaneously but may have to be inducted. To that purpose, the Crow Indian retires to a lonely place in the mountains, and fasts.[16] A Blackfoot medicine man told the story of his initial experience:

When I was about fifteen years old my people were camped near the Sweet Grass Hills. My father was a chief and very rich. My mother was a good provider. Both my parents were good natured. So I thought that my father having been a good man and of some importance, it would be well for me to go out somewhere and sleep and get some power. This was after my parents died. Both of them had advised me to do this. So I went down to the Sweet Grass Hills. Before I went I filled a pipe, took it to a medicine man, telling him that I was poor and that I was going to sleep. The medicine man told me that I would be a great chief some day and that I should have a dream and get some power. So he took some yellow paint and something for a smudge, sang a song, and began to fix me up. His song was: 'The man above hears me. The ground hears me. It is my medicine.' Then this man prayed to the sun saying, 'Look down upon this boy. He is poor. Give him some power, and help him to become a great man. Help him to become a great chief.' Then the man took the paint, painted me, naming all the different animals as he did so. He named all that fly, all that swim, and all that walk, etc. 'Of these one will come to you. You must not be scared away. If you run away you will not get power to become a great man.' Then while the man was painting me he sang this song: 'He hears me. The wind is my medicine. The rain is my medicine.' He rubbed the paint upon the front and the back of my head and on my back and on my shoulders. As he did so he sang, 'Now this man has the sun power.'

The boy went to the hills and when it became dark he was afraid of animals and ghosts and felt like running away. He stayed, however, although he could not sleep that first night. He stayed there seven days and nights and at last had a dream. A raven appeared that brought him to a man.

Now the man said: 'Raven you give him power first, then I will fix him up.' So the raven put some red paint down and made a smudge of sweet pine. Then he sang a song, took up the paint and prayed for me. Then he sang another song and made the sound of a raven. Then the raven said: 'You must not jump or try to dodge bullets for they will not hit you. But you must let no one throw a moccasin at you or hit you with it, you will lose your power.' Now it was the man's turn. He wore a coyote skin for a cap and this he gave to me. He made a smudge out of sage grass. Then he sang a song: 'I want to eat a person,' and made the sound of a coyote. Then he took up some white paint, rubbed it on my body and painted my nose and mouth red, and my head, breast and back yellow. 'Now,' said the man, 'I give you power to doctor men shot by bullets. Power to take out the bullets. Power to take out things sticking in the throat as when people are choked.' Now I have this power.[17]

Whoever was selected or chose to become a medicine man had to acquire supernatural power, power that came from the spirits, the animal gods, the spirits of lightning, thunder, earth, water, wind, and mountains. Since all objects were animated, power might be derived from any of them. The candidate had to acquire songs, prayers, ceremonials, fetishes, and the spirit that gave him the power became his guardian spirit, the constant source of his faculties.

Some obtained supernatural power through their initial experience, like the Blackfoot boy whose story we just read. Others underwent a long period of training to gain control of power, a period during which they lived in retirement, praying, fasting, bathing, bringing sacrifices, suffering self-inflicted torture.[18] Fasting was an important element of training among many tribes, particularly those of the Southern woodland, the Creek, Choctaw, and Chickasaw.[19] But even those men who had been given power in their initial vision usually underwent a subsequent period of training, serving an apprenticeship to an experienced medicine man, living with him and paying him a sometimes high fee. Many songs and prayers were long and ceremonies complicated, and here as in every other religion greatest attention was paid to ritual details. A ceremonial could not be altered, the sequence of words or the melody of a song could not be changed lest they should lose their efficacy. Indeed, their purpose was to enlist the attention and help of certain spirits who, however, would not recognize a ritual if it had been changed, and thus would not be able to honor their pledge. Hence, training was often long and arduous. The Choctaws distinguished four degrees of initiation,[20] and the Blackfoot Indians had one form of training that was known as the 'Seven tents of medicine,' seven stations, each of a year's duration, through which the candidate was led, where his will power was so developed that his mind acquired complete control of the body, and where he learned to master the rituals.[21]

Most ceremonials required the presence of certain objects, fetishes, which the medicine man kept in his medicine bundle, his most treasured possession, one that not only gave power but put obligations on its owner, for the spirits would punish any misuse of it. The bag usually consisted of an animal skin, and contained bones, stones, beads, shells, paints, herbs, all the paraphernalia of primitive religion. Medicine men sometimes sold songs or fetishes to each other.

In everyday life, the medicine men of most tribes lived and dressed like other members of the group, but when performing rituals they wore ceremonial dresses, sometimes very elaborate, hung with amulets and talismans; they had rattles and drums, all the tools needed to call or chase the spirits.

The social position of the Indian medicine man was always a very high one and still is today. Even when he is a farmer, tilling the soil like other farmers, among the Cherokees, he is nevertheless considered different from other people. He is greatly respected because he is learned and skilful, by far the best-informed man of the group. The Cherokees consult him not only in case of sickness but in endless other matters of everyday life, because 'nobody knows so much about fish traps and the way to build them and the wood to be used by preference; none knows more about the best periods for hunting different kinds of game, or all the artifices used to decoy them; nor can anybody make rattles, or wooden masks, or feather wands better than they can.' [22]

Primitive man had a profound respect for knowledge, and Sumner and Keller conclude their discussion of the functions of the shaman with a remark that is so true that it should be quoted literally.

> The savages were too near to the raw struggle for existence to hold in light esteem that which they thought contributed strongly to their insurance against ill; it has been reserved for civilized man, secure behind the bulwarks of which the savage laid the foundations, to play the wanton fool, as no nature-man could or would, with fanciful and perverse floutings of the knowledge—of the science—he ought to reverence. Only civilized man is secure enough, by virtue of the work and thought and suffering of those who gained knowledge for mankind, and for him, to affect contempt and condescension for their indispensable labors.[23]

The medicine man was paid for his labors, and the fee was usually determined by the success of the treatment and by the social status and wealth of the patient. Many Indian medicine men became wealthy and therefore powerful. There was a temptation to use magic for economic exploitation. Among the food-gathering Yokut Indians of California it happened that the medicine man made rich people sick in order to treat them for money, which then was divided with the chief.[24] Successive failures of a medicine man, on the other hand, made him a suspect and frequently the target of persecution.

In populous tribes medicine men were often organized in societies [25] named after an animal. These societies sometimes had special functions. Thus the members of the Omaha Bear Society treated all kinds of disease, while the members of the Buffalo Society specialized in surgical work.[26] In the esoteric societies of the

Pawnees, members of the same society derived their power from the same guardian spirit.[27]

Specialization in medicine is by no means a late phenomenon of civilization but is very frequently encountered among primitives, Indians, and others.[28] Specialization is usually one of power and function. Thus the Takelma of Oregon have two types of medicine man, one who is able to cause and cure disease and one who can only cure it.[29] The Havasupai of Arizona have three types of medicine man, one who has power over the weather, one who cures diseases, and one who treats wounds, fractures, and snake bites.[30] The Chemehuevi who live along the Colorado River have a rattlesnake, an arrow, and a horse medicine man who respectively treat diseases such as are caused by snakebite, injuries due to a fall, or injuries caused by a horse.[31] Among the Apache specialization is highly developed. 'The Apache has help for everything against which he has to contend.' 'We have shamans for all purposes. There is a ceremony for nearly everything in life. There are ceremonies for sickness, love, hunting, war, and so on. All these are recognized.'[32] Equally far-reaching is the specialization among the Blackfoot Indians.

> Treating diseases is not limited to a few individuals in the tribe, but is widely diffused, more especially among the men. Nor does each doctor possess power over any large number of diseases or ailments. The members of the tribe know that for some ailments a certain doctor must be obtained and that for other ills, different doctors should be called.[33]

We mentioned before that a number of American Indian tribes, besides having medicine men, also have herbalists, individuals who are not versed in magic and do not possess songs but have a deeper knowledge of herbs and their medicinal uses than other people and are therefore consulted and paid fees in the case of minor ailments that do not require ceremonial treatment. Similarly there are women in every tribe who are more skilled than others in helping fellow women in childbirth and who therefore act as midwives.

If we now look at Siberia we find a shaman who differs from the Australian or American medicine man in many ways. The Indian medicine man, as we have seen, is quite a sane individual. He has visions, to be sure, and occasionally falls into a trance, but this is nothing unusual in a society that believes that every object is animated by spirits. The Siberian shaman, on the other hand, undoubtedly is psychopathic. Mental illness plays a great part in his life and behavior, as we shall see in a moment.[34]

Shamanism is usually considered a religion, 'the native religion of the Ural-Altaic peoples from Bering Straits to the borders of Scandinavia.'[35] It is a primitive religion that combines polydemonism with nature worship and belief in a supreme god. The shaman is priest, sorcerer, prophet, and physician but, unlike his Indian counterpart, he belongs to the inspirational type. He has close intercourse with the spirits, has the faculty to call them, to have them possess him and speak through him.

There probably was a time of personal shamanism when everybody knew how to protect himself, how to perform the rites, and how to use charms, amulets, incantations. This developed into a family shamanism, as it is still found among the Koryaks and many other tribes, where in every family someone has assumed the responsibility of protecting the family and knows how to handle the spirits. The next step was to be the development of the professional shaman. Family and professional shamanism are encountered side by side.[36]

Shamanism is often hereditary; sometimes a dead shaman selects his successor, who is informed of his vocation in a dream. Or then, a young man may suddenly feel that he has been called. It comes over him like a disease. It is a disease, one that might well kill him if he resisted the call, because the vocation is compulsory; there is no escape from it. Indeed, whatever the mode of selection may be, it works in such a way that the individuals chosen are people of a special type, dreamers, highly nervous and excitable people. They are sick and recover by shamanizing. A Yakut-Tungus shaman told:

When I was twenty years old, I became very ill and began 'to see with my eyes and hear with my ears' that which others did not see or hear; nine years I struggled with myself, and I did not tell any one what was happening to me, as I was afraid that people would not believe me and would make fun of me. At last I became so seriously ill that I was on the verge of death; but when I started to shamanize I grew better; and even now when I do not shamanize for a long time I am liable to be ill.[37]

The period of preparation is filled with great trials. Some candidates are raving mad, run through the woods, jump through fire and into the water of rivers. Great excitement may be followed by a state of deep and protracted unconsciousness. Of the Koryak shaman, Jochelson says: 'I was told that people about to become shamans have fits of wild paroxysms alternating with a condition of complete exhaustion. They will lie motionless for two or three days without partaking of food and drink. Finally they retire to the wilderness, where they spend their time enduring hunger and cold in order to prepare themselves for their calling.'[38]

The preparation is both mental and physical. Living in segregation, the candidate spends long periods sleeping or in meditation, conversing with the spirits, gathering inspiration from them. But he also learns from older shamans to beat the drum, to sing and dance, and even such skills as ventriloquism. The period may last for years and is one of great suffering, until the consecration brings relief and healing.

The Buryats have very elaborate consecration ceremonies, beginning with purification rites.

One such ceremony does not confer all the rights and powers of a shaman; there are, in fact, nine. But very few shamans go through all these purifications; most only undergo two or three; some, none at all, for they dread the responsibilities which devolve upon consecrated shamans. To a fully consecrated shaman the gods are very severe, and punish his faults or mistakes with death.[39]

In the less advanced tribes the professional shaman performed all the duties of a priest, physician, and prophet. He knew the intentions of the gods and thus could tell what sacrifices, ceremonies, and prayers should be offered. He cured patients by driving the evil spirits out, and as a prophet he foretold the future.[40] In the more advanced tribes shamans were frequently specialized. Thus the Chukchee distinguish between the ecstatic shaman who communicates with the spirits, the shaman prophet who foretells the future and prescribes protective ceremonials, and the incantating shaman who is a sorcerer.[41]

Shamans are not equally powerful or equally courageous. Shamanizing is a dangerous vocation which exposes individuals to the wrath of the spirits. According to Sieroszewski [42] the Yakuts distinguished three categories of shamans according to the esteem in which they were held by the people, The Great Shaman, The Middling, The Little Shaman, in other words, a distinction of degree. The Buryats and some other tribes distinguished between white and black shamans. The white ones had power over the good spirits, were healers and in charge of birth, marriage, and similar ceremonies, while the black shamans were in contact with the evil spirits and brought illness and death.[43]

Just as the American medicine man requires his medicine bundle with all it contains for the exercise of his profession, so the Siberian shaman must have a number of accessories. They are not ornaments but essential tools without which he could not perform the ritual properly and thus would lose his power over the spirits. One is the drum that every shaman possesses. With it he calls the spirits, and its sound carries him to the superworld. Perhaps equally important is the shaman's coat, a cowhide hung with a great many objects made of iron and copper, discs, rolls of tin, bells, plates, each of which has a magical connotation. A Yakut shaman's dress has 35 to 40 pounds of iron.[44] The cap of the Buryat shaman is of lynx skin with ribbons, or he wears an iron diadem, according to the degree of consecration he has reached. Many shamans wear masks or cover their eyes with handkerchiefs, because they penetrate the world of the spirits by their inner sight.[45] They also usually have breastplates of iron.[46]

Like other medicine men, the shaman is paid for his services. He was paid in kind in the early days, when he was successful. With a developing money economy, he received in tsarist times among the Tungus and Yakuts from one to twenty-five rubles for a performance, in addition to food.[47]

There has been some speculation with regard to the nature of the initial psychosis that usually precedes the vocation of the shaman. Most writers considered it hysteria; some spoke of epilepsy, which it was certainly not. Ackerknecht ventured the view that the description of the mental symptoms 'would rather fit into our picture of schizophrenia insofar as they fit into one of our pictures at all,' [48] a diagnosis that would explain the manic as well as the catatonic symptoms.

A medicine man similar to the Siberian shaman is found in Africa, particularly among the Bantu. He too belongs to the inspirational type; possessed or at least accompanied by a spirit that speaks through him, he exorcises and prophesies. The Bantu have two types of healers. One is the *bamuri,* the 'men of the trees,' a herbalist, who knows drugs, plants, but animal and mineral drugs as well, knowledge that has been transmitted in the family or some of which he may have purchased from some other herbalist. There are many specialists among them. One has a cure for infants' diseases, another for leprosy, while a third one may treat only abscesses.[49]

The other healer is the diviner, the *inyanga,* the medicine man proper. His vocation is revealed to him in dreams.

> The spirits speak to him and give him no peace. He becomes a 'house of dreams,' as the Zulu say. He begins to wander about the hill-sides and lives for weeks by himself close to some river or other water. He comes back and is often seized by fits which may recur at intervals for months. He is constantly groaning and appears to endure a great deal of mental as well as bodily suffering. He hears voices calling to him in the night and goes out on to the hill-side in the darkness and cold. He may even see the faces of relatives long since dead. These are at first blurred but tend to become clearer until there is no mistaking their identity.[50]

When the family realizes what is happening to the patient, they call a medicine man to train him and thereby to cure him—or her—because women are called just as men, and in some tribes more frequently than men. A long period of training and initiation follows. The candidate has to observe food taboos, must purify his body by taking medicine—vomitives and purgatives—by washing the skin; he must bring prescribed sacrifices, must confess what he sees in his dreams and who the spirit is that talks to him and instructs him. It usually is the spirit of an ancestor of the dead father or the mother's brother, but among the Shangana-Tonga it is an alien spirit from a foreign tribe.[51] The candidate is instructed in dances and songs, in throwing the bones, in the use of drugs, in finding hidden things. He must observe all rules painstakingly, because every infraction would revive the old symptoms. And, at last, the consecration and with it the cure are achieved. The candidate undergoes a final purification, employing the stomach content of a sacrificed animal. He is invested with protective amulets, and a feast and general rejoicing, in which the Bantu are masters, mark the end of a trying period and the beginning of a new career.[52]

The whole process is strangely similar to that which takes place in Siberia. In Africa, just as in Siberia, mental illness is the starting point, and becoming an inyanga or a shaman is the cure. By accepting the career with all its burdens and dangers, the patient makes an adjustment and becomes a useful member of society, while if he refused it he would remain unadapted, psychotic, a burden to society.[53]

In other sections of Africa the medicine man is usually of the non-inspirational type. He is trained in the knowledge of herbs, in the art of magic and in religious rituals by another medicine man, his father very frequently, because a medicine man has the desire to pass his knowledge and power on to the most intelligent of his children. The profession, however, need not be hereditary, and children born under unusual circumstances or others who had strange experiences, such as falling from a tree without being injured, were often considered predestined for the task.

Different as the medicine men are in various sections of the world, they have nevertheless many traits in common. They are learned men, although the content of their learning is very different from what we should expect a physician to know. Their anatomical knowledge of the animal body hardly goes beyond differentiating between which parts are good to eat and which not. There are a few peoples that occasionally perform autopsies of human bodies in an endeavor to find the disease or the witchcraft substance that has killed the patient. It is obvious, however, that these autopsies are not carried out in a spirit of scientific investigation. They are crude openings of the abdomen, and anything that strikes the imagination of the dissector may be considered witchcraft substance.[54] Ackerknecht, who collected the scattered reports on such primitive autopsies, came to the conclusion that they had not contributed in any way to a better knowledge of the human body.[55] This is not astonishing, because such dissections are made for magic and not scientific purposes. Primitive man, as a matter of fact, would not have any use for anatomical knowledge.

The same is true for physiology. The organs may have a name, and the people usually know where they must hit an animal or a man so as to kill him most quickly, but they have no idea in regard to the function of the individual organ. A number of tribes do not even correlate sexual intercourse and pregnancy.[56] And when primitives ascribe the seat of the soul to a certain organ, it may be the heart or the head, but just as well the fat that surrounds the kidneys or the big toe.[57] The body is alive when it is inhabited by the soul, just as a tree and a rock are animated when a spirit resides in them. Man is part of the world and subject to the same mysterious forces.

The medicine man is a learned man because he knows more than other people about the transcendental world, so much that he even has power over it. And another characteristic common trait is that medicine men are sincere. There was a time when anthropologists considered them swindlers and humbugs, who fooled the people with a few tricks for the sake of material gain. Today nobody doubts that they are sincere and believe in what they are doing, just as the patients do. It of course must have happened more than once that a medicine man overstepped his limitations and pretended to have power that he did not possess. Where is the physician today who has not occasionally taken credit for a result that nature achieved and not his treatment? It undoubtedly also happened that the medicine man misused his power to exploit his fellow men in order to gain wealth, prestige, and more power.[58] This too, I am afraid, is not without modern parallels. On the whole, however, the medicine man was honest and sincere and performed a very important function in a society of which he was one of the most prominent members.

NOTES

1. E. Loeb, 'Shaman and Seer,' *Am. Anthrop.*, 1929, 31:61ff.; E. H. Ackerknecht, 'Psychopathology, Primitive Medicine and Primitive Culture,' *Bull. Hist. Med.*, 1943, 14:40f.
2. Rivers, *Medicine, Magic and Religion*, London, 1924, p. 6.
3. *Oxford English Dictionary*.
4. A. W. Howitt, *Native Tribes of South East Australia*, London, 1904, p. 408ff.; by permission of Macmillan & Co.; see also A. W. Nieuwenhuis, *Janus*, 1924, 28:92ff.
5. Howitt, p. 389.
6. About the Arunta see B. Spencer and F. J. Gillen, *The Native Tribes of Central Australia*, London, 1899; *The Northern Tribes of Central Australia*, London, 1904; *Across Australia*, London, 1912, 2 vols.; also A. W. Nieuwenhuis, *Janus*, 1924, 28:173ff.
7. J. P. Kleiweg de Zwaan, *Die Heilkunde der Niasser*, Haag, 1913, p. 36ff.
8. E. H. Ackerknecht, *Bull. Hist. Med.*, 1942, 12:556.
9. E. H. Ackerknecht, *Trans. New York Acad. Sci.*, 1945, II, 8:26ff.
10. M. E. Opler, *An Apache Life-Way*, Chicago, 1941, p. 201.
11. Corlett, *The Medicine-Man of the American Indian and His Cultural Background*, Springfield and Baltimore, 1935, p. 121.
12. Ibid. p. 102.
13. Eric Stone, *Medicine among the American Indians*, New York, 1932, p. 8.
14. John G. Bourke, 'Medicine Men of the Apache,' *Rep. Bur. Am. Ethnol.*, 1892, 9:456.
15. Opler, p. 202.
16. Corlett, p. 115.
17. Clark Wissler, 'Ceremonial Bundles of the Blackfoot Indians,' *Am. Mus. Nat. Hist., Anthrop. Papers*, 1912, 7 (pt. 2):65-298.
18. Sumner, *The Science of Society*, New Haven and London, 1927, 2:1366.
19. Corlett, p. 142.
20. Ibid. p. 142.
21. Ibid. p. 102f.
22. Mooney, *The Swimmer Manuscript* . . . Smithsonian Inst., Bur. Am. Ethnol., Bull. 99, Washington, 1932, p. 89.
23. Sumner 2:1420. By permission of Yale Univ. Press.
24. A. H. Gayton, 'Yokuts-Mono Chiefs and Shamans,' *Univ. Calif. Publ. Amer. Archaeol. Ethnol.*, 1930, 24:398ff. Various examples also in Paul Radin, *Primitive Religion, Its Nature and Origin*, New York, 1937, p. 40ff.
25. *Handbook of American Indians North of Mexico*, Smithsonian Inst., Bur. Am. Ethnol., Bull. 30, 1907, 1:838.
26. Corlett, p. 116ff.; F. La Flesche, 'The Omaha Buffalo Medicine Men,' *Am. J. Folklore*, 1890, 3:215ff.
27. Corlett, p. 120.

28. George Rosen, *The Specialization of Medicine, with Particular Reference to Ophthalmology,* New York, 1944.
29. W. Z. Park, 'Shamanism in Western North America, a Study in Cultural Relationships,' *Northwestern Univ. Stud. Soc. Sciences,* 1938, no. 2:101; Rosen, p. 8.
30. L. Spier, 'Havasupai Ethnography,' *Am. Mus. Nat. Hist., Anthrop. Papers,* 1929, part 3, p. 277; Rosen, p. 8.
31. I. T. Kelly, 'Chemehuevi Shamanism,' *Essays in Anthrop. Presented to A. L. Kroeber,* 1936, pp. 129, 136-9; Rosen, p. 8.
32. Opler, p. 201.
33. Corlett, p. 98.
34. E. H. Ackerknecht, 'Psychopathology, Primitive Medicine and Primitive Culture,' *Bull. Hist. Med.,* 1943, 14:30-67.
35. *Encyclopædia of Religion and Ethics,* New York, 1921, 11:441-6.
36. The literature on shamanism and the shaman is very large. The most important studies were made by Russian ethnologists. A good bibliography of Russian and other works is to be found in: M. A. Czaplicka, *Aboriginal Siberia, a Study in Social Anthropology,* Oxford, 1914; see also G. Nioradze, *Der Schamanismus bei den Sibirischen Völkern,* Stuttgart, 1925; T. K. Oesterreich, *Possession,* London, 1930.
37. W. L. Sieroszewski, *12 lat w Kraju Jakutów,* Warsaw, 1900, p. 396; Czaplicka, p. 173.
38. W. Jochelson, 'The Koryak,' *Memoir of the Jesup North Pacific Expedition,* New York, 1905-8, 6:47.
39. Czaplicka, p. 186.
40. Ibid. p. 191.
41. Ibid. p. 193f.
42. Loc. cit. p. 628; Czaplicka, p. 196.
43. Czaplicka, p. 200f.
44. Ibid. p. 215.
45. Ibid. p. 203.
46. About the shaman's costume see also Nioradze, p. 60ff.
47. Czaplicka, p. 177.
48. Ackerknecht, *Bull. Hist. Med.,* 1943, 14:43.
49. A. W. Hoernlé, in Schapera, *The Bantu-Speaking Tribes of South Africa,* London, 1937, p. 226ff.; H. A. Junod, *The Life of a South African Tribe,* London, 1913, vol. 2, p. 414ff.
50. Schapera, p. 230f., after H. Callaway, *The Religious System of the Amazulu,* London, 1884.
51. Junod, 2, p. 436f.
52. The making and the psychology of a Bantu medicine man are pictured in a striking book by Wulf Sachs, *Black Hamlet: The Mind of an African Negro Revealed by Psychoanalysis,* London, 1937.
53. See Ackerknecht's discussion of the phenomenon, *Bull. Hist. Med.,* 1943, 14:45ff.
54. Evans-Pritchard, *Witchcraft, Oracles and Magic among the Azande,* Oxford, 1937, p. 43ff.

55. E. A. Ackerknecht, 'Primitive Autopsies and the History of Anatomy,' *Bull. Hist. Med.*, 1943, 13:334-9.
56. A. W. Nieuwenhuis, 'Die ursprünglichsten Ansichten über das Geschlechtsleben des Menschen,' *Janus*, 1928, 32:289-314; see also B. Malinowski, *The Father in Primitive Psychology*, New York, 1927, and M. F. Ashley Montagu, *Coming into Being among the Australian Aborigines*, New York, 1938.
57. Ackerknecht, 'Primitive Autopsies . . . ,' p. 334.
58. Examples in Paul Radin, *Primitive Religion, Its Nature and Origin*, New York, 1937.

*

6. Diagnosis and Prognosis

We must now watch the medicine man in action. An individual has fallen ill, seriously ill, so that house remedies would be of no avail. The family crowds together in the hut or in front of it, where the patient has been brought and where he lies moaning. Neighbors come, look at the sick man, and everyone has a word of advice. Finally the medicine man is called. How does he act?

Here we must remember that primitive medicine, within its own orbit, is logical. The premises may seem strange, but once they are known and accepted we soon find that the conclusion is reached by a reasoning that is logical to us also. All medical actions, in other words, are determined by the views held of the nature and causes of disease. We must also be aware that primitive therapy always tends to be not symptomatic but causal. The medicine man's task, therefore, consists in removing the agent that has caused an individual's illness, and in order to be able to do this he must find out what the cause was. He must make a *diagnosis.*

Today, in examining a patient we also try to make a diagnosis, which, to a large extent, will determine our treatment. But since we have different pathological views and have established disease entities, we diagnose first of all the disease from which a patient suffers and find that he has, e.g. typhoid fever, pneumonia, a gastric ulcer, or a tumor of the brain. We are also interested in etiology, in the cause or causes of a disease. Typhoid fever is determined by the bacillus that causes it. In the case of pneumonia our treatment will differ according to whether we are dealing with a pneumonia caused by bacteria or one caused by a virus. But we know very little about the factors that cause a gastric ulcer or a brain tumor, and in dealing with such diseases our actions are determined by the form and seat of the pathological process.

Primitive man thinks differently. To him the cause is the disease, and it is the cause that he must diagnose. To that end he may begin, very much as we do, by interrogating the patient and his relatives or—in technical language—by taking the history of the patient. He will ask him whether he remembers having broken any taboo or having committed any other offense by which he might have incurred the wrath of the spirits. He will ask about dreams, because they might very well give a clue about what has happened. Or did the patient recently notice anything suspicious, a strange object at the entrance or in the roof of the hut that might be a fetish? Or has he enemies that could have wished to kill him through witchcraft? Did he quarrel with his son, or his wife, or his neighbor? If so, they would be suspected. The questions asked naturally depend on the views held in a tribe about the cause of disease.

In some cases the diagnosis may be very simple, because the patient knows what made him sick. He freely confesses that he sinned, and this confession not only provides the diagnosis but is the first step toward recovery.[1] Or he knows that some fellow man bewitched him. In all such cases the medicine man has a lead along which he can work.

The situation is different when the patient was stricken out of a blue sky and neither he nor his family have the faintest idea what causes his illness. In such a case the medicine man must consult the spirits. All primitive peoples and the people in all ancient civilizations believed in oracles, believed that the gods answered questions if they were put in the proper ritualistic way. The gods might answer in words, as Zeus did at Dodona or Apollo at Delphi, or they might answer more enigmatically through signs that had to be interpreted.

Thus the medicine man in order to diagnose the obscure cause of an individual's illness becomes a diviner who consults oracles. The methods employed are numerous. In the Solomon Islands the medicine man comes with an assistant.

> . . . and the two sit down, the wizard in front, the assistant at his back and they hold a stick or bamboo by the two ends. The wizard begins to slap with one hand the end of the bamboo he holds, calling one after another the names of men not very long deceased; when he names the one who is afflicting the sick man the stick of itself becomes violently agitated.[2]

Another method used among the Saoras in India follows the same idea. The patient is requested to hold a saucer filled with oil in which a wick is lighted. The medicine man drops grains into the flame and with every grain he calls out the name of a spirit. The first grain that catches fire indicates which spirit has caused the illness.[3]

With the Loango in French Equatorial Africa, a diviner is called who, when night falls, goes into a trance in front of a fire. His soul has left him and is consulting with the ancestral spirits. When he comes back to earth, he can tell whether the illness has been caused by a wizard, by break of taboo, or by a fetish.[4] The Siberian shaman, similarly, works himself into a frenzy, beating the drum, singing, and dancing until he has summoned his protective spirit, learned from him what is wrong with the patient, and secured the aid of the spirits.[5] Among some American Indian tribes, the medicine man followed a similar procedure. Schoolcraft pictured a hut especially built by the Sioux Indians for consultation with the spirits, which are seen flying around the hut.[6] The Cherokee medicine man, on the other hand, takes resort to 'examining with the beads' when neither the interrogation of the patient nor dreams have given any clue. He takes a black bead between thumb and index finger of the left hand, a white or red bead between the corresponding fingers of the right hand, and names a number of diseases or disease causes. If the disease named is not the one from which the patient suffers, the bead of the right hand remains motionless or is sluggish, but it shows great vitality the moment the correct name is being uttered, thus confirming the diagnosis.[7]

There are many methods of divination employed to find the individual who has produced someone's illness. On Murray Island, north of Queensland, an elaborate shrine is used, which consists of stones and shells arranged so as to represent a plan of the island. In the early morning the experts gather and watch the place. If a lizard comes out of a shell, it means that the culprit is to be found in the hut that corresponds to the shell. And if two lizards should happen to come from two different shells and begin to fight, the victor's shell would be indicative.[8]

The Azande have a highly developed system of divination that has been analyzed in great detail by Evans-Pritchard.[9] The poison oracle is considered the most dependable of all. The poison is an alkaloidal substance related to strychnine that is administered to fowls, and the oracle is consulted not only to ascertain the cause of someone's sickness but whenever an authoritative opinion is desired, 'on all occasions regarded by Azande as dangerous or socially important.' Before consulting the oracle, the individuals involved must observe certain taboos, must abstain from sexual intercourse, from smoking hemp, and from eating certain foods. The poison is forced into the chicken's beak and the reaction is watched. Some die immediately under spasms, others die after having been jerked backward and forward. Some recover and others are entirely unaffected. The test is conducted twice as a double check. The poison oracle is, e.g. asked to kill the fowl if the illness of X was produced by Y. If the fowl dies, poison is given to another chicken and this time the oracle is requested to spare the fowl if the illness of X was produced by Y. If the fowl survives, the question has been answered in the affirmative and Y is considered guilty. If, however, the chicken is killed in this second test also, the verdict is contradictory and therefore invalid.[10]

The poison oracle is expensive because it requires chickens and a supply of poison that not everybody possesses. The Azande, therefore, have a number of other cheaper oracles, such as the termites oracle that everybody can operate. All that is needed is branches of the *dakpa* and *kpoyo* trees and a termite mound that can be found everywhere in the bush. A branch of either tree is stuck into a mound and the oracle is requested to have the termites eat *dakpa* only if e.g. the illness of X has been caused by Y. If it is found on the following morning that the termites have eaten *dakpa* only, the verdict given is in the affirmative. It is negative if the termites have eaten *kpoyo* only and inconclusive if they have eaten both. Double tests are made here also, but the procedure is slow because a night is required for every answer. Or, the verdict of the termites may be corroborated in the poison oracle.

Like other Africans, the Bantu know many methods of divination [11] through which they can discover the cause of someone's illness. They are clever at 'smelling the witch'—when the medicine man, having worked himself into a frenzy, suddenly has an inspiration that tells him who the guilty person is. They have, moreover, a number of methods that can be compared to our throwing dice or reading the future from playing cards. Thus they have six half-shells of a hard fruit, three larger ones, considered male, and three smaller or female ones. They are thrown and conclusions are drawn from their position to one another and from whether their convex side is uppermost or not. Similar use is made of a set of four pieces of carved ivory, two of which are notched or female while the two without notch are male. They are thrown and each of the sixteen possible combinations has a certain meaning that a skilful diviner knows how to interpret.

The most elaborate and most popular method of divination among the Bantu consists in 'throwing the bones.' Every medicine man or diviner of any standing possesses a bag or basket full of bones and some other objects, each of which has a definite symbolic value. Among the Sotho the four principal pieces consist of two large male ones, one old and one young, carved from the hoof of an ox, and two smaller female ones, old and young, made from bone, horn, or ivory. Since the male pieces have four sides each and the female two, sixty-four different combinations are possible. The position of the four principal bones determines the general tenor of the oracle, while the lesser bones, mostly tali and astragali, indicate the details. The symbolism is striking. Junod, who examined the content of many bags among the Shangana Tonga,[12] found that bones of the impala stand for the chief and his wife, those of the baboon for the village, of the wild boar for the medicine man, of the greedy panther for the white man, of the reed buck for the wizard, while shells symbolize man's properties. Bones are always in pairs, male and female, and must come from animals that the diviner has killed himself, so that it takes much time to acquire a complete set. The Bantu's entire world is reflected in these bones. 'It is,' as Junod said,[13] 'a résumé of all their social order, of all their institutions, and the bones when they fall, provide them with instantaneous photographs of all that can happen to them. This system is so elaborate that I do not hesitate to say that together with their folklore, their *lobola* customs, and their burial rites, it is the most intelligent product of their psychic life.'[14] It is obvious that this kind of divination requires a long period of training.

The accusation of black magic is a serious one. The suspected individual, once he is caught, may confess. He did practice magic in order to kill the patient on his own account or for somebody else who paid him for it. Or he denies the charge, either because he feels innocent or because he wants to escape punishment. In such a case, another test is made that is also a form of divination. The suspected person is subjected to an *ordeal* that will reveal his guilt or innocence.[15]

The ordeal as a method of judiciary procedure has been fought by all colonial powers and has become rather rare today, but it used to be almost universal in Africa. Its most popular form was the poison ordeal. An individual suspected of witchcraft was made to drink poison. If he was innocent he vomited; if he was guilty the poison killed him. The belief in the infallibility and justice of the test was such that it was accepted without protest and that people who felt innocent were eager to submit to it. The poison was gathered under observation of certain taboos, and the potion was prepared in prescribed concentration and quality.

Lévy-Bruhl pointed out that the primitive concept of poison was totally different from ours. To us a poison is a chemical substance that is harmful to the organism and destroys it when it is given in a certain concentration. The individual resistance may vary within limits, but given in a certain quantity the poison will invariably kill a person. To the primitive the substance that we consider poison is indifferent in itself. It is guilt that activates it and makes it deadly. Thus the poison acts as a mystic reagent. Poison plus guilt kills an individual while poison given to an innocent person is harmless and is rejected immediately. The next chapter will tell us that in a very similar way drugs that are given for therapeutic purposes are often considered indifferent in themselves and become active only if the right charm, incantation, or prayer are spoken over them.

The ordeal is a final judgment, and the poison by killing an individual serves a threefold purpose. It reveals or confirms his guilt for all the world to see. It punishes the culprit with death and, at the same time, it destroys the evil that has been active in him. The primitive African ordeal is, therefore, different from the medieval 'judgment of God.' It is a simple magical procedure.

I think that a medical remark should be made at this point, one that I have not seen in the anthropological literature so far, namely this: vomiting is a physiological mechanism. It is a defense reaction that tends to liberate the organism of noxious substances, but it is one that has a strong nervous and emotional element. We all know from our own experience that there are situations in which we vomit very easily, at the mere sight or thought of things. It seems very likely to me that an African native who felt innocent and was made to drink the poison cup was so ready to vomit that he ejected the potion immediately and without effort, while one who knew that he was guilty felt so blocked that he could not vomit. As we know that primitives are highly emotional and very suggestible, such a hypothesis is not farfetched, and it would also explain the firm belief in the justice of the test.

The poison ordeal was by no means the only one used. Another method was the water ordeal. The accused was plunged into a river or lake. If he floated, he was guilty; the water had rejected him. But he was considered innocent if he sank down, which meant that the water had accepted him, and the bystanders were quick in rescuing him. The 'ducking of witches' was a popular practice in the Middle Ages.[16]

Other ordeals were with boiling liquids, water, oil, or molten metal, and with hot irons or fire. The suspected person had to plunge his arm into the boiling oil or whatever the liquid was and if he was scalded, it was a proof of guilt. There are observations recorded according to which individuals did plunge their arm into boiling liquid without being scalded.[17] It must have happened more than once because otherwise the test would soon have lost its significance, but the mechanism that prevented scalding has not been investigated. It is possible that suspects had a chance to protect their arm with an ointment or some other preparation. The hot-iron ordeal was widespread also and was applied through the centuries in many variations, but the principle remained the same. Whether a person had to lick a hot iron, or had to carry it or walk on it, guilt was established as soon as the individual was seriously burned. The fire ordeal seems less formidable when we remember that most primitives have leather-like soles.

All these ordeals—and many other forms could be added—differ from the poison ordeal in that they do not punish the guilty person with death and therefore also do not destroy the evil force that was active in him. They merely indicate the guilt, as would another oracle, and it is left to society to mete out the appropriate punishment.

The severity and finality of the ordeal are attenuated in many other ways. In Africa, it happens that the poison is given not to the suspect himself but to a substitute, a slave, a child, a dog, or a chicken.[18] This is done in the case of minor offenses or when the suspect enjoys a certain immunity—if he is a chief or a member of the nobility. Another modification is observed when the poison is given in a dose that does not kill the guilty but merely makes him sick for a while, long enough to purge him of evil thoughts.

Special mention should be made of the Australian form of ordeal, which is one by combat.[19] The accused person is taken out into the open field, is painted in white and left with a shield or two while the other members of the tribe throw spears and boomerangs at him. If he is wounded the guilt is admitted and also atoned. The test is also carried out after the accused has confessed a crime, so that the ordeal has not primarily diagnostic value but a much more composite character.

Widespread as the ordeal was, it was by no means universal. It was never developed by the American Indians, just as it remained foreign to the Chinese and to Greek and Roman law. It was prevalent in Africa and also in India and among the Teutonic people.

Without diagnosis there cannot be any effective treatment. The cause of an illness must be known so that it may be removed. Confession and divination tell the medicine man where to seek the agent that made an individual sick. And if magic was involved, the witch must be caught.

The diagnosis determines all further actions, but there is something else that the patient wants to know, namely, what his chances of recovery are. The medicine man, in other words, must make a *prognosis,* must find out whether the patient will survive or die, and possibly whether his illness will be short or long. To that end the medicine man must again take recourse to divination and must observe and interpret the omens, the signs through which the gods reveal their intentions. The interpretation of omens became a highly developed science in all ancient civilizations, and we shall see later in this volume what a cardinal part it played in Babylonian medicine. The belief in omens, in signs that announce good luck or bad luck, persisted through the ages and is today still widespread. How many people are not afraid of the black cat, the broken mirror, or spilled salt, particularly people who are in danger, such as aviators in wartime who are exposed to hazards over which they have little control? Some of them are found to observe and interpret omens as carefully as any savage might do.

Omens are spontaneous or sought. The flight of birds, their cries, celestial phenomena, abnormal births in animals and man were considered spontaneous signs, while others were sought by inspecting the entrails of victim animals, by dripping oil on water, or similar procedures.

The interpretation of omens plays such a great part in the life of primitives because it is believed that they have not only indicative but also causative value. The comet that terrified medieval man not only announced impending disasters—war, famine, and pestilence—but brought them. The salt that I spill on the table means bad luck and brings it—unless I am skilled in the matter, take some of the spilled salt and throw it over my left shoulder, a magic rite by which I neutralize the evil effect of a bad omen. This very fact, namely that the action of omens is not irrevocable, that it can be neutralized or even changed, keeps primitive man constantly on his toes. If you plan to start out on a journey and the omens are bad, you postpone the trip until you have better auspices. Your knowledge has averted a catastrophe, and you begin your voyage with good chances that it will succeed.

More can be done in the matter, and an evil omen may be changed into a good one. Among the Dyaks of Borneo, it is a good omen to see birds on the right, and when you visit a sick relative or friend you hope to encounter such a sign. When you do, you immediately sit down and chew some betel or tobacco or whatever you happen to have, in order to hold the good luck. You wrap up in a leaf some of the matter chewed under such good auspices and take it to the sick. He will swallow it and will feel greatly benefited since the mixture is impregnated with the mystic force of the good omen.[20] If, however, on your way to the sick you suddenly see birds in a field to your left, a very bad sign, you immediately turn around and retrace your steps, whereby the birds will now be on your right. You walk in a semi-circle around the birds, keeping them always to your right, and thus through your knowledge and skill you have transformed an evil omen into a good one and have brought good luck upon yourself and your sick friend.

Another method of warding off an evil omen consists in destroying it. When a Maori in New Zealand sees a lizard on his path, he knows that it has been sent by an enemy as an evil omen that will cause his death. And so he destroys the omen by killing the lizard.[21]

A similar reaction is observed among primitives to what the Romans called *monstra* and *portenta,* abnormal births and abnormal happenings in men and animals, most of which were considered very bad omens that had to be destroyed. Lévy-Bruhl collected many examples to this point from various sections of the globe,[22] and I should like to quote only a few of them. Thus among the Wasambara of East Africa an infant was killed if it was born with the feet first. And if a goat giving birth for the first time brought forth twins, the goat and the kids were killed. Similarly a dog or a goat were killed if they were found eating their excrements.[23] All these were considered abnormal happenings loaded with magic, and evil omens that must be eliminated.

Thus the observation, interpretation, and control of spontaneous omens are very important to the primitive because they not only permit him to make a prognosis of the patient but also because they greatly influence the course of his illness.

Sought omens are answers of oracles, and all methods of divination discussed previously, even including ordeals, can be used in order to find out whether a sick man will live or die. Most primitive oracles answer with yes or no whatever question is put to them, and an ordeal can be used for prognostic purposes in such a way that e.g. a relative of the patient plunges his hand into boiling water. If it is scalded the sick will die, if not he will live.

NOTES

1. D. M. Spencer, *Disease, Religion and Society in the Fiji Islands,* New York, 1941, p. 66f.
2. R. H. Codrington, *The Melanesians,* Oxford, 1891, p. 210.
3. F. Fawcett, 'On the Saoras (or Savaras), an Aboriginal Hill People of the Eastern Ghats of the Madras Presidency,' *J. Anthrop. Soc. Bombay,* 1:261.
4. Bartels, *Die Medicin der Naturvölker, ethnologische Beiträge zur Urgeschichte der Medicin,* Leipzig, 1893, p. 161.
5. Czaplicka, *Aboriginal Siberia,* Oxford, 1914, p. 228ff.
6. H. R. Schoolcraft, *Historical and Statistical Information Respecting the History, Condition and Prospects of the Indian Tribes of the United States,* Philadelphia, 1851-5.
7. Mooney, *The Swimmer Manuscript* . . . Smithsonian Inst., Bur. Amer. Ethnol., Bull. 99, Washington, 1932, pp. 41, 132.
8. Rivers, *Medicine, Magic and Religion,* London, 1924, p. 30.
9. Loc. cit. pp. 258-386.
10. See the examples in Evans-Pritchard, *Witchcraft, Oracles and Magic among the Azande,* Oxford, 1937, p. 300ff.
11. Schapera, *The Bantu-Speaking Tribes of South Africa,* London, 1937, p. 235ff.
12. Junod, *The Life of a South African Tribe,* London, 1913, 2:496ff.
13. Ibid. p. 521.
14. I had the bones thrown for me once in Transvaal by a *nganga* from Manyikalana. The ceremony began by my putting a coin of two shillings six pence into the bag, a detail that must never be omitted. The bones were then thrown on a mat and the *nganga* contemplated them for a long time. He made a few general statements: that I should beware of colds, that

people were talking about me, etc.; and after a while he declared that he was not in the mood to continue. The situation obviously was a very abnormal one.

15. About ordeal, see Hastings, *Encyclopædia of Religion and Ethics,* 9:507ff.; L. Lévy-Bruhl, *La Mentalité primitive,* Paris, 1922, p. 244ff.; Harley, pp. 153ff.; Schapera, p. 241f.
16. Hastings, 9:509.
17. E.g. J. L. Wilson, *Western Africa,* London, 1856, p. 228.
18. Lévy-Bruhl, p. 263.
19. Ibid. p. 282ff. where the chief literature is given.
20. H. L. Roth, *The Natives of Sarawak and British North Borneo,* London, 1896, vol. I, p. 192.
21. W. H. Goldie, 'Maori Medical Lore,' *Trans. New Zealand Inst.,* 1904, 37:18.
22. Lévy-Bruhl, p. 158ff.
23. A. Karasek-Eichhorn, 'Beiträge zur Kentniss der Waschambara,' *Bässler Arch.,* 1911, 1:188, 103-6. There are tribes, on the other hand, that revere monsters.

*

7. Treatment

Now, at last we have reached the point where we can discuss the primitive treatment of disease, a treatment, as we mentioned before, determined by the views held of the cause and nature of disease.

If we look at Australia first, we remember that there the chief cause of disease was considered to be the intrusion of a foreign object into the victim's body by means of magic. The purpose of treatment, therefore, was to remove the object from the sick man. To that end the Kurnai medicine man inquired where the patient felt a pain. He then touched the sick part, rubbed it gently until he suddenly declared that he felt the object under the skin. He covered the part with a piece of cloth from which after a while he produced a bit of quartz, a splinter of wood, a glass bead, or whatever the object might have been.[1] In other cases he rubbed the sick part energetically and sucked it with his mouth. Then suddenly he spit the foreign object out.[2]

Spencer and Gillen, reporting on the tribes of Central Australia, say:[3]

In case of sickness the natives have implicit trust in the medicine man, and in serious cases two or three, if they are available, are called in, in consultation. No reward of any kind is given or expected. If the patient is cured, then the reputation of the medicine man is enhanced; but if not, the failure is put down to the malignant action of superior magic, exerted by some hostile spirit or individual . . . In ordinary cases the patient lies down, while the medicine man bends over him and sucks vigorously at the part of the body affected, spitting out every now and then pieces of wood, bone, or stone, the presence of which is believed to be causing the injury and pain. This suction is one of the most characteristic features of native medical treatment, as pain in any part of the body is always attributed to the presence of some foreign body that must be removed.

The treatment is more complicated in serious cases when the medicine man finds that the foreign body is an *ullinka,* a short barbed stick attached to an invisible string, the pulling of which by a spirit causes great pain.

While the patient is supported in a half-sitting attitude, the medicine man first of all stands close by gazing down upon him in the most intent manner. Then going a few yards away, he looks fiercely at him, bends slightly forward and repeatedly jerks his arm outwards, at full length, during which performance he is supposed to project some of the Atnongara stones into the patient's body in order to counteract the evil magic at work within him. Going rapidly, with a characteristic prancing, high knee-action from one end of the cleared space to the other, he repeats the movement with dramatic effect. Finally he comes close again, and after much mysterious searching finds and cuts the string which is invisible to everyone but himself. There is not a doubt among the onlookers as to his having really done this. Then once more the projecting of the Atnongara stones is repeated, and after this, crouching down over the sick man, he places his mouth upon the affected part and sucks until at last the *ullinka* is extracted—either in fragments or very rarely, and only if he be a great and very distinguished medicine man—whole—and shown to the wondering audience, the Atnongara stones returning once more into his own body.[4]

The view that disease was caused by object intrusion was widespread also among the American Indians, and sucking was therefore a chief method of treatment there too, but the ceremonial was more elaborate than in Australia. Among the Cheyennes it consisted of purifications, smoking of a pipe, rattling, singing; and the sucking produced buffalo hair, stones, and even lizards.[5] Healing rites of the Zuñi that lasted several days and nights were described by M. C. Stevenson, and there too the final act that brought healing was the sucking of the affected part, from which the medicine men produced pebbles, bits of blanket, and yards of yarn.[6] A method of extraction of a special kind was practiced by the Arapaho and Choctaw Indians, where the medicine man did not suck the skin with his mouth directly but actually drew blood by scarifying the skin and applying a horn cup, whereby the object was found in the blood that filled the cup.[7]

Two points require some discussion in connection with these practices. It is obvious that the objects produced in the course of a treatment did not come from the patient's body but from the medicine man's bag. They belonged to his stock-in-trade, and very adroitly he placed some appropriate ones into his mouth, which he could spit out at the right moment. All early observers agreed that the medicine men were masters of legerdemain, and M. C. Stevenson, who watched Zuñi medicine men many times very closely, could never catch them secreting any objects in their mouth or hands except once, when she saw that an old medicine man who was pressing pebbles from a patient's eyes was actually holding them in the palm of his right hand, but so cleverly that the hand seemed to be held in a perfectly natural position.[8]

Many early ethnologists used these observations as an argument for the insincerity of the medicine men, accusing them of fooling and exploiting the people with cheap tricks. Such a view overlooks the fact that the removal of such an object is a magical and not a rational cure. The object was introduced not physically, but magically on the strength of certain rites, and it is removed in a similar fashion. The medicine man knows very well that he is holding an object in his mouth when he begins the treatment—it may be an important fetish—and by performing the rites, of which sucking is one, he expects his object to attract the foreign body from the patient's parts so that the two become one magically. Thus he can produce the object in all sincerity.

Another point is that while these treatments are purely magical in purpose they nevertheless include elements that are also found in rational therapy. The rubbing that often precedes the sucking is a form of massage, and the sucking itself has the effect of cupping and is, in other words, a method of bleeding. Object intrusion—*Hexenschuss*—is frequently considered the cause of acute rheumatic pains, and there can be no doubt that massage and cupping do relieve such pains. Thus we realize from the very start that primitive therapy is a combination of empirico-rational, magical and, as we shall soon see, religious elements, which are interwoven inextricably, and, while the motivation of a treatment may be primarily magical or religious, it may well be combined with methods that are used in scientific medicine today for totally different reasons.

We mentioned before that the view that attributes disease to loss of the soul is particularly frequent in Siberia, among the Eskimos, the American Indians of the Northwest, in Polynesia and Melanesia. Wherever such a view prevails, the medicine man's task is to find out who took the soul, where it is kept, and to bring it back into the patient's body. The Siberian shaman consults his guardian spirits and in a trance goes out to fetch the lost soul. Or, among the Buryats, he may try to lure the soul back. Into a pail he sticks his arrow and puts in food of which the patient is particularly fond. He carries the pail to the place where he expects the soul to be kept. After a while he returns the pail and if the patient trembles violently and cries tears of joy, it means that the soul has been recovered. The procedure may not succeed the first time and may have to be repeated.[9]

The medicine man of the Eskimos acts very similarly. He too tries to lure the soul back by means of presents; or he prays to the spirits to return it; or he goes to the land of the dead, seeking for it.[10] Among the Eskimos of the northwest coast of America the medicine man

> fasts four or five days and then walks about in the forest looking for the soul. When he sees it, he catches it between the palms of his hands and returns to the sick man, who lies covered by a reed mat. Relatives and friends who are present beat time and sing, and the medicine man puts the soul back into the body. The patient who in the meantime has been dosed with purgatives and deprived of food, is now allowed to eat first the tail and later the chest of a salmon.[11]

The medicine men of the Haida Indians of British Columbia and Alaska have soul-catchers, forklike carved instruments made of bone, with which they capture the lost souls.[12]

On the island of Nias, in Polynesia, the medicine man sits in front of the patient's hut and calls the evil spirit that abducted the soul by beating the drum for hours with his left hand while waving a palm leaf with the right. When he has succeeded in catching the spirit's attention, he requests him to return the soul, and when he suddenly sees a glowworm on a leaf he knows that the spirit has given in. He catches the insect and holds it near the nose or clavicles of the patient so that the soul may re-enter the body.[13]

The Nias islanders also believe that man's shadow is animated, and similar ceremonies are performed to recover the abducted shadow. The medicine man makes an *adu,* an image of wood, that he places near the patient's eating bowl. He then beats the drum and pronounces incantations, and when he sees a ray of the moon on the bowl he knows that the shadow-soul has returned. He takes it carefully, puts it into a quiver and urges the patient to keep it safely locked so that he will never lose it again.[14] If, however, the spirits have devoured the soul, there is no recovery and the patient must die.

Natives of central Celebes believe that the soul may leave the body as the result of a sudden fright. In such a case they whip the patient, hoping that the soul may feel pity for him and return.[15]

Recovery of the soul is an elaborate ceremony among the Menangkabau of central Sumatra. Eight different substances are prepared for sacrifice under observance of certain rites. Benzoin, a balsamic resin, is burned, and the healer, a woman, is covered with blankets. After a while a tremor of her legs indicates that the soul is leaving her body. It flies to the realm of the spirits, seeking allies to recover the lost soul. Renewed tremor under the blanket and the sound of voices indicate that the mission has succeeded. The healer's soul has returned and with it came spirits bringing back the lost soul of the patient. They are invited to partake in a sacrificial meal, and their advice is sought in regard to further treatment of the patient. But if the mission failed, the patient must die.[16]

If illness was the result of sympathetic magic the medicine man's prime endeavor will be to find the sorcerer, to force him to break the spell. Whereupon the community will in all probability punish him for his crime. But if the case remains dark [17] and the culprit is not found in spite of oracles; if black magic seems to be involved and the disease lingers on—in such a case the treatment will consist of general magic-religious procedures.

When disease has been sent by supernatural powers, a spirit, a ghost, or a god, either because the patient has broken a taboo or has otherwise offended a spirit, or simply because he has fallen a victim to the ghost of an unreconciled dead or to the malice of a demon, in all such cases the treatment will be primarily religious.

Whenever an individual has sinned and is stricken with disease as a result of it, confession appears as the first step toward remission. Sumner and Keller very justly called confession a sort of exorcism by ritual.[18] The sin resides, so to say, in the patient and must be driven out by ritual of which confession is the initial step. Other steps to the same end may be purification, propitiation, and supplication of the spirits, sacrifices, prayer and atonement, as elements of a general ritual, while special measures may be required by the specific nature of the disease in question. Thus, if for some reason or other a spirit has entered the patient's body, whether it be a case of plain spirit intrusion or one of true possession, the first task will be to drive the spirit out.

Numerous methods are used for such a purpose. Some are naïvely mechanical. The medicine man rubs the patient violently, trying to rub out the demon through such a protracted massage.[19] Or, among the Koniaga Indians of Alaska, the medicine man throws himself upon the patient, wrestles with him and thus tries to eject the spirit.[20] Among certain tribes of Celebes the sick man is whipped not to call the soul but to make the patient's body an unpleasant residence for the demon so that he may relinquish it.[21] On Samoa as well as on the Nicobar Islands, the medicine man frequently comes armed with a spear with which he wants to catch the demon.[22] All these procedures are usually accompanied by a great deal of noise intended to frighten the spirit; and the medicine man and his assistants may be wearing horrifying masks for that purpose also.

Fumigation is another method widely used to drive out a demon, particularly with substances that have an acrid smell, like hair of buffalo or reindeer, or with cypress needles that are sharp so that their smoke will hurt the spirit.[23] Fumigations were applied frequently in ancient medicine, and particularly in the treatment of gynecological diseases.[24] This is significant because the uterus was originally considered an organ of a special kind, one that was animated and had a life of its own. It seems, therefore, very probable that fumigation as a treatment of somatic diseases was taken over from magico-religious practices.

Throughout South America, the most popular method of driving out a spirit was bleeding through venesection or scarification, and it was believed that the demon escaped with the blood.[25] It may also be, although there is not sufficient evidence to prove it, that primitive trephining was in some cases practiced to create an opening for a spirit to leave the patient's head.

All methods discussed so far tended to extract the spirit mechanically. There is another group of practices the purpose of which was to transfer the demon from the patient to another individual, to an animal, a plant, or some inanimate object. On some islands of the Malay Archipelago, the medicine man makes a doll from palm leaves and puts it over the patient's head with some food in front of the doll and on the sick man's forehead. The spirit lured by food comes out, eats what he sees on the patient's forehead, and then enters into the doll in order to eat the rest of the food. But at that moment the medicine man grabs the doll and cuts its head off.[26] On the island of Timor-Laut, it is believed that epilepsy is caused by intrusion of a spirit that has the shape of a bird, and consequently bird-like dolls are made. Food is sacrificed to them, and when the spirits have entered them they are shot at with arrows.[27] The Yuruna Indians of Brazil transfer the demon into twigs, which are thrown away after the patient has been rubbed with them violently,[28] and on some Malayan islands the spirit is banned into a peppercorn.[29]

By far the most potent method of driving out spirits, however, is exorcism, the expelling of demons through the magic power of the word. As a matter of fact, all other methods are usually combined with incantations. Certain words have to be spoken at the right moment if the spirit is to yield to mechanical pressure or to let itself be transferred. Either these incantations have the form of commands, ordering the demon to relinquish its host; or they are appeals to more powerful spirits for intercession; or they are simply magic formulae, words combined in such a way that a spirit, when it hears them, cannot resist them.

All ancient cults have made a wide use of words, from prayers to hymns and incantations, to propitiate and to appease the deity. They appear as part of every ritual, and the following sections of this volume will show what an important part they have played in the medical systems of the ancient Orient.

This may be the place for us to mention the elaborate healing rituals of certain American Indian tribes. If anywhere, then certainly among the primitives disease was not considered a private matter of the individual. It never is, but primitives were quite outspoken in looking at disease not only as a social sanction but also as a social responsibility. When a tribesman was stricken with severe illness, it was a misfortune that concerned the whole social group, and the family and sometimes the community joined in order to readjust the sick to his environment by common action. This is most graphically expressed in the Indian ceremonials of which those of the Navahos are perhaps the most highly developed.

The Navahos are deeply religious people, and according to the Leightons a Navaho man spends from a fourth to a third of his productive hours in religious activities.[30] The Navahos are also very much concerned about health and disease, and the majority of their thirty-five principal ceremonials deal with disease.[31]

They believe that in the beginning the world was inhabited by supernatural beings who lived and fought monsters with physical and magical weapons, songs, and dances, a mythology such as we also find in other parts of the world. One day the gods decided to leave the earth and to retire to their permanent homes in the East, South, West, North, Zenith and Nadir. But before doing this they created the Navahos and taught them the arts and crafts and the songs and dances that gave them power over spirits and permitted them to fight disease, famine, war, and other calamities.

When a Navaho is sick, feels 'bad all over,' it is because he 'fell out of harmony with the forces of nature'[32] either because he broke a taboo, killing e.g. a totem animal, or because he became a victim of witchcraft, or, for some other reason. The purpose of the treatment must be to reintegrate him into the harmony of nature, and the family and neighbors join means and efforts to that end.

The Navahos have three types of healing personnel: the diagnostician, frequently a woman who finds out what the cause of the disease is; the curer, who knows drugs and fragments of ceremonials and who attends to minor ailments; and finally the singer or chanter, who is priest, magician, and physician, a man who has undergone years of training and who knows entire ceremonials. How highly his services are valued is evidenced by the fact that he is paid amounts up to $500 in cash or kind for his services.[33] He is called in case of serious illness or whenever the people can afford him.

Ceremonials are lengthy affairs that last from two to nine days. The excitement is great when one is being prepared. The hogan, or hut, is cleaned. The family of the sick stocks up food and retrieves the jewels from pawn at the trader's store. The following timetable will give an idea of such a program.[34] It is that of the 'Night Chant,' a ceremonial performed to cure diseases of the head such as blindness, deafness, facial paralysis, headaches, but also crippled legs:

First night: Circle kaytahns[35] are made and four masked gods use them.

Second day: A.M. A sweat-house is built and the patient treated to a sweat-bath.[36] Cigarette kaytahns[37] are made and offered to the gods.
P.M. Small sand-painting sometimes made.
Evening. Patient dressed in spruce boughs. Songs.
Third day: Second sweat-bath in morning.
Two sets of kaytahns made. Morning and night.
Fourth day: Sweat-bath in morning. Kaytahns.
Yucca-root bath in afternoon.
Rites of tree and mask in evening.
All-night vigil over masks. Hozonji songs[38] at dawn.
Fifth day: A.M. Sweat-bath and kaytahns. Sand-painting.
Initiation ceremonies at night.
Sixth day: Whirling Logs sand-painting. Five to seven hours.
Gods in costume beg gifts.
Evening. Summit songs. Practice dancing.
Seventh day: A.M. Naakai dancers. Sand-painting. Rites. Five to six hours.
Evening. Singing and practice dancing.
Eighth day: A.M. Fringe Mouth sand-painting. Very elaborate.
Evening. Second initiation rites. Dance rehearsals.
Ninth day: A.M. Kaytahns and masks prepared.
P.M. Crowd arrives. Rites. Rehearsal of first dance.
Early evening. First dance. *Atsalei.*
7 P.M. or later. Second dance. *Naakai.* All night.
At dawn, the Blue Bird Song.

The sand-paintings play an important part in all such ceremonials, and the Navahos are justly famous for the skill with which they execute them. They are made with sand and ground rock of different colors, and represent the sun, the moon, the winds, the rainbow, human and animal figures, and a great many other symbols in different combinations. Their size varies from two inches to twelve feet in diameter. The patient is placed in the middle, and it is believed that the spirits are attracted by the magic power of the allegories represented. They look at the painting critically, and if they find faults they turn away and the sick man is left to himself. If, however, they find that the painting is correct they stay on and can be appeased with songs. They forgive the patient and stop troubling him. The devils that caused his illness are now banned in the symbols of the painting, which the singer erases with a wand of eagle plumes, thus erasing the disease.

A ceremonial like the one we just outlined combines all elements of primitive medicine. It is religious first of all, with its prayers, hymns, and sacred dances, but it includes all the paraphernalia of magic, with its sand-paintings, sacrificial sticks, and cigarettes. And it combines all of this with certain rational treatments, massage, sweat-baths, drugs, namely emetics and purgatives, inhalation of incense, and similar therapeutic measures.

There can be no doubt that treatments carried out for nine days and nights on such a high emotional pitch must give results in many cases, and not only of hysteria. The very unity of primitive medicine, the fact that it never addresses itself to either body or mind but always to both, explains many of its results also in the somatic field. That a ceremonial in the course of which the patient comes into complete harmony with nature and the universe must have a strong psychotherapeutic value goes without saying.[39]

Since the character of primitive medicine is primarily magico-religious, we have discussed magical and religious treatments first, but from whatever angle we approached the problem we always also found rational treatments applied in some way or other. And when we use the word 'rational' we must be aware that we are using it for simplicity's sake, meaning physical, dietetic, and pharmacological treatments that are not mystical in themselves, although they may very well be worked into a magico-religious system. The following examples will illustrate this very convincingly.

We mentioned before that most primitives know disease conditions that they consider 'natural,' that is diseases that need not be explained. They come of themselves and people know how to treat them.[40] If they need advice they seek it from the herbalist, not from the medicine man. It is primarily the minor ailments of everyday life, the colds and coughs and upset stomachs and minor wounds that are treated in such a way by the patient himself or by members of his family or neighbors, particularly women. But then there are also more serious diseases that are sometimes not explained but considered 'natural' and treated accordingly, such as malaria, venereal diseases, tuberculosis, filariasis, skin eruptions, diseases that are very common in certain regions. When everybody has them, they seem obvious and, of course, do not call for special investigation and explanation. This is also sometimes true for diseases imported by the white man. Here too the cause seems to be known, so that one need not seek further.

These 'natural' diseases are treated 'rationally,' and among the rational treatments are some that are almost universally found with primitives, namely poulticing, bloodletting, massage, vapor baths, and counter-irritation. Rivers used the universality of these treatments as an argument for the single origin of culture.[41] While there is no doubt that some diffusion must have occurred, it seems to me equally certain that these methods must have been developed independently from instinctive actions in various parts of the world, as I pointed out in the beginning of this section.

These treatments are rational in our sense of the word, that is, experience tells that they relieve pain and other disease symptoms, but we frequently find them combined with magico-religious procedures.

A poultice made of certain leaves, or of leaves beaten to pulp, or, occasionally, of cow-dung [42] amount to a local application of heat, which in a number of ailments has a beneficial effect. A poultice, however, may also be applied to an aching limb in order to extract a foreign body believed to have been introduced by magic. The medicine man after a while will demonstrate the object in the poultice.

Bleeding through scarifications, venesection, or cupping is practiced by most primitive peoples in the treatment of pneumonia, pleurisy, and other diseases, particularly those that are combined with fever. It brings a certain relief by decongesting the system, as primitives found out empirically. We just saw, however, that the South American Indians practice it in order to drain out a spirit.

Whoever has suffered from lumbago or other rheumatic pains knows what a help a good thorough massage is. This too is a universal treatment that primitives use, just as ancient civilizations did from Greece and Rome to the Far East, where it was brought to rare perfection. If ever a treatment was developed from instinctive actions it was this, but primitives also used it to drive a spirit out or in preparation for sucking out a magic object.

The vapor-bath or sweat-bath undoubtedly has a history of diffusion. Our Turkish bath is the old Roman bath that was popular with rich and poor all over the Roman empire; it was taken over by the Moslems and spread by them as far as their conquest reached and beyond. It seems very likely, however, that it originated independently in other parts of the world also. It is quite general with American Indians, North and South, and is found today from Finland to Africa. The steam-bath certainly is a method of general hygiene as well as of physical therapy, but like other baths it may be used also as a religious purification rite.

Most astonishing is the sometimes very considerable knowledge of drugs that primitives possess. All observers agree that there is hardly a tribe, primitive as it may be, that does not use at least some medicinal plants, and more highly developed peoples may well apply hundreds of them in the treatment of disease.[43] It is not always easy to find out what the drug lore of a tribe is, because many remedies are kept secret; they are the treasured possession of a family or of an individual herbalist or medicine man, who may have purchased the secret for much money and is using it now as his chief working capital. Once we have succeeded in obtaining a native drug, we may have a handful of dried roots or leaves and may find it still very difficult to identify the plant. Even if we succeed, our task is not ended, because now we want to know whether it is pharmacologically active or not, and if it is, what its active substances are chemically. For that purpose we need large quantities of the drug so that extracts can be made in sufficient amounts for analyses. Colonial countries rarely have the laboratories and personnel to undertake these difficult examinations and experiments competently, so that the drugs have to be shipped home, where the pharmacologists have other problems to attend to and usually show very little interest in exotic drugs of doubtful merit. And yet we should remember that we owe many effective drugs to primitive and folk medicine, such as opium, coca, cinchona, ephedrine, caffeine, cascara sagrada, chaulmoogra, digitalis, ipecacuanha, podophyllum, pyrethrum, and squill, to mention only a few.[44]

Without indulging in undue expectations we should, therefore, survey primitive drug lore carefully. This was well done in South Africa, where Karl P. Thunberg identified 24 medicinal herbs as early as 1780.[45] T. E. Bowditch in 1819 described 37 indigenous drugs,[46] and Andrew Smith published in 1888 a study of South African materia medica in which 137 plants were identified.[47] In 1932, J. M. Watt and M. G. Breyer-Brandwijk presented the results of many years of study, during which they had examined 1,713 species experimentally, had isolated 667 chemical substances, and had found that at least 449 of these plants were active drugs and poisons.[48] Two years later D. G. Steyn published a toxicological study in which 164 species of plants were described as being poisonous, 42 of which were used as drugs by the Bantu.[49]

South Africa has been singled out as an outstanding example in this field of study. Having an Institute of Medical Research, three Medical Schools, and several efficient public-health laboratories, the country was well prepared to investigate its indigenous drugs and native drug lore. Excellent work has, however, been done for other sections of Africa also. The often-quoted George Way Harley and his wife gathered in Liberia a herbarium of over 1000 plants which they identified and many of which they found to have medicinal uses.[50] The materia medica of peoples that possess a literature presents a somewhat different problem and will be discussed in other parts of this work, although the early pharmacological literature obviously reflects mostly primitive empirical knowledge.[51]

Primitives prepare drugs in very much the same way as was done by all civilized peoples for thousands of years, that is, until the advent of the modern pharmaceutical industry.[52] They make decoctions and sometimes infusions of leaves, bark, roots, or flowers; or mixing the powdered drug with oil or animal fats they prepare salves and ointments; or burning dried plants, they produce fumes that are inhaled or to which the skin is exposed. Drugs are given internally *per os* or in the form of enemas. The Chiricahua Apache pour the liquid through an enema tube made of carrizo or elderberry wood, and after the pouring is done, they blow into the tube.[53] The natives of Liberia and other Africans use a gourd for the purpose, inserting the stem into the rectum.[54]

Primitive drug lore is very rich and includes much sound rational medicine, but here as in the case of other rational treatments the application of drugs is frequently combined with magico-religious rites. A drug is administered with a charm or while an incantation is sung, and it is believed that the holy words give the drug its power. Thus the Cherokee medicine man treated with ginseng a headache that radiated into the back of the neck. The patient had to chew it and hold it in his mouth. The medicine man, while rubbing the patient's forehead gently with the palm of his right hand, sang:

The men have just passed by, they have caused relief,
The wizards have just passed by, they have caused relief,
Relief has been rubbed, they have caused relief. Sharp!

After finishing the song, the medicine man took a sip of water and blew the water mixed with ginseng juice on the patient's head wherever the pain was most acute. This and the singing were repeated four times, and if necessary the whole ceremony was repeated four times.[55]

Or, to make a patient vomit bile, the Cherokee medicine man gave a decoction of the inner bark of black gum, white alder, red alder, and hazelnut, but before giving it he invoked the Spirit of the Weasel:

Now then! Ha, now thou hast come to listen, Weasel, thou powerful wizard.
Now then! Ha, now thou hast come to put the feet upon the white cloth. Now thou hast come and pulled out the bile. Ha, now thou hast come to take it far away, and to scatter it in the Great Lake.
Thou art a wizard indeed. Relief has been caused. Sharply!

The patient then drank the potion and the ceremony was repeated four times, whereupon the sick man was given warm water to drink.[56]

The more highly developed primitive peoples have as a rule good craftsmen and good artists, in other words, people with imagination and with skilful hands. Hence, ethnologists have sometimes wondered why surgery remained undeveloped technically and limited in scope. It is not difficult to answer this question when we remember that surgery, although technical in character, is determined in its scope by the concept of disease prevailing in a given society. Since surgery aims at removing the disease by cutting out the diseased part or at restoring disturbed anatomical conditions, it seems quite obvious that surgery could not fully develop before the nineteenth century, that is, before medicine had accepted an anatomical concept of disease. The fact that today we think primarily in terms of function or physiology has opened up new vistas and new possibilities to surgery, but our physiology remains based on anatomy.

As long as medicine conceived disease in terms of philosophy and looked upon it as a disturbance in the equilibrium of the body's humors, surgery could not be more than a last resort to which physicians had recourse when dietetic and pharmacological treatments failed. And this was still more the case wherever the prevailing concept was magico-religious. It is highly characteristic that the chief major operation performed occasionally by primitives is trephining of the skull—and sometimes of other bones [57] —an operation the intention of which may well be to create an opening for spirits to escape.[58]

Other major operations are mentioned rarely, and when we find them described we must evaluate the sources very carefully. Thus we read that the natives of Tumale in Central Africa performed amputations with great skill.[59] The patient was given an alcoholic beverage until he was practically unconscious. Skin and muscles were cut through and the bare bone, placed on a block, was cut with a hatchet. The hemorrhage was controlled by having the parts cauterized with hot butter or a redhot stone, after which the stump was tightly dressed. This sounds interesting, but the source is a dissertation of 1845 written by a man who had never been in Africa and merely reported what had been told him by a Negro whom a Bavarian prince had brought to Munich.[60] There is no doubt that surgical amputations were performed occasionally by primitives, although undoubtedly very rarely.[61] Punitive mutilations, the cutting of a hand or of a foot, were frequent enough, but this cannot be considered surgery any more than it is dentistry when somebody knocks out his neighbor's teeth. Nor are the ritual mutilations, such as the extremely widespread circumcision, surgery in the strict sense of the word, and neither are such interventions as tattooing, the production of ritual scars, the splitting of lips, the perforation of the nose or the lobes of the ear, and similar magico-cosmetic operations.

One major operation, a Caesarean section, was witnessed in 1879 in Uganda by a British physician, Robert W. Felkin, who described it in great detail and even made a few sketches of what he saw.[62] This is very startling indeed, particularly since the operation—a very dangerous operation in the pre-aseptic era—was apparently fully successful. The patient, a primipara of twenty years of age, was given plenty of banana wine and was tied to the bed. The surgeon, assisted by two men, washed his hands and the patient's abdomen with wine, then with water. After having first pronounced an incantation he gave a shrill yell that was answered by the crowd outside, whereupon he made a quick incision from the navel to the symphysis pubis, cutting through the abdomen as well as through the uterus wall. The amniotic fluid immediately escaped and bleeding points were touched by an assistant with a red hot iron. The child was taken out quickly and turned over to an assistant. The cord was cut and the placenta was removed by hand. The uterus was not sutured. The abdominal wound was covered temporarily with a porus grass mat, and the patient was raised to let the fluid out. Then the wound was closed with seven thin nails and string, very much as a chicken is trussed with skewers and string. The child was alive and the wound was healed on the eleventh day. A strange story indeed, almost too good to be true.

Major operations are very rare among primitives, and their surgery practically boils down to the treatment of wounds, fractures, and dislocations.[63] Wounds were frequently not treated at all, or an incantation was sung over them, a procedure that undoubtedly must have given better results than many active treatments. The American Indians were known to keep the wounds clean, and in their clashes with the white man their wound treatment often gave better results than that of their enemies. Eric Stone justly pointed out that the Indians treated their wounded in isolated lodges, while the white soldiers were kept in hospitals where they were exposed to hospital gangrene and other infections.[64] The Australians of Victoria sucked wounds, and other primitives dressed wounds with leaves, salves, and other substances.[65]

Hemorrhage presented an acute emergency that called for action, and while some primitives were helpless and let the patient bleed to death, others developed effective methods to control the bleeding. Thus the Indians packed the wound tightly with hot sand, with eagle's down, or with scrapings from the inside of tanned hides.[66] The Melanesians applied a bandage of tapa cloth tightly to the bleeding part,[67] and the cautery was widely used for the control of hemorrhage in many sections of the world.

The suturing of wounds was practiced by few primitive peoples. According to Schoolcraft [68]—a not too reliable source—the Winnebago, Dakota, Tuscarora, and some other Indian tribes sutured with threads of sinew on bone needles, the same kind of skewer method that we encountered in Uganda. Very strange is a method of suturing abdominal wounds with termites that has been found in such widely separate places as India, East Africa, and Brazil. The method is one of India's classical surgical procedures and is described in Suśruta's work.[69] It consists briefly in bringing the edges of the intestinal wound close together, having termites bite through them, whereupon their heads are cut off. They act like pincers or like the serres-fines of modern surgery.[70]

Fractures and dislocations also present an emergency that calls for action, and primitives developed some very clever methods of immobilizing a fractured limb. Thus the Shoshone Indians made a splint of fresh rawhide that had been soaked in water. It could be adjusted very accurately and when it had dried it made an effective cast.[71] Other tribes used strips of bark in a similar way, and in case of a compound fracture cut windows into the cast.[72] Some South Australian tribes made splints of clay which, when they had dried, were as good as casts of plaster of Paris.[73] Others simply applied slats of wood fastened by thongs. If in spite of these good splints results were often unsatisfactory, it was primarily because the initial reduction of the fracture was not accurate enough. Lack of anatomical knowledge was also a handicap in the reduction of dislocations. Manipulations were purely empirical and consisted in pulling and jerking the dislocated limb and in exerting pressure on the head of the articulation. Bone setters were specialists in many tribes.[74]

Primitive medicine is timeless and we had the choice to discuss it either here in the beginning of this book, or much later, at the end. It seemed more logical to do so here, because, although we had to base our discussion primarily upon conditions prevailing among contemporary primitives, we know that the elements of primitive medicine may be found in all societies, at all times, in the ancient Orient as well as in Greece, in the Middle Ages as well as in the midst of our modern industrial society. It is the emphasis only that changes.

In primitive medicine magical, religious, and empirico-rational views and practices are blended so as to form an inseparable whole, as we have seen on every page. The same elements occur in higher civilizations and even today, but are separate as a rule. From the Greek period on, a system of medicine developed that was based on experience and excluded the transcendental. It became our scientific medicine of today, which dominates the picture. But side by side with it healing cults persisted through the ages. Whatever the accepted religion happened to be, it always appealed to a group of people who put faith before reason, and in case of sickness had more confidence in the intervention of a god than in the forces of nature, so that they put their trust in the priest rather than in the physician. And at all times there were people who sought security in the performance of magic rites.

This timelessness and ubiquity of the elements of primitive medicine made it necessary for us to discuss it here in an introductory way. And now, at last, we are prepared to lift the veil of history. We look eastward to watch the dawn and first flowering of civilization.

NOTES

1. A. W. Howitt, *Native Tribes of Southeast Australia,* London, 1904, p. 379.
2. Ibid. p. 408.
3. B. Spencer and F. J. Gillen, *Across Australia,* London, 1912, pp. 339-41.
4. Similar treatments can still be seen in Australia today: see W. L. Warner, *A Black Civilization,* New York, 1937, p. 217; but today the medicine man is paid, at least among the Murngin, although the fee in the case reported—a stick of tobacco and some nut bread—was not high.
5. J. B. Grinnell, *The Cheyenne Indians,* New Haven, 1923, vol. 2, p. 130.
6. M. C. Stevenson, *30th Ann. Rep.,* 1908-1909, *Bur. Amer. Ethnol.,* Washington, 1915, p. 40.
7. See Clements, *Primitive Concepts of Disease,* Univ. of Calif. Publ. Amer. Archaeol. Ethnol., 1932, p. 216.
8. Loc. cit., p. 40.
9. Nioradze, *Der Schamanismus bei den Sibirischen Völkern,* Stuttgart, 1925, p. 95.
10. Corlett, *The Medicine-Man of the American Indian and His Cultural Background,* Springfield and Baltimore, 1935, p. 84.
11. Ibid. p. 93.
12. Bartels, *Die Medicin der Naturvölker* . . . p. 203, where illustrations are given.
13. Kleiweg de Zwaan, *Die Heilkunde der Niasser,* Haag, 1913, p. 47.
14. Ibid. p. 45f.
15. Bartels, p. 201, after J. G. F. Riedel, *De Topantunuasu of oorspronkelijke volksstammen van Central Selebes,* s'Gravenhage, 1886.
16. Bartels, p. 201f., after J. L. van der Toorn, *Het animisme bij den Minangabauer der Padangsche Bovenlanden,* s'Gravenhage, 1890.
17. It would be a mistake to believe that all cases of illness are properly diagnosed in primitive society. As many remain undiagnosed with them as do with us today.
18. Sumner, *The Science of Society,* New Haven and London, 1927, 2:1142.
19. Bartels, p. 187.
20. Ibid. p. 190, after H. H. Bancroft, *The Native Races of the Pacific States of North America,* vol. I, New York, 1875.
21. Bartels, p. 190.
22. Ibid.
23. Ibid. p. 191f.
24. E.g. Hippocrates, ed. Littré, 7:315ff.
25. For the literature see Clements, p. 220.
26. Bartels, p. 195.
27. Ibid. p. 196.
28. Ibid. p. 194, after K. von den Steinen, *Durch Central-Brasilien. Expedition zur Erforschung des Schingú im Jahre 1884,* Leipzig, 1886.
29. Ibid. p. 195.

30. Alexander H. Leighton and Dorothea C. Leighton, *The Navaho Door, an Introduction to Navaho Life,* Cambridge, Mass., 1944, p. 30. About the Navahos and Navaho medicine see also: Dane Coolidge and Mary R. Coolidge, *The Navajo Indians,* Boston, 1930; Frank Cushing, 'Sand-paintings of the Navajos,' *Tenth Ann. Rep. Bur. Am. Ethnol.*, 1888-1889; Franc J. Newcomb and Gladys A. Reichard, *Sand Paintings of the Navajo Shooting Chant,* New York, 1937; Leland C. Wyman, 'Navaho Diagnosticians,' *Am. Anthrop.*, 1936, 38:236-46. Further literature in Kluckhohn and Spencer's *A Bibliography of the Navaho Indians,* New York, 1940.
31. Leighton, p. 26.
32. For this and the following see Leighton, pp. 25ff., 55ff.
33. Ibid. p. 28.
34. Coolidge, pp. 190-91.
35. *Kaytahns* are painted sticks that are offered to the gods. They are made of willow, pinyon, cedar, or some other wood and are prepared under prescribed ritual.
36. A sweat-house is a low hut in which steam is produced by pouring water on heated stones. After the sweat bath the patient plunges into cold water and dries himself in sand.
37. Sacrificial cigarettes made by loading pieces of the carrizo cane with tobacco. They are painted and decorated, and are offered to bird and other animal spirits. See Coolidge, p. 235f.
38. Good luck songs.
39. See A. H. Leighton and D. C. Leighton, 'Elements of Psychotherapy in Navaho Religion,' *Psychiatry,* 1941, 4:515-23; and also E. H. Ackerknecht, *Bull. Hist. Med.*, 1942, 11:511ff.
40. See E. H. Ackerknecht, 'Natural Diseases and Rational Treatment in Primitive Medicine,' *Bull. Hist. Med.*, 1946, 19:467-97.
41. Rivers, *Medicine, Magic and Religion,* London, 1924, p. 81ff.
42. Harley, *Native African Medicine*, Cambridge, Mass., 1941, p. 67.
43. Practically every ethnological monograph that mentions medical practices lists a number of drugs.
44. McKenzie, *The Infancy of Medicine,* London, 1927, pp. 182-4, gives very good lists of 'modern botanical remedies emanating from folk-medicine' and groups them, (1) undoubted, (2) probable, and (3) questionable remedies, with (4) a list of poisonous herbs recognized as such by folklore.
45. Described in Karl P. Thunberg, *Travels in Europe, Africa and Asia Made between the years* 1770 *and* 1779, London, 1795, 4 vols.
46. T. E. Bowditch, *Mission from Cape Coast Castle to Ashantee,* London, 1819.
47. Andrew Smith, of St. Cyrus, *A Contribution to South African Materia Medica,* Lovedale, South Africa, 1888.
48. J. M. Watt and M. G. Breyer-Brandwijk, *The Medicinal and Poisonous Plants of Southern Africa,* Edinburgh, 1932.
49. D. G. Steyn, *The Toxicology of Plants in South Africa,* Johannesburg, South Africa, 1934.
50. G. W. Harley, p. viiif.; see also his botanical list, pp. 267-75. Some other books on African materia medica are: H. Pobéguin, *Les Plantes médi-*

cinales de la Guinée, Paris, 1912; J. M. Dalziel, *The Useful Plants of West Tropical Africa,* The Crown Agents for the Colonies, 1937.

51. Where a literature is available the philological and historical interpretation of the texts must precede the botanical and pharmacological investigation. Hence the importance of having medico-historical research centers in such countries as India. See H. E. Sigerist, 'The Need for an Institute of the History of Medicine in India,' *Bull. Hist. Med.,* 1945, 17:113-26.
52. About the primitive preparation of drugs see Bartels, p. 119ff.
53. Opler, p. 221.
54. Harley, pp. 54f.; illustrations in Bartels, p. 121.
55. Mooney, *The Swimmer Manuscript* . . . Smithsonian Inst., Bur. Amer. Ethnol., Bull. 99, Washington, 1932, p. 171. The book contains a splendid collection of Cherokee sacred formulae.
56. Ibid. p. 217f.
57. Primitive trephining is practiced particularly in Melanesia, on the islands of New Caledonia and Uvea where it is performed not only on the skull but also on bones of the extremities. See Bartels, p. 301ff. In North Africa and the Balkans trephining is a practice of folk medicine.
58. Trephining was considered a major operation because it had a high mortality. The opening of the skull is actually not a difficult operation, and is one that can be performed with most primitive tools, a shark's tooth or a bit of glass. It does not cause much bleeding and the pain is tolerable.
59. E. Gurlt, *Geschichte der Chirurgie und ihrer Ausübung,* Berlin, 1898, vol. 1, p. 211.
60. Lorenz Tutschek, *Medicinische Zustände in Tumale (Central Africa),* Inaug.-Abhandlung, Munich, 1845.
61. The Masai, the best primitive surgeons, did practice amputations in emergencies; see H. H. Johnston, *The Uganda Protectorate,* New York, 1902, vol. 2, p. 829.
62. Robert W. Felkin, *Über Lage und Stellung der Frau bei der Geburt auf Grund eigener Beobachtungen bei den Negervölkern der oberen Nilgegend,* Marburg, 1885.
63. McKenzie, p. 345.
64. Eric Stone, *Medicine among the American Indians,* New York, 1932, p. 78.
65. See Bartels, p. 282ff.
66. Stone, p. 79.
67. McKenzie, p. 346.
68. H. R. Schoolcraft, *Historical and Statistical Information Respecting the History, Condition and Prospects of the Indian Tribes of the United States,* Philadelphia, 1851-5.
69. An English translation of the Suśruta Samhita, ed. by Kaviraj Kunja Lal Bhishagratna, vol. II, Calcutta, 1911, p. 400f. (section on therapeutics, chap. 14).
70. The Arabic surgeon Abu'l-Qasim (died 1013) knew the method and did not consider it reliable. It seems probable that it originated in India, in antiquity, was taken over in the Middle Ages by the Arabs, and was spread

by them to Africa and to Asia Minor, where it was still practiced in the 19th century. This leaves open the question how the method reached Brazil.

71. Stone, p. 82.
72. Ibid. p. 83.
73. Bartels, p. 290.
74. E. H. Ackerknecht gave a very good critical and well-documented survey of primitive surgery in *Am. Anthrop.*, 1947, 49:25-45; see also his 'Contradictions in Primitive Surgery,' *Bull. Hist. Med.*, 1946, 20:184-7.

III. ANCIENT EGYPT

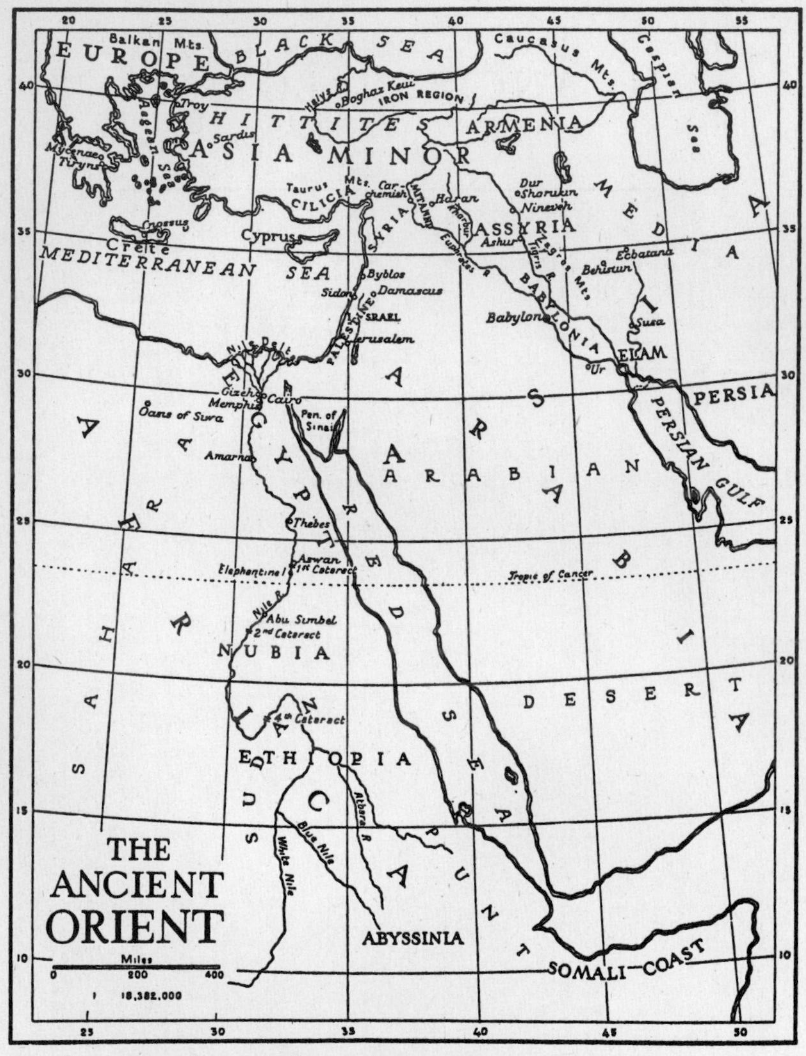

Based on map from *Outlines of European History* by Robinson and Breasted. Used by permission of Ginn and Company.

*

1. The Setting

GEOGRAPHY

Praise to thee, O Nile, that issuest forth from the earth and comest to nourish the dwellers in Egypt. Secret of movement, a darkness in the daytime.

That waterest the meadows which Re hath created to nourish all cattle.

That givest drink to the desert places which are far from water; his dew it is that falleth from heaven.

Beloved of the Earth-God, controller of the Corn-God, that maketh every workshop of Ptah to flourish.

Lord of fish, that maketh the water-fowl to go up stream without a bird falling.

That maketh barley and createth wheat, that maketh the temples to keep festival.

If he is sluggish the nostrils are stopped up, and all men are brought low;

The offerings of the gods are diminished, and millions perish from among mankind;

The greedy man causes confusion throughout the land, and great and small are brought to naught.

When he arises earth rejoices and all men are glad; every jaw laughs and every tooth is uncovered.

Bringer of nourishment, plenteous of sustenance, creating all things good.

Lord of reverence, sweet of savour, appeasing evil.

Creating herbage for the cattle, causing sacrifice to be made to every god.

He is in the underworld, in heaven and upon earth,

Filling the barns and widening the granaries; giving to the poor.

Causing trees to grow according to the uttermost desire, so that men go not in lack of them.[1]

It is no wonder that the Nile was worshiped as a deity from remote antiquity because Egypt truly was 'a gift of the river' as Herodotus put it,[2] and Egyptians were all those from Elephantine to the sea who drank its water.[3] Egypt is an oasis in the desert, a narrow corridor of fertile land, extending some 600 miles from the first cataract at Aswan to the apex of the Delta north of Cairo. It is here the valley opens up and the river separates in branches—seven in antiquity, two today with a network of canals—thus forming the Delta, a very fertile plain, 100 miles in length from Cairo to Alexandria.

The Nile determined the division of Egypt into two sections: Upper Egypt, the southern part, from Aswan to Cairo today, from Elephantine to Memphis in antiquity, a valley from a few to 30 miles wide bordered by bluffs; and Lower Egypt, the northern section, the Delta.

The country has little rain. Only the Delta can count on regular rainfall during the winter months, on an average of 42 days. Cairo has an average of only 26 rainy days, and there is hardly any precipitation in Thebes. The country, therefore, depended for irrigation entirely on the Nile and its inundation. This periodic flooding of the land by the rising waters of the river was a great mystery to the people of antiquity. The sources of the Nile were unknown to them and actually remained unknown for thousands of years. The Egyptians believed that the river came from Heaven or from the Underworld, and what caused the floods if not the tears of Isis weeping over the loss of her husband, Osiris?

From the time of the Greek travelers and philosophers from Thales rational explanations of the inundation have been sought.[4] Some believed that the north winds blowing against the mouth of the river hindered the flow of the water into the sea. Others thought that the inundation was due to the fact that the river flowed from the Ocean, 'which flows round all the world' and that the inundation was actually nothing else but a movement of the Ocean. A third speculation, that the phenomenon was caused by the melting of the snow and by heavy summer rains in Ethiopia, was close to the truth, yet it appeared to critics as the most unlikely: how could there be snow in a country where the heat was so great that the people had become black?

Today we know the sources of the Nile as well as the mechanism that causes its flood. North of Khartum, in the Sudan, the White Nile and the Blue Nile flow together, two very different rivers. The White Nile comes from the lake region of central Africa and for thousands of miles flows slowly through plains, carrying large quantities of clear water. The Blue Nile, on the other hand, is a tempestuous mountain river which like the Atbara, another affluent, comes from the Ethiopian highland and brings not only water but also mud: the mud that has created the arable soil of Egypt, and has filled the Valley and the Delta with a layer of humus, 30 to 40 feet deep in Upper Egypt, 55 to 70 and in places even more feet deep in the Delta; the mud that has made Egypt the 'Black Land,' so different from the 'Red Land' of the desert.

As the subsoil is rocky and there is little infiltration of water from the river, without the inundation the cultivable area would have been very small and the layer of humus, moreover, would have been used up very soon. The inundation not only irrigates the country but brings every year new mud and thus restores the soil. The Nile not only created Egypt but is re-creating it every year.

The inundation is caused by the winter rains in the lake region of central Africa and by the melting of snow in the mountains of Ethiopia. The beginning of the flood becomes noticeable in Khartum early in April, when the White Nile swells and carries loads of vegetable materials brought from tropical swamps. One month later the Blue Nile begins to rise, carrying mud. Combined, they start flooding the land from the middle of June and the waters continue to rise to 40 and even 45 feet in the Valley, to from 20 to 25 feet in the Delta, until the middle of September when the inundation reaches its peak. The water then falls rather rapidly from the middle of October on, leaving the country irrigated and covered with a new layer of good earth.

This unique phenomenon exerted a profound influence upon the life and destinies of the Egyptian people. Cities and villages as well as isolated farm houses had to be built on artificial mounds.[5] All farm labor ceased when the land was flooded, and we believe Diodorus when he says that the masses of the people, relieved of their labors during the entire time of the inundation, turned to recreation, 'feasting all the while and enjoying without hinderance every device of pleasure.'[6] But the rise of the river was watched with great attention and not without anxiety. The government had constructed a Nilometer at Memphis, a well on the bank of the river with lines on the wall that indicated the stage of the Nile,[7] and permitted them to measure accurately how many cubits and fingers it had risen. Messages were sent out to the other cities carrying the information, and when the season was reaching its height, the whole nation held its breath until the information came that the river had begun to fall. At that moment everybody knew how large the next harvest would be, whether the year would be a prosperous or a poor one. If the river did not rise sufficiently, the water did not reach far enough. It also happened that the inundation did not take place at all, for several years in succession. The result was famine and general misery.[8] If, on the other hand the river rose too much, the flood became destructive, tearing down dykes and dwellings. Sixteen cubits at Memphis was considered the optimum.

An economy that is entirely at the mercy of such a natural phenomenon obviously contains an element of insecurity; and civilization began in Egypt—in the fourth millennium B.C.—when people joined their efforts for the social control of the water supply in order to reduce this factor of insecurity, by holding the water when it was scarce and by damming it up and channeling it when there was too much of it. A. Moret and G. Davy, in a stimulating book,[9] have pointed out how an organized collective effort was required to build the system of basins, dykes, sluices, and canals that determined the administrative structure of the country. It was work that called for leadership, and each great basin of irrigation was the nucleus of an agricultural district that developed into a nome or province. Since, moreover, the water was by necessity passed on from the higher districts in the south to the lower in the north, the system called for far-reaching co-operation between the groups and for discipline under the authority of a supreme ruler. Thus the Nile not only created the land and fed the people of Egypt but it welded them into a nation and determined its organization.

It had also other far-reaching effects. The calendar year began when the flood set in, and this was at about the time of the heliacal rising of Sothis or Sirius, that is, the first day when the Star was seen rising in the East above the horizon after its conjunction with the sun. The year was one of three seasons, each of four months, the season of the inundation, that of sowing and growing, and that of harvesting. The month had 30 days, the year therefore 360 days, plus five extra days, the so-called epagomenal days on which the birthday festivals of the five chief deities were held. The Egyptians, however, soon found that the solar year was not 365 but 365¼ days long. The farmer whose rhythm of life was set by the Nile could not follow a calendar under which the seasons changed constantly, small as the change was during an individual's lifetime.[10] He therefore followed the solar calendar that began every year with the rising of Sirius. This, at least, was the case from the XIIth Dynasty on.[11] The other, the sliding calendar of 365 days, however, was preserved side by side with the solar calendar down to the Roman period. This was done, according to J. W. S. Sewell, because it provided 'an automatic record of the passage of years in an era.' Indeed, the opening day of this calendar fell on one and the same solar day every 1460 years.

Flood control also presented the Egyptians at an early time with a number of engineering problems. The building of dams, water basins, canals, and similar structures undoubtedly required expert knowledge, but it must be remembered that considerable engineering feats were performed throughout the ancient world empirically without higher mathematics.

We may also expect that the floods erasing the borderlines of fields made it necessary to re-survey the land frequently, an operation that requires geometrical knowledge. Herodotus thought that the Greeks learned geometry, the art of measuring land, from the Egyptians. He said:

Sesostris[12] divided the country among all the Egyptians by giving each an equal square parcel of land, and made this his source of revenue, appointing the payment of a yearly tax. And any man who was robbed by the river of a part of his land would come to Sesostris and declare what had befallen him; then the King would send men to look into it and measure the space by which the land was diminished, so that thereafter it should pay the appointed tax in proportion to the loss.[13]

Here again the knowledge required was rather elementary, but it is remarkable, nevertheless, that the Egyptians had a decimal system of numeration as early as the Ist Dynasty and that they knew how to compute the area of a triangle, a rectangle, a trapezium, and even a circle. In the latter case they figured the square of eight-ninths of the diameter, which gives for π a value of 3.1605.[14]

The geography of Egypt also determined to a very large extent the pathology and morbidity of the country. Herodotus was impressed by the good health conditions he found. 'The Egyptians,' he said, 'are the healthiest of all men, next to the Libyans; the reason of which to my thinking is that the climate in all seasons is the same; for change is the great cause of men's falling sick, more especially the change of seasons.'[15]

Today, health conditions are appallingly bad. With a high birth rate of 43.4 per 1000 inhabitants in 1938, the general death rate was 26.4, one of the highest death rates recorded anywhere in the world. The infant-mortality rate, that is the number of deaths of children under one year per 1000 live births, was 163 in 1938, and the average expectation of life at birth was only 31 years for males, 36 years for females, in the period 1917 to 1927.[16] How can we reconcile these terrifying figures with the optimistic report of Herodotus? Must we assume that health conditions deteriorated in the course of 2500 years, or was Herodotus wrong, or were standards so very different?

There can be no doubt that general economic conditions did deteriorate, and very considerably, particularly during the Turkish period. Such a brilliant observer as Napoleon made the very pertinent remark:

In no other country has the administration so much influence on public prosperity. If the administration is good, the canals are well dug and well kept up, the regulations on irrigation are carried out justly, and the inundation reaches far. If the administration is bad, corrupt or weak, the canals are blocked with mud, the dykes are badly kept up, the regulations on irrigation are disobeyed, and the principles of the system of irrigation are thwarted by the sedition and private interests of individuals and localities. The Government has no influence on the rain or snow which falls in Beauce or Brie, but in Egypt the Government has direct influence on the extent of the inundation which takes their place. That is what makes the difference between the Egypt governed by the Ptolemies and the Egypt already decaying under the Romans and ruined by the Turks.[17]

And Napoleon might have added that when the country's economy decayed the people's standard of living dropped and health conditions deteriorated.

Herodotus on the other hand formed his judgment not on the basis of statistics but on general impressions, and whoever has traveled in foreign lands knows how deceptive such impressions often are. The people we see in the streets of the city or on the fields of the farm are the people in good health, while the weak and the sick are in the house. A superficial traveler in South Africa is apt to admire the splendid physique of the Bantu he sees in the native reserves and to declare them the healthiest people on earth. On inquiring, however, he soon learns that a woman needs twelve pregnancies on an average in order to have two surviving children. Eight pregnancies end in miscarriage while four children are born of whom two die during the first years of life.

It is quite possible that general health conditions were better in ancient than in modern Egypt, for a number of reasons. The population was probably one-half of what it is today. Diodorus calls Egypt a densely populated country, which it certainly was according to ancient standards. 'The total population, they say, was of old about seven million and the number has remained no less down to our day.'[18] In 1938 the population was estimated at 16,237,000.[19] The same area, in other words, cultivated as primitively as it was in antiquity, had to feed twice as many people, at a time when export crops such as cotton were greatly increased. The obvious result was impoverishment of the population and lowered standards of health. This might have been offset by the greater efficiency of modern public-health and medical services, but Egypt is extremely backward, with only 1.6 physicians and 2.7 hospital beds per 10,000 population in 1929.[20]

Herodotus was a native of Halicarnassus in Caria, which, like the whole coast of Asia Minor and the Aegean islands, was infested with malaria in the fifth century B.C.[21] When he traveled in Egypt, he must have been struck by the absence or at least rarity of intermittent fevers, and this must have been an important factor in his favorable judgment about health conditions. Four hundred years later, Strabo was astonished to find that Alexandria, in spite of the dampness of its site, was free from marsh fevers.[22]

There is malaria in Egypt today although the disease does not constitute one of the major health problems of the country.[23] The inundation of the Nile provides breeding places for mosquitoes, but, on the other hand, the proximity of the desert and the complete absence of woods are conditions not conducive to the development of mosquitoes in large numbers.[24] Whenever the land was cultivated intensively and whenever the canals were well kept, the incidence of malaria was low, but it was bound to rise when agriculture deteriorated and the system of irrigation was neglected. Hence it is no wonder that the disease was rare in antiquity and became more frequent during the Turkish period.

Today the diseases encountered most frequently in Egypt are the infectious diseases carried by water, food, and innumerable flies, the diseases of filth and poor sanitation. The Nile is at the same time the source of water supply and a drainage canal. When it floods the country it brings not only fertile mud and water but also carries germs of disease: larvae of ankylostoma, which cause the hookworm disease, long known as 'Egyptian chlorosis' or 'Egyptian anemia'; or cercariae, parasites that cause the Bilharzia disease from which perhaps as many as 40 per cent of the male population suffer.[25] The various forms of diarrhea and enteritis are the most common diseases and by far the chief causes of death, playing havoc particularly with young children.[26] Eye diseases and resulting blindness are very frequent—first of all, trachoma, purulent conjunctivitis, and primary glaucoma.[27]

There can be no doubt that all these diseases occurred in antiquity also. We have the testimonies of paleopathology that we have discussed previously, and we have those of the medical papyri that we shall analyze later. It is impossible, however, to determine how frequent these diseases were in the various periods of antiquity, with the few exceptions we have mentioned before. The materials available, bones, mummies, and texts, rarely permit any quantitative conclusions.

There is one last point we must bring up when we talk of the geography of Egypt. We are inclined to think of Egypt as a large country because it played a great part in the history of human civilization for several thousand years, and because its rulers had grandiose visions and a hunger for survival that made them erect gigantic monuments, pyramids, sphinxes, obelisks, large statues of the gods and of themselves. And yet in square miles of cultivated land, Egypt was not larger than Belgium is today or the State of Maryland, covering an area of about 12,000 square miles.

We mentioned the natural borders of Egypt, and we must realize that with deserts in east and west, rocks in the south, and a coastline in the north which made it difficult for ships to land, Egypt was a closed country. To the ancient writers it seemed 'fortified on all sides by nature.' [28] It was; and this peculiar geography is responsible for the fact that Egyptian civilization was a closed civilization. While the language of Babylonia was spoken at times all over the Near East, and Babylonian views and techniques spread all over Asia, perhaps as far as China, the Egyptian language was spoken in Egypt alone and the Egyptian hieroglyphs were never used for writing any other language. Egypt obviously had trade relations with other countries, and we shall see that there was a time when Egyptian physicians were in great demand in foreign lands. Objects produced by Egyptian industry have been found in neighboring countries, but Egyptian civilization as a whole remained self-sustained and introverted. To the Greek visitors, Egypt was a land of mystery, with its huge monuments covered with pictorial inscriptions. It remained a land of mystery until the beginning of the nineteenth century; a captain of artillery in the expeditionary corps of Napoleon dug up, in 1799, the Rosetta stone, a basalt block with a bilingual inscription in Greek and Egyptian, the latter in hieroglyphic and demotic characters; and the genius of Champollion succeeded in deciphering it and laid the foundation for the study of the Egyptian language, literature, and archaeology.

CHRONOLOGY

An oasis in the desert of northeastern Africa, created and re-created by the Nile—this locates Egypt in space. We must now try to locate Egyptian civilization in time.[29]

Egyptian and Greek traditions agree that Menes, the founder of the Ist Dynasty, united Upper and Lower Egypt. This must have been around 3000 B.C.[30] Before that time, Egypt had been inhabited for thousands of years. Tools of flint of paleolithic man have been found. Villages and cemeteries of a chalcolithic period have been excavated, revealing tools of polished stone, pottery, textiles, and objects of copper and gold. People began to till the soil, to domesticate animals, living in clans protected by fetishes or totems.[31] The uniformity of climate and geographic conditions in general created a very homogeneous civilization, but the soil was more fertile in the Delta, the country was more wide-open there than in the Valley, and it seems that in the predynastic era civilization developed more rapidly in the north.

As we mentioned before, in Egypt flood control and irrigation were at the basis of all social organization. They called for collective efforts and induced the people to accept the leadership of a chieftain who assumed control over the dykes, basins, and canals of the region, protected the people against enemies, and in exchange exacted taxes in kind and services from them.

Such a system of irrigation makes the people sedentary, bound to a patch of land, the one that gets the water from a certain canal; and the time came when the clans had settled down in nomes, or provinces, each of which had its local deities. There must have been competition and fights between the nomes, but the fact that the welfare of all depended on the same source, the waters of the Nile, forced them to unite at an early date. In Lower Egypt one of the local chiefs assumed power over the others and became the country's King. And a similar process took place in Upper Egypt. This was a heroic age that was remembered later as the time when the gods were still living and ruling on earth.

Menes came from the south and united the two kingdoms by conquering Lower Egypt. He founded the city of Memphis on the border of his conquest. The period of the first two or Thinite Dynasties, frequently called the *Protodynastic Age,* lasted from about 3000 to 2600 B.C. It was a period of great cultural advances of which the most significant undoubtedly was the development of the Egyptian alphabet from pictorial signs and also the invention of suitable writing material. A reed that grew along the river, cut into thin strips pasted together crosswise, provided a vegetable membrane on which it was easy to write with a pointed reed dipped into a mixture of water, gum, and soot. Thus were invented pen, ink, and paper, writing materials that were infinitely easier to handle than the clay tablets of Babylonia.

The invention of writing affected the social structure. Writing was necessary for the administration of the country, for the keeping of records; and the scribes, the men who could read and write, who could compose a document, could write a book and knew the literature, became men of importance to the king. Heretofore, society had consisted of two classes, the nobles, a landed aristocracy, descendants of the local chieftains, now officials at the court, governors of nomes and warriors in times of war; and on the other side of the scale, the farmers and craftsmen. Now a new class began to develop, that of the literati, one that was the more prominent when the country was at peace and not in need of warriors. Many members of that class were made high officials; physicians sprang from it and, in competition with it, the nobility was forced to send its children to the court school.[32]

Property and the crafts were still free to a certain extent, but from the IInd Dynasty on, a census of immovable property and of movable goods—the latter assessed in gold—was held every two years to determine the amount of taxes and labor due the crown.[33]

The next period of Egyptian history may justly be called the *Pyramid Age.* It covers the four Memphite Dynasties, III to VI, and runs from about 2600 to 2200 B.C. It was a period of great art and great endeavors. The kings built for themselves tombs that were considered wonders in antiquity and are still most impressive monuments today, still visited by thousands every year: the pyramids, built in the necropolis of Memphis, outside of today's Cairo. The oldest is the step-pyramid at Sakkara, built for King Zoser of the IIIrd Dynasty, with a beautiful temple at its foot. It is the oldest monument of hewn stone known to the world, and it was built by a man of genius, Imhotep, the first universal scholar, architect, engineer, statesman, physician, and sage, of whom we shall have to say more because he was deified and in the course of time became the hero of medicine, so that the Greeks identified him with their own Asclepius.

The pyramids of Gizeh, tombs of Cheops, Chephren, and Mycerinus of the IVth Dynasty represent tremendous engineering feats. The largest consists of 2,300,000 blocks of limestone, weighing, on an average, two and a half tons each.

The pyramids are a most appropriate symbol of the absolute monarchy that had developed in Egypt. The king was not *primus inter pares* but was now king by divine right, was Horus among men, heir to Osiris, and at the same time son of Ra.[34] He was priest, judge, and commander of the army. He owned the land of Egypt, and the census was now limited to livestock. He could entrust land to people of his choice, but it remained his. He ruled with an army of officials and scribes and lived surrounded by the members of his family and the high officials that constituted his court in life as well as in death, for the members of the court built their tombs around the pyramids as they had built their villas around the royal palace.

All resources of the country were mobilized to carry out the gigantic building program and to supply luxuries to the court. The quarries of the neighborhood were exploited to provide stone for building, the copper mines of the Sinai peninsula yielded metal for tools, and expeditions sent to the South on the land and sea routes brought ivory, ebony, aromatic gums, ostrich feathers, and other similar luxury products.

Thanks to the necropolis of Memphis we know the period quite well, because it was the custom to decorate the funeral chambers with carved paintings representing scenes of everyday life. They depict not only the life of the king and noblemen but also that of the people who worked for them, the farmers, the craftsmen, the sailors and soldiers. And from the end of the Vth Dynasty on, tombs were decorated not only with pictures but also with texts, the so-called Pyramid Texts, hymns and magic formulae written in archaic language, religious poetry concerned with the blessed dead and his life in the hereafter.

The Pyramid Age was followed by what is commonly called the *First Intermediate Period,* which includes the time from the late VIth to the late XIth Dynasties, or from about 2200 to 2000 B.C. The central power weakened and some local monarchs made themselves independent. Cities in the Delta also claimed independence, and whenever in Egypt the central authority was weak, the country was open to civil strife and to foreign invasion from Asia. The irrigation system suffered immediately, and as a result agricultural production decreased sharply and the country was impoverished. Absolute monarchy broke down and was followed by an oligarchic authority carried by a feudal aristocracy. The kings of Thebes and those of Heracleopolis contended for power. Anarchy was rampant at times and deep pessimism is reflected in the literature of the period.[35]

A social revolution took place. The people rose:

> The nobles are in mourning; the common people exult; every city says, 'Come, let us put down the mighty among us.' The country is in revolution turning like the potter's wheel. Thieves become owners of goods and the rich are robbed. The townspeople are put to the corn-mills, and those who are clad in fine linen are beaten. Ladies who had never seen the light, go out of doors. The land is full of factions; the man who goes to till the soil carries a shield . . .[36]

Order was restored by the barons of Thebes toward the end of the XIth Dynasty in the twenty-first century B.C. Again the two Egypts were united under one rule. A new period of great prosperity began, that of the *Middle Kingdom.* Around 2000 B.C. Amenemhet I founded the brilliant XIIth Dynasty, which ruled for two hundred years and under which literature, the arts and crafts, mathematics, and also medicine flourished as never before. It was

Egypt's classical age, what the fifth century B.C. was to be to Greek civilization. The irrigation system was restored and improved. The Fayyum that had become swampy was drained, and Lake Moeris, that greatest irrigation basin, was completed by Amenemhet III, who was buried in the Labyrinth, a building that greatly puzzled the Greeks. The natural frontiers were reinforced with forts and a wall built across the isthmus of Suez, but the might of Egypt was extended to the north of Phoenicia and the royal fleet sailed to Crete and the Aegean islands. A canal was built that connected the Nile with the Red Sea.

Unity of the land had been restored, but the government was not an absolute monarchy, not the bureaucratic state it had been at the time of the Old Kingdom. It was a feudal age and the noble families resided on their estates, loyal to the king but without being his officials. The people too had gained certain rights, such as admission to the Osirian mysteries, amounting to religious equality.[37] A middle class developed. In the cemetery of Abydos were hundreds of tombs of individuals who had no title of either office or rank, commoners who had become rich as landowners, artisans, or tradesmen, who were carefully embalmed and buried with the paraphernalia that formerly only the nobility was thought to require in after-life.[38] The career of a scribe was glorified more than ever, and graduation from a court school opened the doors to office and honor. The peasants and most artisans were serfs but not slaves. They were attached to the soil or to the shop, and when a farm or workshop changed ownership the people had a new lord, but they could not be sold individually. There were slaves also, most of them foreign prisoners of war.

The flowering of a culture never lasts very long. One or two centuries is usually all that we may expect, because the many factors required for such a condition rarely occur in combination. That does not mean that culture breaks down after a short few centuries, on the contrary; once the period of bloom is over, many centuries are needed for the fruit to ripen. Ideas that had been conceived are now developed and applied to life. Techniques that had been invented are worked out and used on an increasing scale. Literary and artistic forms and styles are elaborated until all the possibilities they offer have been exploited. In science and medicine the period of flowering is not that of greatest achievements but rather that of greatest findings and concepts, which, developed and applied in the following age, lead to practical achievements, to decreased mortality, and generally better health conditions.

Egypt was no exception to the rule. The Middle Kingdom did not last long, but the New Empire continued civilization during the course of half a millennium. In Egypt the situation was, however, complicated by the fact that there was not a steady development but that the country around 1750 B.C. during the reign of the XIIIth Dynasty experienced another breakdown, one more invasion from the east, the *Later Intermediary Period.* History repeated itself. Weak kings were unable to maintain the unity of the country. Anarchy resulted and the low lands, fertile and vulnerable, attracted the foreign invader. Walls and fortresses are useless where there is not the power and determination to man and hold them. The invaders were the Semitic Hyksos, who occupied Lower Egypt and built their fortified capital Avaris near Memphis. But Egypt, although defeated militarily, was at the height of its cultural development, and at such a stage a country can not be subjugated permanently. Its assimilating and regenerative force is tremendous. The Hyksos endeavored to become Egyptians and identified their god Baal with the Egyptian Seth. The names of their kings include that of Re, and they maintained the State organization they had encountered. Ultimately, they were driven out, back into Asia whence they had come. The restoration had its origin in the South, with Thebes as its given headquarters. The XVIIth Dynasty was still tributary to the Hyksos, but it took up the struggle against them and Ahmose, founder of the glorious XVIIIth Dynasty, defeated them definitely, conquered their capital, drove them beyond the eastern desert, and pursued them right into Palestine.

Ahmose ascended the throne around 1580 B.C. and this marks the beginning of a new period in Egyptian history, the period of the *New Empire.* It is called 'empire' and not merely 'kingdom' because Egypt now extended its power far beyond its natural borders. The Hyksos domination had destroyed feudalism, the power of local sires; and the new state, born from war, was and remained for centuries a military state. Pharaoh was now, first of all, supreme commander of a great army of archers and of war chariots, for the horse had been introduced from Asia. And while the king in the past used to be pictured worshiping the gods, he is now depicted fighting the enemy in his chariot at the head of an army.

The XVIIIth Dynasty produced brilliant rulers, men and women: Amenhotep I, who fought campaigns in Nubia, Libya, and Syria and consolidated the empire; Thutmose I, who pushed the southern frontier to the fourth cataract and claimed the Euphrates as his northern borderline; Hatshepsut, a great queen, the first woman to wear the crown of the two Egypts, the 'female Horus,' who erected magnificent buildings, reopened the copper mines of Sinai, revived foreign trade, re-established the sea route to Punt. Her husband, Thutmose III, ruled after her death for over half a century, from 1501 to 1447 B.C., and is remembered as the greatest general that Egypt ever produced. In six Asiatic campaigns he defeated a league of rebellious princes and consolidated for over a century Egypt's domination over Western Asia. His warships cruised in the Eastern Mediterranean and an Egyptian governor administered the Aegean isles.

Never was Egypt stronger and never wealthier. The wars brought large numbers of slaves to the country, thus increasing the resources of manpower. From north and east and south every year tribute was poured into the treasury in the form of gold, precious stones, woods, textiles, and drugs, and on New Year's Day Pharaoh presented the members of his court with gifts, not land that had to be tilled, as in the past, but luxuries.[39] The tomb of Tutenkhamon, found untouched and excavated recently by the Earl of Carnavon and Howard Carter, has given the best possible picture of the arts and crafts in the fourteenth century B.C.[40] It is a highly developed, refined art that reveals the full mastery of techniques, but it cannot be denied that it shows the early signs of decadence.

A great religious movement must be mentioned here that took place during the XVIIIth Dynasty, the attempt of Amenhotep IV to establish a monotheistic religion. In the Old and Middle Kingdoms priesthood had, as a rule, been an office held incidentally by laymen [41] much as it used to be in ancient Rome. At the time of the

New Empire, however, priesthood became a profession and a very influential one, because the temples became extremely wealthy. The gods had originally been local deities and their importance was to a large extent determined by the part played by a given locality. Thus when Thebes became the brilliant capital of a great empire, Thebes' god Amon became the supreme deity, and the High Priest of Amon was as influential a man as the highest army commander or state official. His wife was called the god's chief concubine, just as the queen was the Divine Consort.

Amenhotep IV abolished the cult of Amon and all local cults and established instead as religion of the state a solar monotheism, the worship of the Sun god, of Re-Aton:

> Thou shinest beautiful on the horizon of heaven,
> O Living Disk, who didst live from the beginning.
> When thou risest in the Eastern Horizon
> Thou fillest every land with thy beauty.
> Thy rays embrace the lands even to the limit
> Of all thou hast created. Thou art Re.
> Thou reachest unto every land, uniting all
> For thy beloved son Ikhnaton.[42]

Ikhnaton was the name that Amenhotep adopted and he built a new residence Akhetaton. He was only eleven years old when he ascended the throne and he died in his twenties. He is represented with a strangely elongated skull and rather feminine features.[43] There has been some speculation about his personal part in the movement, whether he himself was the great reformer or whether he was the tool of forces behind the throne.[44] However that may be, the new religion never became universal. It was a product of the court and never took hold of the masses. Albright also pointed out that it did not lay any stress on social justice, on the welfare of the people,[45] but, first of all, antagonized the vested interests of a hierarchy that had become extremely powerful. After Ikhnaton's death the reaction set in from Thebes and was carried through with great violence. Every vestige of the heretic king was wiped out except in Lower Egypt, where the cult must have persisted for some time. And it left profound traces in art and literature.

Ikhnaton had only daughters. His son-in-law and successor, Tutenkhaton, under the pressure of the reaction changed his name to Tutenkhamon. He too died young, and soon thereafter, around 1350 B.C., the dynasty that had seen Egypt's greatest expansion died out. The rulers of the next, the XIXth Dynasty, traced their ancestry back to the Hyksos. A general of Ikhnaton, Harmhab, founded the dynasty whose most forceful kings were Seti I and Ramses II. They succeeded in holding the empire together in spite of the interplay of strong disintegrating forces, and we still can see the colossal portrait statues and other monuments that they erected to themselves. Palestine was tributary to Ramses II, and he is believed to be the Pharaoh who in the thirteenth century B.C. enslaved the Hebrews. But he was unable to drive the Hittites out of Syria. Bronze and iron clashed for the first time. The Egyptian troops armed with bronze weapons faced soldiers who fought them with iron. The Bronze Age was coming to an end.

The decline of the Egyptian Empire was now steady and inevitable. Life continued, of course, for many centuries. Frankincense was burned and gods were worshiped in gigantic temples now as before. Walls were covered with pictures, and books were written. The dead were embalmed and their mummies were kept in painted sarcophagi. And every year in June the Nile began to rise and flooded the land in eternal rhythm. But Egyptian civilization had spent its momentum; it had lost its creative power. Artistic, literary, and scientific production amounted to a mere repetition of formulae. Wars were fought with foreign mercenaries hired for the purpose. From the tenth century on and for almost three thousand years Egypt was no longer an independent country. Pharaohs continued to rule the people, but they became tributaries to foreign powers, to the Libyans in 945, the Ethiopians in 712, the Assyrians in 670, the Persians in 525; and in 332 B.C., the country was conquered by Alexander the Great.

NOTES

1. Translation by T. Eric Peet in *A Comparative Study of the Literatures of Egypt, Palestine, and Mesopotamia*, London, 1931, pp. 77-8. This and

other quotations from this book by permission of the Oxford University Press.

2. Δῶρον τοῦ ποταμοῦ, Herodotus, II, 5.
3. Ibid. II, 18.
4. The views are summarized and discussed by Herodotus, II, 20-27, and Diodorus, I, 38-41.
5. Diodorus, I, 36, 8.
6. Ibid. I, 36, 10.
7. Strabo, 17, 1, 48.
8. See the famous 'Famine Stele' of Doser in G. Roeder, *Urkunden zur Religion des alten Aegypten*, Jena, 1915, p. 177ff.; also Genesis, 41.
9. A. Moret and G. Davy, *Des Clans aux empires, l'organisation sociale chez les primitifs et dans l'orient ancien*, Paris, 1923 (*From Tribe to Empire*, London, 1926).
10. Namely 1 day every 4 years, or 10 days in 40 years.
11. See one of the most recent discussions, J. W. S. Sewell, 'The Calendars and Chronology,' *The Legacy of Egypt*, edited by S. R. K. Glanville, Oxford, 1942, pp. 1-15. For further literature on chronology see note 30.
12. Ramses II.
13. Herodotus, II, 109.
14. About Egyptian mathematics see T. E. Peet, *The Rhind Mathematical Papyrus*, Liverpool, 1923; Chace, Bull, Manning, and Archibald, *The Rhind Mathematical Papyrus*, Math. Assoc. of America, Oberlin, Ohio, 1929 (with photographic reproduction of the papyrus and a most complete bibliography of Egyptian mathematics); W. W. Struve, 'Mathematischer Papyrus des Staatlichen Museums der Schönen Künste in Moskau,' *Quellen und Studien zur Geschichte der Mathematik*, Abt. A 1, Berlin, 1930; O. Neugebauer, *Die Grundlagen der ägyptischen Bruchrechnung*, Berlin, 1926; K. Vogel, *Die Grundlagen der ägyptischen Mathematik*, Munich, 1929; T. E. Peet, 'Mathematics in Ancient Egypt,' *Bull. John Rylands Library*, 1931, 15:409-41; Max Simon, *Geschichte der Mathematik im Altertum*, Berlin, 1909; Abel Rey, *La Science orientale avant les Grecs*, Paris, 1930; O. Neugebauer, *Geschichte der antiken mathematischen Wissenschaften*, vol. 1: *Vorgriechische Mathematik*, Berlin, 1934.
15. Herodotus, II, 77.
16. The figures are those of the League of Nations, Health Organisation, *Annual Epidemiological Report, Corrected Statistics of Notifiable Diseases for the Year* 1938, Geneva, 1941; and *Statistical Year-Book of the League of Nations*, 1942-44, Geneva, 1945. Health conditions are worse than the figures indicate, because reliable statistics are available only for a third of the population, namely that living in cities and towns that have Health Bureaus.
17. Quoted from Moret and Davy, loc. cit. p. 34.
18. Diodorus, I, 31. According to Herodotus, II, 177, the number of 'inhabited cities' at the time of Amasis (6th century B.C.) was 20,000. Diodorus, I, 31, refers to over 30,000 villages and cities at the time of Ptolemy Lagus, the general of Alexander who reigned in Egypt from 323 to 283. Josephus in

his *Jewish War*, II, 385, writing about a century after Diodorus, refers to the population of Egypt as numbering 7,500,000 exclusive of Alexandria.

19. League of Nations, Health Organisation, *Annual Epidemiological Report . . . for* 1938, Geneva, 1941, p. 60.
20. League of Nations, Health Organisation, *International Health Year Book*, 1930, vol. VI, Geneva, 1932, pp. 194-5. Conditions are improving through the efforts of the government which has recently created 182 rural health centers.
21. We are well informed about the occurrence of malaria at that time through the Hippocratic writings, most of which were written in that very region.
22. Strabo, 17, 1, 7.
23. The number of reported cases in 1937 was 36,238 with 141 reported deaths; in 1938 it was 17,511 with 68 deaths. See League of Nations, Health Organisation, *Annual Epidemiological Report . . . for* 1938, Geneva, 1941, p. 51.
24. T. W. Kirkpatrick, *The Mosquitoes of Egypt*, Cairo, Government Press, 1925, p. 168.
25. 'Ankylostomiasis and Bilharziasis in Egypt,' *Reports and Notes of the Public Health Laboratories*, no. 6, Cairo, Government Press, 1924; for these and other diseases see also F. M. Sandwith, *The Medical Diseases of Egypt*, London, 1905.
26. The annual number of deaths from diarrhea and enteritis per 100,000 population is around 1000. In other words 1 per cent of the population dies every year from these—preventable—diseases. See League of Nations, Health Organisation . . . loc. cit. p. 71.
27. Max Meyerhof, 'A Short History of Ophthalmology in Egypt,' *Bull. Ophth. Soc. Egypt*, 1927, 20:33-52; 'Cinquante Ans de progrès ophtalmologique en Egypte,' *Folia ophthalmologica orientalia*, 1932, 1:1-25.
28. Diodorus, I, 31, 6: Ἡ μὲν οὖν Αἴγυπτος πανταχόθεν φυσικῶς ὀχύρωται.
29. About general history of ancient Egypt see *The Cambridge Ancient History*, vols. I-II, Cambridge, 1923-4; J. H. Breasted, *History of the Ancient Egyptians*, New York, 1913; *History of Egypt*, 2nd ed., New York, 1924; H. R. H. Hall, *The Ancient History of the Near East*, 7th ed., London, 1927; Eduard Meyer, *Geschichte des Altertums*, Stuttgart, 1925-34, 7 parts in 4 vols.; A. Moret, *L'Egypte pharaonique*, Paris, 1932.
30. From 2000 B.C. on the chronology of Egypt is well established but there is no unanimity of opinion for the preceding periods. Breasted and Meyer (*Die ältere Chronologie Babyloniens, Assyriens und Aegyptens*, Stuttgart, Berlin, 1925) assumed that the unification of Egypt by Menes took place around 3360 or 3315. J. W. S. Sewell, in *The Legacy of Egypt*, Oxford, 1942, p. 11, sets the reign of Menes at 3188-3141. Since Scharff's studies (*Hist. Zschr.*, 1939, 161:3-32) Egyptologists are inclined to date the beginning of the Ist Dynasty around 3000 or even later. See also W. F. Albright, *Ann. Am. Sch. Or. Res.*, 1926, 6:72f.
31. A. Moret, *The Nile and Egyptian Civilization*, London, 1927, p. 465.
32. H. Schneider, *Kultur und Denken der alten Aegypter*, Leipzig, 1907, p. 39ff.

33. Moret, *The Nile and Egyptian Civilization*, London, 1927, p. 139f.
34. Ibid. p. 188.
35. Ibid. p. 220ff. and an excellent discussion in W. F. Albright, *From the Stone Age to Christianity*, Baltimore, 1940, p. 135ff.
36. Fragments from *Admonitions of an Old Sage*, quoted from Moret, *The Nile and Egyptian Civilization*, p. 225. Quoted by permission of Routledge & Kegan Paul, Ltd.
37. See Moret's lengthy discussion of the subject, loc. cit. p. 252ff.
38. J. H. Breasted, *A History of Egypt*, 2nd ed., New York, 1924, p. 168f.
39. See J. H. Breasted in *Cambridge Ancient History*, Cambridge, 1924, vol. II, p. 98ff.
40. Howard Carter, *The Tomb of Tut-ankh-Amen*, London, 1923-33, 3 vols.
41. See Breasted, loc. cit., II, pp. 49ff.
42. The beginning of Ikhnaton's famous 'Hymn to the Sun' in the adaptation of J. Mayer and T. Prideaux in *Never to Die, the Egyptians in Their Own Words*, New York, 1938, p. 162.
43. See F. Proskauer, 'Zur Pathologie der Amarnazeit,' *Zschr. ägypt. Sprache*, 1932, 68:114-19; E. Snorrason, 'Cranial Deformation in the Reign of Akhnaton,' *Bull. Hist. Med.*, 1946, 20:601-10; P. Ghalioungui, 'A Medical Study of Akhenaten,' *Annales Serv. Antiqu. Egypte*, 1947, 47:29-46, 11 figs.
44. W. F. Albright, *loc. cit.* p. 166f.
45. Ibid. p. 168.

*

2. Social and Economic Conditions

In giving this brief outline of the setting of ancient Egyptian civilization in time and space, we were not concerned with medicine but with the people who created Egyptian medicine and with the country in which they lived. In discussing the geography of the land, however, we have already obtained an idea of the diseases, of some at least, that plagued the people, because the prevalence of disease is largely the result of geographic factors. Another set of such determining factors is to be sought in the social and economic conditions under which the people live. After having discussed the physical environment in which Egyptian life unfolded itself, we must now examine the equally important social environment. This will bring us much closer to the medical field because we shall hear not only of conditions conducive or inimical to health but also of man's reaction to these conditions, of his attempts to promote health and prevent illness.

Before we enter into a discussion of living and working conditions in ancient Egypt, however, we must be aware of one possible objection that might be made to such a presentation. Ancient Egypt has a history of over 3000 years and many conditions obviously changed in the course of time. Is it, therefore, permissible to discuss such aspects of Egyptian life as nutrition, housing, clothing as a whole without specifying each time whether we mean a condition prevailing under the Old Kingdom, or the Middle Kingdom, or the New Empire?

Such an objection is very justified in view of the fact that our sources are very uneven and haphazard. Egyptian life must be reconstructed from an infinity of scattered archaeological and literary sources [1] and while they are abundant for certain periods they are very scarce for others. We also know from our own experience how rapidly living conditions can change, how different our present diet, clothing, and housing are from those of our grandparents.

This is undoubtedly true, but we must remember that in the pre-industrial age living conditions were much more static than they are today. And the Orient is still in the pre-industrial age, so that many techniques, customs, and habits have remained unchanged for thousands of years. This is particularly the case in a country like Egypt, where the people live on a small area that has an unchanging strong natural rhythm set by the river. H. R. Hall very justly remarks: [2]

> So far as the life of the common people is concerned, Egypt is the most amazingly unchanging country in the world, it has changed less even than China. The life of the fellah of the XIIth or even of the IVth Dynasty is much the same as it is to-day. The change of religion to Christianity and then to Islam has altered nothing but the form of prayer: the changes of political allegiance have mattered nothing at all. The agricultural and urban classes were differentiated just as they are to-day.

If life has changed so little we are certainly justified in making use of such late sources as Herodotus and even Diodorus.

DAILY LIFE

A child was to be born, and the prospective mother felt the first pains of labor.[3] She was very young; Egyptian girls married at the age of 12 or 13, as they still do today; and their husbands were hardly more than 15 or 16. All over the East people did and still do marry very young, as soon as puberty has set in, and women age very rapidly. Today with the spread of education the upper classes marry somewhat later, but child marriage remains the rule with the common people. Colonial governments, in order to protect the young people's health, have repeatedly tried to raise the legal age for marriage. Thus in British India the Sarda Act of 1930 made fourteen years the minimum age for marriage for girls, but such laws are difficult to enforce.

Child marriage, therefore, was not peculiar to ancient Egypt, but we do find a custom that was almost unique among civilized peoples, namely, marriage between brother and sister.[4] It must have been a very old custom, because Isis married her brother, Osiris, and Nephthys her brother, Seth. Marriage with the sister was very frequent in the ruling house, and it is not astonishing that the king, being an incarnation of the deity on earth, followed the divine example and adopted a custom that kept the divine royal blood pure. In the course of time the court and the lower classes did as their ruler did, and in Ptolemaic and Roman days marriage with the sister was the rule in Egypt. In the second century after Christ fully two-thirds of the inhabitants of the city of Arsinoe were married to brother or sister.[5] This condition seemed strange to the Greek observers, who called it 'contrary to the general custom of mankind.'[6] Indeed, the question must be raised whether such close consanguineous marriage must not necessarily lead to degeneration. The legislation of all modern countries forbids marriage with the sister or half-sister, and until recently the common view was that such unions were sterile, or when there were offspring, that the children were usually weak, inclined to have symptoms of deaf-mutism, idiocy, or other mental diseases.

Marc Armand Ruffer in one of his finest studies examined the physical effects of consanguineous marriages in the royal families of ancient Egypt [7] and came to the conclusion that no evil effects could be noticed. He pointed out that the XVIIIth Dynasty, in which consanguineous marriage was the rule, produced nine distinguished rulers, the greatest figures in Egyptian history. The Ptolemies provide a good field of study because the first four kings issued from non-consanguineous marriages while from Ptolemy V to Ptolemy XV marriage with the sister was the rule. No difference could be found between the two groups, and the average age of the Ptolemies—not counting those who were murdered—was 64 years, a remarkable record.

These findings are in accordance with the experience of the geneticists. After all, the best race horses and dogs are bred through incestuous union, and it is only when hereditary diseases occur in an individual that close inbreeding becomes inadvisable. At any rate there is no indication whatever for the assumptions that the downfall of Egyptian civilization might have been due to degeneracy of the race resulting from consanguineous marriage.

Monogamy was the rule in Egypt as everywhere, for economic reasons, because few people could afford to support more than one household; but there was no legal barrier to a man's having several wives and, of course, an unlimited number of concubines. The king and the noblemen had their harems then as they had them in Mohammedan times.

Whenever we study ancient civilizations, we must always keep in mind that their sex life and sex morals were different from ours. Sexual intercourse was not considered a sinful act that had to be excused and justified. There were taboos, to be sure, and Herodotus relates that 'it was the Egyptians who first made it a matter of religious observance not to have intercourse with women in temples, nor enter a temple after such intercourse without washing,' [8] and we shall find more taboos in the Old Testament. The attitude toward sex, nevertheless, was infinitely freer than under Christianity. Since people of all classes married young, they had normal sex relations from the time they felt the urge, and thus escaped frustrations that many young people experience in modern society. Slave girls were probably available in all wealthier households and were ever ready to satisfy the desires of the lord or his sons. There was no fear of having many children. Infant mortality was probably high [9] and reduced their number automatically; in an agrarian and in a feudal society, moreover, children are never unwelcome because they represent cheap labor. Ramses II had at least 170 children, and an official of the Middle Kingdom by name of Baba had 60.[10] Prostitution was an accepted institution that served primarily the needs of men who were away from their homes, travelers and soldiers.

If a married couple had no children, who was responsible, the husband or the wife? When was a woman pregnant and when not? And if she was pregnant, would she give birth to a boy or to a girl? These are questions that parents have asked at all times and it is no wonder that methods had been devised very early in order to find an answer to them. The measures applied may seem strange today but we should not simply label them 'most absurd superstitions,' as W. Wreszinski did in the case of birth prognoses of the Berlin Papyrus 3038,[10a] because, after all, there is a sound idea behind all these prescriptions. It is perfectly correct to assume that the body of the woman who has conceived is different from what it was before and that this difference should manifest itself in the early stages, if not in the general appearance of the woman then perhaps in her urine. Since Aschheim and Zondek this does not seem absurd at all but, of course, the Egyptian method was not scientific:

> . . . you shall put wheat and barley into purses of cloth, the woman shall pass her water on it every day—it being mixed with dates and sand. If both sprout she will give birth; if the wheat sprouts, she will give birth to a boy; if the barley sprouts, she will give birth to a girl; if they do not sprout, she will not give birth at all.[10b]

When the young woman felt the first pains of labor, she called for a few fellow women, usually two, to assist her, members of her household or neighbors. She retired to a corner of the house where in anticipation of the event she had placed statuettes of Bes and Thoeris.[11] She knew that she would need their protection, because a woman in childbirth is weak and preoccupied and thus falls an easy prey to evil spirits unless she is protected. And who could do this better than Bes and Thoeris? Bes, an African deity by origin, was an ugly fellow, and this was the very source of his power. He was a dwarf with short limbs, a big belly, an animal-like face with bulging eyes. He was frequently clothed with a panther skin with claws, had a wild headdress, and wore a metal disc around his neck. This made him a veritable collection of apotropaic implements, and he was better equipped than anybody else to frighten and chase off the evil spirits and to catch and neutralize the evil eye. People therefore had him around whenever they felt particularly exposed to the spirits, at night when sleep had obliterated all vigilance or during the ecstasy of love. At the time of the New Empire the figure of Bes appears sometimes carved on the headrest. He is also found on the handle of mirrors, because a woman provokes the envy of the spirits when she admires her beauty in the mirror, and adds to it by painting eyebrows and lips. It is no wonder that Bes was ever present when a woman was in childbirth.

Thoeris, on the other hand, was the special protectress of pregnant women. She herself had given birth to the world. She appears with the features of a pregnant hippopotamus standing on her hind legs. Sometimes she holds the hieroglyph that means 'protection' in one paw and the sign of life in the other. Her statues are usually small, having been used as amulets, but there are also larger ones. Two of them in the Berlin Museum are hollow, and pregnant women praying to the goddess put bits of their clothes into them. Another statue also in the Berlin Museum could be filled with milk that dripped out of the breasts, probably the votive offering of a mother who was afraid that her milk would give out.[12]

When the pains of labor set in, the woman knelt down, sitting on her heels. She knelt on two or four flat stones or bricks so that there would be more room under her for the child to come out. One helping woman held her back while the other knelt in front ready to receive the child. Cephalic presentation was considered the normal position of the child, as indicated by the hieroglyph that serves as determinative for 'to give birth to.' Another hieroglyph represents the highly pregnant woman kneeling, and a third, later and even more realistic, shows the woman kneeling on the stones while the child is just delivered.[13] 'To sit on bricks' or 'on stones' became synonymous with 'to give birth to,' [14] and when the parallel bricks were connected by a transversal one, a kind of parturition chair was constructed, ancestor to the *Kursie el-wilada* that Egyptian women often use today.

Women of wealth had more than two helpers, and goddesses or the queen-goddesses gave birth in houses specially constructed for the purpose. The reliefs in Hatshepsut's temple at Deir el-Bahri give a splendid picture of the queen's birth from the moment her mother Ahmes conceives to the moment the royal child is given the breast by a divine nurse.[15] Only women of the aristocracy had wet nurses; the overwhelming majority of all mothers nursed their children themselves and usually did it for a long time, up to three years, as is still the case today. This long period of nursing was owing to economic reasons on one side, because mother's milk was the cheapest and simplest food to provide for the child; and on the other hand nursing prevented conception, and although children were welcome, the long period of nursing was a natural protective mechanism that prevented mothers from having a child every year. The desire for contraceptives did actually exist, although it must have been limited to very small social groups. The recipes preserved consist of fumigations or irrigations of the vagina with certain drugs, but the texts are mutilated and it is difficult to decide whether the measures were effective or not.[16] Other recipes have come down to us telling how to cause abortion, because in Egypt as everywhere situations must have arisen under which it was undesirable for a woman to have a child.[17]

Egyptian boys were circumcised probably between the age of 6 and 12, or just before adolescence. It is a strange ritual operation that became highly characteristic of the Jewish and Mohammedan religions and is widespread among the Negroes of Africa. It is still controversial how general circumcision was in Egypt and what meaning it had. The archaeological and literary sources, scenes representing the operation,[18] pictures and statues of nude circumcised figures, the evidence of classical writers and of papyri of the Roman period, and, last but not least, the mummies of undoubtedly circumcised individuals are not too numerous and not always unequivocal.[19] It seems certain that at no time was circumcision practiced on all males as is the casė in Judaism and Islam. It also seems that it was not a rite limited to and distinctive of the priesthood, because mummies of kings have been found that showed no trace of circumcision, and on the other hand there are pictures of shepherds, fishermen, sailors, and other common people from the Old Kingdom who were clearly circumcised. From all evidence, we may conclude that the rite, although never universal so that it never assumed the significance it had later in other civilizations, yet was widespread at times; and in the Roman period it was practically required for the priests. The Romans tried to discourage circumcision but could not suppress it, because certain religious acts could be performed only by officiants who were circumcised.[20]

This also clearly reveals the religious character of the rite. Herodotus thought that it was practiced for reasons of hygiene when he wrote: 'They practise circumcision for cleanliness' sake; for they set cleanliness above seemliness,'[21] a statement that is obviously wrong. The operation was performed in temples, not by physicians but by priests,[22] with a stone knife and not a bronze one, a detail that shows that the custom was old. It may be that it was an initiation particularly into the cult of Re, as Foucart pointed out,[23] because an old tradition related that blood fell from the phallus of the god when he performed his own mutilation. Circumcision thus would be an imitation of the god's mutilating operation. However it may be, there can be no doubt in regard to its religious character.

Strabo relates that the Egyptians 'circumcise the males and excise the females.'[24] By ἐκτέμνειν he apparently means the resection or 'cutting out' of the clitoris and labia minora or at least of parts of them. There are no early sources to this operation but it is very probable that it was practiced long before Strabo's time. It is still practiced today among the poorer classes of Egypt[25] and particularly also in Nubia, where it is combined with infibulation.[26]

'Most of the children are reared without shoes or clothing because of the mildness of the climate of the country,' Diodorus said,[27] and this was true for Egypt as it still is for the entire tropical and subtropical East. Indeed the climate did hardly require more than a blanket at night and possibly a headdress to protect one from insolation. Whatever clothing the Egyptians wore was for the purpose of decoration or to increase the sex stimulus or for magical ends. Modesty in the Christian sense was entirely unknown, and a nude body was certainly less alluring than one clad in a diaphanous slip.

Herodotus tells us that in Egypt 'every man has two garments, every woman only one,' [28] which was basically correct, although fashions changed in Egypt as they do everywhere. The dress was the tropical one derived from the girdle. It consisted for men of a loincloth, which, according to the prevailing fashion, was worn tight or loose, short or long, and of a second garment that was a kind of shirt or tunic that varied a great deal in style and was by no means worn all the time. Egyptians, particularly of the Old Kingdom, are usually represented wearing only one piece of clothing. Laborers at work never wore more, if they wore that much. They frequently had nothing but a simple girdle tied in front with a knot which originally undoubtedly had magical significance.

The women's single garment was a slip that reached from under the breasts to the ankles and was held up by bands over the shoulders. It was worn very tightly during the Old Kingdom, became somewhat looser later, but even so did not permit much motion; women at work, maidservants, and dancers wore like the men a loincloth or girdle. Sandals and a kerchief for women, a linen cap for men completed the costume.

The material of all clothing was linen, usually worn white. Cotton and silk were unknown and the woolen mantles, mentioned by Herodotus,[29] seem to have come into use only in Greek times.

The costume that had remained relatively simple for two thousand years became very elaborate during the New Empire. The loincloth developed into a ruffled or pleated skirt and the ample tunic had flowing sleeves. Women of the upper classes now frequently had a second garment also and, when formally dressed, men and women wore heavy wigs.

This is not the place to discuss the history of the Egyptian costume [30] and the vagaries of fashion, since our interest lies primarily in the hygienic aspect of clothing; from this point of view the Egyptian dress was undoubtedly sound. It left enough surface free and did not impede the movements of the body. The only objectionable part was the wig, which was heavy and hot and hard to keep clean; but it was used only by a small upper class and only on formal occasions. Nor is this the place to discuss the exquisite jewelry, the bracelets and anklets, the collars, necklaces, and girdles, the pins and rings, that rich Egyptians wore and of which the tomb of Tutenkhamon has given us such an excellent picture. Jewels, in Egypt as everywhere, served not only esthetic purposes but were first of all amulets intended to protect their bearers.

It is a general rule that the less clothing a people wears, the cleaner it keeps the body. The Egyptians were no exception to this rule, and rich and poor washed frequently, morning and evening and before every meal. The richer houses had bathrooms, not with tubs like ours,[31] but more like the Greek bath, a place where hot water was poured over the bather. Soap was still unknown and soda was used as cleansing material. And a wide use was made of ointments to prevent the skin from becoming too dry. Ointments and aromatic oils were considered an absolute necessity for all classes of society. The Proverbs of Ptahhotep recommending marriage say: 'If thou be wise, marry. Love thy wife sincerely. Fill her belly and clothe her back. Oil is the remedy for her body. Make glad her heart all thy life. She is a profitable field for her lord.'[32] Ointments were part of the wages paid to workers, and at the time of Ramses III workers of the necropolis of Thebes struck and the complaint they addressed to their employers, the priests, said: 'We have come because we are hungry and thirsty. We have no clothes, we have no ointments, we have no fish, we have no greens.'[33]

The Egyptian lady washed her body, shaved it with a bronze razor, used tweezers to remove reluctant hair, anointed her skin, made a wide use of perfumes, painted her lips and her cheeks, and took particular care in painting her eyes. In the days of the first Dynasties, the lower lid was painted green and the upper lid black.[34] Later both lids were kept black so that the white of the eye would be the more brilliant. The most common eye paint was lead sulphide.[35] The great emphasis placed on the painting of the eyes makes it probable that it had not only cosmetic but also magic significance.[36]

In Egypt as in every civilized country, women took great care of their hair, washed it, anointed it, wore it longer or shorter, in plaits. in curls, or straight, according to the prevailing fashion. Men were shaven as a rule, and certain categories of priests, in the later periods at least, shaved the head also.[37] We mentioned before that members of the court and the nobility wore wigs on formal occasions, and we may add that they, and particularly the king, also wore artificial beards. These strange customs are undoubtedly parts of a ritual, reminiscences of a costume that had been given up in daily life centuries before but preserved in the cult.[38]

The Egyptians' hair was black, and women as well as men disliked its turning gray, indicative of old age, and also disliked losing hair and becoming bald. The doctors had remedies.[39] Against grizzling, they recommended anointing the head with oil that contained blood of a black calf or of a black ox, or fat of a black snake. More complicated was a prescription that consisted of the womb of a she-cat, raven's egg, oil, and laudanum, boiled and applied to the head. Rare fats were used 'to make the hair of a bald-headed person grow,' namely fat of a lion, fat of hippopotamus, fat of crocodile, fat of cat, fat of serpent, and fat of ibex, mixed together. For spotted baldness the head was anointed with oil that contained the burnt quills of a hedgehog.

It would be interesting to examine such recipes in detail. Many are purely magical, but at the same time reflect certain biological views. The animals whose blood is used against graying hair must be black, but it is not their skin or hair that is used; it is their blood. In other words, it is believed that the blood possesses the black-making property. Other recipes are purely empirico-rational, like the one that prescribes anointing of the head with oil and turpentine to make the hair grow.[40] All in all, these ancient Egyptian remedies were probably as effective and ineffective as our present innumerable hair tonics.

The Greek travelers were struck by the Egyptians' cleanliness. 'They drink from cups of bronze which they cleanse out daily,' Herodotus wrote,[41] adding, 'this is done not by some but by all. They are especially careful ever to wear newly washed linen raiment.' In Hellenistic times—and this may well have been a very old custom—the Egyptians tried to be clean not only externally but also internally, by evacuating the intestinal tract with emetics and enemas on three consecutive days every month, according to Herodotus,[42] or 'sometimes at intervals of three or four days,' according to Diodorus.[43] The Greek observers and probably also the Egyptians who gave them the information explained the custom rationally, saying that the people believed that diseases were engendered by superfluities of the food. It may well be, however, that the origin of this custom was religious, like that of many other precepts of purity.

The Greek travelers were amused to find that Egyptian customs were often contrary to their own. Herodotus wrote: [44]

> Among them, the women buy and sell, the men abide at home and weave, and whereas in weaving all others push the woof upwards, the Egyptians push it downwards. Men carry burdens on their heads, women on their shoulders. Women make water standing, men sitting. They relieve nature indoors, and eat out of doors in the streets giving the reason that things unseemly but necessary should be done in secret, things not unseemly should be done openly.

Egypt was a fertile country and food was plentiful, unless the land had been hit by a drought because the inundation had failed. In normal years large quantities of grain were grown that provided the staple food of the people, bread and beer. Three to four loaves of bread and two jars of beer were considered a good daily ration, not counting the onions that went with it.[45] Bread was baked in a great variety of kinds and shapes. Funeral lists speak of the kinds of bread and cake that had been given the dead on his journey to the Netherworld.[46] Some varieties were even imported from Asia.[47] The bread of the common people was very coarse. It was made from barley, spelt, or bearded wheat that was ground very primitively between two stones or in a handmill so that the flour still contained large quantities of husks and even straw and unbroken grains of cereals.[48] The teeth of Egyptian skulls show a high degree of attrition. In the Delta a kind of bread was made from dried lotus.[49]

Next to bread, fish was probably the most popular food and the chief source of protein to the common people. It was consumed in great quantities raw, roasted, or boiled, sun dried or pickled.[50] A great variety of birds was found along the river and in the marshes, ducks, quail, small birds. Hunting was an elegant pastime of the rich, who are sometimes represented hunting birds with a kind of boomerang.[51] Of domestic birds the goose was a great favorite and appeared roasted not only on the rich man's table.[52] Cattle were raised in the very beginnings of Egyptian history, and at the time of the New Empire the country had an abundance of cattle that provided meat, milk, and animal power. Sheep and goats were also kept, primarily for food, as there was not much demand for woolen fabrics. It seems that the pig was taboo, for it was not eaten.[53] To slaughter an ox or a cow, it was turned on its back and the arteries of the throat were cut with a metal knife. The blood was collected and examined to make sure that the animal was not possessed by a spirit, after which it was poured away.

Vegetables and fruits were plentiful, particularly onions, leeks, and garlic, various beans, melons, watermelons, cucumber, olives, dates, figs, and grapes.[54] The chief fat used for cooking was olive oil,[55] and honey was served for the sweetening of dishes.

The Egyptians, attached as they were to their river, thought that Nile water was the best water on earth, and when a princess married abroad she had Nile water sent to her from home.[56] The water was carried in goat-skin bags and cooled in the houses in porous clay jars. Milk was a popular drink in a country that was so rich in cattle. But the most popular beverage was beer, which was consumed by rich and poor. It was not like our beer, but rather like the so-called caffre-beer of which the Bantu are so fond today, or the Russian kvas or, as a matter of fact, the beer that the Egyptian farmers brew today. Barley or any other cereal was moistened and dug into the soil until it began to sprout. It was then ground coarsely; a dough was made with leaven added, and shaped into loaves, which were baked for a short time so that the interior remained raw. The loaves were then broken into pieces and put into a vat covered with water; the mixture was allowed to ferment for about a day, whereupon it was strained and the beer was ready.[57] It was a pale, foamy, and slightly acidulous drink. Hops were unknown but by adding other flavoring substances different brands of beer were produced.

While beer was everybody's drink, wine appeared probably only on the table of the rich. The vine had been cultivated in Egypt since pre-dynastic days, and Egyptian wines were famous until Islam destroyed vineyards here as all over the Near East. We shall see later that wine was widely used in medicine as a vehicle for drugs.

Drunkenness was apparently not rare and seems to have occurred in all layers of society, from the farmers to the gods. Banquets frequently ended with the guests, men and women, being sick, and this did not in any way seem shocking. But there were moralists who raised their voice against abuse of alcoholic drinks, and in the *Wisdom of Ani,* a late didactic book, it is said: [58]

> Take not upon thyself to drink a jug of beer. Thou speakest, and an unintelligible utterance issueth from thy mouth. If thou fallest down and thy limbs break, there is none to hold out a hand to thee. Thy companions in drink stand up and say: 'Away with this sot!' If there then cometh one to seek thee in order to question thee, thou art found lying on the ground, and thou art like a little child.

People also knew magic formulae that were intended to ward off the evil effect of intoxication.[59] Herodotus tells us that at rich men's banquets, after dinner 'a man carries round an image of a corpse in a coffin, painted and carved in exact imitation, a cubit or two cubits long. This he shows to each of the company, saying: "Drink and make merry, but look on this; for such shalt thou be when thou art dead." Such is the custom at their drinking-bouts.' [60]

The people had three meals a day; [61] the king and the court, however, five.[62] All in all, the Egyptian diet, with its coarse bread, milk, vegetables, fish, and occasional meat, was a well-balanced one, conducive to health, provided the people had enough to eat. This must have been the case as a rule, since the Nile Valley was fertile by nature and independent of local rainfall.

In a country that has the climate of Egypt, housing conditions are not so important a factor in the maintenance of health as they are in a northern climate, because life unfolds itself mostly in the open air. People frequently work, eat, and sleep out of doors. The house is a shelter that protects against the rays of the sun during the summer heat at the time of the siesta. It is the storehouse of the poor, in which the family keeps all its property. It is the seat of a self-supporting economic unit in the case of the rich man who owns enough land and people to produce all the food and basic commodities that the household may need.

Tombs, temples, and the gigantic statues of the gods were built of stone for all eternity. Many have survived the millennia—eloquent testimonies of Egyptian culture. But the dwellings of ordinary mortals were built of more perishable materials, and if we have some information about housing conditions in various periods of Egyptian history it is because houses and gardens were sometimes pictured on the walls of tombs, because clay models of dwellings were placed in tombs, and because archaeologists were able to excavate cities such as Kahun and El Amarna, cities that were abandoned or destroyed after having been inhabited for a century or less, so that their original ground plans are still recognizable today.[63]

In Egypt as in many other countries, the round hut built of poles and reed was the earliest form of dwelling. It was followed by the square hut made of the same materials. Diodorus is undoubtedly correct when he writes that 'traces of these customs still remain among the herdsmen of Egypt, all of whom, they say, have no other dwelling up to this time than one of reeds, considering that with this they are well enough provided for.'[64] The next step was the mud hut, the adobe house built of bricks baked in the sun, a porous building material very appropriate to the climate.

An ancient Egyptian city was probably not very different from the native section of an Oriental town today, with streets kept narrow to hold the sun out, with bazaars, with high walls behind which the houses of the rich were hidden. The workers' dwellings in Kahun were built back to back in long double rows. They were small, one-story units, with a front of only 20-32 feet, containing a few rooms, while the houses of the rich, built in a special section of the town, had up to 70 rooms.

Ikhnaton's city was to be a monument to the glory of Aton. It had broad avenues planted with trees. Workers' houses were not very different from those of Kahun, yet a little more spacious, and the better ones even had a bathroom and sometimes a toilet that could be flushed. Material civilization had undoubtedly progressed. The sewage was drained into the street, into a gutter built in the middle of the street.

In the course of time, with the development of the cities, houses grew in height and Diodorus reports that houses in Thebes had four and even five stories.[65] The advantage of the block house was that many people could live on a relatively small space. The rich, however, preferred the court house, a dwelling in which rooms opened into a court, the atrium of the Romans, the patio of Spain. Such a house was entirely oriented toward the interior. When balconies were added, they were built not toward the street but toward the court or garden. Rooms were ventilated by clerestory windows, which, of course, had no glass, and sometimes special ventilators were constructed on the roof so as to catch the north wind, the same device that is still being used today and is known as *malkaf*.[66] There was no need for heating in that climate; as fuel for cooking, dried cow dung and straw were used, more rarely also wood and charcoal.

The houses of the rich in town and country contained not only living and sleeping rooms and quarters for the servants, but also granaries and other storerooms, and workrooms for the craftsmen that belonged to a feudal household. Greatly valued in Egypt as in every desert country was the garden. It seemed to be the height of luxury to have a rich garden with ponds and many trees—sycamore, palm, fig, pomegranate, tamarisk, and others—and, of course, vines and many flowers with which to decorate the table.

Furniture, except in the palaces, was relatively sparse and simple, because such a large part of man's life took place out of doors. Poor people slept on the floor or on clay bunks along the wall, dressed and with a bundle of clothes as pillow. Rich people had beds of interlaced cord with piles of folded sheets as mattresses and a wooden headrest. And under the bed a chamber pot was kept for use during the night. Chairs were used from the first dynasties on, a fact that is remarkable when we remember that many Oriental people still squat. Chests and baskets were the containers that took the place of our cupboards, and mats sometimes covered the floors.

The houses were dark as a rule because windows were few. They were lit by lamps that consisted of saucers filled with salt impregnated with castor oil and on which a wick floated. The Egyptians were proverbially fond of pet animals and many had dogs, cats, tame monkeys, or ichneumons.

A warm country with periodic floods where organic material decomposed rapidly and water puddles stayed on for a long time obviously had many insects. We all know what a plague flies are in Egypt today, and it seems that the ancient Egyptians chased them away with the same kind of fly flaps used now. But they had an effective method of protecting themselves against mosquitoes and gnats. According to Herodotus,[67]

. . . gnats are abundant; this is how the Egyptians protect themselves against them: those who dwell higher up than the marshy country are well served by the towers whither they ascend to sleep, for the winds prevent the gnats from flying aloft; those living about the marshes have a different device, instead of the towers. Every man of them has a net with which he catches fish by day, and for the night he sets it round the bed where he rests, then creeps under it and so sleeps. If he sleep wrapped in a garment or cloth, the gnats bite through it; but through the net they do not even try at all to bite.

LABOR AND RECREATION

The worm hath taken half his corn, the hippopotamus the rest. Mice abound in the field, and the locust has descended. The cattle devour and the sparrows pilfer. Alas for the husbandman!

The remainder that lieth upon the threshing-floor, the thieves have made away with it. The ploughshare of copper hath perished, and the yoke of horses hath died at the threshing and ploughing.

And now the scribe landeth upon the embankment to register the harvest. His bodyguard carry sticks and his negroes palm-switches. They cry, Give up your corn. And there is none there. He is stretched out and beaten, he is bound thrown into the canal. His wife is bound before his eyes and his children put in fetters. His neighbors run away to look after their own corn.[68]

Situations such as the one described here in a text of the New Empire must have occurred endless times, since the lot of the Egyptian farmer was a hard one, in antiquity as it still is today.[69] Egypt was primarily an agricultural country and the overwhelming majority of the population consisted of farmers. They, together with the artisans whose status was at all times very much the same as that of the farmers, were the Egyptian people. Their toil created the wealth of the nation and it is highly regrettable that we do not know more about their life. The beating of a serf, the eviction of a free farmer, the working day of a weaver, and the wages of a miner were not matters to be recorded in hieroglyphs on the temple walls. If we know about them at all it is through incidental remarks, and it is little enough we do know. The only profession about which we are well informed is that of the scribes, because they wrote a great deal about themselves and glorified their estate on every opportunity.

It is very regrettable that we do not know more about labor conditions in ancient Egypt, because at all times and everywhere work is one of the chief determining factors of health and disease. Man by necessity spends the greater part of his conscious life working and it obviously makes a great difference under what conditions this work is done. Work in itself is not harmful to health; it is, on the contrary, essential to its maintenance, because it determines the chief rhythm of our life, balances it, and gives it meaning and significance. An organ that does not work atrophies and the mind that does not work becomes dumb. There is no greater joy than that of creation. The farmer who after months of labor and expectation sees the grain germinate, grow, and ripen with heavy ears, the craftsman who has just completed a beautiful piece of furniture, pottery, or cloth, both feel a satisfaction that is an important factor of health, mental and physical.

But work, on the other hand, may also be harmful to health, may become a chief cause of disease, when there is too much of it, when it is too hard, exceeding the capacity of an individual, when it is not properly balanced by rest and recreation, or when it is performed under adverse circumstances. The working conditions that make labor beneficial or harmful are not only the physical ones, the many factors that constitute the hygiene of labor, but also the relation of the worker to his raw materials and tools. It obviously makes a great difference whether farmers or artisans work as free men who own their means of production, or whether they are in the service of an employer; in the latter case it makes a difference whether they are hired under a contract or whether they are serfs or slaves.

It seems, although our information on the subject is rather scanty, that throughout the earlier part of Egyptian history the great majority of all farmers and artisans had the status of serfs, that is, that they were bound to the soil or to the shop.[70] Under the absolute monarchy of the Old Kingdom they were serfs to the king, who owned the land, or to one of the king's favorites who had been given some land. In the feudal state of the Middle Kingdom they were serfs to the king, to the nobility that owned large domains, and later also in increasing measure to the temples. The farmers tilled the soil, raised cattle and other animals, and delivered the product of their labor to their lords, retaining as wages a portion of the crop. How large this was we do not know; it was probably just enough to feed the family.

Herodotus, speaking of the Delta, makes the remark,[71]

> . . . there are no men, neither in the rest of Egypt, nor in the whole world, who get in their produce with so little labor; they have not the toil of ploughing up their land into furrows, nor of hoeing, nor of any other work which other men do to get them a crop; the river rises of itself, waters the field, and then sinks back again; thereupon each man sows his field and sends swine [72] into it to tread down the seed, and waits for the harvest; then he makes the swine to thresh his grain, and so garners it.

There is no doubt that the fertility of Egypt must have greatly impressed Greek travelers, who remembered the rocky soil of their homeland; but they overlooked the fact that a great deal of hard labor was required to keep the irrigation system functioning. Canals and dykes had to be repaired constantly, and in antiquity just as today many fields had to be irrigated by hand with water drawn from a well, the Arabic *shadūfa,* that can be seen today all over North Africa.

Thus the peasant was not only a farmer but a navvy as well, and he was, moreover, liable to forced labor at any time. He never knew when the king's overseers would come, take him away from the farm, press him into a gang to supplement slave labor in the building of pyramids, temples, roads, or other public construction. In spite of the fertility of the soil, the life of the farmer, therefore, was by no means an easy one; he was, on the contrary, very much exploited.

Conditions probably improved somewhat under the New Empire. In the bureaucratic state that developed at that time farmers who were not directly attached to the court or to the temple were allotted land by the state. They may have had the status of free tenants, as Moret believes,[73] but they remained heavily taxed and liable to forced labor. Their lot seems to have been better, however, than in the past: they had a legal status, and it is also probable that they were less frequently called upon for forced labor, since the number of slaves available for public works was very much greater in a period of extensive foreign conquests that brought in many prisoners of war.

Farm labor with primitive tools is always hard work, and the working day in the seasons after the inundation was, in all probability, from sunrise to sunset. The productivity of labor must have been as low then as it is today all over the Orient. High productivity can never be expected when working time is long and wages are very low. The farmer instinctively counteracted the evil effects of hard labor by slowing down and by dividing the work among as many people as possible. Next to the farmers who tilled the soil were the herdsmen who guarded the cattle in the pastures. They are usually depicted as wild people of rough manner, who let their hair grow; they were bird hunters and fishermen at times and were skilful in making mats.[74]

The craftsmen, as we mentioned before, had very much the same status as the farmers, that is, they also were serfs, attached to a shop that belonged to the king, a nobleman, or, later, a temple. The product of their labor they delivered to their lord and received in exchange as wages food for themselves and their families. They probably were also permitted to keep a portion of their products, which they traded on the market. They too were liable to forced labor; and, like the farmers, many of them became independent during the New Empire.

An interesting literary document from the beginning of the Middle Kingdom, which has been preserved in two manuscripts,[75] describes the hardships of the various trades. It is part of the so-called wisdom literature and is usually referred to as the *Instruction of Dwauf*. A father bringing his son to the capital where he is to study in the writing school exhorts him to work hard so as to be able to embrace the greatest of all professions, that of a scribe, and as a matter of contrast he pictures the various trades in darkest colors. It obviously is a satire and working conditions were not so bad as they were here described—just as the French physicians of the seventeenth century were not so stupid as Molière pictured them in his comedies. And yet Molière did not invent the character of his physicians, he simply exaggerated certain particular traits that he saw in them and to which he objected. Similarly the author of the *Instruction of Dwauf* did not invent the hardships of the various trades. They were real enough. He simply exaggerated certain aspects so that by contrast the profession of the scribe would stand out the more gloriously. If we keep in mind that we are dealing with a satire, we may use this document as a source to labor conditions in the Middle Kingdom. A few passages may be quoted as illustration.[76]

Never have I seen the stone worker sent on an embassy or the goldsmith dispatched on an errand. But I have seen the metal worker at his task at the mouth of his furnace. His fingers were like the hide of crocodiles; he stank worse than fish spawn.

Every workman who holds a chisel is wearier than he who hacks the ground; wood is his field and his hoe is the metal. At night when he is supposed to be free, he still toils more than his arms can do. In the night he burns a light.

The stone mason seeks work in every hard stone. When he has finished, his arms are destroyed and he is weary. When he sits down at dusk, his thighs and his back are broken.

The barber shaves till late in the evening. He goes from street to street seeking for men to shave. He strains his arms to fill his belly and works as indefatigably as a bee.

The boatman who carries his goods down to the Delta to get their price, works more than his arms can do; the gnats kill him.

The weaver in the workshop is worse off than the women [who also must always sit in the house]. He squats with his knees to his belly and does not breathe fresh air. He bribes the doorkeeper with bread that he may see the light.

The cobbler is very wretched; he is forever begging; he has nothing to bite but leather.

The fuller washeth upon the river bank, a near neighbor of the crocodile.

This certainly is a very dark picture that is exaggerated in many ways, although conditions must have been bad enough. Long hours of industrial work are backbreaking and there is no doubt that some of it was performed in ill-ventilated and dark rooms, until late into the night. We also know that the overseer was all too ready to activate the work with a whip of hippopotamus hide or a palm switch. Egyptians were beaten a great deal, not only the slaves and serfs but also the children at home and at school and adults in court. On the other hand, we must remember that industry was carried out on a small scale as house and handicraft industry. Much of it was undoubtedly performed in the open air, as we see it today in an Arabian *sūq* or bazar. This all reduced health hazards although it did not reduce the exploitation of labor inherent to the system. The best a working man could hope for was to feed his family. The number of those who succeeded in joining the small middle class or in obtaining posts in the administration could not have been large.

The gigantic buildings of the Pharaohs required an enormous supply of labor. One source, as we have seen, consisted of farmers and craftsmen, serfs and others, called up for forced labor. But this source was not unlimited, because the land could not be depleted of workers without dire consequences for the whole national economy. Another source of cheap labor was provided by the wars. Throughout antiquity prisoners of war and other foreign captives became slaves; they belonged to the state and were assigned from one administration to another wherever they were needed most urgently. Or it might happen that some of them were given away, to a general as a reward, or to a temple together with cattle and other goods.

These public workers, if we may call them thus, were organized in semi-military fashion, usually in gangs of 5, 10, and 100, with foremen of different ranks. The gangs worked and lived together and the foreman kept a record of his men. One very interesting such document has been preserved, in which a foreman kept a list of his 43 workers and indicated on which days some of them had been missing and for what reason. Illness was by far the chief cause of absenteeism.[77]

The laborers were housed close to their working place. The building of a pyramid took many years and in a city's necropolis construction never ended, so that it was worthwhile building mud huts for the workers. They lived with their families and were paid wages in kind, food mostly and a few other basic commodities such as firewood, a piece of linen for clothing, or ointments. They lived from hand to mouth without any reserves and when wages were not paid in time they simply starved. As the administration was frequently corrupt or at least inefficient, this happened quite often. The workers sometimes struck for their wages [78] and such strikes were not merely demonstrations; having no food the laborers had not the strength to work.

By far the hardest lot was that of the mine workers, particularly in the gold mines of Nubia, which were operated almost exclusively with convict labor. The journey to the mines was an ordeal in itself. Diodorus has given us a terrifying picture of working conditions as they existed there at the time of the Ptolemies and there is no reason to assume that they were any better in the days of the Pharaohs. He writes: [79]

In the extremities of Egypt, on the frontiers of Arabia and Ethiopia, there is a country with many and large mines of gold, which is recovered by much hard labor and expense. There the earth is of a black color and is full of streaks and veins of a remarkable whiteness, the lustre of which surpasses the most brilliant natural products. From this earth those who have charge of the mining operations obtain the gold by means of a large number of workers, for the kings of Egypt collect condemned prisoners, prisoners of war and others who, beset by false accusations, have been in a fit of anger thrown into prison; these, sometimes alone, sometimes with their entire families, they send to the gold mines; partly to exact a just vengeance for crimes committed by the condemned, partly to secure for themselves a big revenue through their toil.

Those who have been thus consigned are many, and all are fettered; they are held constantly at work by day and the whole night long without any rest, and are sedulously kept from any chance of escape. For their guards are foreign soldiers, all speaking different languages, so the workers are unable either by speech or by friendly entreaty to corrupt those who watch them. The hardest of the earth that contains the gold is exposed to a fierce fire, so that it cracks, and then they apply hand labor to it; the rock that is soft and can be reduced by a moderate effort is worked by thousands of the luckless creatures with iron tools that are ordinarily used for cutting stone. The foreman, who distinguishes one sort of rock from another, instructs the workers in the whole business and assigns their tasks. Of those who are condemned to this disastrous life such as excel in strength of body pound the shining rock with iron hammers, applying not skill but sheer force to the work, and they drive galleries, though not in a straight line, but in the direction taken naturally by the glistening stone; these then, on account of the windings of these passages, live in darkness, and carry around lamps attached to their foreheads. In accordance with the peculiarities of the rock they have to get into all sorts of positions and throw on the floor the pieces they detach. And this they do without ceasing, to comply with the cruelty and blows of an overseer. The young children make their way through the galleries into the hollowed portions and throw up with great toil the fragments of broken stone, and bring it outdoors to the ground outside the entrance. . . As these workers can take no care of their bodies and have not even a garment to hide their nakedness, there is no one, who seeing these luckless people would not pity them because of the excess of their misery, for there is no forgiveness or relaxation at all for the sick, or the maimed, or the old, or for women's weakness, but all with blows, are compelled to stick to their labor until worn out they die in servitude. Thus the poor wretches ever account the future more dreadful than the present because of the excess of their punishment and look to death as more desirable than life.

We admire the great artistic productions of ancient Egypt, the tombs, the temples, the statues, and obelisks. We are enchanted with the exquisite work of their handicrafts, the potteries, the jewels, the furniture, the thousands of bronze statuettes that fill our museums. We like the reliefs and paintings that adorned the interior of tombs and temples and give such a vivid picture of Egyptian life. But we often forget that these creations, great and small, are the result of the labor of millions of anonymous people, slaves and serfs and small freemen, who toiled for a bare living, who often sacrificed their health and their life for the enjoyment of a small upper class.

Work must be followed by rest. The energy spent in the process of production must be re-created. Rest and recreation are important factors of health, and sleep and food alone are not enough to restore a human being, because man is endowed with a mind and he experiences hopes and fears, joys and sorrows, love and hatred. Man must have emotional outlets; and hope and joy are as necessary for his well-being as sunshine is to the life of the plant. How did the Egyptians fare in this respect? [80]

We are much better informed about the amusements of the rich than about those of the poor. This is not only a matter of sources but is also owing to the fact that in antiquity and for many centuries thereafter the rich had all possible recreational facilities available to them while the poor had not. The Egyptian of means had his country house to which he retired at every opportunity, where he enjoyed the shade of his garden and the coolness of the pond. When he felt like having exercise and excitement he went hunting or fishing. Standing on a flat boat he had it pushed into the thickets of papyrus reed in the swamps along the river and shot birds with an old-fashioned boomerang-like instrument, or speared fish. Hunting remained the favorite sport of the noble and rich throughout the ages.

When the wealthy Egyptian felt like being entertained at home or wished to entertain visitors, he asked for musicians and dancers. A harpist and a flutist came, and a group of scantily dressed girls performed dances with great precision while others were beating the measure. Or a *tableau vivant* was cleverly staged. A large harem had great resources of talent, girls who could dance, sing, play instruments, play ball games, or juggle. Or professionals were hired for the purpose from outside. In the New Empire musicians and instruments were imported from Syria and orchestras became much more elaborate. If the lord was in the mood for some rougher entertainment, he ordered his people to wrestle in front of him. But when he wished to spend a quiet evening he played *senet* with a friend or *hounds and jackals,* games played on boards with various figures and knuckle bones.

It was easy for the rich to find relaxation but much more difficult for the poor, who worked long hours and were exhausted in the evening. Until very recently the people who worked hardest and needed recreation most could rarely hope for more than the satisfaction of some animal instincts with food, sexual intercourse, and sleep, and whatever spiritual satisfaction religion was able to give them.

The lot of the farmer was always a little better in this respect than that of the industrial worker. The latter labors the year around while farm work is seasonal. After months of uninterrupted work, the farmer has quiet periods. We already quoted Diodorus as saying that in Egypt 'the masses of the people, being relieved of their labors during the entire time of the inundation turn to recreation, feasting, all the while and enjoying without hindrance every device of pleasure.'[81] The feasting probably did not consist in much more than the consumption of bread, fish, and plenty of beer, and 'every device of pleasure' was probably just singing and dancing, but there is no doubt that to the farmer the inundation was not only in the days of Diodorus, but at all times, a period of rest and rejoicing.

Otherwise it was religion that interrupted the monotony of the common man's life. Religion created holidays, days of rest dedicated to the worship of the gods. They were days commemorating some event in a god's life, days on which the temple was open to the people, who, if they happened to live in the capital, could see Pharaoh in person, he, a god and son of a god, worshiping with his subjects. Sometimes processions took place; the god left his house and was carried through the city. Or episodes of the god's life were recreated in mystery plays. Food was sacrificed to the gods on such days in enormous quantities and some of it was distributed among the people.

The church took a great deal from the people because it was they who created the wealth that went to the temples. It gave them in exchange holidays, emotions, the illusion that they had a part in the wealth and pomp of the church, and the hope that life would not end with death, although the hereafter did not promise to be any better than the life on earth.

NOTES

1. This has been done in several books such as A. Erman, *Aegypten und ägyptisches Leben im Altertum,* neu bearbeitet von H. Ranke, Tübingen, 1923; and A. Wiedemann, *Das alte Aegypten,* Heidelberg, 1920.
2. *Cambridge Ancient History,* vol. I, p. 317.
3. About childbirth see A. Müller von Stwolinski, *Die Geburtshilfe und Gynäkologie bei den alten Aegyptern,* Diss., Munich, 1904; F. Weindler, *Geburts- und Wochenbettsdarstellungen auf altägyptischen Tempelreliefs,* Munich, 1915; I. Menascha, 'Die Geburtshilfe bei den alten Aegyptern,' *Arch. Gynäkol.,* 1927, 131:425-61; I. Harvey Flack, 'The Pre-History of Midwifery,' *Proc. R. Soc. Med.,* 1947, 40:713-22; Wiedemann, p. 70ff.
4. It occurs among primitives such as the Veddahs of Ceylon.
5. Erman-Ranke, loc. cit. p. 180.
6. παρὰ τὸ κοινὸν ἔθος τῶν ἀνθρώπων, Diodorus, I, 27, 1.
7. *Proc. Roy. Soc. Med.,* Sect. Hist. Med., 1919, 12:145-90; reprinted in *Studies in the Paleopathology of Egypt,* Chicago, 1921, pp. 322-56.
8. Herodotus, II, 64.
9. Skeletons and mummies of children are very frequent in Egyptian cemeteries, see Wiedemann, p. 74.
10. Wiedemann, p. 73f.

10a. *Pap. Berlin,* p. xiv.

10b. See Erik Iversen, *Papyrus Carlsberg No. VIII with Some Remarks on the Egyptian Origin of Some Popular Birth Prognoses* (Kgl. Danske Videnskabernes Selskab. Hist.-fil. Meddelelser XXVI, 5), Copenhagen, 1939.

11. W. A. Jayne, *The Healing Gods of Ancient Civilizations,* New Haven, 1925, p. 55f.; H. Epstein, 'Gott Bes, ein Beitrag zur Deutung seines Wesens,' *Arch. Gesch. Med.,* 1919, 11:233-55.
12. Erman-Ranke, p. 311.
13. Weindler, loc. cit. p. 31f.
14. Menascha, p. 449.
15. Described in great detail with very good pictures in Weindler, loc. cit.
16. The chief recipes are *Pap. med. Kahun* (Felix Reinhard, 'Gynäkologie und Geburtshilfe der altägyptischen Papyri,' *Arch. Gesch. Med.,* 1917, 10:147-

61), xxi-xxiii; *Pap. Ebers,* 93; *Pap. Berlin* 3038, 192. For a discussion of these prescriptions see N. E. Himes, *Medical History of Contraception,* Baltimore, 1936, pp. 59-68.

17. *Pap. Ebers,* probably 94.
18. Only two scenes representing the operation are known, one from the Theban temple of Khonsu (XXIst Dynasty), first published by F. Chabas, 'De la Circoncision chez les Egyptiens,' *Rev. archéol.,* 1861, pp. 298-300. The upper part of the relief is destroyed, but enough is preserved to permit a reconstruction of the scene. A second such scene was found by Loret in 1899 at Sakkara. It is very important because it dates from the VIth Dynasty and is well preserved. It has been reproduced many times, e.g. J. Capart, 'Une Rue de tombeaux à Saqqarah,' *L'Art égyptien,* Brussels, 1908, p. 51, plate lxvi; or E. Holländer, *Plastik und Medizin,* Stuttgart, 1905, p. 485.
19. An excellent survey and analysis of the sources are given by G. Foucart in Hastings, *Encycl. of Rel. and Ethics,* New York, 1911, vol. iii, pp. 670-77.
20. Δεῖν αὐτὸν περιτμηθῆναι διὰ τὸ μὴ δύνασθαι τὰς ἱερουργίας ἐκτελεῖν εἰ μὴ τοῦτο γενήσεται, *Tebt. Pap.,* 1907, vol. ii, no. 293.
21. Τά τε αἰδοῖα περιτάμνονται καθαρειότητος εἵνεκεν προτιμῶντες καθαροὶ εἶναι ἢ εὐπρεπέστεροι, Herodotus, ii, 37.
22. By 'servants of the Ka,' see Erman-Ranke, pp. 368 and 410.
23. Loc. cit. p. 676.
24. Καὶ τοῦτο δὲ τῶν μάλιστα ζηλουμένων παρ' αὐτοῖς τὸ πάντα τρέφειν τὰ γεννώμενα παιδία καὶ τὸ περιτέμνειν καὶ τὰ θήλεα ἐκτέμνειν, ὅπερ καὶ τοῖς ἰουδαίοις νόμιμος, Strabo, Geogr., 17, 2, 5.
25. Menascha, loc. cit. p. 434f.
26. W. G. Fröhlich, 'Sitten und Gebräuche der Nubier, insbesondere die Mädchenbeschneidung und ihre Folgen,' *Schweiz. med. Wschr.,* 1921, 791-6.
27. Diodorus, i, 80, 6.
28. Herodotus, ii, 36.
29. Ibid. ii, 81.
30. The Egyptian costume is discussed in Erman-Ranke, pp. 231-62; Wiedemann, pp. 117-28; for pictures see the attractive pamphlets of the Metropolitan Museum of Art: *The Private Life of the Ancient Egyptians,* New York, 1935, and Nora E. Scott, *The Home Life of the Ancient Egyptians,* New York, 1945.
31. Our bathtub in which the bather lies or sits came to us from Rome.
32. Translation by T. Eric Peet in *A Comparative Study of the Literatures of Egypt, Palestine, and Mesopotamia,* London, 1931, p. 103.
33. See Erman-Ranke, p. 141, after *Turin Pap.,* 42-8.
34. Erman-Ranke, p. 257.
35. Of 58 black and green eye paints analyzed, 37 were galena or lead sulphide, while the rest included 2 of lead carbonate, 1 of black oxide of copper, 5 of brown ochre, 1 of magnetic oxide of iron, 6 of oxide of manganese, 1 of sulphide of antimony. Of the green pigments 4 were malachite and 1 chrysocolla. J. R. Partington, *Origins and Development of Applied Chemistry,* London and New York, 1935, p. 143; A. Lucas, *Ancient Egyptian Materials*

and Industries, London, 1934, pp. 79ff. The face paint was red oxide of iron or hematite, Lucas, p. 84f.

36. If the painting of the eyes had any medical purpose it was certainly to protect the eyes by magic means, not by disinfecting the eyelids, as is frequently written. Lead sulphite that has antiseptic and astringent qualities is a white powder, while the black powder used as eye paint is lead sulphide, which is not antiseptic.
37. Wiedemann, p. 134; Herodotus, II, 37. According to Herodotus, priests shave their bodies every third day, ἵνα μήτε φθεὶρ μήτε ἄλλο μυσαρὸν μηδὲν ἐγγίνηταί σφι θεραπεύουσι τοὺς θεούς.
38. Wiedemann, p. 140.
39. *Pap. Ebers*, 65-7. Quotations from Papyrus Ebers are from the translation by B. Ebbell, *The Papyrus Ebers, the Greatest Egyptian Medical Document*, Copenhagen, 1939. All quotations by permission of Ejnar Munksgaard, publishers, Copenhagen.
40. Ibid. 67.
41. Herodotus, II, 37.
42. Ibid. II, 77.
43. Diodorus, I, 82, 1.
44. Herodotus, II, 35.
45. The sources for this statement are in Erman-Ranke, p. 219.
46. Ibid.
47. Wiedemann, p. 289.
48. M. A. Ruffer examined a number of specimens of Egyptian bread; see his study 'Abnormalities of Ancient Egyptian Teeth,' in *Studies in the Paleopathology of Egypt*, Chicago, 1921, p. 288f.
49. Herodotus, II, 92; Diodorus, I, 43, 5.
50. Herodotus, II, 77.
51. E.g. on the wall painting reproduced in *Wall Decorations of Egyptian Tombs*, London, British Museum, 1914, plate 3.
52. Wiedemann, p. 292f. The goose is the poor man's pig in that like the pig it eats all kinds of left-overs.
53. Herodotus, II, 47; Wiedemann, p. 285.
54. See among others Numbers, XI, 4-6; Diodorus, I, 34, 3ff.; also K. Hintze, *Geographie und Geschichte der Ernährung*, Leipzig, 1934.
55. Castor oil was widely used for lighting and for medicinal purposes.
56. Wiedemann, p. 296.
57. Ibid. p. 299.
58. A. Erman, *The Literature of the Ancient Egyptians*, transl. by A. M. Blackman, New York, n.d. [1927], p. 236f. By permission of Methuen & Co. Ltd.
59. Pleyte, *Etude sur un rouleau magique du Musée de Leide*, Leiden, 1866, p. 142.
60. Herodotus, II, 78.
61. Pyramid Texts, 404.
62. Ibid. 717.
63. About the Egyptian house see Wiedemann, pp. 157-96; Erman-Ranke, pp. 194-230. The sites of most ancient cities are still inhabited today so that

excavations are difficult and it is well-nigh impossible to reconstruct in detail the original plans. Kahun, however, near the entrance to the Fayyum was built by Senusret II, was inhabited primarily by the workers who built the king's pyramid at Illahun, and was abandoned after about a century. Excavated by Flinders Petrie it is a good example of housing at the beginning of the Middle Kingdom. The city unearthed by L. Borchardt at the site of today's Tell el-Amarna was Ikhnaton's residence Akhetaton, which was destroyed after his death. It is an example of housing during the New Empire.

64. Diodorus, I, 43, 4.
65. Ibid. I, 45, 5.
66. Wiedemann, p. 168.
67. Herodotus, II, 95.
68. *Pap. Anastasi,* v, 15, 6ff.; *Pap. Sallier,* I, 6, 1ff., in the translation of T. Eric Peet, loc. cit. p. 106.
69. We must not take this particular description too seriously. It is part of a didactic text that glorifies the profession of the scribe who 'directeth the work of all men. For him there are no taxes, for he payeth tribute in writing, and there are no dues for him.'
70. See G. Dykmans, *Histoire économique et sociale de l'ancienne Egypte: L'organisation sociale sous l'Ancien Empire,* Paris, 1937, vol. III; A. Moret, *The Nile and Egyptian Civilization,* London and New York, 1927, p. 260ff.
71. Herodotus, II, 14.
72. Sheep were used for that purpose in the earlier days, see Erman-Ranke, p. 517.
73. Moret, loc. cit. p. 267.
74. Erman-Ranke, p. 525f.
75. *Sallier* II and *Anastasi* VII of the British Museum. The text in both manuscripts is very corrupt.
76. The following is a free adaptation of some passages from A. Erman, *Die Literatur der Aegypter,* Leipzig, 1923, p. 100ff.; English edition by A. M. Blackman, New York, n.d., p. 67ff.; A. Moret, loc. cit. p. 268f.; J. Mayer and T. Prideaux, *Never to Die,* New York, 1938, p. 120.
77. The text is published in *Inscriptions in the Hieratic and Demotic Character from the Collections of the British Museum,* London, 1868, plate 20f.; see Erman-Ranke, p. 139f.
78. Examples in Erman-Ranke, p. 140ff.
79. Diodorus, III, 12ff. Translated by G. Booth, London, 1814.
80. See the very good discussion of amusements in Erman-Ranke, pp. 263-93; also Wiedemann, pp. 371-86.
81. Diodorus, I, 36, 10.

*

3. Magico-religious Medicine

So far we have studied the setting of Egyptian civilization in space and time and we have tried to find out how the people lived and worked and what they did to maintain their health and to prevent illness. We are now prepared to discuss how they acted once health had broken down and disease had taken hold of an individual.

In the preceding section of this book we have seen that in primitive medicine magical, religious, and empirico-rational elements are inextricably combined. In Egyptian medicine we encounter all these elements also; they are frequently combined but a separation has taken place. The physician is not a medicine man or a shaman. *The Secret Book of the Heart* distinguishes between three types of healers, the physician, the priest of Sekhmet, and the sorcerer.[1] And the love-sick boy laments that neither the master-physician nor the magicians can cure him.[2] Magic and religious and rational medicine run side by side, overlapping here and there, yet they are different systems of medicine. Some patients consulted physicians, others went to see a priest, while still others sought healing in magical formulae. And we can well imagine that cases occurred when one and the same patient tried one system after another.

It has often been said that Egyptian medicine was sober and empirico-rational in the beginning, during the Old Kingdom and far into the Middle Kingdom, and that it then gradually became mystical and got more and more into the hands of priests and exorcists. This view is probably based on the fact that a powerful professional clergy arose during the New Empire who had the tendency to monopolize all branches of science and learning. It is also true that the two youngest papyri that deal with illness and its cure are mostly magical[3] while the older medical papyri contain few incantations. This does not mean much, however, since the total number of medical papyri preserved is very small and new findings may easily change the picture. It is very likely that the religious element became stronger during the New Empire. Wherever there is a numerous clergy that has a firm grip on the people, magico-religious medicine flourishes at the expense of rational medicine, as we can see today in a number of countries. I think, however, that it would be a mistake to assume that Egyptian medicine started out empirically, developed along rational lines, and then degenerated into a prayer and incantation medicine. The Egyptians were always a religious people, as is evidenced by their burial customs, their earliest literature, and entire civilization. Spells and incantations for the cure of disease can be found formulated in literature as early as the Pyramid Texts.[4] There probably was a shift in emphasis in the course of the centuries but magico-religious and empirico-rational medicine could be found in Egypt at all times side by side and we are therefore justified in discussing them separately.

Paradoxically, one may say that Egyptian society consisted of the gods, the dead, and the living.[5] The gods and the dead were considered ever present, influencing man's destinies at every moment, with needs that the living had to satisfy. They needed homes, temples, and tombs, and they got the best homes of the country. They needed food, and received it in the form of sacrifices. They required constant attention and it was given to them by means of prayers and manifold rites. The house had a shrine in front of which a lamp was kept burning. Shrines could be found on the wayside and along the river. And the traveler stopped for a moment, offering a prayer and a few flowers. Days of public worship, with processions, dances, and general rejoicing, marked the eternal rhythm of nature, celebrating the fertility of the soil or the completion of the harvest, or commemorating events in the life of the gods.

It was a rich pantheon that called for the people's worship: local gods, many in animal form, whose importance rose and fell with the importance of the nome or city they represented; cosmic gods, like Re, the sun, or Osiris, who died and was reborn like nature. In the course of time groups of gods such as Isis, Osiris, and Horus were universally worshiped even beyond the boundaries of Egypt. The scribes paid special tribute to Thoth, their patron, inventor of the script: 'Come to me, Thoth, thou lordly ibis, thou God, for whom yearneth Hermopolis. Letter-writer of the Nine Gods, great one in Unu . . . Come to me and care for me; I am a servant of thine house. Let me tell of thy mighty works in whatsoever land I be.'[6] We shall have to say more about Imhotep and his functions as a healing god.

In addition to the gods, the dead, and the living, the world was inhabited by spirits, demons, evil forces that made the crocodile bite you when you expected it least, that threatened women in childbirth, infants, the weak, and the careless. You had to be on guard all the time. The gods and the dead could be reached directly with prayers or you could write them letters. The way to control the world of spirits was magic, a series of actions, rites that had to be performed, of objects that had to be worn, and of formulae that had to be recited at the right moment. Magic was the chief means of protection an individual had, but he also possessed spells that were able to produce desirable conditions, a girl's love, easy delivery, or the restoration of health. And magic obviously could also be used for evil purposes, to make a fellow man weak and sick or to kill him altogether.

In our Western capitalist societies an individual's security is determined by his bank account, by his savings at large. With money he can buy whatever he needs to satisfy his material needs, food, shelter, clothes, but he can also purchase books, concert and theater tickets, higher education for his children, in other words, means to satisfy his and his family's spiritual needs. Money will also buy him the services of a physician and medicines when he is sick. Organized charity tries to satisfy minimum needs when an individual for some reason or other is unable to work and possesses no savings; in more recent time, social insurance, a form of compulsory saving, endeavors to guarantee the wage earner a certain amount of security.

In ancient Egypt as in most early civilizations, the common man felt secure when he was at peace with the transcendental world.

Whether he would eat or not was in the hands of the gods anyway, and the best method to keep socially adjusted and safe was by keeping the gods and the dead benevolent and by restraining the spirits with religious and magical means. To that end a certain amount of knowledge was required, which was handed down by tradition. One had to know prayers, sacrifices, rites, spells, what amulets to wear, when and at what places the presence of Bes or Thoeris or other protective deities was needed. The traveler preparing to set out on a hazardous journey had to be supplied not only with food but also with magic formulae to protect him against wild animals in the desert, against shipwreck, and other accidents.[7] Everybody had to be familiar with the lucky and unlucky days, because such knowledge determined a man's actions. Papyrus Sallier IV of the British Museum lists such days as follows:

> 1st day of Hathor. The whole day is lucky. There is festival in heaven with Ra and Hathor.
>
> 2nd day of Hathor. The whole day is lucky. The gods go out. The goddess Matchet comes from Tep to the gods who are in the shrine of the bull, in order to protect the divine members.
>
> 3rd day of Hathor. The whole day is lucky.
>
> 4th day of Hathor. The whole day is unlucky. The house of a man who goes on a voyage on that day comes to ruin.
>
> 6th day of Hathor. The whole day is unlucky. Do not light a fire in thy house on this day, and do not look at one.
>
> 18th day of Pharmuthi. The whole day is unlucky. Do not bathe on this day.
>
> 20th day of Pharmuthi. The whole day is unlucky. Do not work on this day.
>
> 22nd day of Pharmuthi. The whole day is unlucky. He who is born on this day will die on this day.
>
> 23rd day of Pharmuthi. The first two-thirds of the day are unlucky, and the last third lucky.[8]

When an individual fell sick he dropped out of society. The subtle balance maintained painstakingly between him, the gods, the dead, and the spirits was suddenly upset, and he found himself out of harmony with the world. He was the victim of the spirits, of evil magic, was the object of the wrath of the gods; and the most logical way to restore the lost balance and to regain security was by religious or magical means, with prayers, incantations, rituals similar to those encountered in primitive medicine.

This could be done on a very high ethical level, as in the case of the man who was stricken with blindness because he committed the sin of swearing falsely by Ptah, Lord of Truth, and who in a poignant prayer begged for mercy: [9]

I am a man who swore falsely by Ptah, Lord of Truth;
And he caused me to behold darkness by day.
I will declare his might to him that knows him not and to him that knows him,
To small and great.
Be ye ware of Ptah, Lord of Truth.
Lo, he will not overlook the deed of any man.
Refrain ye from uttering the name of Ptah falsely;
Lo, he that uttereth it falsely,
Lo, he falleth.
He caused me to be as the dogs of the street,
I being in his hand:
He caused men and gods to mark me,
I being as a man that has wrought abomination against his Lord.
Righteous was Ptah, Lord of Truth, toward me,
When he chastised me.
Be merciful to me; look upon me, that thou mayest be merciful.

A prayer, an invocation of the gods, is included in one of the recitals that open the Ebers Papyrus: [10]

Oh Isis, great in sorcery! Mayst thou loosen me, mayst thou deliver me from everything bad and evil and vicious, from affliction (caused) by a god or goddess, from dead man or woman, from male or female adversary who will oppose me, like thy loosening and thy delivering with thy son Horus. For I have entered into the fire and have come forth from the water, I will not fall into this day's trap. I have spoken (and now) I am young and am . . .

Oh Re, speak over thine (Uraeus) serpent! Osiris, call over what came out of thee!

Re speaks over his (Uraeus) serpent, Osiris calls over what came out of him. Lo, thou hast saved me from everything bad and evil and vicious, from afflictions (caused) by a god or goddess, from dead man or woman, etc.[11]

Worship of the gods and of the dead was primarily the realm of religion. Magic, on the other hand, provided the means to force an event that seemed desirable to man, or to avert threatening evil. Since spirit intrusion or at least affliction by a spirit—demon or ghost of the dead—was considered the chief cause of disease in the magico-religious medicine of Egypt, the means for prevention and cure consisted in the wearing of amulets, the reciting of incantations, and the performing of certain rites, all intended to keep off or to drive out the spirits. The exorcist was either a specialist in the subject, a sorcerer, or he was a priest. Magic in all early civilizations was a perfectly legitimate science in its own way, and there is no reason why Egyptologists should consider the use of charms a superstition or why they should feel apologetic when they encounter an incantation in an otherwise for the most part rational medical manuscript.[12]

Texts of incantations and descriptions of other magic procedures are encountered scattered all over the literature of Egypt. We find them in the religious literature, where they form an integral part of the legends of the gods.[13] But we also find them in the form of narratives relating the wonderful deeds of the great magicians of the past.[14] Collections of magical prescriptions occur in a number of papyri of the New Empire [15] and on such monuments as the Metternich stele.[16] They obviously all contain incantations for the treatment of sick people because disease was one of the great evils that had to be fought by magic. But in addition to these texts we have two manuscripts that deal almost exclusively with medical matters and their magical treatment.

One is a relatively short piece of papyrus [2.17 x 0.157 meters] with 9 written pages on the recto and 6 on the verso, owned by the Berlin Museum [P. 3027] and usually referred to as *Zaubersprüche für Mutter und Kind*, the title given it by its editor, A. Erman.[17] It was written at the end of the Hyksos period or at the beginning of the New Empire, that is, in the sixteenth century B.C., and is a compilation from two sources. The first [including the charms A-E] was a collection of incantations against two diseases of infants, *nšw* and *tmjt,* diseases that we cannot identify because the words are unknown and the symptoms mentioned, when they are mentioned at all, are too vague.[18] The second [F-V] was a book that began with charms to facilitate childbirth[19] and continued with prescriptions[20] and incantations for the protection of infants in the morning and in the evening, when an amulet was made, or in order that the mother might have sufficient milk. This fascinating text makes it possible for us to look into the Egyptian nursery. Just as a mother today knows lullabies with which she puts her crying babe to sleep, the Egyptian mother was skilful in making amulets and knew the right words to be spoken when the child was sick and restless and threatened by evil forces. Some writers on Egyptian medicine do not include this papyrus in their discussion because of its magic content,[21] an attitude that is certainly not justified. Medical history must pay attention to all measures employed to help women in childbirth and to protect infants, whether such practices are rational or not.

The other medical papyrus that is predominantly magical is today in the British Museum in London [No. 10059]. It was written at the end of the XVIIIth Dynasty, that is, in the middle of the fourteenth century B.C.[22] Many of the prescriptions are obviously older[23] inasmuch as the papyrus is the copy of a scribe who did not always understand what he wrote. The papyrus is 2.10 meters long, 0.175 high, has 9 pages on the recto, 10 on the verso, and is in a bad state of preservation.[24] It contains 61 prescriptions, most of them magical,[25] for the treatment of a variety of diseases, and it ends with two prayers to Amon that have been appended by the scribe and have no connection with the book.

Magic religious treatments were used primarily in the case of magic religious diseases to counteract the magic that had taken hold of an individual in a general way or, more commonly, to drive out a spirit. Afflictions were caused 'by a god or goddess, by all kinds of whdw,'[26] 'by dead man or woman, etc.'[27] The evil spirits of Egypt that caused disease had not the outspoken individuality of Babylonian demons, who had names and whose ways of life were depicted in numerous texts. They were anonymous ghosts or demons who sometimes 'arrived in darkness, gliding in, the nose backwards and the face turned' [28] so that they might not be recognized as what they were. They arrived under the pretension that they wanted to kiss an infant, to quiet the crying babe, but they actually intended to harm it and to snatch it away.[29] Or they shot arrows at the victim [30] or took possession of him or of parts of his body, of a bone [31] or some other organ. Or the evil spirit was believed to be a foreign woman, Asiatic or a Negress,[32] who had come to harm the children of Egypt. All gods could send disease, obviously, but some were more inclined to do so than others, such as Sekhmet, the 'lady of pestilence,' who sent the plagues over the land; or Seth, who had slain his brother Osiris.[33]

Magic religious treatments, however, were used not only to drive out a spirit, not only to fight evil magic, but in the treatment of other diseases, of poisoning caused by the sting of the scorpion [34] and the bite of the snake,[35] and of all other diseases that we call somatic: diseases of the eyes,[36] of the skin,[37] burns,[38] 'to quiet the heart when the legs tremble,' [39] hemorrhoids,[40] aneurism,[41] diseases of the penis,[42] gynecological diseases,[43] to stop menstruation,[44] to get milk in the mother's breasts,[45] and many other conditions.

Incantations represented a perfectly legitimate form of therapy that could be applied at any time in all cases of illness, just as magic was a perfectly legitimate cause of disease, and possibly a disease itself that might be treated, not only with incantations but also with drugs. Thus the Ebers Papyrus prescribes in order to expel 'magic in the belly,' not spells but: 'The interior of hmm, the interior of w*ḏ*ᶜjt, frankincense, colocynth, sweet beer, are rubbed together and drunk by the man.' [46] A mixture of various flours combined with yeast from date wine was applied to drive out from the patient's body the evil effects of the male and female ghost.[47] To the same purpose a paste made from bread, various fats, honey, natron, salt, dough, and several other ingredients was applied as a poultice to the sore parts.[48]

We must now examine the character and style of the incantations used in the treatment of disease. It is common to all magic procedures that they must be performed accurately. One word left out, one gesture omitted, may easily render the spell ineffective. Magic, therefore, requires a vast knowledge of rites and these rites are oral or manual. Both are frequently combined, as we shall see.

The sorcerer whose task it was to drive out or to keep away a spirit from the body of a man through the magic power of the word had various means of doing it. The simplest was the command. Addressing himself to the spirit he ordered it to get out: 'Get thee hence, thou female breaker of bones, thou crusher of stones, who enters into the vessels.'[49] Or the disease was addressed: 'Spit, vomit, perish as thou arosest.'[50] Or the command had the form of a prohibition:

> Art thou come to kiss this child? I will not suffer thee to kiss him.
> Art thou come to quiet him? I will not suffer thee to quiet him.
> Art thou come to harm him? I will not suffer thee to harm him.
> Art thou come to take him away? I will not suffer thee to take him away from me.[51]

It was important for the magician to know who his opponent was. Knowing his name gave him particular power with which he could threaten the spirit. 'I know thy name . . . do I not know thy name? . . .' was said repeatedly in an incantation for the eye.[52] Or if he was not sure he considered various alternatives:

> Art thou a servant? Come in the vomit.
> Art thou a noble? Come in his urine.
> Come in the sneeze of his nose.
> Come in the sweat of his limbs.[53]

Threatening and scaring the ghost was a good method employed very frequently. The worst that could happen to a spirit was to be forced to eat excrements. Hence the threat:

> O ghost, male or female, thou hidden, thou concealed one, who dwelleth in this my flesh, in these my limbs—get thee hence from this my flesh, from these my limbs. Lo, I brought thee excrements to devour! Beware, hidden one, be on your guard, concealed one, escape! [54]

Or the conjurer simply said as a protection against the pest of the year: 'I am the abomination that came forth out of Buto. O Meskhenet, that came forth out of Heliopolis; O men, O gods,

O dead, be ye far from me. I am the abomination.'[55] How could a spirit care to take possession of an abomination?

Or he threatened: 'I will go up to heaven and see what is done there, for nothing is done in Abydos to expel afflictions caused by a god or goddess . . .'[56]

Cajoling the demon by pretending to be healthy, to be 'immunized,' was another method and it was said at the time of pest: 'I am the healthy one in the way of the passer by. Shall I be smitten while I am healthy? I have seen the great disaster. O this fever, do not assail me, for I am the one who has come forth out of the disaster. Be thou far from me.'[57]

Spirits were supposed to react very much like humans and were, therefore, cursed, threatened, warned, given orders, or entreated just as a man would do to his fellow man.

In many incantations one or more gods were summoned by the sorcerer. He knew how to invoke them and at his request they came and drove the spirits away and protected the sufferer. An incantation of the London Papyrus against a woman's disease says: 'Recede thou who comest on the arrows; the gods who rule at Heliopolis keep thee off.'[58] Anubis and Thoth are the helpers in another spell of the same papyrus.[59] Sometimes the god was greeted with praise and flattery:

> Hail to thee, Horus, thou that art in the town of Hundreds, thou sharp-horned one, who shootest at the mark . . . I come to thee, I praise thy beauty: destroy thou the evil that is in my limbs.[60]

In such a case it is impossible to tell whether we are dealing with an incantation or a prayer but there are no sharp borderlines between the two. The same applies to a certain extent to several spells in the Berlin Papyrus in which Re is invoked, texts of great beauty such as:

> Spell to read in the early morning over an infant.
>
> Thou risest, O Re, thou risest. When thou hast seen this dead one as he cometh to N.N. born of N.N.,[61] and the dead, the woman . . . She shall not take the infant in her arm. Re saveth me, my Lord, says the woman N.N. I shall not turn her over, I shall not turn over the infant.

My hand lies on thee, the seal is thy protection. Re riseth. Lo, I protect thee.[62]

It happened not infrequently that he who pronounced the incantation, the exorcising sorcerer or the mortal seeking protection, identified himself with a god. This is the case in several charms against the pest on the verso of the Edwin Smith Papyrus, such as the following:

Withdraw, ye disease demons. The wind shall not reach me, that those who pass by may pass by to work disaster against me. I am Horus who passes by the diseased ones of Sekhmet, Horus, Horus, healthy despite Sekhmet. I am the unique one, son of Bastet. I die not through thee.[63]

And in a spell of the Berlin Papyrus the magician addresses the sick child with the words: 'Thou art Horus and thou awakest as Horus. Thou art the living Horus; I dispell the disease that is in thy body and the ailing that is in thy limbs . . .'[64]

But not only the exorcist and patient identified themselves with a god, every organ was sometimes identified with a deity and we possess a number of interesting texts to that effect. Thus an incantation of the Berlin Papyrus lists the parts of the body as follows:[65]

Thy vertex is Re, thou healthy child, thy occiput is Osiris, thy forehead is Sathis, Lady of Elephantine, thy temple is Neith, thy eyebrows are the Lord of the East, thy eyes are the Lord of Mankind, thy nose is the Nourisher of the Gods, thy ears are the two Royal Serpents, thy elbows are Living Hawks, thy arm is Horus, the other is Seth, thy . . . is Sopd, the other is Nut, who gives birth to the gods . . . thy lung is Min . . . thy spleen is Sobk, thy liver is Harsaphes of Heracleopolis, thy intestines are Health, thy navel is the Morning Star, thy leg is Isis, the other is Nephthys . . . no limb of thee is without its god, each god protects thy name and all that is of thee . . .

This view that every limb was a god or rather was ruled by one must have prevailed throughout the course of Egyptian history because we find it mentioned in the Book of the Dead[66] and millennia later in Origen's treatise against Celsus.[67] Origen wrote in the third century of the Christian era that the Egyptians divided the human body into 36 parts—some into more—and that each part was under the care of a god. 'And they cure the ailments of the parts by invoking these'[68] namely the corresponding gods. This was a view that was almost universal in antiquity and, since the gods were also identified with parts of the universe, planets, rivers, mountains, the possibility was given for the development of a mythological anatomy on one side and of astrological medicine on the other side. The human body appeared as a microcosm that reflected the macrocosm, the universe. Traces of this mythological anatomy are still preserved in our nomenclature. We still call the first cervical vertebra that carries the skull Atlas, after the Greek demigod who carried the world. We speak of a Mons Veneris, of a Labyrinth, hidden in the depth of the rocky bone, the *os petrosum*. These are not poetic images but reminiscences of an old system of mythical anatomy.[69] And as to astrological medicine or iatromathematics we shall have to say more about it in this and other volumes because it was developed into a forceful system that played an important part in the Middle Ages and Renaissance and is not dead today.

Returning to the incantations of ancient Egypt we find that many of them consist of tales of the life of the gods, of crucial episodes, the recalling of which in the right words assumes magic power. As a matter of fact, many mythological details have been preserved in such incantations. A few texts may serve as illustrations. For the treatment of a burn it was said:[70]

> As young Horus was in the swamp, fire fell on his body—it did not know him[71] and he did not know it—his mother was not present to recite an incantation over him and his father had gone away. Horus called Duamutef, Kebehsenuf, Hapi, and Amset: 'My young sons, the fire is violent and there is nobody here to drive it from me. Do ye that Isis cometh forth . . .'
>
> 'Come with me, my sister Nephthys,[72] walk with me . . . I know how to extinguish the fire with my milk, with the wholesome flood that is between my legs. When it is given over his body, his vessels are healthy. I do that the fire recedeth from him . . .'

A similar but somewhat shorter charm against burns in which Isis also comes to the rescue of Horus is found in Papyrus Ebers:[73]

Thy son Horus is burnt in the desert. Is water there? There is no water there. There is water in my mouth and a Nile between my thighs; I come to extinguish the fire. Is recited over milk of a woman who had borne a male child, gum and ram's hair, is applied to the burn.

Another such story was recited when the patient felt suffocating: [74]

Suffocation, suffocation. Osiris is sick in the nose. 'Nothing shall happen to him, nor shall he raise his arm; [75] "perish!" shall not be said to him,' said Isis.

'I give that his limb shall be protected with that which cometh out of my son,' said Atum . . .

'Run out ye . . . that are in the face of my son Horus! I place this my lock upon him,' said Isis. . .

An invocation of gods and demons with many dark mythological implications is the substance of an incantation against the plague: [76]

O Flame-in-His-Face! Preside over the horizon, speak thou to the chief of the Hemesut-house, who makes Osiris, first of the land, to flourish. O Nekhbet, lifting the earth to the sky for her father, come thou, bind the two feathers around me, around me, that I may live and flourish because I possess the White One. The first is the Great One dwelling in Heliopolis; the second is Isis; the third is Nephthys; while I am subject to thee.

O Seizer-of-the-Great-One, son of Sekhmet, mightiest of the mighty, son of the Disease-Demon Dened, son of Hathor, mistress of the crown, and flooder of the streams; when thou voyagest in the Celestial Ocean, when thou sailest in the morning barque, thou hast saved me from every sickness.

Incantation against this year, with the breath of every evil wind.

Horus, Horus, healthy despite Sekhmet, is around all my flesh for life.

Speak the words over two vulture feathers, with which a man has covered himself, placed as his protection in every place where he goes. It is a protection against the year, expelling sickness in the year of pest.

The following charm, finally, may be quoted as an example of sympathetic magic. Its purpose was to arrest the menstrual flow: [77]

Anubis has come forth to prevent the Nile from entering the sanctuary of . . . so that she who is in it, be protected.

This charm shall be spoken over a band of flaxen threads. A pad is made from it and put into her flesh.

Another group of incantations is characterized by the fact that their text is not in the Egyptian but in some foreign language. The London Papyrus has four charms in a Semitic dialect,[78] one in the language of Crete.[79] They were obviously imported spells used originally perhaps against foreign demons but then also because words that are not understood appeared as particularly potent. Many parallels could be cited from our medieval magic literature.

The oral rite was all important. The correct choice of words to frighten a spirit, to enlist the help of the gods, the intonation probably also in which a spell was recited or sung, this all must have had a profound effect upon the patient. We know the power of suggestion and know how highly responsive religious individuals are to such rites. I should not be astonished if the sorcerer with his spells had had better results in many cases than the physician with his drugs. Magician and priest were able to put the sick in a frame of mind in which the healing power of the organism could do its work under the best conditions. They gave him peace and confidence and helped him to readjust to the world from which disease had torn him.

The mere oral rite, however, was not enough but was usually combined with manual rites. First there was the time factor to be considered. Just as the Navaho Indian sang his chants at sunrise or sunset or any other prescribed time of the day or night, so did the Egyptian his incantations. A spell 'for the protection of the body' was 'to be read over a child when the sun rises' and began with an invocation of Re.[80] Another in the same collection was 'to be read over a child in the early morning.' This particular charm was 'to be spoken over a seal and over a hand. One makes an amulet of them, knotting them into seven knots, that is, one knot in the morning, another in the evening until they are seven.'[81] Another spell was recited 'in the evening when Re sets in the land of life.'[82]

Prescriptions were also sometimes made about the dress that the magician must wear. 'He who pronounces this incantation shall be dressed in a wrapper of finest linen and shall be holding a stick.'[83] Such indications, however, are not very frequent because it was obvious that the magician, who as a rule, certainly during the New Empire, was a priest, must be pure. Purity was an essential requirement for all religious actions in antiquity and we may accept as a matter of course that he who pronounced an incantation was washed, clean shaven, dressed in pure linen, had not approached a woman, and possibly also observed certain food taboos.[84]

The manual rites performed in the course of an incantation appear in infinite variety from the simplest to the most elaborate and complicated. The rite may have consisted of nothing but putting one's hands on the patient, the classical gesture of protection so familiar to us from the Bible. After having exorcised a demon the magician said: 'My hands are on this child, and the hands of Isis are on him, as she puts her hands on her son Horus.'[85] Or the magician held his seal over the child and such a seal was obviously a powerful fetish: 'My hand is on thee and my seal is thy protection.'[86] Simple enough but somewhat more elaborate was the rite in the course of which a magic circle was drawn around the house of the individual who was to be protected against the pest. One of the incantations of the Edwin Smith Papyrus gives the following directions: 'Let the words be spoken by a man having a stick of des-wood, while he comes forth into the open and goes around his house. He cannot die by the pest of the year.'[87] Or the incantation was said 'before a nefret-flower, bound to a piece of des-wood, and tied with a strip of linen. Let them be passed over the things; the pest will be exorcised. . .'[88] Or the words were spoken over images of the gods, 'Sekhmet, Bastet, Osiris, and Neheb-kau, written with frankincense on a band of fine linen and attached to a man at his throat.'[89] Incantations sometimes were combined with sacrifices to the gods. A charm to ease childbirth was spoken over the two bricks on which the woman in labor knelt and it was said furthermore that a sacrifice should be brought to the goddess Nut, by placing meat, geese, and frankincense on a fire.[90]

More complicated manual rites were performed as an expression of sympathetic magic. 'To cause the womb to go to its place: an ibis of wax is placed on charcoal, and let the fume thereof enter into the interior of her vulva.'[91] The ibis was the bird of Thoth, the inventor of medicine, and wax frequently used for making such magic images was produced by bees which, as Gardiner pointed out, sprang from tears shed by Re.[92] Another incantation 'to drive out the blood from a wbn' was spoken 'over an ibis made of excrements whose beak was filled with . . . seeds. Put the beak into the opening of the wbn. It was effective at the time of Amenhotep III.'[93] Excrements, as we mentioned before, were particularly hateful to spirits. A disease of the male genital organ caused by an enemy, man or spirit, was to be thrown back to its author by having a mythological incantation spoken over 'a fresh phallus made of dp-t cake, inscribed with the name of the enemy, his father's name and his mother's name. To be put in the midst of fat meat, to be given to the cat.'[94]

Incantations were transitory matters. The magician came or the patient was brought to him. After some preparation, some purifications, the magic words were spoken, some rites were performed, and all was over. In many cases this was probably enough for the patient who was under great nervous tension to feel suddenly improved or even cured. We all have seen such miracle cures since there is still a great deal of magic religious medicine in our present Western world and our knowledge of psychiatry makes it possible for us to understand the psychological processes involved much better than in the past. There is no doubt, however, that most patients were not suddenly improved and that they felt a strong desire to hold the magic force and have it act on them for a longer period of time. This could be done by charging an object with it, making it thus a powerful amulet or talisman.

We have encountered such amulets in various previous examples. Some amulets were simple yet sufficient to carry the charm, a band of fine linen over which the words were spoken or on which they were written,[95] a braid of hair with four knots attached to a child's throat,[96] a fish abhorrent to ghosts on a string tied with a knot;[97] or 'one had the child or his mother eat a cooked mouse; the bones in a bag of fine linen are attached to his throat and one ties seven knots.' [98] Knots, as we see, played a very important part in the making of such amulets. They were believed to have the faculty of binding forces and in addition seemed to present obstacles, as Gardiner pointed out,[99] quoting to that effect an interesting passage from a magical papyrus:[100] 'If the poison pass these seven knots, which Horus has made on his body, I will not allow the sun to shine.'

The number of knots was also considered very important. They were four or seven, as a rule, just as some incantations had to be recited four times or seven times.[101] These were the two cosmic numbers which we shall encounter throughout antiquity not only in magic but in philosophy also.

Some amulets charged with the magic power of incantation were complicated and costly. In one case the charm had to be spoken over three beads, one of lapis lazuli, one of jasper, and one of malachite. A necklace was made of them for the sick child.[102] Still more elaborate was another amulet made by having the incantation spoken over beads of gold, rings of amethyst, and a seal on which a crocodile and a hand were pictured. Strung on a very fine string they were attached to the child's neck.[103] These were amulets for the children of rich parents. The choice of stones and metals was by no means arbitrary, and the selection was not made primarily because the materials were precious, although this was a factor since it implied the idea of sacrifice. The choice was rather determined by the fact that in Egypt as in all ancient civilizations minerals, metals, plants, every object, animate and inanimate, were attributed certain magic virtues. The correct choice and combination of materials were therefore extremely important.

The next amulet is one that leads us to another group of prescriptions. Addressing the demons that threatened a child, the magician said: [104] 'I have made for him a protective charm against thee consisting of evil-smelling herbs, of garlic which is harmful to thee, and of honey which is sweet for men but horrible to ghosts, and of a fish tail and of a rag and of the backbone of a perch.' There is no doubt that this is a true amulet; the herbs, garlic, and honey were not eaten but mixed with the other ingredients and perhaps wrapped in the rag and put next to the child. But in other cases herbs, garlic, honey over which a spell had been spoken were consumed by the patient. In other words, not only bands of linen, beads, rings, and seals were charged with magic power but also vegetable, animal, and mineral substances, what we usually call drugs. A prescription of drugs thus charged became an internal amulet that exerted its power from inside. The preparation and mixing of the drugs was a manual magic rite. Not the drug in itself was effective, but the words spoken over it made it so. But just as gold, amethyst, or lapis lazuli had inherent magic virtues so had plants and animal parts and minerals used as drugs. The art of medicine consisted in selecting the right drugs, preparing them in the magically correct way, and speaking the appropriate words over them. I think we touch here the origin of the pharmacological therapy of Egyptian medicine. Many, perhaps the majority, of Egyptian drugs used had no perceptible effect according to modern pharmacological standards. They became part of the materia medica and remained part of it for thousands of years for magic reasons. In many instances this is easily apparent. We mentioned in some other connection a recipe in which blood of a raven was used to prevent hair from becoming gray too soon. This was a simple case of sympathetic magic.[105] Such a system, however, was able to include a great amount of sound empirical knowledge. Since every object of nature had its inherent magic virtue it might well happen that this virtue coincided with the pharmacological effect. The virtue of castor oil taken internally, whether magical or empirical, was always a cathartic one. The day came when drugs were prepared and given without incantation and this was the moment when magic and medicine separated, when physician and magician-priest became different individuals.

The texts illustrative of this intimate relation between magical and empirical medicine are very numerous and a few examples will suffice. Some prescriptions are general, such as the following 'spell when a medicament is applied to all sick parts of the body':

> I have come forth from Heliopolis with the Great Ones from the temple, the Lords of Protection, the Rulers of Eternity; they protect me.
>
> I have come forth from Sais, with the Mother of the Gods and they have granted me their protection . . .

God keepeth alive him whom he loveth. I am one who is beloved by his God. This is why He keepeth me alive.[106]

Such an incantation could be used to charge magically any external remedy that was applied to any part of the body irrespective of what drugs the remedy consisted of and irrespective of its form, whether it was an ointment, a poultice, or anything else. This is equally true for the next spell, which was recited in a general way 'on drinking a remedy': [107]

Come, remedy! Come thou who expellest evil things in my stomach and in these my limbs! The spell is powerful over the remedy. Repeat it backwards! Dost thou remember that Horus and Seth have been conducted to the big palace at Heliopolis when there was negotiated of Seth's testicles with Horus, and he shall get well like one who is on earth. He does all that he may wish like these gods who are there . . .

This mythological incantation was fit to charge any potion but other such spells were more specific. Thus on applying a remedy to the sick eyes the Eye of Horus was invoked and the following charm had to be recited four times: [108]

This Eye of Horus created by the spirits of Heliopolis, which Thoth has brought from Hermopolis—from the great hall in Heliopolis,—in Pe,—in Dep,[109]—sayest thou to it: 'Welcome, thou splendid Eye of Horus,—thou content of the Eye of Horus—brought to drive out the evil of the God, the evil of the Goddess, the demon, male and female, the dead, male and female, the enemy, male and female, who have insinuated themselves into the eyes of the sick under my fingers.—Protection, behind me protection, come, protection!'

Other incantations were spoken over certain prescriptions of drugs. We mentioned before a mythological spell from Papyrus Ebers against burns [110] that was to be spoken over 'milk of a woman who has borne a male child, gum and ram's hair,' to be applied to the burn. Another such charm against burns that we quoted [111] was to be spoken over a combination of 'acacia . . . barley cake, cooked . . . seed, cooked deret fruit, cooked. . . Mix, stir with the milk of the mother of a boy. Apply to the burn until it is healed. Bandage it with a ricinus stalk.'

One of the safest methods to charge remedies with magic power consisted in reciting incantations over their basic ingredients. Beer was one of the chief vehicles for drugs given as potions; honey was the sweetening substance that took throughout antiquity the place of our sugar; grease was used for salves; barley went into many remedies, barley water in the form of πτιϐάνη was one of the chief dietetic foods of the Greeks and must have been prescribed long before them. And finally, a measuring cup had to be used in the compounding of drugs. The Hearst Papyrus has a most interesting series of chapters with incantations for the measuring cup, the barley, the grease, the honey, and the beer.[112] The first may be quoted as a sample:

> Spell for the measuring cup, when it is taken to measure a remedy.
>
> This measuring cup in which I measure this remedy is the measuring cup in which Horus has measured his eye and it was measured correctly; and thus life, happiness and health were restored.
>
> This remedy is measured in this measuring cup, in order to drive out with it all diseases that are in this body, etc.

And finally we must mention one element that figures most frequently at the end of incantations, namely the recommendation. It may be very simple, consisting of a word or of a few words added as marginal notes by somebody who used the charm and found it satisfactory. Later, as happened usually in such cases, the note became part of the text. Thus we find recommendations like 'good,' [113] or 'very good,' [114] or 'really excellent, proved many times,' [115] or 'I saw its good effect,' [116] or 'really proved, I saw its effect on myself,' [117] and similar remarks undoubtedly made by the user of the charm. Simple as these words were they increased the suggestive power of the text.

A different type of recommendation is presented by those in which reference is made to some divine authority or to the antiquity of the charm. Papyrus Ebers [118] and Papyrus Hearst [119] have a series of remedies consisting of charms and drugs 'made by Re on his own behalf, made by Shu for Re himself, made by Tefnut for Re himself, by Geb for Re himself, by Nut,' and finally a sixth remedy 'made by Isis for Re himself to expel illness in his head.' Remedies made by gods for gods had to be good. Other incantations were transmitted in a book [120] that 'was found in the night, having fallen into the court of the temple in Khemmis, as secret knowledge of this goddess,[121] by the hand of the lector of this temple. Lo, this land was in darkness, and the moon [122] shone on every side of this book. It was brought as a marvel to the majesty of King Khufu.'

Such a story that relegated a book to remotest antiquity and gave it an almost divine origin was the obvious invention of some priest, while other references to earlier days may well have been genuine. Three recipes of the London Papyrus [123] were said to have been found effective at the time of Amenhotep III, a statement that may well be true.

We cannot conclude this chapter without adding a few more words about the healing gods of ancient Egypt.[124] We may be very brief, however, because the preceding pages have told us a great deal about them. We have seen them in action interfering in the destinies of man. We saw how episodes of their lives when recalled at a crucial moment exerted a profound influence on the life and welfare of mortals. The faculty to send disease when provoked, or to relieve from illness when placated or invoked in the correct way, was one that all ancient deities possessed. Yet in the course of time a certain specialization took place. Some gods were more apt to send plagues over the land while others were especially sought and worshiped as healers and magicians.

We encountered Thoth as the god to whom the scribes prayed because he had revealed to man the art of writing. But he had revealed other arts and crafts also, among them the healing art. He was the physicians' patron to whom they prayed for guidance. In the introduction to the Ebers Papyrus [125] Re, the sun god, said:

> I will save him from his enemies, and Thoth shall be his guide, he who lets writing speak and has composed the books; he gives to the skillful, to the physicians who accompany him, skill to cure. The one whom the god loves, him he shall keep alive.

He was a great physician and magician himself, physician to the gods. When Horus was bitten by a scorpion, Re sent him to cure the god, son of gods, because he knew the words to be spoken; [126] and in protecting Horus he protected every sick man.[127] The Greeks identified Thoth with their Hermes and the books that were supposed to contain the wisdom of Egypt were, therefore, called the Hermetic Books.

From the few magic texts we have quoted it is apparent that Isis held an important place in the pantheon of healing deities. Her legend is full of episodes of magic cures [128] and over and over again she appears as the great magician 'whose counsel is the breath of life, whose sayings drive out sickness, and whose word gives life to him whose breath is failing.' [129] It is well known that in Roman days the cult of Isis spread all over the ancient world and at a time when people were pining for healing, physical and spiritual, and for redemption, these very functions of Isis acquired particular significance. To Diodorus she was a healing goddess, discoverer of drugs, versed in the art of curing people who flocked to her temples, lying down in the halls, expecting to be relieved of their ailments by the goddess in their sleep.[130]

Horus, the child of Isis and Osiris, appeared frequently in the incantations we quoted. Stung by a deadly scorpion he was saved by the powerful spells of the gods and thus acquired himself special faculties to cure people bitten by venomous animals. On the Metternich Stele and on many amulets he is pictured standing on two crocodiles, holding scorpions, serpents, a hippopotamus, and other dangerous animals in his hands. His charms had power over them. The Greeks and Romans worshiped him as a healing god also who had been instructed in the healing art by his mother Isis and whose oracles were sought by sick people.[131]

Hathor, Mistress of Heaven, an old cosmic deity, was the protectress of women who invoked her in childbirth, as they also did Heket, goddess of fertility, and her consort Khnumu, who on the potter's wheel molded the child and his ethereal double, his Ka.[132] We encountered Sekhmet as the Lady of Pestilence who sent plagues over the land. Pictured with the head of a lioness surmounted by a solar disc she was a fierce-looking and mighty goddess who destroyed beings and seemed to enjoy destruction. But she who was able to send evil could also relieve from it. Consort of Ptah, she was worshiped together with him, and her priests are repeatedly mentioned as healers together with magicians and physicians.[133] Whether they actually were surgeons, as Ebbell believes,[134] is a question we shall discuss later.

If we should mention all the healing deities of Egypt we should have to list the entire pantheon, and this is obviously impossible. But there is one god we must not omit because the Greeks identified him with their own Asclepius, namely Imhotep, or 'Ιμούθης as they called him. His cult was very popular in Graeco-Roman times and the chief centers of worship were Memphis, where according to tradition he was buried, and the island of Philae, where Ptolemaeus V Epiphanes had erected a temple to him. He was worshiped as a healing god, and sick people and barren women came to sleep in the precinct of his temples as they did in those of Isis. The same kind of miracle cure was attributed to him as to the Epidaurean Asclepius.[135] Imhotep was a newcomer to the Egyptian pantheon and his history presented a number of puzzles. In his own and other temples of a late period he was pictured with all the attributes of dignity becoming to a deity, with a beard, holding a scepter in one hand, the sign of life and happiness in the other.[136] But numerous earlier statuettes have been preserved in which he appears like a human being, like a priest, with clean-shaven head, dressed in a short skirt and sandals, and reading a book.[137] This is very unusual for a god. The Ptolemies, furthermore, in their inscriptions to him addressed him not in the style customary in the invocation of gods but with formulae used in addressing one of the blessed dead.[138] In the *Song of the Harper,* that famous poem from the Middle Kingdom on the eternal theme, be merry today for tomorrow you will be dead, Imhotep is referred to as a well-known sage of old together with another wise man who lived during the IVth Dynasty. 'I have heard the discourses of Imhotep and Harzozef with whose words men speak everywhere. Where are their places now? Their walls are destroyed, their habitations are destroyed as if they had never been.'[139] And in the Hermetic writings Imhotep is considered a deified man.

It was Kurt Sethe who was able in a splendid study to reconstruct the history of Imhotep as that of a great man who in the course of time became a healing god.[140] As we now know he was a contemporary of King Zoser of the IIIrd Dynasty, at whose court he held important posts and played a leading part.[141] He was the king's vizier and a legend relates how it was because of his advice that a seven-years' famine was ended. He was chief architect to the court and built his master's tomb, the step-pyramid at Sakkara, and the temple at Edfu. A lector-priest he was also, according to tradition, astrologer, magician, and undoubtedly a physician of great renown. We have no early documents relating to his medical activities. Yet they must have been considerable and must have impressed his contemporaries even more than his general learning because they determined his later fate. He was heroized, became a demigod, and ultimately the healing god identified with Asclepius.

It is difficult to tell at what time these various processes took place. He certainly was worshiped as a demigod in the beginning of the New Empire. During the reign of Amenhotep III the scribes invoked him, pouring a libation out of their water bowl and saying: 'Water from the water bowl of every scribe to thy Ka, O Imhotep.' [142] It is the demigod that the many statuettes represent. A late Greek papyrus mentions that the cult of Imhotep was restored by King Mycerinus, a fact that would imply that he was deified rather soon after his death, during the IVth Dynasty. This, however, is a statement that cannot be substantiated from any other source and bears all the marks of late fiction.[143] Imhotep entered the Egyptian pantheon as a regular god very late, not before the Persian period and perhaps even as late as the Greek, or at least under Greek influence,[144] and it is easy to understand that there must have been a strong tendency to increase his authority by tracing the cult back to remote antiquity.

Imhotep is popular with doctors today because Sir William Osler referred to him as to 'the first figure of a physician to stand out clearly from the mists of antiquity.' [145] Medicine like any other craft must have heroes to worship, examples to follow; and little as we know about Imhotep's medical activities, yet he will always be one of our heroes because he is probably the first physician whom we know by name and certainly the first whose reputation was such that he was paid divine honors.

NOTES

1. Thus in *Pap. Ebers,* 99, 2. The parallel passage in *Pap. Edwin Smith* 1, 6 mentions only the first two. (Quotations from Papyrus Ebers are from the translation by B. Ebbell, *The Papyrus Ebers, the Greatest Egyptian Medical Document,* Copenhagen, 1939; quotations from Papyrus Edwin Smith are from the translation by James Henry Breasted, *The Edwin Smith Surgical Papyrus,* Chicago, 1930. For a full description of these papyri see chapter IV, 'Medical Literature.')
2. Seven days from yesterday I have not seen my beloved,
   And sickness hath crept over me,
   And I am become heavy in my limbs,
   And am unmindful of mine own body.
   If the master-physicians come to me,
   My heart hath no comfort of their remedies,
   And the magicians, no resource is in them,
   My malady is not diagnosed. . .
   Better for me is my beloved than any remedies . . .

   Translation by A. H. Gardiner in *The Legacy of Egypt,* Oxford, 1942, p. 77.
3. *Pap. med. London,* Brit. Mus. No. 10,059, and *Berlin* No. 3027.
4. See Kurt Sethe, *Die altaegyptischen Pyramidentexte,* 4 vols., Leipzig, 1908-22; *Übersetzung und Kommentar,* 4 vols., Glückstadt, 1935-9, where a number of spells and other magic rites may be found.
5. About Egyptian religion in general see W. M. Flinders Petrie in *Encyc. Rel. Ethics,* vol. v, and A. H. Gardiner's article on magic, ibid. vol. VIII; Günther Roeder, *Urkunden zur Religion des alten Aegyptens,* Jena, 1915; J. H. Breasted, *Development of Religion and Thought in Ancient Egypt,* New York, 1912; A. Erman, *Die Religion der Aegypter, ihr Werden und Vergehen in vier Jahrtausenden,* Berlin and Leipzig, 1934.
6. A. Erman and A. M. Blackman, *The Literature of the Ancient Egyptians,* London and New York [1927], p. 305.
7. E. A. Wallis Budge, *The Literature of the Ancient Egyptians,* London, 1914, p. 253.
8. Ibid.
9. T. Eric Peet, *A Comparative Study of the Literatures of Egypt, Palestine, and Mesopotamia,* London, 1931, p. 89.
10. *Pap. Ebers 1.*
11. The final paragraph shows that the text is an incantation because it announces the result of the invocation.
12. J. H. Breasted speaks of 'rolls of ancient hocus-pocus, like the medical papyrus of the British Museum, or the "Charms for Mother and Child" in the other well-known roll at Berlin. Such primitive superstition dies hard.' See also his remarks about the 'unsavory magical hodge-podge' on the back of the Edwin Smith Papyrus, p. 19.

13. Thus in the story of Isis betraying Re into telling her his secret name, a story which itself became part of incantations against snakebite. See Pleyte and Rossi, *Les Papyrus de Turin*, Leiden, 1869-76, plates 31, 77, 131-8; also *Zschr. ägypt. Sprache*, 1883, 21:27-33.
14. Thus in *Papyrus Westcar*, edited by A. Erman, *Mitteil. a. d. Orient. Samml. d. kgl. Museen*, vols. v and vi; translation in Erman and Blackman, loc. cit. p. 36ff.
15. A list of them may be found in I. A. Pratt, *Ancient Egypt, Sources of Information in the New York Public Library*, 1925, p. 257ff.; *Ancient Egypt* 1925-1941, New York, 1942, p. 193ff.
16. W. Golenischeff, *Die Metternichstele*, Leipzig, 1877; German translation in G. Roeder, loc. cit. p. 82ff.
17. Facsimile of the text in *Hieratische Papyrus aus den Königlichen Museen zu Berlin*, Bd. iii, 10. Heft, Leipzig, 1911; transcription, translation, and commentary by A. Erman, *Zaubersprüche für Mutter und Kind. Aus dem Papyrus 3027 des Berliner Museums*, Berlin, 1901. [From Abhdl. kgl. Preuss. Akad. Wiss. Berlin, 1901.] In the following the papyrus will be cited as *Mother and Child.*
18. The disease tmjt might be a gastro-intestinal disease because in one of the incantations [B] the text says, 'because the stomach of this infant, born by Isis, is sick,' although the interpretation is not quite certain. Nšw may perhaps be a disease with convulsions since it is one that may attack all members [E].
19. The first [F] begins with an old mythological hymn and was to be spoken over the bricks on which the woman in childbirth knelt.
20. In the midst of this purely magical papyrus are two ordinary recipes prescribing simple drugs against the disease b^{ee} [H, I].
21. Thus e.g. H. Grapow, who speaks of only 7 medical papyri, *Untersuchungen über die altägyptischen medizinischen Papyri*, part I, Leipzig, 1935, p. 1ff.
22. Thus Grapow, loc. cit. p. 2, a date that has now been generally accepted. Wreszinski (see note 24) assumed that the papyrus had been written around 1200 B.C.
23. Three prescriptions [No. 14, 44, 51] refer to the reign of Amenhotep III.
24. The papyrus was published in facsimile; transcription and translation with commentaries by Walter Wreszinski, *Der Londoner medizinische Papyrus und der Papyrus Hearst*, Leipzig, 1912. In the following the papyrus will be cited as *Pap. med. London.*
25. There are some prescriptions of drugs, particularly in the treatment of burns, e.g. 15-21.
26. About the very important concept *whdw* see Paul Richter, 'Ueber uhedu in den ägyptischen Papyri,' *Arch. Gesch. Med.*, 1909, 2:73-83, and particularly the brilliant study of R. O. Steuer, 'whdw, Aetiological Principle of Pyaemia in Ancient Egyptian Medicine' [Suppl. Bull. Hist. Med. 10], Baltimore, 1948. Steuer was able to demonstrate that *whdw* was the pus-making principle, a magical concept originally which, however, gradually evolved and is encountered in a biological sense in a number of texts.

27. *Pap. Ebers,* 30.
28. *Mother and Child,* C.
29. Ibid.
30. *Pap. Leyden* 346, 1.5 and perhaps also *Pap. med. London,* 45.
31. *Pap. med. London,* 4.
32. *Mother and Child,* D and E.
33. Gardiner in *Encyc. Rel. Ethics,* VIII, p. 264.
34. *Pap. Turin,* 31 and 77.
35. The most famous spell against snakebite is the one mentioned before that relates how Isis made Re reveal his secret name, preserved in the Turin Papyrus; translations in T. Eric Peet, *A Comparative Study of the Literatures of Egypt, Palestine, and Mesopotamia,* London, 1931, p. 19ff.; Günther Roeder, *Urkunden zur Religion des alten Aegyptens,* Jena, 1915, p. 138ff.
36. *Pap. med. London,* 34.
37. Ibid. 6, 8.
38. Ibid. 46-8.
39. Ibid. 14.
40. Ibid. 37.
41. *Pap. Ebers,* 108.
42. *Pap. med. London,* 38.
43. Ibid. probably 1-3, 13, 40, 45.
44. Ibid. 41, 42.
45. *Mother and Child,* O.
46. *Pap. Ebers,* 34, where a number of recipes are given for the same illness.
47. *Pap. Hearst,* 73.
48. Ibid. 74.
49. *Mother and Child,* B.
50. *Pap. Ebers,* 30.
51. *Mother and Child,* C.
52. *Pap. med. London,* 23.
53. *Mother and Child,* D.
54. *Pap. Hearst,* 85.
55. *Pap. Edwin Smith,* verso, 3rd incantation.
56. *Pap. Ebers,* 30.
57. *Pap. Edwin Smith,* verso, 4th incantation.
58. *Pap. med. London,* 40.
59. Ibid. 36.
60. *Pap. Leyden* 347, 3. 10-13, after Gardiner, *Encyc. Rel. Ethics,* VIII, p. 265.
61. Here the name of the patient and the mother were to be inserted.
62. *Mother and Child,* Q.
63. *Pap. Edwin Smith,* verso, 2nd incantation. See also the 7th incantation. Sekhmet was the goddess of pestilence. Breasted is much impressed by the mention of wind and thinks that 'we have here doubtless the earliest occurrence of the notion of pestilential or disease-bearing winds.' This may be although it is by no means certain since wind appears also as a cause of disease in the veterinary papyrus of Kahun.

64. *Mother and Child,* E.
65. Ibid. U. See also E. The text is corrupt in various passages and I have quoted only those parts of the text that seem well established.
66. Chap. 42.
67. Contra Celsum VIII, 58. *Patrologiae Graecae,* vol. XI, cols. 1604-5.
68. Καὶ δὴ ἐπικαλοῦντες αὐτοὺς ἰῶνται τῶν μέρων τὰ παθήματα.
69. See Eberhard Hommel, 'Zur Geschichte der Anatomie im alten Orient,' *Arch. Gesch. Med.,* 1919, 11:177-82.
70. *Pap. med. London,* 46.
71. The idea is that if the fire had known that it was dealing with the great god Horus it would not have assailed him. See Wreszinski's comments, p. 204f.
72. Isis is now speaking.
73. *Pap. Ebers,* 69.
74. *Pap. med. London,* 36.
75. Namely in lament.
76. *Pap. Edwin Smith,* verso, 1st incantation.
77. *Pap. med. London,* 41.
78. Ibid. 27-30.
79. Ibid. 32.
80. *Mother and Child,* S.
81. Ibid. Q.
82. Ibid. S.
83. Ibid. F.
84. See examples in Gardiner, *Encyc. Rel. Ethics,* VIII, p. 267.
85. *Mother and Child,* D.
86. Ibid. S.
87. *Pap. Edwin Smith,* verso, 2nd incantation. The stick that the magician carries in this and other incantations was a symbol of authority.
88. Ibid. 7th incantation.
89. Ibid. 5th incantation.
90. *Mother and Child,* F.
91. *Pap. Ebers,* 94.
92. *Encyc. Rel. Ethics,* VIII, p. 266.
93. *Pap. med. London,* 44.
94. Ibid. 38.
95. Ibid. 39 *et passim.*
96. *Mother and Child,* N.
97. Ibid. M.
98. Ibid. L.
99. *Encyc. Rel. Ethics,* VIII, p. 266.
100. *Pap. Turin,* 135.8.
101. Examples for the recitation four times *Pap. med. London,* 6, 22, 29-31, 34; *Pap. Hearst,* 170. Seven times is not quite so frequent but see *Pap. med. London,* 1.
102. *Mother and Child,* A.

103. Ibid. P. See also G. Roeder, *Urkunden zur Religion des alten Aegyptens*, Jena, 1915, p. 119.
104. Ibid. B; Roeder, loc. cit. p. 116.
105. This is equally true of case 9 of *Pap. Edwin Smith,* where the egg of an ostrich was prescribed for a fracture of the skull and a charm had to be spoken over the recipe. The use of liver of beef, pig, turtle (e.g. *Pap. med. London,* 35, 40), and other animals undoubtedly has magic origin also and it would be a mistake to consider it the anticipation of modern treatments.
106. *Pap. Hearst,* 78; the incantation is long and I have quoted only beginning and end.
107. *Pap. Ebers,* 2.
108. *Pap. med. London,* 22.
109. Wreszinski (ibid.) draws attention to the fact that the various cities named as origin of the Eye of Horus were inserted by individuals who used the book and whose local patriotism made them assume that the Eye had come from their home town. Written first as marginal notes, the various names were put together and made part of the text by some scribe.
110. *Pap. Ebers,* 69.
111. *Pap. med. London,* 46.
112. *Pap. Hearst,* 212-16.
113. *Mother and Child,* P.
114. *Pap. med. London,* 25c.
115. *Pap. Ebers,* 1, also 30.
116. *Pap. med. London,* 26.
117. Ibid. 12.
118. *Pap. Ebers,* 46-7.
119. *Pap. Hearst,* 71-5.
120. *Pap. med. London,* 25b. English translation by Breasted, *Pap. Edwin Smith,* p. 5.
121. Uto of Khemmis, whose attribute was the serpent.
122. I.e., Thoth, the god of learning and medicine.
123. 14, 44, 51.
124. See Ernst Bloch, 'Die medizinischen Gottheiten der alten Aegypter,' *Arch. Gesch. Med.,* 1911, 4:315-22; Walter Addison Jayne, *The Healing Gods of Ancient Civilizations,* New Haven, 1925; and in general the literature about Egyptian religion.
125. *Pap. Ebers,* 1; also *Pap. Hearst,* 78.
126. Waldemar Golenischeff, *Die Metternichstele,* Leipzig, 1877; see G. Roeder, *Urkunden zur Religion des alten Aegyptens,* Jena, 1915, p. 91.
127. Ibid. p. 83.
128. Thus in the story how Isis betrayed Re into telling her his secret name; see Roeder, loc. cit. p. 138ff.
129. T. Eric Peet, *A Comparative Study* . . . p. 20.
130. Diodorus, I, 25.
131. Ibid.

132. See, e.g. the reliefs in the temple of Hatshepsut at Deir el-Bahri, in F. Weindler, *Geburts- und Wochenbettsdarstellungen auf altägyptischen Tempelreliefs,* Munich, 1915, fig. 4.
133. Thus *Pap. Ebers,* 99.
134. Ibid. p. 14.
135. See, e.g. the story in F. L. Griffith, *Stories of the High Priests of Memphis,* Oxford, 1900, pp. 42, 143.
136. Thus, e.g. in the temple at Philae and in the temple of Ptah at Karnak; see J. F. Champollion, *Monuments de l'Egypte et de la Nubie,* 1835-45, vol. 1, pl. 78; R. Lepsius, *Denkmäler aus Aegypten und Aethiopien,* Berlin, part IV, vol. 9, pl. 15.
137. Every Egyptological museum possesses such statuettes. The Wellcome Historical Medical Museum in London has a large collection of them. Small statuettes of Imhotep were used as amulets.
138. See Sethe [note 140], p. 6f.
139. T. Eric Peet, *A Comparative Study . . .* p. 58f.
140. Kurt Sethe, 'Imhotep der Asklepios der Aegypter, ein vergötterter Mensch aus der Zeit des Königs Doser,' *Untersuchungen zur Geschichte und Altertumskunde Aegyptens,* 1902, vol. II, no. 4, pp. 95-118; also published separately with special pagination 1-26; references are to this edition. A monograph in which the literary and archaeological sources on Imhotep have been brought together carefully is Jamieson B. Hurry, *Imhotep the Vizier and Physician of King Zozer and Afterwards the Egyptian God of Medicine,* Oxford Univ. Press, 2nd ed., 1928.
141. Sethe's assumption that Imhotep was a contemporary of Zoser was based on the interpretation of three late sources which, however, put together presented convincing evidence. His conjecture was confirmed later by an inscription of the IIIrd Dynasty in which Imhotep is mentioned with his titles on a statue of Zoser; see B. Gunn, *Annales du service des antiquités de l'Egypte,* 1926, 26:177ff.
142. H. Schäfer, *Zschr. f. ägypt. Sprache,* 1898, 36:147; A. H. Gardiner, ibid. 1903, 40:146.
143. B. P. Grenfell and A. S. Hunt, *The Oxyrhynchus Papyri,* 1915, part XI, p. 221ff. The papyrus was written at a time when Imhotep was a recognized deity and the priests were obviously interested in assigning the origin of the cult to early days of Egyptian history.
144. F. W. von Bissing, *Deutsche Literaturzeitung,* 1902, Sept. 13, col. 2330.
145. Sir William Osler, *The Evolution of Modern Medicine,* New Haven and London, 1921, p. 10.

*

4. Empirico-rational Medicine

If this book had been written before 1922 I should never have thought of discussing Egypt's magico-religious and empirico-rational medicine in separate chapters. We knew at that time, of course, that there was more to Egyptian medicine than incantations and amulets, that in addition to the magician there was a physician who treated his patients primarily with drugs. We also had some evidence of surgical interventions, literary as well as paleopathological. We knew, moreover, that the Egyptians had made a first attempt to explain the phenomena of health and disease philosophically rather than mythologically. Yet this entire rational sector was limited. The materia medica seemed extremely rich at first sight but a great many recipes that looked rational could be understood only as manual rites of magic procedures. The common origin of all Egyptian medicine in magic and religion seemed apparent—at least to me—and the logical way to present it was to discuss it as a whole and to develop how the rational element branched off and to a certain extent assumed a life of its own.

But then in 1922 James H. Breasted published two preliminary accounts of the Papyrus Edwin Smith, which created a sensation among students of ancient medicine.[1] We suddenly heard of a very old text that was almost entirely rational, revealed a keen observation of nature, and reflected a great amount of sound empirical knowledge and practices. It was a surgical papyrus, to be sure, and surgery was at all times a craft in which little could be achieved with magic, but there could be no doubt about the importance of this papyrus. It was a great document in itself and at the same time it made the other papyri appear in a different light, integrating our picture of the rational aspect of Egyptian medicine.

I still believe in the common origin of all Egyptian medicine, one in which magic, religious, and empirical elements were interwoven inextricably as they are in primitive medicine. But the Papyrus Edwin Smith makes it evident that the empirico-rational element was stronger than we had assumed and that the split between magic, religion, and medicine proper occurred rather early. This may justify the discussion of these various aspects in separate chapters although I should like to repeat that there are no sharp borderlines. The magician did not hesitate to prescribe drugs at times as part of his ritual, just as the most rational physician in certain cases took recourse to prayer and magic then as he sometimes does today.

The Papyrus Edwin Smith taught us another great lesson. It demonstrated how very careful we must be in interpreting archaic medicine. Our material is very scanty and we may have to draw far-reaching conclusions from less than a dozen texts. We usually do not know how important these books had been at the time when they were written, whether they were characteristic of the official medicine of the day or whether they represented side lines, the peculiarities of a certain school. This does not mean that we should resign ourselves merely to listing a few facts without attempting to interpret and evaluate them. In the case of Egypt we shall see in a moment that we have books preserved not in one but in several of the few manuscripts, a fact that permits conclusions. We shall also see that different as the texts may be they nevertheless reveal a very definite pattern, one that became clearer through the Papyrus Edwin Smith but that was known before. Excavations, however, may bring forth new books at any moment, and we must be prepared to revise our views whenever new material requires it, as we did after 1922.

MEDICAL LITERATURE

We have seen the magician in action protecting people with charms and amulets, treating patients with all kinds of oral and manual rites, which we have studied in detail. Our task now is to look at the physician and to find out how he acted when a sick man was brought to him, what he saw, what he did, and what thoughts guided his actions.

Before we can do this, however, we must be familiar with the sources from which we derive our knowledge. We have discussed those medical papyri that were primarily magical and we must now briefly describe those of which the content is mostly if not exclusively empirico-rational.

There can be no doubt that medical books were written at an early date, nor is this particularly astonishing since medical books appear among the early documents of literature in all ancient civilizations. Apart from religious texts required for the cult of the gods and of the dead, the need is greatest for practical books in which may be found how to arrange the calendar, how to measure a piece of land, and how to prepare a medical prescription. Much technical knowledge is transmitted by word of mouth but prescriptions, whether magical or rational, have to be filled accurately and it is impossible to remember them all. Hence the need for writing them down as soon as sufficient knowledge has been accumulated.

We have no papyri from the Old Kingdom nor do we know of any medical texts written on walls, but there is plenty of indirect evidence of medical books having been composed at that time. We need not necessarily believe the stories that serve as introduction to some of the books preserved and tend to link them up with the gods and with the early rulers. We mentioned such a story before, which sounded like a fairy tale.[2] Another less colorful one introduces the *Book on the Vessels of the Heart* and tells that it was found under the feet of Anubis at Letopolis and brought to his Majesty the King of Upper and Lower Egypt Usephais, one of the rulers of the Ist Dynasty.[3] Another version of the same anecdote relates that after the death of Usephais the book was brought to King Sened of the IInd Dynasty, because it was so excellent.[4] This story was probably invented, like the previous one, in order to give more authority to the book, and yet the brilliant Egyptologist Kurt Sethe found that the language of this particular book was very archaic and showed peculiarities not encountered after the Old Kingdom.[5] This merely shows that some such stories may be true after all. Manetho's statement that medical books were attributed to a king of the Ist Dynasty, Athotis, son of Menes,[6] sounds incredible but may be based on true tradition. Breasted has drawn attention to an inscription from the VIth Dynasty that testifies to the existence of medical books at that time. King Neferirkere was inspecting a building under construction in the company of his vizier and chief architect Weshptah when the latter suddenly suffered a stroke. He was carried back to the palace; priests and physicians were called. The text, Weshptah's mortuary inscription, then says: 'His majesty had brought for him a case of writings . . . They said that he was unconscious.'[7] The writings in the case were undoubtedly medical books but we obviously cannot tell what their character was.

The most forceful argument for the antiquity of some medical texts is linguistic. A book such as is encountered in the Papyrus Edwin Smith contained a number of terms that were antiquated long before our present copy was written. They had to be explained. What did the recommendation mean to have a patient 'moored to his mooring stakes'?[8] We should expect it to mean that he should be kept quietly in bed. But no, the commentator who still was familiar with these old terms said that it meant that the patient should be 'put on his accustomed diet and do not administer to him any medicine.' The papyrus has sixty-nine such commentator's glosses, which form a dictionary of technical terms.

The earliest medical literature of Egypt,[9] so far as we know it, consisted of monographs, each of which was devoted to one particular subject. Later such monographs were frequently combined to form compendiums. It happens that the three oldest papyri preserved are examples of just such monographs. Unfortunately we have nothing but small fragments of the first two consisting of a few leaves only, found in the ruins of Kahun. They are fragments of books written in the middle of the XIIth Dynasty, that is around 1900 B.C.

One of them is known as the *Veterinary Papyrus of Kahun.*[10] It is a short and mutilated fragment which strangely enough is not written in the hieratic writing customarily used for textbooks but in the same cursive hieroglyphics in which religious texts were written at that time. Short as the fragment is it is nevertheless extremely important because it gives us documentary evidence of the existence of veterinary medicine at an early date. This in itself is not astonishing since we know from other civilizations such as, e.g. that of India that veterinary medicine developed parallel to and in close relation with human medicine.[11] Cattle were wealth and people were attached to their pet animals then as they are now. The loss of a cow or of a bull affected their owner sometimes more than the loss of an infant, which could be replaced without financial sacrifice. I know countries today where veterinary services are much better organized than medical services. Ancient Egypt, moreover, like India, held many animals sacred, embalmed them like humans when they had died, and attended to their health while they were alive. We know nothing about the veterinarian, but we may assume that some herdsmen were more skilful than others in the treatment of cattle diseases and that priest-magicians were called for incantations and looked after sacred animals. It may also be that a physician attached to the court of a nobleman treated not only the members of the household but also the animals that were part of it.

However this may have been, the short veterinary fragment of Kahun is important because it teaches us not only that there was veterinary medicine but that it had the same character as human medicine. The fragment deals with diseases of various animals, particularly the dog and the bull.[12] One case may be quoted here as example:

Treatment for a bull with wind.[13]

If I see a bull with wind, he is with his eyes running, his forehead wrinkled, the roots of his teeth red, his neck swollen:

Repeat the incantation for him. Let him be laid on his side, let him be sprinkled with cold water, let his eyes and his hoofs and all his body be rubbed with gourds or melons, let him be fumigated with gourds . . . wait herdsman . . . be soaked . . . that it draws in soaking . . . until it dissolves into water: let him be rubbed with gourds of cucumber.

Thou shalt gash him upon his nose and his tail, thou shalt say as to it, "he that has a cut either dies with it or lives with it." If he does not recover and he is wrinkled under thy fingers, and blinks his eyes, thou shalt bandage his eyes with linen lighted with fire to stop the running.

The text follows a certain pattern that we shall find again in a similar way or more elaborated in other medical papyri. It begins with a title indicating the disease, which is named after its chief symptom. Then the other symptoms that the examining veterinarian perceives are indicated, whereupon prescriptions for the treatment are given in some detail. Reference is made to an incantation the text of which is not given here, either because it could be found in some other passage of the book now lost to us or because it was the obvious charm to be spoken in such a case, one the knowledge of which could be assumed. All such technical books presupposed a certain amount of knowledge and we must never expect them to describe every single procedure in full detail. Most of the treatment is fully rational: the animal is sprinkled with cold water, rubbed with the juice of gourds or melons, fumigated, and, most important of all, venesection is performed on it in two places. This undoubtedly must be the meaning of 'gash him,' particularly since nose and tail have always been and still are today favorite places for venesection on cattle. If this general treatment fails, then the eyes are to be treated locally. The sentence, 'he that has a cut either dies with it or lives with it,' must be considered a kind of prognosis, meaning that the outcome is uncertain when the illness has reached the point at which venesection must be practiced.

Neffgen, who studied the papyrus with the knowledge of a veterinarian, thought that the disease described in this case was malign catarrhal fever, a cattle disease that has a high mortality. I have dealt with this fragment in some detail because we shall disregard it in our future discussions. It has an interest of its own but is too short to contribute in any way to our knowledge of general Egyptian medicine.

Much more important for our study is the other fragment, the *Gynaecological Papyrus of Kahun.*[14] It is better preserved than the previous one and larger, consisting of three pages. It is also a fragment from a monograph devoted to a special subject, in this case Diseases of Women. The text on page three has a different character and style from that on the first two pages and it may be that the scribe copied from different sources, although the language is the same. The seventeen cases presented on page one and two follow a rather rigid schedule. Each one begins:

'Remedy for a woman who suffers from . . .' followed by a list of symptoms.

The next section is pathogenetic rather than diagnostic, introduced by the formula:

'Thou shalt say concerning it . . .' and here the cause of the symptoms is indicated: the uterus has gone up or down, is biting or starving or restless.

And finally the treatment is indicated, beginning with the words: 'Thou shalt do against it . . .'

This pattern is not maintained on the third page of the fragment, where we find a variety of prescriptions intended to enable one to find out whether a woman is fertile or barren, whether she has conceived, what the sex of the fetus in utero is, with recipes for promoting or preventing conception. In other words this entire section does not deal with women's diseases but with matters of pregnancy. As some of the prescriptions occur, although not literally, in the Berlin Papyrus 3038 [15] they must have been common knowledge. We shall discuss the content of these fragments in a later chapter.

Proceeding chronologically we now come to *Papyrus Edwin Smith* which together with the Ebers Papyrus undoubtedly represents our most important source of Egyptian medicine. The papyrus was purchased in 1862 at Luxor from a native dealer by Edwin Smith, one of the early pioneers of American Egyptology. It was in all probability found in a tomb in the necropolis of Thebes. Smith was aware of the importance of the manuscript but at that time it would have been practically impossible to prepare an adequate translation of such a highly technical text. After Smith's death his daughter presented this priceless document to the New-York Historical Society, in 1906, and in 1930 James H. Breasted published the papyrus with facsimile, transcription, translation, commentary, and introductions, certainly one of the most accomplished editions that has ever been made of an ancient text.[16] The great expectations aroused by Breasted's preliminary announcements were more than justified when the full text became known, and all over the world medical historians and Egyptologists joined forces to study and evaluate the book.[17]

Whenever such a new and unexpected document is discovered, there is a certain tendency to overrate its importance and to underestimate the texts previously known. This was decidedly the case here and Breasted was not always fair toward such books as Papyrus Ebers, which I consider as important as Papyrus Edwin Smith although along a different line. The Smith Papyrus appeals to the modern reader on account of its clear disposition and its absence of magical and speculative elements, but we should always keep in mind that it is a monograph on wounds, hence a surgical text, while Papyrus Ebers is a collection of medical books dealing primarily with internal diseases, and that most of its constituent parts, moreover, are mere collections of recipes.

The Smith Papyrus is a fragment like the papyri previously discussed, but a large one, 4.68 meters long, while the Ebers Papyrus with 20.23 meters is considerably longer. All in all it has 21.5 columns, 17 on the recto with 377 lines and 4½ on the verso with 92 lines. In comparison the Ebers Papyrus has 108 paginated columns. Both papyri were written at the end of the Hyksos period or at the beginning of the XVIIIth Dynasty, that is, around 1600 B.C., but both are copies of much older texts that may go back to the Pyramid Age.[18] The beginning of the Smith Papyrus consists of fragments from the *Book on the Vessels of the Heart*. The verso, which has no connection with the text of the recto except that the beginning was written by the same scribe, contains eight incantations against pest from which we have quoted repeatedly in the previous chapter, a prescription for a woman's disease, cosmetic recipes, one for an ailment of the anus, and one of great magic to transform an old man into a youth.

The bulk of the papyrus, however, the entire recto with exception of the few initial fragments, is taken up by the beginning of a *Book on Wounds*, and it is this book that gives the papyrus its unique position in the literature of archaic medicine. The seventeen columns contain the description of 48 cases, injuries, wounds, fractures, dislocations, tumors, in other words the kind of troubles that fall into the realm of the surgeon. Unlike other medical books this monograph is arranged according to a system, the cases being listed in the order which later was to become the traditional one, namely, *a capite ad calcem* in the following way:

- Head (27 cases, the first incomplete)
  - Skull, overlying tissues and brain, cases 1-10
  - Nose, cases 11-14
  - Maxillary region, cases 15-17
  - Temporal region, cases 18-22
  - Ears, mandible, lips and chin, cases 23-7
- Throat and neck, cases 28-33
- Clavicle, cases 34-5
- Humerus, cases 36-8
- Sternum, overlying soft tissue and ribs, cases 39-46
- Shoulders, case 47
- Spinal column, case 48 (incomplete)

The book breaks off abruptly in the midst of the discussion of the treatment of an injury of the spine and we shall never know what induced the scribe to interrupt his work in the middle of a sentence. It is, of course, a great pity that we do not possess the entire book, as it undoubtedly dealt with injuries, fractures, and dislocations of the pelvis and the lower extremities, and it would have been interesting to know whether the discussion also included abdominal wounds, bladder stones, and similar conditions, and if so how Egyptian surgeons acted in such cases. Nevertheless even in its fragmentary form the book is extraordinarily important not only because it is the oldest surgical manual we possess [19] but also because it enriches our knowledge of Egyptian medicine considerably.

We saw that in the Gynaecological Papyrus of Kahun the cases discussed on the first two pages followed a certain pattern. Each case had a title followed by a list of symptoms. Then came the diagnosis of the pathogenesis and finally the treatment. In the Smith Papyrus we encounter this pattern again but in a more elaborated form. The title is brief as a rule, named after the chief symptom, such as:

> *Instructions concerning a perforation in his cheek* (case 15) or
> *Instructions concerning a gaping wound in his head, smashing the skull* (case 5).

In a few cases the title lists more symptoms, e.g.:

Instructions concerning a gaping wound in his head, penetrating to the bone, smashing his skull, and rending open the brain of his skull (case 6).

The next part is probably the most interesting, namely, the *examination,* introduced with the words, 'If thou examinest a man having . . .' whereupon the title is repeated. And then come detailed instructions to the surgeon, advising him how to examine the case, palpating the wound, probing it; it tells him what symptoms he should look for, listing, describing, and evaluating them in a way not encountered in any other archaic medical book, one about which we shall have to say more in a later chapter. The examination is so important because it gives us the disease picture such as the Egyptian surgeon had observed it. It is followed by the *diagnosis,* which as a rule is a repetition of the title introduced by the words, 'Thou shouldst say concerning him: one having . . .' whatever the injury had been. Then follows, as a new element that we have not met with before, the *verdict,* which may be one of three:

An ailment which I will treat
An ailment with which I will contend
An ailment not to be treated

The verdict is in itself not a prognosis. The surgeon after having examined a case and after having diagnosed the nature of the injury makes a decision about his further course of action. Shall he treat the case or not? What are his chances of success? Here for the first time we encounter the view that was widespread in antiquity, that hopeless cases were not to be touched,[20] while today the physician endeavors to alleviate symptoms to the very end even when the patient has no chance of recovery. Although the verdict is not a prognosis it implicitly includes one, because it obviously is the anticipated course of the ailment that determines the verdict, and the three types of verdict correspond to the logical three types of prognosis, favorable, uncertain, and unfavorable. In three cases (6, 8, 34) the verdict takes the place of the diagnosis; in other words the title is not repeated and the surgeon goes on immediately to determine his course of action. In two cases the verdict appears as part of the treatment: 'An ailment which I will treat with the fire-drill. Thou shouldst burn for him over his breast . . .' (39); 'An ailment which I will treat with cold applications to that abscess which is in his breast.' (46). This merely shows that the scheme was not followed rigidly.

Breasted claims that Papyrus Edwin Smith is the only one that has negative verdicts, while favorable and uncertain verdicts occur in other papyri also,[21] a statement that seems strange because Papyrus Ebers undoubtedly has negative verdicts in the surgical section although they are worded somewhat differently.[22] The Smith Papyrus has more negative verdicts, which may be owing to the fact that it describes many very serious wounds.

In 14 cases after careful examination and discussion of the symptoms the surgeon came to the conclusion that he would not treat such an ailment.[23] Breasted has greatly emphasized this fact and considered it conclusive evidence for the purely scientific interest of the Egyptian surgeon. He wrote:

> One of the most important observations [24] in appraising this surgical treatise is the fact that out of 58 examinations the surgeon recommends treatment in 42 instances, leaving 16 without treatment. This latter group evinces the surgeon's interest in the human body quite apart from any thought of healing or treating it . . . This group of 16 injuries described but not treated in our surgical treatise is without parallel in Egyptian medical literature . . . These discussions demonstrate the surgeon's scientific interest in the human body as a field of observation and disclose him to us as the earliest scientific mind which we can discern in the surviving records of the past.

I must confess that I do not understand this reasoning. The book in all probability is a textbook,[25] a manual of surgery written for the instruction of other surgeons. A number of typical injuries are discussed and the surgeon is told which ones respond to treatment and what this treatment should be. How could the instructor make clear which injuries are fatal and should not be touched by the surgeon unless he discussed them in detail? The unfavorable verdict was a very severe one, since it left the patient without treatment, and no conscientious surgeon made it unless he had examined the case very carefully; but he had to be taught what symptoms he had to look for and what they meant before he could reach a correct verdict. Hence I fail to see why this group of cases should have a significance different from the others. Its purpose is just as practical. I do not mean to belittle the very remarkable power of observation and reasoning expressed in this papyrus and there is no doubt that we can find in Egypt attempts to explain the phenomena of life, of health, and disease rationally, but I do not think that the unfavorable verdicts are an example.

Diagnosis and verdict are followed by the indication of the *treatment*, that is, the surgical treatment proper, the manipulations of which are frequently described as part of the examination[26] while the treatment that follows the verdict consists mostly of the application of dressings and of general nursing and dietetic measures. This separation of the manual treatment from the others is strange and we shall have to say more about it later.

In a number of cases a second examination is described, which is followed by a different diagnosis. These are actually differential diagnoses as a rule and the examinations describe symptoms found in different types of the same injury. Repeated examinations may, however, also refer to the same case, taking place at different stages of the illness. Such is case 7, 'concerning a gaping wound in his head, penetrating to the bone and perforating the sutures of his skull,' where three examinations are given and the verdict is changed. Case 47 'concerning a gaping wound in his shoulder' has even five examinations and the various possibilities that the course of such a wound may take are considered carefully.

And finally in 29 of the 48 cases the book contains glosses, 69 in all, which constitute a most valuable dictionary of technical terms welcome not only to the philologist but also to the historian who has to interpret these cases medically. These glosses are partly a commentary to the text. We know what splitting a skull is (case 4), but the commentator is more specific about it and wants us to know that 'it means separating shell from shell of his skull, while fragments remain sticking in the flesh of his head, and do not come away.' He had other surgical books available from which he drew for his explanations. Thus specifying what 'smashing his skull' (case 5) means he said: 'The "Treatise on What Pertains to His Wounds" states: "It means a smash of his skull into numerous fragments, which sink into the interior of his skull."' These glosses greatly enrich the text of the book. They were added by a man who was fully familiar with the subject and had a contribution to make to it.

Other glosses intend primarily to elucidate terms that had become obsolete and hence might be misunderstood. We mentioned in some other connection the term 'moor him at his mooring stakes' which according to the commentator meant 'putting him on his customary diet without administering to him a prescription,'[27] an interpretation that we should never make if we did not have the gloss. All Oriental languages are very vivid and full of images, of which some are obvious and others not.[27a] Every technical language develops terms that are obvious at the time but not so centuries or millennia later. Glancing through a modern American textbook I find expressions like 'electrolytic pattern,' 'a Weir-Mitchell routine,' 'Dieulafoy's erosion,' terms that every physician understands, but five hundred years from now may require explanatory glosses.

A word of caution should be said here applying not only to the glosses of Papyrus Edwin Smith but to commentaries at large. The man who wrote the glosses was an expert without any doubt, but he was not infallible; he wrote down what things in his opinion meant but in some case or other he might have been wrong. This is a possibility that should always be kept in mind. Commentators, moreover, as we know from later medical literature, have a marked tendency to pretend that they know everything.

The glosses of Papyrus Edwin Smith are not a unique phenomenon in the medical literature of Egypt because Papyrus Ebers has twenty-seven glosses also. Unfortunately through the carelessness of one of the scribes the individual glosses were not attached to the case which they are intended to interpret but have been collected into two groups and appear now misplaced in the *Book on the Vessels of the Heart.*[28]

I think it is futile to raise the question of authorship in the case of a book such as the one contained in the Papyrus Edwin Smith. Most archaic books like most archaic works of art are anonymous and the custom of having the author's name attached to his creation is relatively young. In his first enthusiasm Breasted voiced the opinion that the book might have been written by Imhotep himself. He mentioned this very cautiously as a pure conjecture,[29] and actually refuted it himself when he said that the book was the work of a surgeon who 'had followed an army in time of war.'[30] It is not very probable that the vizier of a great Pharaoh would have acted as an army surgeon. There is good internal evidence, however, that the book was a manual of war surgery or rather that the experience it reflects was gained to a large extent from war injuries. The fact that patients are designated as a rule as men and not as women is not so important. Women who stayed in the homes were less exposed to injuries than men anyway, and besides in most cases discussed, the sex of the patient was irrelevant and the treatment was the same whether a man or a woman was concerned. It is rather the type of wounds that points to war, particularly the many wounds of the head that impress me as having been caused by weapons. There certainly were other causes of injury, accidents that must have been very frequent in the construction of the pyramids and other buildings, beatings, and the accidents of everyday life.

The Papyrus Edwin Smith in the splendid edition of Breasted was so surprising and so impressive that for a while it completely overshadowed the other Egyptian medical books that had been known for a long time, and particularly the *Papyrus Ebers,* which until 1922 had been our chief source of Egyptian medicine. Today we can look at the material more objectively and I have no hesitation to say that I consider the Papyrus Ebers at least as important if not more important than the Papyrus Edwin Smith. It has not the same appeal to the modern physician because it has a magic element, because much of its materia medica is obsolete, and because it has not the systematic arrangement of the Smith Papyrus, but it is invaluable for the wealth of information it contains in many different fields of medicine.

As we now know, the papyrus was once in the hands of Edwin Smith[31] but it was purchased at Luxor by the German Egyptologist Georg Ebers in 1873, who only two years later published it in a splendid facsimile edition with introduction, analysis of content, and a glossary contributed by L. Stern.[32] At that time it would have been impossible to give a complete translation of a text that contained so many technical terms and names of drugs. It was the first Egyptian medical papyrus ever published and it had been preceded only by a few short notes by H. Brugsch on the Berlin Papyrus[33] and by a note of S. Birch on the London Papyrus.[34] In other words there had not yet been a chance to study the medical language of Egypt and the best that could be done was to add a glossary. A first translation was attempted by H. Joachim in 1890,[35] a Berlin physician who had learned Egyptian and was advised by the Scandinavian Egyptologist J. Lieblein, who himself had published a number of studies on the subject.[36] Though Joachim's translation had all the weaknesses of a first attempt, it was very welcome because it made the content of this important papyrus accessible to readers who were not trained Egyptologists, and it remained the only version available[37] until 1937, when B. Ebbell published a new translation which showed a great improvement over the previous one.[38] This was possible since in the meantime the other papyri had been published and the Egyptian Dictionary launched by Erman was available.[39]

Papyrus Ebers, as we mentioned before, is closely related to Papyrus Edwin Smith. They were probably found in the same tomb or whatever the place was where they survived the millennia, and were written in the same language and script, at about the same time. Papyrus Ebers may have been written a little later but they both date from the beginning of the XVIIIth Dynasty, that is, from the first half of the sixteenth century B.C., and the content of both is much older. Yet they differ in many ways. Papyrus Ebers is almost five times longer, measuring 20.23 meters and having 108 columns of 20 to 22 lines.[40] It is not a fragment but a complete compendium of medicine with a well-defined and dignified beginning, which we have quoted in another connection.[41]

The chief difference, however, lies in the fact that in Papyrus Edwin Smith we have, apart from the opening fragment and the miscellaneous materials on the verso, large sections of one monograph, a 'Book on Wounds,' while Papyrus Ebers is a collection of monographs and excerpts devoted to a variety of subjects. How many monographs have been put together and how the original compiler inserted individual recipes or groups of them from other sources are hard to tell. When a section is opened with the words, 'The beginning of remedies prepared for women,' [42] or with the title 'The beginning of the physician's secret: knowledge of the heart's movement and knowledge of the heart,' [43] and these titles are followed by substantial passages pertinent to the subject, we know that the compiler was copying definite treatises. In other cases he or a physician who used the book added recipes here and there. Sometimes also we find well-defined sections beginning abruptly without Incipit, such as the very important surgical section which begins without any general title with a case 'Instructions concerning an enlarged gland on the neck of a man.' [44] Grapow divided the text into 45 sections and subdivided many of these still further, leaving only such recipes together that belong to one another without any doubt or that appear in the same combination in other papyri.[45] I think that for practical purposes we may accept Ebbell's rough division into the following nine groups of texts, but it must be understood that most of them are not homogeneous and consist of parts derived from different sources:

1. Invocation of the gods and recitals to be spoken when treating a patient (1,1-2,6)
2. Internal diseases and their treatment (2,7-55,20)
3. Prescriptions for diseases of the eyes (55,20-64,5)
4. Prescriptions for diseases of the skin (64,5-76,19)
5. Prescriptions for diseases of the extremities (76,19-85,16)
6. Miscellaneous prescriptions (85,16-93,5)
7. Diseases of women and their treatment; [45a] matters concerning housekeeping (93,6-98,21)
8. Two treatises on the heart and vessels and [misplaced] glosses (99,1-103,18)
9. Surgical diseases and their treatment (103,19-110,9)

The Papyrus Edwin Smith contained a book on wounds, a manual for surgeons with treatments consisting of manipulations, diets, and drugs. This papyrus contains a compendium for physicians. It deals primarily with internal diseases and with specialties that at some time must have been handled by the physician also. The very fact that these special monographs were put together in one and the same papyrus roll seems evidence for the fact that not all Egyptian physicians were specialists. Even the surgical section may possibly be addressed to physicians rather than surgeons. Its subject matter is not wounds, fractures, and dislocations of the bones, but enlarged lymphatic glands, abscesses, all kinds of swellings. And the operations mentioned—but with few exceptions [46] not described because they apparently were taken for granted—may well have consisted of simple incisions and application of the cautery, in other words, operations the general practitioner could perform.

As far as style is concerned we have three different types of books combined in this papyrus. The surgical section just mentioned and a book on 'Diseases of the Cardia' (36,4-43,2) contain descriptions of disease syndromes with instructions for their treatment. They are collections of cases that are fully discussed very much in the same way as those of the Edwin Smith Papyrus and following more or less the same pattern, with title, examination and sometimes re-examination, diagnosis, verdict, and treatment. These books obviously all belong into the same category of didactic medical literature and those of the Ebers Papyrus reveal the same keen sense of observation and acute reasoning as we had found in the Smith Papyrus.[47] To this group also belongs the collection of glosses (99, 12-100,2 and 100,14-102,16).

The second group of texts is represented by the two extremely important theoretical treatises on the heart and vessels, which we shall have to discuss in detail later. They represent nothing less than a first attempt to explain the phenomena of life in health and disease, not mythologically but in terms of a speculative philosophy of nature. Fragments of the first treatise [48] occur on the first page of the Smith Papyrus while the complete second treatise is also found in the Berlin Papyrus.[49]

The third and by far largest group of texts consists of collections of recipes with prescriptions for the treatment of internal diseases, of diseases of the eyes, of the skin, of women, and other ailments. When the Smith Papyrus became known it was pointed out repeatedly how superior it was over the Ebers Papyrus in that it had descriptions of disease and not only indications in regard to treatment,[50] an argument that was entirely beside the point. Not only did the Ebers Papyrus have descriptions of disease in two important sections, but as a manual for physicians it was intended to be primarily a collection of recipes. Our modern pharmacopeias and manuals of pharmacological therapy have no descriptions of disease either.

A picturesque little detail is that the gynecological section is followed by a number of recipes 'to expel fleas in the house, to prevent a snake from coming out of its hole, to prevent a fly from biting, to sweeten the smell of the house or the clothes,' and other similar household remedies.[51] I do not think that this order is accidental; it rather shows that the physician who was an expert on drugs was consulted by the women of the house not only about their sex life and female ailments but also about matters that today would be handled by an 'exterminator,' matters, however, of great hygienic significance.

There are more incantations in the Ebers than in the Smith Papyrus, obviously, because one is surgical and the other medical. You cannot heal a broken leg properly or reduce a dislocated jaw with spells, but you can cure or improve a great many internal diseases with incantations, that is, with religious or magic means you can place the patient in a frame of mind that will activate the natural healing forces of the organism. If we are honest we must admit that until very recently much of our internal therapy was not so very different from magic, although the language of science was used. In a religious society such as the Egyptian was, religious and magical elements will never be entirely absent from medicine and we should not be astonished that books on internal medicine contain spells but rather that there are so few of them. Actually, in the entire Papyrus Ebers treatment by incantation is recommended in only twelve cases, most of which were regarded hopeless.[52] In one case, which may be one of aneurysma arterioso-venosum, it is explicitly said that the physician should not put his hands to it but should instead prepare 'the healing of vessels in all limbs of a man' which according to Ebbell might be a special ointment,[53] and should in addition recite four times early in the morning a spell the text of which is given. This obviously is a hopeless case where neither surgery nor drugs will help and it is one of those few cases with negative verdict where something is done to relieve or to cheer the sick man.

It may well be that not a few of the recipes were originally manual rites of incantations, but as we discussed in the previous chapter such manual rites may be perfectly rational in our sense of the word. The verbal rite gave the drugs their power in the Egyptian's belief, and in many cases the words had been dropped and the drugs were given without special ceremony, or some general prayer was said such as we find in the beginning of the papyrus. This scarcity of spells decidedly places Papyrus Ebers in a totally different category from the London Papyrus or the one for Mother and Child.

Whenever such an important document comes to light its editor shows a very understandable tendency to attach a label to it. Breasted played with the idea that Papyrus Edwin Smith might after all be the work of Imhotep, and Ebers declared that his papyrus was one of the Hermetic Books referred to by Clemens of Alexandria.[54] Clemens, a Christian scholar who died in the beginning of the third century of this era, wrote that six of the forty-two sacred books of the Egyptians—called Hermetic because Thoth, whom the Greeks identified with Hermes, had revealed them—were devoted to medicine.[55] One of them was περὶ φαρμάκων, a Book on Drugs,[56] and Ebers assumed that his papyrus was this very book. Today we know more about the Hermetic Writings,[57] and the Ebers Papyrus, besides, contains infinitely more than a book on remedies, as we have seen before.

We can be very brief with the next two papyri, *Papyrus Hearst* and the *Berlin Papyrus* 3038, because they do not add anything basically new to our knowledge of Egyptian medical literature. They complete Papyrus Ebers in a most fortunate way, transmitting a considerable number of remedies that otherwise would have remained unknown to us. They differ from the Ebers Papyrus in format and general arrangement. Not only is Ebers considerably longer, having 108 columns while Papyrus Hearst has 18 and the

Berlin Papyrus 24, but the pages are larger. The pages of Ebers are 30 cm. high; those of Hearst 17 cm.; and those of the Berlin Papyrus 20 cm. This is probably not an accident but means that Papyrus Ebers had a library format and was used for teaching purposes while the others were practitioners' handbooks.[58] This view is corroborated by the fact that Papyrus Ebers is arranged much more systematically than the other two.

Papyrus Hearst, which now is kept at the University of California, was written at about the same time as Papyrus Ebers, that is, during the first half of the sixteenth century B.C.[59] It is a collection of 260 recipes, of which 96, over a third, are duplicated in Papyrus Ebers.[60] It contains one description of a disease that may be a panaris and has a favorable verdict.[61] The number of spells is small and they are similar or even identical with those of Papyrus Ebers, but Hearst has an interesting series of charms—or should we rather call them benedictions—to be spoken when preparing remedies over the measuring cup, the barley, the honey, the beer, and other basic ingredients.[62] We have given an example in the previous chapter. This papyrus also includes groups of remedies and even the beginning of the important 'Treatise to mitigate all ailments, Remedies to quiet the vessels,'[63] most of the recipes of which are also in Ebers. The majority of the prescriptions, however, are listed without any particular order. They are excerpts from various books, the kind of collection that a practitioner would like to have near at hand all the time and that physicians today are still compiling for their own use.[64]

Papyrus 3038 of the Berlin Museum has very much the same character.[65] It is a well-preserved manuscript that was found at Sakkara in a jar ten feet under the ground. It has 25 pages, three of which are on the verso written by a second hand, with 279 lines all in all and 204 recipes. Five cases of illness are described, two of them in detail,[66] the others in a more abbreviated way.[67] Otherwise we have very much the same type of prescriptions as in the preceding two papyri, Ebers and Hearst.[68] A good many recipes are new, particularly a series of fumigations.[69] Interesting also are the tests to be used in order to find out whether a woman will have children or not,[70] which were added on the verso of the manuscript. Why label them 'most absurd superstitions,' as Wreszinski does?[71] If we used them today it would be the result of superstition, but at that time these tests were in line with a certain speculative physiology, which was not more 'absurd' than the people's religion.

The most valuable feature of the papyrus undoubtedly is that it contains a good version of the 'Book on the Vessels,' which also occurs in the Ebers Papyrus.[71a] The beginning is more detailed here and more solemn and also has a physician's name attached to the book:

> The beginning of the collection of the removal of wehedu, found in ancient writings in a chest containing documents under the feet of Anubis in Letopolis in the time of the majesty of King Usephais, deceased; after his death it was brought to the majesty of King Sened, deceased, because of its excellence . . . It was the scribe of sacred writing, the chief of the excellent physicians, Neterhotep [who made] the book.[72]

The Berlin Papyrus is younger than Ebers and Hearst and was in all probability written at the time of the XIXth Dynasty, which began around 1350 and lasted until about 1200 B.C. The three manuscripts, however, are very closely related and the texts they contain are much older, going back to the Middle Kingdom and some of them even earlier to the Hyksos period or even the Pyramid Age.

To these papyri that have been known for some time must be added another short one that was published with hieroglyphic transcription in 1935 with a group of other texts by Alan H. Gardiner,[73] and was translated and examined in great detail by F. Jonckheere in 1947.[74] It is a fragment of a monograph on 'Remedies for Diseases of the Anus.' Written at the time of the XIXth or XXth Dynasty, that is, in the thirteenth or twelfth century B.C., it consists of 8 columns of 14 lines each. Beginning and end are missing and we do not know how long the book was originally. There is no doubt, however, that the text is considerably older than the present copy. This is the very type of monograph that we find incorporated in Papyrus Ebers. It is interesting to have such a book because we know that among the many medical specialists there was one who was designated as 'Guardian' or 'Shepherd of the Anus' and this text gives us an idea of the kind of medicine he practiced. It is the recipe-type of book and contains 41 prescriptions with one incidental description of disease followed by a diagnosis and a favorable verdict.[75] Only one recipe is duplicated in Papyrus Ebers,[76] which, as a matter of fact, has a number of treatments for diseases of the anus. We shall have to say more about the content of the papyrus.

Our three earliest papyri, those of Kahun and Edwin Smith and one of the youngest, namely, Chester Beatty, were monographs, while three other important papyri were collections of monographs or contained excerpts from such. Some of these compiled monographs were well defined and had their own title. Others were not and consisted mostly of groups of recipes for the same disease or for diseases of one organ. We also saw that some monographs or fragments of such and numerous recipes could be found not in one but in two papyri, sometimes in identical words, sometimes not, but revealing nevertheless a common origin.

The papyri that have come down to us, like all ancient manuscripts, are not originals but copies of copies with all the mistakes and changes, additions and omissions, that a tradition of many centuries necessarily involves. The first task obviously was to publish, translate, and interpret the papyri and this was difficult enough. The next task now will be to re-arrange the texts not according to papyri but according to content, in other words, to edit the monographs from the various manuscripts. It will never be possible to reconstruct the archtype because the number of manuscripts is far too small, but a new collection of the entire Egyptian medical literature known will consist of a series of texts dealing with such subjects as the treatment of internal diseases, of surgical diseases, namely wounds, fractures, and dislocations, of tumors, of gynecological ailments, diseases of eyes, ears, teeth, of cosmetics and a number of similar texts, finally of theoretical writings. H. Grapow did the pioneering work in this field and outlined a new arrangement of the prescriptions, case histories, and spells, about 1200 altogether, contained in these papyri.[77]

MEDICAL PRACTICE

We have seen that the medical literature of Egypt that has come down to us is not large, but that it is rich enough to allow us to form an opinion on the practices of those physicians who were not primarily magicians. I am sure that they all used incantations or prayers at times just as the medieval physician invoked the name of Allah or of Christ or some saint.[78] But there can be no doubt that Egypt had physicians and surgeons who treated their patients primarily with methods that we consider rational. This is evidenced by the papyri as well as numerous other documents.[79]

When Herodotus visited the country he was struck by the fact that there were so many specialists. In a very important passage of his second book he says: [80] 'Medicine with them is distributed in the following way: every physician is for one disease and not for several, and the whole country is full of physicians; for there are physicians of the eyes, others of the head, others of the teeth, others of the belly, others of obscure diseases.' This far-reaching specialization was interesting indeed, particularly since it was not a new phenomenon but had been in existence ever since the Pyramid Age. Egyptologists are inclined to assume that as early as the Old Kingdom medical knowledge was so highly developed that the individual physician could no longer embrace it and specialization became unavoidable.[81] In doing this they project modern experiences into the past. Our present specialization is the result of accumulated knowledge and of a highly complex technology, but we discussed in the previous section of this book that there is also a primitive specialization, a stage at which every doctor knows one disease, or the diseases of one part of the body or one treatment and nothing else, and I think that there can be no doubt that whatever specialization we encounter in archaic civilizations belongs to this type.

The sources about Egyptian physicians and the kind of practice in which they engaged are not numerous, but again we are fortunate in having a sufficient number of inscriptions and literary references to be able to form an opinion on the subject. We obviously are best informed about conditions at the court, because court physicians were high officials and very important ones, since life and well-being of the royal family were entrusted to them. They were buried in style and had their statues made so that posterity knows more about them than about the rank and file practitioner.

Thus a funeral stele found at Gizeh gives us interesting information about such a court physician by name of Irj, who lived around 2500 B.C.[82] He was a very important man, not only a palace doctor but Superintendent of the Court Physicians. In other words, the court was served by a whole collegium of doctors, probably all specialists, of whom Irj was the chief. He was a specialist himself but one who combined several specialties. Indeed, the funeral inscription designates him as 'palace eye physician' and 'palace physician of the belly,' namely, 'one understanding the internal fluids' and 'a guardian of the anus.' The royal anus required as much care in those days as it did at the time of Molière, and in Papyrus Chester Beatty we encountered a manual for the Guardian or Shepherd of the Anus.[83]

Among the court specialists were also physicians of the teeth, dentists, who like other doctors sometimes combined specialties.[84] Thus Hawi at the time of the Old Kingdom attended to both ends of the gastro-intestinal tract by being physician of the teeth and guardian of the anus.[85] Another palace dentist was chief of the collegium of the court physicians.[86] Dentistry was a medical specialty without any doubt.

There was a strict hierarchy among physicians not only at the court but in general. Jonckheere in a very enlightened study [87] has shown that doctors had ranks like officials or priests and that the four major ranks were (1) *Physician,* without special attribute, (2) *Chief of Physicians,* (3) *Inspector of Physicians,* and (4) *Superintendent of Physicians.* The palace doctors, moreover, had a *Senior Physician;* and at the head of the whole medical corps was a doctor who had the title *Greatest Physician of Lower and Upper Egypt,*[88] a title found on inscriptions from the Pyramid Age to the XXXth Dynasty so that it must have occurred universally throughout Egyptian history. Jonckheere thinks that the man who had this exalted title was the chief medical officer of the country, who supervised the activities of the profession and might also have served as intermediary between the practitioners and an office at the head of which was the *Administrator of the House of Health and Chief of the Secret of Health in the House of Thoth* which might have been a kind of Ministry of Health.[89]

This extreme hierarchization may seem strange to us, but we should not forget that we have it also, perhaps not quite so rigidly but nonetheless quite tangibly and not only in our public-health system. We have general practitioners, specialists certified by Boards of Specialties, doctors who control hospitals, others who are university professors, medical politicians at the head of professional organizations, and all these factors automatically create a hierarchy too.

The best physicians of Egypt were attached to the king's court. They were the most highly remunerated, had their own boat that would bring them without delay wherever they might be needed,[90] and it must have been the highest ambition of a doctor to be able to add to his titles that of palace physician. The noblemen who surrounded the king, who administered provinces in his name, or the feudal landlords of the Middle Kingdom had households that were small courts in their own way and there can be no doubt that they had their physicians-in-ordinary also, attached to the household, giving their services not only to the lord and the members of his family but to all those who belonged to the household, the servants, the serfs in workshop and farm, and the slaves. Groups of laborers working on great building projects or groups of miners sent to the copper and turquoise mines of Mount Sinai were accompanied not only by clerks and officers of the commissary but also by physicians who were an integral part of such a labor group.[91] Some physicians must also have been attached to temples. They were probably the ones who served the general public, that is, those people who did not belong to a household that included its own doctors.[92] A widower who was haunted by the spirit of his deceased wife wrote a letter and deposited it with offerings at her tomb. In this letter he reminded her of all he had done for her and said among other things: 'And when you fell sick with the disease which you have suffered, I had a Chief of Physicians called. And he prepared a remedy and did all you said he should do.' [93]

When did a patient call a physician and when a priest-magician? This is difficult to tell. The complaint, the illness, may have been the determining factor. When a man suddenly raved or said strange words in a delirious condition an incantation seemed the most appropriate treatment. Or a patient in certain cases may have consulted both, first the physician then the priest or vice versa.[94] How often does it not happen today that a sick man whom scientific medicine failed to cure seeks aid from sectarian healers or goes on a pilgrimage to a holy place. It may also be that economic considerations played a certain part in the choice of healer. Remedies often contained rare drugs that were costly, while an incantation could be paid for with a modest offering to the temple. In some younger civilizations magico-religious medicine was the poor man's medicine while the scientific medicine of the day was available primarily to the people of means. For a while I was inclined to believe that this was the case in ancient Egypt also. It seems to me, however, that in the archaic civilizations of the East, where religion and magic dominated all aspects of life, both systems of medicine prevailed side by side and were equally sought by rich and poor. And just as there were simple remedies within the reach of everybody and very costly ones, in the same way we also heard of simple amulets made of fishbones, a linen bag, or similar cheap materials and others for the rich consisting of beads of gold and precious stones.

This all brings us to the question of the remuneration of physicians. What was a doctor's income? What was the cost of medical care? Here we must remember that ancient Egypt had no money economy. Trade was by barter and services were remunerated in kind. The numerous physicians attached to the royal palace were supported from the budget of the court and received gifts the amount of which must have varied according to rank and pharaoh's pleasure. In other words they fared exactly like other court officials. Conditions must have been similar with the doctors attached to the household of a nobleman. As members of the household they had board and lodging and received gifts on special occasions. Doctors working with a group of laborers must have been remunerated in kind like all other members of the group, and physicians attached to temples received in all probability their livelihood from the temple budget. We know that at the time of the New Empire many temples had very considerable incomes. If such doctors went out to see 'private patients' they undoubtedly received gifts and this added to their income.

As the sources on that subject are very scanty, much of what we just said is conjectural; but judging from the way scribes and other officials were remunerated it seems more than probable that doctors earned their living in the manner described. In other words, most physicians if not all enjoyed a fair amount of social security and their income was not determined by the amount of ill health of their fellow men. They could afford to treat both rich and poor, and hence we believe Diodorus when he says that in Egypt many people had free medical care,[95] a fact which to a Greek was anything but obvious.

Different as physicians were in regard to specialty, rank, and position they were united by their common worship of Thoth, their patron god. Inventor of medicine, as we mentioned before, physician himself, 'physician of the eye of Horus,'[96] he was accompanied by the doctors who worshiped him and to whom he gave the skill to cure.[97] He was the physicians' god in more than one respect, because he was also the god of learning 'who lets writing speak and has composed the books.'[98] And the physicians naturally were skilled in the art of writing and reading and had gone through the scribes' training. Iwti, a physician of the XIXth Dynasty, on his funerary statue was called 'royal scribe, chief of physicians,'[99] and this combination of titles was by no means unusual.[100]

After having attended the schools of the scribes the young man who wished to become a physician needed specialized instruction. There may have been a time when doctors were trained as apprentices but we have no sources to that effect. We know, however, that special schools existed for the training of doctors in connection with temples. We possess a very important document on this subject from the sixth century B.C. At that time Darius I of Persia was ruling over Egypt and, great statesman that he was, he restored many Egyptian institutions that had decayed. Thus he sent one of his functionaries, an Egyptian priest who was also chief physician by name of Uzahor-resenet, to Saïs with the mission to restore the House of Life, a school for the training of physicians and probably also of priests, which had flourished there in the past. On his statue he reports what he did and the document sheds such important light on medical conditions that we must quote parts of it: [101]

His Majesty King Darius commanded me to come to Egypt, while His Majesty was in Elam as Great King of every country and Chief Prince of Egypt, in order to establish the Hall of the House of Life, the house . . . after their decay. The barbarians brought me from country to country, and conducted me to Egypt as the King had commanded.

I did as His Majesty had commanded me. I equipped them (the two houses above) with all their students from among sons of men of consequence, no sons of the poor were among them. I placed them under the hand of every wise man . . . for all their work.

His Majesty commanded to give them every good thing in order that they might do all their work. I equipped them with all their needs, with all their instruments which were in the writings, according to what was in them (the houses) afortime.

His Majesty did this because he knew the value of this art, in order to save the life of every one having sickness, and in order to establish the names of all the gods, their temples and their revenues, that their feasts might be celebrated forever.

This document, of course, is very young, dating as it does from the sixth century B.C., but it was an old school that was being restored, and tradition-bound as Egyptians were at that time there can hardly be any doubt that the school was re-established along the old pattern. Interesting is the social origin of the students, who all came from 'good families'; also the fact that every convenience was extended to them. The mention of instruments points to surgery. We can well imagine that similar schools existed in other great centers, such as Thebes, Memphis, On. The fact that the schools were connected with temples does not mean that students were instructed in magico-religious medicine alone. The inclusion of surgery in the curriculum clearly points to the contrary. The temples were the centers of learning, ecclesiastical and lay, particularly at the time of the New Empire. In this connection we should always remember that one of the chief roots of our Western university was the cathedral school and that although theology was considered the mother of all learning there was still room for empirico-rational sciences in our medieval universities. Conditions must have been similar in ancient Egypt.

Darius was not the only Persian king who appreciated Egyptian medicine. Before him Cyrus liked to be surrounded by Egyptian physicians.[102] The reputation of Egyptian doctors was great all over the ancient world. We read in the *Odyssey* that 'in medical knowledge the Egyptian leaves the rest of the world behind.'[103] Egyptian doctors were frequently called abroad or pharaoh lent his personal physicians to foreign rulers as a token of friendship.[104] A court physician of Amenhotep II treated a Syrian prince,[105] and it would be easy to give other similar examples.

A word must be said about the priests of Sekhmet. What was their place among the medical personnel of Egypt? Sekhmet, as we saw, was the lion-headed Lady of Pestilence. In Papyrus Ebers, in the beginning of the 'Book on the Vessels of the Heart,' where it is said that the heart speaks out of the vessels of every limb, the text has the significant passage: 'when any physician, any priest of Sekhmet or any magician puts his hands or his fingers upon the head, upon the back of the head' or any other limb, 'then he examines the heart.'[106] In other words, the text distinguishes three categories of medical personnel who all may be feeling the pulse. Papyrus Edwin Smith, which has the beginning of the book in one of the glosses, omits the magician altogether and has the priest of Sekhmet in the first place: 'Now if the priests of Sekhmet or any physician put his hands . . .'[107] Ebbell expressed the opinion that the Sekhmet priest was probably the surgeon and that the Smith Papyrus put him in the first place because it was written for such priests.[108]

Jonckheere has drawn our attention to another important document on this subject.[109] On a monumont of the XIth Dynasty a man is pictured with a legend that says: 'I was a priest of Sekhmet, strong and skillful in the art, one who puts his hand upon the sick and thus finds out, one who is skillful with his hand.' This may well point to the kind of surgeon whose activities are described in the Smith Papyrus, who examines the sick with his hand 'to find out' and who must be skilful with his hand. But the passage may also point to a diagnostician, a specialist in feeling the pulse and in the treatment of diseases attributed to the vessels. We know that Sekhmet was fond of the blood of man and that she was the Lady of Flame.[110] The surgeon had to deal with blood and treated certain wounds with fire, cauterizing them. It may well be that Sekhmet was the patron goddess of the surgeons, but our sources are not sufficient to permit a definite answer.

Auxiliary personnel is very important in medicine. Egypt had the most skilful dressers in the embalmers' shops. The way they bandaged a mummy was a work of art[111] and it may be that the surgeons made use of them.[112]

We also hear of workers being excused from work because they were nursing fellow laborers.[113] In every large group of workers there must have been some individuals who had some knowledge of first aid and nursing and liked this kind of work. They were useful to the employer then as they are today.

And now we should like to see the physician in action. A patient was brought to him or he was called to a sick bed: How did he act? What did he do? It is interesting to find that in ancient Egypt, at the dawn of medical history, the basic procedure when patient and physician met was very much the same as it is today. The patient had a complaint, said what he was suffering or the members of his household did it for him, and whoever has watched such a scene in the East knows how lively it can be when everybody is talking at the same time. Meanwhile the physician looked at the patient and asked a few questions. There is little literature about the questions he did ask because they were taken for granted. It is only very much later that a Greek physician, Rufus of Ephesus, wrote a treatise, the first preserved of its kind, on *The interrogation of patients.*[114] There is no doubt, however, that the Egyptian doctor asked questions also in order to ascertain the history of the sick man to the moment when he first saw him, and we have documentary evidence on the subject. A passage in Papyrus Edwin Smith reads: 'if thou ask of him concerning his malady and he speak not to thee.'[115] Indeed, the physician did ask questions and in the dialogue that ensued he learned from the patient that he was 'too oppressed to eat,'[116] that 'all his limbs' were 'heavy for him.'[117] He learned particularly what pains the sick man felt, that he had 'pains in both his sides,'[118] that it was painful when something entered his stomach,[119] that he had 'pains in his arm, in his breast and in one side of his cardia.'[120] He learned of many more symptoms in such a way, symptoms that could not be seen but had to be told and that formed the complaint that brought patient and physician together.

Even today with all our laboratory tests *inspection* is still one of our chief methods of examination. The physician who is a good observer looking at a patient will see a great deal that may not yet permit him to make a diagnosis but will guide him in his further examination. *Saper vedere,* to know how to see things, Leonardo da Vinci's postulate for the artist, applies to the physician also and was essential to the doctor of antiquity who did not possess the arsenal of instruments and apparatuses with which we are able to supplement our senses.

The Egyptian physicians were keen observers. They looked at the patient's face, found it sometimes abnormally pale or ruddy,[121] looked at the eyes and found them bloodshot,[122] or burning, or having a grain or white spots, or dribbling or drooping,[123] or askew.[124] In some cases the jaw was found contracted[125] or the mouth open[126] or the phallus erected.[127] We cannot possibly list all the symptoms of disease that Egyptian physicians noticed when inspecting the various parts of the patient's body, since this would fill many pages and would be frightfully boring, but I should like to point out the picturesque way in which some symptoms were described. Thus a patient was said to be 'weak like a breath that passes away';[128] another 'has it on his back like the trouble of one who has been stung';[129] and still another's 'face is as if he wept.'[130] In the case of a patient with an obstacle in his cardia the doctor finds that 'his belly is narrow and he is miserable to go like a man suffering from burning in the anus.'[131] In another case the doctor is examining a patient with an enlarged gland and he finds it 'like a fruit of calotropis procera, a decaying bubo whose skin is hard but not very.'[132]

We also compare tumors with fruits all the time and describe one as having the size of an orange, another as being like a small cantaloupe. In antiquity when medical matters had to be described in everyday language such comparisons were quite unavoidable and much more frequent than today.

The physician inspected not only the sick man's body but also what came out of it, urine, feces, 'what is lifted by cough,'[183] or blood, which in the case of an intestinal hemorrhage is described very graphically as being 'like pig's blood after it is fried.'[184] It seems, however, that Egypt never developed a system of uroscopy such as we find it in its most rigid form in Byzantine medicine or in our Western medieval medicine.

While the physician looked at the patient he also noticed abnormal smells. Thus we read that a gaping penetrating wound in the head after a while when it had taken a turn to the worse gave off an odor 'like the urine of sheep.'[185]

Palpation, the tactile examination, played an extremely important part also, then as it does today. The surgeon laid his hand upon the wound, palpated it, probed it with a finger.[136] This may not seem a very sterile procedure, but we may assume that the strict rules of cleanliness to which priests were subjected applied to physicians and surgeons also. We have no documents about it but these may well have been measures that were taken for granted. The Papyrus Edwin Smith was not a treatise of general surgery but a collection of cases. The surgeon palpated the wound in order to discover how deep it was, and whether the skull was broken. Sometimes he found 'something disturbing' under his fingers[137] or he found 'that smash which is in his skull deep and sunken.'[138] In another case of fractured skull he found 'that smash which is in his skull like those corrugations which form in molten copper and something therein throbbing and fluttering under thy fingers, like the weak place in an infant's crown before it becomes whole.'[139] Palpating fractures of the nose, of the maxilla, and of the humerus, he found them crepitating under his fingers.[140] In a desperate head wound the surgeon found the patient's countenance 'clammy with sweat.'[141] This clamminess of the surface was also encountered in the case of an abscess of the breast, where palpation revealed 'a very large swelling protruding on his breast, oily, like fluid under thy hand.' [142] Swellings and tumors of very different origin were palpated very carefully and Papyrus Ebers has graphic descriptions of some of the findings. Thus it is said of a cystoid swelling that it 'goes and comes under thy fingers and it is as separated things by thy hand when it is fixed.' [143] Palpating the stomach of a patient 'suffering from a resistance in his cardia,' the physician found that it went and came under his fingers 'like oil in a leather bag.' [144] 'An enlarged gland on the neck of a man' felt 'as if there were cloth in it, it is soft under thy finger.' [145]

With their hands the physician and the surgeon tested the sensibility of a patient [146] and also the temperature of parts or of the body as a whole. In a case of illness of the stomach the doctor found the sick man's 'breast-side warm and his belly cool.' [147] An abscess of the breast felt 'very hot therein, when thy hand touches him.' [148] Examining 'a man with an obstacle in his cardia' the doctor found 'that his body all through is shivering when thy fingers are applied to him.' [149] Fever is mentioned frequently in our texts, and the way to estimate its degree undoubtedly was by putting the hand on the patient's forehead or some other part of the body.

The Egyptian physician did feel the patient's pulse and, as we mentioned before, the priest of Sekhmet may even have been a specialist in the field. We shall see later what great emphasis was placed on the heart and on the vessels that go from the heart to every part of the body. Hence it was natural for the physician to evaluate a patient's general condition from the quality of the pulse. 'His heart beats feebly' [150] was an alarming symptom. The doctor knew that if he applied 'the hands or his fingers to the head, to the back of the head, to the hands, to the place of the stomach, to the arms or to the feet, then he examines the heart, because all his limbs possess its vessels, that is: the heart speaks out of the vessels of every limb.' [151] The question is whether the doctor not only evaluated the quality of the pulse but also counted it. Breasted thinks that this was probably the case and even goes so far as to assume that the Egyptian surgeon 'was surprisingly near recognition of the circulation of the blood.' [152] I do not think that there is any evidence or even any probability for such an assumption because the 'circulation' of the blood was not and could not be discovered before quantitative methods were used in the solution of biological problems. Breasted's idea that the pulse might have been counted is based almost entirely on one highly confused and mutilated gloss of Papyrus Edwin Smith,[153] where it is said that examining a man is like counting things with a bushel or counting something with the fingers. The same gloss then has the passage from the 'Book on the Vessels of the Heart' which we just cited. Quite apart from the fact that I do not consider this text in any way convincing I also doubt that the Egyptians had instruments for measuring very small units of time.[154] Even in the seventeenth century the Italian physician Santorio found that the length of a pendlum synchronized with the pulse was a better measure for describing the pulse quantitatively than time, and this is not astonishing when we remember that watches in those days had no hand indicating seconds. Even if the Egyptians had counted the pulse it could not have meant much to them since their knowledge of the cardio-vascular system was necessarily primitive. They undoutbedly knew that the heart beat and hence the pulse was accelerated in physical exertion, fear, and fever, and even without counting the pulse by merely feeling it they could easily determine whether it was slow or fast.

Examining the patient by inspecting him, palpating him, and smelling what seemed abnormal was not all; the Egyptian surgeon also made functional tests. In the case of an injury in a vertebra of the neck he said to the patient: 'Look at thy two shoulders and thy breast.' The diagnosis was determined by the reaction. If the patient was able to move his head to the left and right and down although it was painful, the case was one of mere strain,[155] but if he could not move his head the surgeon diagnosed a displacement in a vertebra.[156] The same test was made in a number of injuries of the head that caused stiffness of the neck.[157] Or the surgeon asked the patient to lift his face in order to see whether he could bend his neck backward,[158] or to open his mouth to find whether it was painful.[159] In the case of an injury of the spinal column he said: ' "Extend now thy two legs and contract them both again." When he extends them both he contracts them both immediately because of the pain he causes in the vertebra of his spinal column in which he suffers.'[160] Making the patient walk a few steps was also revealing in many ways. One with a smash in his skull was found to walk 'shuffling with his sole, on the side of him having that injury which is in his skull.'[161] These are all very fine observations and a system of medicine must be highly developed before the physician is able to make such functional tests.

Using all his senses and taking advantage of his own experience and of that of others as related in the literature, the physician examined the patient and on the basis of his examination made a diagnosis—diagnosis of what?[162] To answer this question we must discuss the Egyptian concept of disease as it appears in the empirico-rational medical literature. What the physician[163] saw, felt, smelled on the patient were pathological symptoms, changes on the surface of the body, changed secretions and excretions, abnormal functions. But at the dawn of medical history Egyptian physicians had observed that certain symptoms occur in combination as syndromes. We find such particularly good descriptions in Papyrus Edwin Smith[164] but some excellent ones also in Papyrus Ebers.[165] One must be very careful, however, in attempting to recognize recently established disease entities in ancient descriptions. When we read that a patient has 'pains in his arm, in his breast and in one side of his cardia' and that 'it is death that threatens him,'[166] this may very well refer to a case of angina pectoris but not necessarily so.[167]

We have established disease entities characterized by cause, pathogenesis, clinical course, anatomical, physiological, chemical, serological, and other changes from the norm. All findings of medical science and the clinical experience of centuries have been drawn upon in establishing these entities, and the statistical evaluation of innumerable case histories in many large hospitals have added color to these disease pictures, strengthened the entities, and at the same time shown that they are not rigid but occur in variations also.

The Egyptians with their primitive knowledge of the structure and function of the human body could obviously not correlate symptoms and explain them from one common origin. They could ascertain empirically that in the case of a dislocated vertebra of the neck a man's extremities were numb, his phallus erected while urine dropped from it, or that in other cases he had an *emissio seminis*,[168] but could not possibly know what caused these symptoms since they were unaware of the function of the spinal cord. It is remarkable enough that they did see all these symptoms and that they connected them with the injury.

To the Egyptian physician the symptom, as a rule, was the disease, and when several symptoms were observed on the same patient the disease was named after the chief symptom. Or, in other cases, the cause was the disease. And sometimes, finally, the illness was simply located in some organ without further characterization. We must illustrate this with a few examples.

Fever, to us a symptom of a great variety of diseases, in ancient Egypt and long thereafter was the disease itself and we have many recipes for its treatment.[169] Other such diseases were coughing,[170] the urge to vomit,[171] 'a swelling of matter that runs in his body,'[172] a suppurating enlarged gland,[173] the fact that a patient had not enough or too much urine,[174] pains in one side of the head,[175] an ear that emits a fetid humor,[176] an ear the hearing of which is poor,[177] a fetid nose,[178] weakness of digestion,[179] a swelling of the male genital organ;[180] diseases of the knee occur when the knee is sick or hard or weak or when it swings backward.[181] Hematuria, again a symptom to us, was a disease in Egypt and must have occurred frequently in the past, as it does today. Although our literature is very fragmentary, the disease is mentioned not less than fifty times.[182] Since hematuria is one of the chief symptoms of schistosomiasis, the Bilharzia disease, and since paleopathological findings confirm the occurrence of the disease in antiquity,[183] we may well assume that the passages preserved refer to this disease, particularly as some other symptoms, namely the cardiac and abdominal, had not escaped the attention of the Egyptian physicians.

In a number of other cases not the symptom but the cause of symptoms was considered the disease. A man had a worm and the worm was the disease. Intestinal worms must have occurred very frequently, as they still do in tropical and subtropical regions. Two kinds are mentioned in the texts, one that is designated with the same word as the snake and hence must be a round worm, probably

Ascaris lumbricoides; and another that was probably the tape worm.[184]

The cause was the disease when the patient had 'a blood nest which has not yet attached itself,' [185] or 'a seizure of purulency which has not yet attached itself,' [186] or when 'it is putrefaction of his phlegm, his phlegm not having descended to his sacral region,' [187] or 'closing of an accumulation,' [188] or similar conditions. I believe that we have the same kind of concept in the gynecological Papyrus of Kahun. The pathogenetic statements according to which the uterus is restless, biting, hungry, thirsty, moving upward or downward, actually mean that these conditions are the disease the symptoms of which are indicated in the title.

And finally we have many prescriptions for the treatment of diseases characterized neither by symptom nor cause but merely by the part of the body affected. Thus Papyrus Ebers has a number of recipes 'to expel diseases in the belly' or 'illness of the belly.' [189] What diseases, what illness, we are not told. It is like the belly ache of our children, a vague ailment located somewhere between chin and knees. Many recipes in this section of the papyrus are designated specifically as evacuants, 'to open the bowels, to cause evacuation, to empty the belly,' or they are remedies against diarrhea, 'to stop evacuations,' but many appear without any specific indication. The same papyrus has prescriptions 'to expel illness in his [Re's] head,' or 'to expel afflictions in the head.' [190] In other cases the breast is ill,[191] or illness has come about in the lips of a woman's vagina.[192] In all such cases the physician's task was to diagnose and to treat the organ affected.

The Egyptian concept of disease was necessarily different from ours, which is the result of developments from the Renaissance on, but the diseases were very much the same that we know today and that still plague the country. Paleopathology provides the only reliable method of ascertaining with a fair degree of certainty what these diseases were, but the material, as we saw, is very limited. Hence we should like to supplement our knowledge from the medical literature and this can be done to a certain extent. It is most difficult in the case of internal and gynecological diseases because all the physician saw was a few external symptoms and he could only speculate about processes that were taking place inside the patient's body. Most of Ebbell's attempts at identification [193] are highly conjectural, as he very frankly admits; and Reinhard, who made a thorough study of the gynecological and obstetrical content of the Egyptian papyri, could identify only a very small number of disease conditions, mostly those which appeared on the surface, like ulcers.[194] It is no wonder that internal and gynecological diseases more than any others were in the realm of magico-religious medicine.

The task is somewhat easier with diseases of organs located on the surface of the body. This is particularly true with the very frequent diseases of the eyes. As early as 1889 Georg Ebers translated the important monograph on the subject included in Papyrus Ebers,[195] and its content has been studied repeatedly by competent ophthalmologists; [196] according to them the Egyptians have known and treated such eye diseases as blepharitis, chalazion, trichiasis, ectropion, pinguecula, pterygium, night blindness, inflammation, hemorrhage, leucoma, iritis, cataract, granulations probably due to trachoma and perhaps also hydrophthalmus and staphyloma. Blindness occurred as the result of various diseases; whether of gonorrhea is very uncertain.[197] Spiegelberg found a beautiful document, the pathetic letter of a painter, contemporary of Ramses II: [198]

> News from the painter Poi to his son, the painter Pe-Rahotep: Do not abandon me, I am in distress! Do not cease to deplore me, for I am in darkness. My God Amon has abandoned me. Bring me some honey for my eyes and some fat . . . and real eye-paint, as soon as possible. Am I not your father? Yes, I am weak. I want to have my eyes and they are missing.

Diseases of the skin appear on the surface also but we cannot expect any accurate descriptions; dermatology is a very young science and, moreover, still has many unsolved problems. Rash, itching, pustules, and similar symptoms rather than diseases are all we can find and most recipes of Papyrus Ebers considered dermatological are actually cosmetic; many of them deal with the scalp, 'to preserve the hair, to make it grow, to expel grizzling and to treat the hair,' recipes that we mentioned before in some other connection. Diseases of the anus were the subject of a specialty and it is obvious that hemorrhoids, prolapsus recti, inflammation and pruritus of the anus did not escape attention. The field, however, that lent itself best to the observation of disease pictures was that of wounds and external injuries, which could be seen, palpated with the hands, and described much better than the often vague symptoms of internal diseases. In discussing Papyrus Edwin Smith we found that the surgeon observed so many symptoms and described them so graphically that from the symptoms indicated we are able to diagnose today not only such simple conditions as an acute mammary abscess (case 39) or a traumatic deviation of the septum (case 12), but such very complicated injuries as fractures of the base of the cranium (cases 3 and 6), and conditions following injuries, such as septic cerebral thrombosis (case 7), or lateral sinus thrombosis (case 20).[199] Thus by interpreting the literature carefully we may increase our knowledge of the diseases prevalent in Egypt in antiquity; but I repeat, we must proceed with great caution.

We were watching the Egyptian physician in action and found him examining the patient, making use of all his senses, whereupon he diagnosed the ailment and named it after the dominating symptom, the cause, or the organ affected. The next step for the physician was to decide whether he would treat the case or not, and we discussed before the three customary types of verdict which were determined by the prognosis tacitly made. Verdicts, however, were passed in all probability only in the case of more serious illnesses. The great majority of all patients who called upon doctors suffered then as they do today from minor ailments, which were treated as a matter of course.[200] The physician's goal in all his actions was to restore the patient's health by treating him, and we now must examine the various methods of treatment used.

The methods of treatment applied at any time are necessarily limited. They consist basically in having chemical, physical, biological, and psychological forces act on the patient, and this may be done in a variety of ways and combinations. In Hippocratic medicine dietetics was in the foreground of all therapeutic activities, the regulation and correction of a man's δίαιτα, of his entire mode of living. Drugs were given to enforce a diet, and surgery was the last resort, except in the case of wounds, fractures, and dislocations. This prominent position given to dietetics was the result of theories that prevailed in Hippocratic medicine and also of long clinical experience. Dietetics is a difficult art, even today when we possess the scientific foundation for it, because more than any other treatment it requires far-reaching adaptation to the individual's constitution and condition. All our norms and standards are based on average figures, and what may be good for one patient may have a totally different effect on another.

We cannot expect much dietetic treatment in ancient Egypt and so far as we may judge from the literature preserved pharmacotherapy was by far the most popular method of treatment. It is certainly not by accident that the majority of the medical books that have come down to us are collections of recipes. This does not mean that the patient's diet was neglected altogether. We saw that the surgical patient was frequently 'moored at his mooring stakes,' that is, kept on his customary diet without being given any drugs. A prescription of the Berlin Papyrus for a man suffering of a not identified disease consists of a preparation of barley which must be given every day. And the recipe adds: 'Prevent him from eating anything hot.' [201] Similar indications can be found incidentally in most of our papyri and it is quite possible that certain diets were taken for granted so that special instructions were not necessary. There is no doubt, however, that drugs were the chief therapeutic agents in Egypt's empirico-rational medicine. The country was famous for its drugs and poisons all over the ancient world, 'for the fertile soil of Egypt,' we read in the *Odyssey*,[202] 'is most rich in drugs, many of which are wholesome in solution, though many are poisonous.'

The interpretation of Egyptian prescriptions and the identification of drugs present considerable difficulties.[203] The name of a plant is meaningless unless it has survived in the Coptic and possibly in the Arabic or some other Semitic language. Sometimes the hieroglyphic determinative points out whether the drug is a leaf, a root, a tree, a gum, or some similar part of a plant. But even when we are able to translate the ingredients of a recipe we are never quite sure that the literal rendering gives the correct meaning. 'Ass's head' and 'pig's tooth,' which occur in recipes of Papyrus Ebers,[204] may well be what the name implies, but not necessarily so; just as in our language buttercups are not necessarily recipients for butter and snapdragons are not wild animals.

When we read the hundreds of recipes preserved in the papyri it strikes us that at the dawn of history the Egyptians developed the style in which we continue to write prescriptions and also the forms in which most of our drugs are given today.[205] We have added subcutaneous, intramuscular, and intravenous injections but little else. The Egyptian prescription is given in the books under a title that indicates the disease against which it is to be used: 'To expel diseases in the belly,[206] To improve the sight by means of something applied to the eyelids,[207] Remedies to fasten a tooth,' [208] and similar headings. Then comes the inscription listing name and amount of each ingredient. The amount is sometimes indicated very carefully, and Chauncey D. Leake has pointed out that this was the case particularly with costly drugs such as frankincense, or with mineral substances that might be toxic.[209] The measures were given according to different systems but they all seemed to be fractions of the bushel, which corresponded to 4.785 liters. The smallest fraction of the bushel was the *ro* or 1/320 of a bushel or approximately 15 cubic centimeters, which is equal to about the content of a tablespoon.[210] In many recipes the dosage was given in *ros*. Sometimes we find instead of measures a red vertical line which probably meant that the ingredients were to be given in equal parts, what we today indicate by the sign $\overline{aa}$.

Next followed indications for the preparation of the remedy. The drugs were boiled and strained or pounded in a stone mortar.[211] Internal remedies were usually given as potions with beer, sweet beer, wine from grape or date, or milk of cow, ass, or woman as vehicles. Sometimes they were formed into a candy with honey or baked into cakes or shaped into cakes with grease. Or pills were made with bread dough: 'malachite is ground fine, put into bread dough, made into 3 pills and swallowed by the man and gulped down with sweet beer.'[212] Sometimes instructions were kept very vague, for it could be assumed that the physician knew how to prepare the remedy; sometimes they were very precise. A remedy to expel fever read:[213]

Powder of dates	5 ro
Powder of *d*3rt	5 ro
Paste fluid	40 ro

Are boiled until 30 ro liquid remain.

Thou shalt give it to a man or woman at agreeable warmth, till he is restored.

One remedy for the belly was left overnight in the dew, whereupon it was strained and taken for four days.[214]

External remedies were applied in a great variety of ways. Ointments were made with oil of olive, balanites, or ricinus; salves with the grease of various animals. Ointments and salves were either rubbed in or applied with dressings. The topic application of an astringent against prolapsus of the rectum is described in an interesting passage of Papyrus Ebers:[215]

For a dislocation in the hinder part: myrrh, frankincense, rush-nut from the garden, mhtt from the shore, celery, coriander, oil, salt, are boiled together, applied in seed wool and put in the hinder part.

Suppositories were used in the treatment of rectum and vagina, and there was not a liquid, from oil to milk to beer, that they did not absorb *per rectum.* Enemas were usually from one to three pints and contained all kinds of mild drugs, so that in a number of cases the intention must have been to have them kept and absorbed rather than to have them cause an evacuation. In the days of Pliny the story was told that the ibis had taught the use of the enema because with its curved beak it washed that part 'through which it is most wholesome to evacuate the residues of the food.'[216] The anus was also treated with heat by having a hot brick or hot sand, probably wrapped in linen, applied to it.[217] An eye remedy was instilled 'by means of a vulture's feather.'[218]

Fumigations were not infrequently used in the treatment of anus and vagina and a recipe of the Berlin Papyrus tells us what the technique was.[219] Seven bricks were heated, and the cold drug was poured over one after another while the patient was held over the developing fumes. We also have an interesting description of an apparatus used for inhalations.[220]

> Thou shalt fetch seven stones and heat them by fire, thou shalt take one thereof and place a little of these remedies on it and cover it with a new vessel whose bottom is perforated, and place a stalk of a reed in this hole; thou shalt put thy mouth to this stalk so that thou inhalest the smoke of it. Likewise with all stones.

The principle, in other words, was the same as for the fumigation treatments of the lower parts.

The prescriptions also include directions for the patient. Remedies should be drunk or eaten 'when finger-warm,' [221] or 'at an agreeable warmth,' [222] or should be 'taken lukewarm.' [223] A remedy to expel 'magic in the belly' must be taken 'by the woman at bedtime.' [224] Some medicines were given once but very many must be taken on four consecutive days. The number four played a very important part in Egypt's pharmacotherapy and must be of magic origin. The seasons played a part in the choice of remedies. One, 'to kill roundworm,' must 'remain during the night in the dew in summer and is drunk in the morning'; [225] another to expel dilated blood vessels in the eye 'is used from the third wintermonth to the fourth wintermonth'; [226] still another, to improve the sight, is prepared from the first till the second wintermonth.[227] Papyrus Hearst has recipes against the evil smell of sweat in the summer,[228] and the Berlin Papyrus has a prescription against an unidentified disease 'which affects all members in the winter.' [229]

A recommendation, 'really excellent, proved many times,' is found occasionally at the end of a prescription,[230] but not as often as in the case of magic spells.

Remedies of a different kind were frequently given in combination. Thus against 'rose [?] in the belly' an ointment consisting of wax, turpentine, and four other ingredients was rubbed in, and a laxative containing among others colocynth and senna was given at the same time; [231] combinations of potion and enema are rather frequent in Papyrus Chester Beatty.[232]

The ingredients of the recipes, in other words the Egyptian materia medica, consisted of substances from the vegetable, animal, and mineral kingdoms. Many of them were house remedies, substances that could be found in every kitchen or could be picked without difficulty in the nearest garden—fruit and vegetables and ordinary spices.[233] Fruits and berries frequently used were grapes, raisin, dates, watermelon, figs, fig-mulberries, fruits of sycamore, of tamarisk, juniper, willow, pistachio, and piñons. Among the vegetables and spices mentioned very often we find cucumber, onions, leek, garlic, beans, peas, celery, lotus, flaxseed, dill seed, mustard, coriander, anise, fennel, cumin, saffron, cinnamon. Cereals such as wheat, spelt, and barley gave flour and bran, and the flour was worked into dough or a porridge was made from it. Chips of ebony, and sawdust of pine, willow, sycamore, and acacia appear as part of recipes; and of the acacia, fruit, juice, and gum were also used. Of resinous materials, many of which have antiseptic qualities, we find the following prescribed: frankincense, myrrh, storax, benzoin, turpentine, sagapen, manna, ladanum.[234] These resins undoubtedly had pharmacological effects; for thousands of years they remained a standing part of the materia medica, and they are still in most pharmacopeas today. Equally effective were some laxatives the Egyptians introduced into Western medicine, which are still universally used, such as, colocynth, senna, and particularly castor oil.

Papyrus Ebers has a very interesting passage on the ricinus plant,[235] which is quite unique in the medical literature of Egypt. It discusses the properties and medicinal uses of the plant very much in the style of the herbals of Graeco-Roman days. W. R. Dawson in a very important paper has pointed out that the book of which this passage is a fragment represents the earliest known herbal of the Mediterranean world, and I should like to quote it in Dawson's free translation: [236]

> List of the virtues of ricinus: it was found in an ancient book concerning the things beneficial to mankind.
>
> If its peel is brayed in water and applied to a head that suffers, it will be cured immediately as though it had never suffered.
>
> If a few of its seed are chewed with beer by a person who is constipated, it will expel the faeces from the body of that person.

The hair of a woman will be made to grow by means of its seeds. Bray, mix into one mass, and apply with grease. Let the woman anoint her head with it.

Its oil is made from its seeds. For anointing sores with a foul discharge (the trouble will depart as though nothing had occurred). It will disappear by anointing thus for ten days. Anoint very early in the morning in order to expel them (the sores). A true remedy (proved) millions of times.

Today castor oil is used not only as a cathartic remedy but it also is an ingredient of lotions for the scalp and of ointments applied in the treatment of pressure sores such as bed sores. In other words, we still use it for the same purposes as the Egyptians did. Other effective remedies were root of pomegranate given as vermifuge,[237] or gallnut of acacia, which contains tannic acid, used in the treatment of burns;[238] and others might be listed in a similar way. Opium was produced in Egypt in Roman times, particularly in Thebes, from where it was exported all over the Mediterranean world as *opium thebaicum;* but there is no evidence that *papaver somniferum* was cultivated before the Greek period. The poppy flowers found on royal mummies, those pictured in a palace of the XVIIIth Dynasty, and the poppy seeds discovered in tombs of the Fayyum are those of another species named *papaver rhoeas.*[239]

Thus Egyptian medicine certainly possessed some valuable vegetable drugs. How much effect could be attributed to the fruits and vegetables mentioned before remains for pharmacologists to decide.[240] Figs and dates were mild laxatives, spices had an appetizing action, and in recent years it has been found that leek, garlic, onions, and similar bulbs contain pharmacologically active substances.[241] Many remedies had probably no effect whatever except perhaps a psychological one. They were given as a result of traditions or possibly *ut aliquid fiat.* We should be careful, however, not to deny the action of a drug solely because we cannot explain it or because we have no experience with it.

In addition to vegetable drugs, animal parts were used in the treatment of diseases, although not so frequently. We mentioned before the various milks that served as vehicles in potions, the fats with which ointments and salves were made. They were fat of ox, ass, ram, goose, antelope, hippopotamus, and other animals. There must have been some idea that dictated the choice of fat—consistency, costliness, or possibly some magic thought.

The animal of whom almost every part was used in medicine was the ox, man's chief friend, who labors for him, supplies him with food, fuel, and hides, and in ancient Egypt also with drugs. Of the ox, brain, liver, gall, spleen, blood, marrow, meat, and fat were used for medicinal purposes. Pig's brain was also given, and the 'brain of silurus fish which is found in the midst of its head.'[242] While the ox's liver was the one most frequently prescribed we also have a recipe which reads: 'dried liver of a swallow is pounded with viscous fluid of fermented drink and applied to a woman for whom abortion has come about, on her breasts, on her belly and on all her limbs.'[243] Gall of tortoise was applied with honey to the eyelids 'to expel white spots in the eyes.'[244] Blood of various animals, ox, ass, pig, goat, hound, bat, lizard, was used particularly in ophthalmology, as was also the dung of different animals, from crocodile's dung to the excrements of the pelican. Fly's dirt with sap of sycamore was 'applied to the mouth of a bubo until it breaks of itself.'[245] Cat's dirt and dog's dung were used with some vegetable drug in a bandage against some purulent affection.[246] A burnt frog in oil was supposed to make a good ointment against a disease which might have been shingles, and so was the burnt head of a certain unidentified fish.[247]

These latter recipes decidedly belong to the so-called *Dreckapotheke,* one which is encountered in all civilizations and is still popular today in folk medicine, where spider webs are used to stop bleeding and hot cow dung is applied in a variety of diseases.[248] These are the home remedies of peasants who live close to the cattle. Others, however, are undoubtedly of magic origin, such as the prescriptions of Papyrus Ebers 'to expel grizzling and to treat the hair'[249] which include shell of tortoise, backbone of raven, womb of a she-cat, raven's egg, blood from the horn of a black ox, tadpole from a pool, horn of gazelle, burned hoof of ass, vulva of a bitch, fat of a black snake, or burnt quills of a hedgehog to make the hair grow.

In the days of hormone therapy and the liver treatment of anemias we are inclined to assume that people of remote antiquity instinctively sought animal parts that we prescribe knowingly today. This, however, was not the case; and Chauncey D. Leake rightly sounded a warning and pointed out that such animal parts were given 'with little evidence of rationality in the light of modern knowledge.' [250]

The number of mineral drugs used was not very large. Antimony sulphide, copper acetate, copper sulphate, copper carbonate, and sodium carbonate were frequently applied in the treatment of diseases of the eyes. Red and yellow ochre were given internally as well as externally.[251] Stibnite, salt, alum, magnetite, powder of alabaster, lapis lazuli were other mineral substances prescribed for their astringent or antiseptic action. Carbon was given in the form of soot from the wall [252] or of ink powder consisting of charcoal and gum.[253]

There was no pharmacist in ancient Egypt. The physician himself compounded his remedies or his servants did it under his supervision, just as he and his assistants probably gathered the necessary ingredients and stored them in the house. Most Egyptian museums possess special containers of collyria, drugs used in the treatment of the eyes. One container in the Louvre has the inscription 'good stibium, good for the eyesight, to expel the blood, to expel the pain.' [254] Drugs imported from abroad were probably stored in royal warehouses, whence the physicians could obtain them.

Egypt had not only physicians who treated patients with drugs but, as we saw, also surgeons. Whoever reads the Edwin Smith Papyrus hoping to find descriptions of elaborate operations will, however, be greatly disappointed. The papyrus is a surgical book, to be sure, because it deals with wounds, fractures, and dislocations, but it contains very little operative surgery. And in the surgical section of Papyrus Ebers we read that in a number of cases an operation should be performed, but there are no indications of the technique of the operation—it was taken for granted, because in Egypt as everywhere else surgery was a craft transmitted from father to son, from master to pupil. It was not learned from books but from practical experience. In Egypt as in other countries the young man who intended to become a surgeon must serve a master as apprentice.

In spite of the fact that we have little direct information about operative techniques there can be no doubt that the Egyptians did practice surgery. Dislocations were reduced; fractures were very common occurrences. Breasted pointed out [255] that in one excavation campaign, which brought to light between 5000 and 6000 skeletons, 3 per cent were found to have had fractures, the result of accidents, possibly of war wounds and perhaps also of beatings. In the case of fractures, the ends were adjusted and immobilized with some kind of splint, either a brace of wood padded with linen or a piece of wood wound with linen or a bandage made stiff with glue such as was used in the preparation of mummies. Papyrus Hearst has a series of recipes for the treatment of a broken bone.[256] After it had been reduced, a bandage with flour of bean or barley, cream, honey, and similar glutinous ingredients was applied, which when it had dried might very well have become a case similar to a plaster cast.[257]

We are well informed about the treatment of wounds. A piece of fresh meat was applied to a wound the first day—a very sensible treatment, because the meat acted as a cushion thus stopping hemorrhage by means of pressure. Fresh meat, moreover, has hemostatic properties. Cauterization was another method of hemostasis. Or a poultice was made consisting of wax, grease, balanites oil, honey, roasted barley, and another unidentified ingredient.[258] On the following days a mixture of oil and honey was applied with an absorbent lint.[259] As a rule, no attempt was made to effect healing by first intention,[260] and suppuration was considered the normal healing mechanism. The wound was filled with plugs or swabs of linen and if the secretion was too profuse some drying remedy such as sour barley bread was applied, but if it was too dry it was bandaged with grease and turpentine.[261] 'To make the flesh grow' stibium was given with grease of ox, chip of malachite, and honey.[262]

If the wound was wide open the surgeon tried to bring the edges closer together. This was done with adhesive plaster, 'two bands of linen which one applies upon the two lips of the gaping wound in order to cause that one join to the other.' [263] Whether the Egyptians sutured wounds or not is still a controversial question. Breasted thought they did and translated the word *ydr,* which occurs six times in Papyrus Edwin Smith, with stitching, sewing, stitches, or suture.[264] Ebbell on the other hand thought that the word rather designated a clamp, what the Greeks called ἀγκτήρ, the Romans' fibula, an instrument they occasionally used to close wounds.[265]

There is no evidence, archeological or literary, of trephining of the skull or the amputation of arms or legs or similar major operations. Superficial tumors and cysts were removed and in the latter case it was observed that the swelling consisted of a viscous humor and wax-like substance contained in a kind of pouch, and 'if anything remains in its pouch, it will return.'[266] An abscess was opened through incision and drained, whereupon 'thou shalt treat it as one treats a wound in any limb of a man.'[267] Ebbell thinks that the Egyptians operated on patients suffering from hernia, hydrocele, and even aneurysm,[268] but I am afraid that the texts are not clear enough to permit such bold conclusions.[269] I have no doubt, however, that there was much more surgery in Egypt than we know about, because, as I said before, many more operations were performed in all early civilizations than were recorded in literature.

Operative treatments were usually combined with the application of drugs, and many surgical cases were treated with drugs exclusively or even with incantations, particularly when the case was hopeless.[270] It is strange that in Papyrus Edwin Smith manipulations are indicated as a rule as part of the examination, while the treatment proper is pharmacological or possibly dietetic. It seems that in this papyrus the examination was primarily a manual affair, so that all that was done with the hands was listed in the same section. This, by the way, is not the case in Papyrus Ebers, where the advice to perform an operation is given and the ensuing treatment is indicated after the presentation of examination, diagnosis, and verdict, as we should expect.[271]

The only instrument mentioned in the surgical literature was the fire drill used for cauterization,[272] but it is perfectly obvious that the Egyptian surgeons possessed a whole arsenal of knives, lancets, hooks, probes, pincers, and other instruments without which they could not have performed their operations. I am convinced that every museum has such instruments, but they have never been studied in any way systematically in regard to the possibility of their having been used for surgical purposes.[273] The chief difficulty is that unless a whole set of instruments of undeniably surgical nature is found together it is almost impossible to decide with any degree of certainty that a knife was employed in the operating room rather than in the kitchen. And instruments that impress us very strongly as being surgical, like those pictured on a relief of the temple of Kom Omboi, may just as well have been the tools of a goldsmith.[274] A systematic exploration of our museums would nevertheless be very desirable.

We mentioned before that dentistry was a medical specialty, and like all other specialties it must have had its own literature. Fragments from a dental monograph are preserved in Papyrus Ebers, 'The beginning of remedies to fasten a tooth,' [275] and a few recipes also in Papyrus Hearst.[276] From what little literature we have it seems that in Egypt as in all ancient civilizations most dentistry consisted of pharmacological treatments. To fasten a tooth yellow ochre, powdered millstone, malachite, frankincense, and similar drugs were applied with honey. Ulcerated gums were treated with an application of cinnamon, gum, honey and oil, or with fruit of sycamore, beans, honey, malachite, and yellow ochre. Or a mouthwash, consisting of cow's milk, fresh dates, and manna, had to be used for nine days. Another contained fruit of sycamore, honey, frankincense, and water in addition to several unidentified drugs. The gums were also treated with remedies that had to be chewed and then spit out. Such remedies consisted of celery, bran, sweet beer, and some unknown drugs. 'To treat a tooth which grows against an opening in the flesh' cumin, frankincense, and another drug were given. And against 'blood-eating in the tooth' the patient rinsed his mouth for four days with a remedy that contained gum, fruit of sycamore, water, and three unidentified drugs.

We know practically nothing about dental operations. A mandible from a tomb at Gizeh possibly from the IVth Dynasty shows an abscess area in the region of the right first molar and below two holes which may have been drilled to drain the pus.[277] It was also in a tomb of the IVth Dynasty at Gizeh that H. Junker found two teeth, a second and third lower left molar, linked together by gold wire, in other words, a retentive prosthesis. One of the teeth must have been loose and was fastened to its neighbor.[278] Similar but more elaborate work was found in Sidon by Renan's mission to Phoenicia,[279] and since the same grave contained Egyptian objects it was assumed that the dental prosthesis was of Egyptian origin, particularly as a second set was found under very similar circumstances.[280] Who but an Egyptian dentist could have made such prostheses? This is quite possible but by no means certain. The Phoenicians had excellent craftsmen and were clever inventors. It is strange, moreover, that only one of the more than 20,000 skulls excavated in Egypt had such a wire attachment of teeth. If prosthetic work had been performed generally we certainly could expect more specimens.[281]

In a highly religious society such as the Egyptian was, psychotherapy was practiced as a matter of course, if not consciously then as part of the cult with its many religious and magic rites which tended to keep the individual adjusted to his world or to readjust him if necessary. We have discussed this aspect of Egyptian medicine in such detail that we need not come back to it now. Suggestion played an important part in all forms of treatment, even those that seem most rational to us. Religious people always felt that the daily bread they ate, which sustained life and re-created it constantly, was a great mystery. And how much more mysterious were drugs.

Greek and Roman visitors were particularly impressed by the Egyptian cults and eagerly adopted them, the more so the less they understood them. But one thing they did understand: that all these cults promised healing of mind and body. Diodorus reported that over the holy library of the Ramesseum at Thebes was written: 'healing place of the soul.'[282]

Magico-religious therapy was primarily etiological; its aim was to remove the cause of the disease by driving out a demon or the ghost of a dead person, or by reconciling the patient with the transcendental world. Empirico-rational therapy, on the other hand, was for the most part symptomatic. The symptom was the disease, and drugs were given or an incision was performed to relieve the sick of a symptom or of a group of symptoms. We also find etiological treatments, however, in rational medicine. We saw that sometimes the cause was considered the disease. A patient had worms; a vermifuge relieved him of the cause and thereby also of the symptoms of his illness. We find in the literature, moreover, a number of treatments that are probably not of empirical origin but are determined by theoretical considerations, which brings us to a discussion of medical theories.

MEDICAL THEORY

The starting point of all physiology lies in a few elementary observations. Man knew only too well that he could not live without food, that food sustained life, and his labor was devoted to provide the food which he and his family required. But man must have observed very soon also that another substance was equally necessary to life, namely the air that was breathed in and out as long as life existed. Where there was no air, man choked, and with the last breath life abandoned the body. In other words, two substances of the outside world—food and air—were essential to life, of which one entered the body through the mouth and the other through the nose. The fact that excrements were discharged from the body must have been related early to the intake of food, as soon as man began to reflect about these matters. The connection was apparent and it was found that a large quantity of food consumed increased the bulk of the feces and that certain foods liquefied them.

On the other hand, man observed that there was a substance inside the body that must be necessary to life also, because it was found everywhere and because life ceased when it left the organism. Wherever you scratched the skin blood came out, and the best way to kill animals or enemies was to hit them in such a way that they would lose their blood. Early also the blood was related to the heart, the mysterious organ that was in perpetual motion as long as life lasted, that beat wildly in your breast when you were running or afraid or feverish. We saw how paleolithic man painted the heart of a mammoth because it must have struck him as an organ of a special kind.

Physiology began when man entered into speculations about these substances, when he tried to guess what their purpose was and to correlate the action of food, air, and blood. And pathology, in the modern sense of the word, began when it was assumed that deviations from the normal functions caused disease, and man speculated about the nature of these abnormal functions.

It is extraordinarily interesting that in ancient Egypt, at the dawn of history, we find in the oldest medical literature two theoretical treatises, one of which deals primarily with physiology and the other chiefly with pathology. The basic idea of both was that in the human body there was a system of vessels [283] originating in the heart, connecting it with all other parts of the body, and carrying air and liquids such as blood, urine, tears, sperm, and solid matters such as feces, all believed to come from the heart. The heart was considered the central organ and its beat was felt in the pulse; it also was the seat of thinking, feeling, and all other nervous functions.[284]

The significance of connecting canals was obvious to the Egyptians who had covered their land with a network of them in order to bring the water and mud of the Nile to the remotest places. But they also knew that the land suffered when the canals were out of order, just as disease resulted when the canals of the human body, the *metu*, did not function as they should.

We must have a closer look at these two treatises. The one dealing primarily with physiology is preserved in Papyrus Ebers [285] and a fragment of it is in Papyrus Edwin Smith.[286] The text is sometimes dark and also confused by the fact that a collection of old glosses found its way into it. The treatise was named *The Physician's Secret: Knowledge of the Heart's Movement and Knowledge of the Heart.* After an introduction, which we have quoted in another connection and which says that vessels go from the heart to every limb, and that by feeling the pulse you feel the heart that 'speaks out of the vessels of every limb,' the text then proceeds to list 46 vessels. Divested of the glosses it reads in Ebbell's translation:

There are 4 vessels in his nostrils, 2 give mucus and 2 give blood.

There are 4 vessels in the interior of his temples which then give blood to the eyes; all diseases of the eyes arise through them, because there is an opening to the eyes.

There are 4 vessels dispersing to the head which effuse in the back of the head . . .

There are 4 vessels to his 2 ears together with the (ear) canal, 2 on his right side and 2 to his left side. The breath of life enters into the right ear, and the breath of death enters into the left ear . . .

There are 6 vessels that lead to the arms, 3 to the right and 3 to the left; they lead to his fingers.

There are 6 vessels that lead to the feet, 3 to the right foot and 3 to the left foot, until they reach the sole of the foot.

There are 2 vessels to his testicles; it is they which give semen.

There are 2 vessels to the buttocks, 1 to (the right) buttock and the other to (the left) buttock.

There are 4 vessels to the liver; it is they which give to it humor and air, which afterwards cause all diseases to arise in it by overfilling with blood.

There are 4 vessels to the lung and to the spleen; it is they which give humor and air to it likewise.

There are 2 vessels to the bladder; it is they which give urine.

There are 4 vessels that open to the anus (rectum?); it is they which cause humor and air to be produced for it. Now the anus opens to every vessel to the right side and to the left side in arms and legs when (it) is overfilled with excrements.

This is speculative physiology, to be sure, based upon a speculative anatomy about which we shall have to say more in a moment, and yet this very old short text represents in my opinion a grandiose attempt to explain the phenomena of life not mythologically but in a rational way. At the same time it lays the foundations for a speculative but rational interpretation of disease, a theme that is developed further in the second theoretical treatise and in a not inconsiderable number of recipes.

The second treatise is preserved in two versions, one in Papyrus Ebers [287] and one in the Berlin Papyrus.[288] It is primarily pathological in that it deals with the system of vessels of the human body as the seat of origin of all diseases. It is entitled *The Collection on the Expelling of the Wehedu* and we mentioned before that according to recent investigations of Steuer, *wehedu* designated a pus-making principle.[289] The book is the one that we quoted as having been 'found in ancient writings in a chest containing documents under the feet of Anubis in Letopolis in the time of the majesty of King Usephais, deceased,' etc. It describes not 46 but 22 vessels, in other words, follows another system than the treatise mentioned before.[290]

Combining the two versions we get about the following text:

There are 22 vessels in man; they carry the air to his heart and also carry the air to all his limbs.

There are 2 vessels in him to his breast; they make burning in the anus. What is done against it: fresh dates, leaves of . . . of sycamore, water, pounded together, strained, to be taken by the patient for 4 days until he is well.

There are 2 vessels in him to his thigh; if he is ill in his thigh or his feet ache (?), then thou shalt say concerning it: it is that the vessel šrtjw of his thigh has received the illness. What is done against it: viscous fluid . . . natron, are boiled together and drunk by the man for 4 days.

There are 2 vessels in him to his neck. If he is ill in his neck and his eyes are dimsighted, then thou shalt say concerning it: it is that the vessels of his neck have received the disease. What is done against it: myrtle (?), washerman's slops, piñon, fruit of . . . are mixed with honey, applied to his neck, and it is bandaged with it for 4 days.

There are 2 vessels in him to his arm; if he is ill in his arm or his fingers have . . . then thou shalt say concerning it: one suffering from . . . What is done against it: let him vomit by means of fish with beer and . . . or meat, and his fingers are bandaged with water melon until he is healed.

There are 2 vessels in him to the back of his head.

There are 2 vessels in him to his forehead.

There are 2 vessels in him to his eyes.

There are 2 vessels in him to his eyebrows.

There are 2 vessels in him to his nose.

There are 2 vessels in him to his right ear, the breath of life enters into them.

There are 2 vessels in him to his left ear; the breath of death enters into them.

They together go to his heart, divide at his nose, and unite at his hinder parts, and illnesses of the hinder parts arise through them; it is excrements that are carried, it is the vessels of the feet that begin to die.[291]

These two short treatises are supplemented by glosses and prescriptions. The glosses do not fit the text as those of Papyrus Edwin Smith do, that is, the terms explained do not occur in the treatise to which they had been attached. Yet there is a certain connection in that many of the glosses reflect the same theoretical views. Thus we read:

As to 'the breath which enters into the nose': it enters into the heart and the lung; these give to the whole belly.[292]

Or the very picturesque gloss:

As to 'faintness': it is that the heart does not speak or that the vessels of the heart are dumb, there being no perception of them under thy fingers; it arises through the air that fills them.[293]

Thus we also learn from the glosses that a patient's mind passes away because the vessels of the heart carry feces,[294] or that heat from the anus causes debility of the heart.[295]

Papyrus Hearst contains a number of very important prescriptions for the treatment of the *metu.*[296] The purpose was to quiet the *metu* when they were irritated,[297] to soften them when they were stiff, to animate and refresh them when they were inert and tired, to cool them when they were too hot, or to remove swelling and pain. In other words abnormal conditions of the *metu* caused disease. They also were believed to take in disease and to carry it into certain parts of the body, just as they also took in remedies. Treating the *metu* was etiological therapy. If excrements ascended the body, causing illness in another part, it was advisable to treat the *metu* of the anus. It was important for the physician 'to understand the internal fluids.'

Scanty as the material is, it nevertheless gives us an idea of what rational medical theories prevailed at the time when this medical literature was written, that is, at about the end of the Old Kingdom, but also at the time when it was still used, that is, for a score of centuries. Since our system of medicine is based on anatomy, as modern Western physicians we are inclined to believe that it is not possible to practice medicine effectively without an extensive knowledge of the structure of the human body. We should keep in mind, however, that this is a recent development that was initiated as late as the Renaissance. The Greeks had much knowledge of anatomy, to be sure, but they made little use of it in their medical systems, as we shall see in our next volume.

In ancient Egypt as in all archaic civilizations the chief sources of anatomical knowledge were the kitchen and the cult. All ancient people noticed the analogy between the structure of man and that of certain animals. There was a heart that beat, lungs that breathed the air in and out, sexual organs with which they copulated, a liver, a spleen, kidneys, and other analogous organs. The cook who prepared an animal for the table knew well enough that the gall bladder had to be removed very carefully because its content was bitter, and that the kidneys had to be washed thoroughly lest they have an unpleasant taste of urine. The priest who sacrificed an animal to the gods knew where the blood came from and which parts were edible and which not. All people, primitive and archaic, had names to designate the chief parts of the body. The fact that a word for brain occurs in Papyrus Edwin Smith for the first time means very little.[298] It is pure accident; the content of the cranial cavity must have been known and named long before that time. Neolithic men who in Western Europe and Africa trephined skulls knew not only the brain and its membranes but also its venous sinuses. The cooks must have known the brain, but they did not write books. In the early days, moreover, little attention was paid to the brain. The chief organ was the heart, a view that is still found in our language when we speak of somebody being of good heart, or as losing his heart, or as recovering heart, or of 'bread which strengtheneth man's heart,' or of a city being located in the heart of the country.[299] The brain for a long time was at best considered an organ that produced mucus which came out of the nose when somebody had a cold.

We mentioned before that the embalming of corpses was not a

source of anatomical knowledge because organs were taken out of the body roughly and brutally. There is, moreover, no evidence of any kind that dissections were performed in Egypt before the Hellenistic period. We sometimes hear that surgery could not have been practiced unless surgeons had had extensive anatomical knowledge. But we saw that actually very little operating was done, and as long as the field of surgery was limited all the surgeon needed was some experienc in topographical anatomy. Whoever reduced a dislocated jaw or a dislocated humerus obviously had some empirical knowledge of the bones and articulations involved, but at the same time he might be convinced that air entered the body through the nose, passed through the heart, and left the body through the anus.[300] Or he assumed that there was a direct connection between eye and ear, for in order to cure blindness he ground the humor of pig's eyes with stibium, red ochre, honey, and 'poured it into the ear of the man, so that he may be cured immediately.' This was considered 'really excellent,' but it was good in addition to recite a spell twice: 'I have brought this which was applied to the seat of yonder and replaces the horrible suffering.'[301]

The religious origin of anatomy is particularly evident among the ancient Egyptians for whom life on earth was a mere episode and who so anxiously preserved the bodies of the dead. This was done not only physically through embalming but also through a religious ritual by which the chief parts of the body were identified with organs of the sungod.[302] This is why we have lists of organs in early religious texts and also in incantations, some of which we quoted before. It is noteworthy that in all such texts the organs are listed in the order *a capite ad calcem*, and this may well be the origin of an arrangement of materials that was customary in the medical literature for thousands of years. Papyrus Edwin Smith follows this order and so do many medieval books, an order that is by no means obvious because it would be just as logical, if not more so, to begin with the feet and to go up to the top of the head. The plant germinates on the soil and then grows up, and animals and man are first close to the earth and then grow up.

The anatomical nomenclature is interesting.[303] Some organs have several names, older and younger ones, some used in everyday life, others used in poetry, and finally the names invariably found in the medical literature. Some names are picturesque. The shoulder blade was called the razor because it looked like an Egyptian razor. The convolutions of the brain were compared to the corrugations of metallic slag.[304] The fork at the head of the ramus of the mandible was compared to the claw of a two-toed bird,[305] and a segment of the skull reminded the surgeon of a turtle's shell.[306]

Thus the major organs were known, had names, and it was believed that they were all connected with one another either directly or via the heart through a system of canals or vessels, which ran in pairs or in groups of three and carried air, blood, all that was necessary to life and also the refuse that was ultimately discharged. It is futile to guess whether these vessels were arteries or veins or nerves or anything else, because we are dealing with speculative anatomy and physiology. The heart was the central organ but the nose was considered essential also because it was the entrance gate to the air. 'Thy eyes are the lord of mankind, thy nose feeds the gods, thy ears are the two royal snakes,' we read in an incantation,[307] and the average Egyptian had no doubt that a woman could become pregnant through the mouth.[308] Equally speculative was the pathology based on these anatomical and physiological concepts. Throughout this kind of medical theory we encounter the view that the major organs, the heart, the uterus, the stomach, the vessels, and others, had some life of their own. They were able to wander around in the body, had appetites, whims, moods, and had to be satisfied and pacified. This was a left-over of mythological views which persisted for a very long time.

Speculative as these theories are I find them nevertheless very impressive, as they represent the beginning of medical science, a science which was different from our sober natural science but still one which endeavored to explain the phenomena of life and death, of health and disease, rationally without having recourse to the gods. It was a way of thinking in terms of a philosophy of nature, and in doing it the Egyptians anticipated views and methods of the pre-Socratic philosophers of Greece. It is probably not by accident that the first of them, Thales of Miletos, traveled in Egypt, where he had experiences that influenced his philosophy in a decisive way, as we shall see in our next volume.

*

Epilogue

Long before Egypt lost its political independence it had lost its creative power. The great tradition was no longer inspiring but had become stifling. Artists and writers copied established patterns and the lack of originality in art was believed to be compensated by having buildings and statues erected in gigantic size. Religion, once a source of inspiration, had become rigid and formalistic and was administered by a rich and powerful clergy.

Egyptian medicine, however, was more famous than ever. We have no evidence of new creative ideas having come forth during the last period of Egyptian history, but in medicine as in all technical and scientific fields experience accumulated with every century. Physicians knew more symptoms of disease, could probably evaluate them better, and had more drugs available than in the past. There can be no doubt that magical and religious medical practices flourished, but I am equally convinced that the old classical empirico-rational system of medicine had not been forgotten. The Hermetic books to which Clemens of Alexandria refers were not collections of incantations, but discussed the human body, diseases, instruments and appliances, drugs, diseases of the eyes, and gynecological ailments.[309] And it was certainly not for the sake of charms that Egyptian doctors were called to all the courts of the ancient world.

Egyptian medicine was known and must have exerted considerable influence far beyond the borders of the country. We mentioned before how the Amarna letters tell us of physicians' being loaned to foreign courts to Syria and Assyria. A. S. Yahuda claims on the basis of a linguistic study of the Pentateuch that the Hebrews 'had a wide knowledge of Egyptian medicine, of its methods and practices.'[310] Cyrus of Persia liked to be surrounded by Egyptian physicians and Darius always had some of them at his court because at that time they were still considered the best in the world;[311] we saw how anxious he was to restore medical education at Saïs. At his court Egyptian and Greek physicians clashed and Herodotus tells us in his inimitable style how Democedes of Croton proved his superiority over the Egyptians in treating the king's foot.[312]

Greek and Egyptian physicians must have met and exchanged information long before that time and there can be no doubt whatsoever that the Greeks learned a great deal from Egypt. This is perfectly obvious with respect to the Hellenistic period, when Alexandria was the center of Greek science and learning. Materia medica as reflected in the works of Dioscorides and Galen was undoubtedly greatly enriched from Egypt. But the influence must have set in very much earlier. We should be careful, however, in appraising such influences, and I think that Breasted has given a very good example of how easily mistakes are made by philologists who are not familiar with the subject of their texts.

Papyrus Edwin Smith describes the reduction of the dislocated mandible in the following words:[313]

> Thou shouldst put thy thumbs upon the ends of the two rami of the mandible in the inside of his mouth and thy two claws [meaning two groups of fingers] under his chin, [and] thou shouldst cause them to fall back so that they rest in their places.

The Hippocratic treatise *On Articulations* describes exactly the same operation although in greater detail,[314] and the commentary to this treatise by Apollonius of Kitium gives an illustration of it that must go back to the first century B.C.[315] Breasted concludes that the treatise of Papyrus Edwin Smith, 'or some other old Egyptian book of surgery containing our surgeon's directions for reducing a dislocated mandible must have been known to the early Hippocratic practitioners.'[316] The mistake lies in the fact that there is no other method of reducing a dislocated jaw and that this is a most unpleasant and painful accident, leaving the patient with wide-open mouth, unable to take any food; wherever and whenever this happened an attempt must have been made to succor the unfortunate fellow man. And if the surgeon, or blacksmith, or neighbor, or whoever it was who tried to help the victim, was lucky he discovered the only anatomically possible method of reducing the dislocated mandible, the one that the Egyptian and the Hippocratic surgeons used and that we still practice today.

In other words, I do not think that this is a good example to demonstrate Egyptian influence upon Greek medicine. There are much more convincing ones, such as the birth prognoses of Papyrus Berlin and of Papyrus Carlsberg No. VIII, some of which occur almost literally in the Greek medical literature and are found again centuries later in the popular medical literature of Western Europe.[317] An Egyptian prescription that in substance reads: 'put wheat and barley into separate containers, add the pregnant woman's urine, and if the wheat sprouts she will have a boy but if the barley sprouts it will be a girl,' is so specific that if we find the same instruction in some later literature we are justified in assuming an Egyptian origin of it.

Egyptian medical literature did not end abruptly. Collections of prescriptions continued to be written, namely in the Coptic language of the Egyptian Christians. It was not pure Egyptian medicine, to be sure, and was strongly influenced by the Greeks and later by the Arabs; but it carried on Egyptian traditions nevertheless and was written in a language that was a continuation of the old Egyptian, thus preserving many words that would have been lost otherwise. It is very probable that every monastery had such a book of recipes from which the monks learned how to treat their brothers and guests. The fragment of such a book containing 45 recipes against skin diseases was found and published in 1810 by G. Zoëga.[318] A shorter fragment with 11 prescriptions for the treatment of diseases of the breasts from the monastery of Deir el-Abiad was published by M. U. Bouriant,[319] and finally in 1921 E. Chassinat published in an excellent edition a large manuscript of the ninth or tenth century of this era found by Bouriant at Meshaikh.[320] This manuscript has 237 recipes, almost 100 of which are against disease of the eyes, which remained the curse of Egypt through the centuries and millennia, and many against the also very frequent diseases of the skin. The prescriptions follow very closely the pattern found in the ancient Egyptian papyri, and the drugs are in many cases the same.

When the Meshaikh manuscript was written, Greek medicine had completed its course and Arabic medicine was just bursting into full bloom. Much time had passed since Imhotep had built the pyramid of Sakkara for his Lord. Memphis was gone and Cairo was founded and mosques were being built to the glory of Allah, the Merciful, the Clement. The desert had charitably covered the ruins of a great civilization with a thick layer of sand and only the tallest buildings remained visible, testimonies of a great past, full of mystery and strangely attractive.

But Egyptian culture was by no means dead. The impetus it had given in the arts and crafts, in literature, medicine, and science, was carried into the younger civilizations of the neighboring countries where it proved to be a strong stimulus. And the day came when the genius of Champollion and the spade of the archaeologist lifted the veil and we stood looking in deep reverence at the great and manifold achievements of Egyptian culture.

NOTES

1. J. H. Breasted, 'The Edwin Smith Papyrus,' *Quart. Bull. New-York Hist. Soc.*, 1922, 6:1-31; 'The Edwin Smith Papyrus, Some Preliminary Observations,' *Recueil d'études Egypt. dédiées à la Mémoire de Jean-François Champollion*, Paris, 1922, pp. 385-429.
2. See p. 287.
3. *Pap. Ebers,* 103.
4. *Pap. Berlin,* 163a.
5. Sethe, *Imhotep,* p. 21.
6. Quoted by Sethe, ibid.
7. J. H. Breasted, *Ancient Records of Egypt,* Chicago, 1906, vol. I, §§ 242-6.
8. *Pap. Edwin Smith,* 3 d.
9. By far the best discussion of the Egyptian medical papyri as a whole is Hermann Grapow, 'Untersuchungen über die altägyptischen medizinischen Papyri,' *Mitteilungen der Vorderasiatisch-Aegyptischen Gesellschaft,* vol. 40, no. 1, 1935; vol. 41, no. 2, 1936 [quoted in the following as Grapow I and Grapow II]. I wish to acknowledge here my great indebtedness to

these two books; they are the foundation for all present and future work on Egyptian medical literature. A very good analysis of character and style of archaic medicine at large is presented by O. Temkin, 'Beiträge zur archaischen Medizin,' *Kyklos,* 1930, 3:90-135.

10. Published with English translation by F. L. Griffith, *The Petrie Papyri. Hieratic Papyri from Kahun and Gurob,* London, 1898, Kahun LV, 2, pp. 12-14, plate VII.
11. H. Neffgen, *Der Veterinär-Papyrus von Kahun, Ein Beitrag zur Geschichte der Tierheilkunde der alten Aegypter,* with German translation from the English; important for its comments by a veterinarian.
12. The beginning of our fragment dealing with diseases of fish or bird is so mutilated that little can be made of it. Otherwise the fragment contains three cases, one dealing with a dog disease (according to Neffgen, encephalitis), the two others discussing a disease of cattle.
13. Griffith read *Treatment for the Eyes of a Bull with Wind* to which see Grapow I, p. 20; the disease is obviously not an eye disease.
14. Published by Griffith, loc. cit. Kahun VI, 1, pp. 5-10, plates V and VI, also with English translation. A German translation from the English with discussion of the contents in Felix Reinhard, 'Gynäkologie und Geburtshilfe der altägyptischen Papyri,' *Arch. Gesch. Med.,* 1917, 10:147-61. [Cited in the following as *Pap. med. Kahun.*]
15. E.g. *Pap. med. Kahun* 26 = *Pap. Berlin* 196.
16. *Edwin Smith Surgical Papyrus, in Facsimile and Hieroglyphic Transliteration with Translation and Commentary,* edited by James Henry Breasted, 2 vols. (The University of Chicago Oriental Institute Publications, vols. III and IV), Chicago, 1930. [Cited as *Pap. Edwin Smith,* with numbers referring to the cases.] In 1949 the Papyrus was presented to the New York Academy of Medicine.
17. In preparing his edition Breasted consulted with Arno B. Luckhardt, physiologist of the University of Chicago. The distinguished medical historian Max Meyerhof studied the text with the Egyptologists L. Borchardt and S. Schott and published a very detailed analysis and a German translation. ['Ueber den Papyrus Edwin Smith, das älteste Chirurgiebuch der Welt,' *Deut. Zschr. Chir.,* 1931, 231:645-90.] O. Temkin and I gave a joint seminar about the papyrus with the Egyptologist Walther Wolf at the University of Leipzig in 1931. Abel Rey in his book *La Science orientale avant les Grecs,* Paris, 1930, gave the papyrus a dominant place in Egyptian science. J. G. De Lint, a physician who was also a student of Egyptology, translated the papyrus into Dutch, 'Chirurgische tekst van den Papyrus Edwin Smith,' *Bijdragen tot de Geschiedenis der Geneeskunde,* 1931, 11:211-32; 'De achterzijde van den Papyrus Edwin Smith,' *Nederl. Tijdsch. Geneesk.,* 1935, 29:880-89. Finally in 1939 B. Ebbell translated the Papyrus Edwin Smith and the surgical sections of Papyrus Ebers into German with a very good commentary: *Die alt-ägyptische Chirurgie,* Skrifter utgitt av Det Norske Videnskaps-Akademi i Oslo, II. Hist.-Filos. Klasse, 1939, no. 2.

18. On the basis of paleographic evidence Breasted thinks that the Edwin Smith Papyrus is slightly older than the Ebers Papyrus, see pp. 25-9 and 593-5.
19. There may be just as old Chinese books but the chronology of the early Chinese medical literature is still very uncertain.
20. There were exceptions to the rule and Papyrus Edwin Smith in three hopeless cases (6, 8a, 20) still had some alleviative treatment.
21. *Pap. Edwin Smith,* p. 47.
22. Favorable verdicts occur sixteen times in Papyrus Ebers, twice in Papyrus Berlin (154, 161), once in *Pap. Hearst* (174), and once in *Pap. Chester Beatty* (12). The uncertain verdict is found twice in *Pap. Ebers* (105). What else but a negative verdict is it when it is said in *Pap. Ebers,* 'Thou shalt not do anything to it' (109, 110), or 'Thou shalt not put thy hand to any likeness of this' (109), or 'Thou shalt not put thy hand to such a thing' (108), whereupon in the latter case the recital of a spell is recommended since other treatment seems hopeless?
23. Case 17 shows a contradiction. It has an unfavorable verdict but at the same time indicates a treatment to be pursued until the patient recovers. There obviously must be a scribal error somewhere. The case is not clear. Named 'a smash in his cheek,' it actually is much more serious and may concern a fracture of the basis of the skull, in which case the unfavorable verdict would be more than justified and the error would have to be sought in the treatment.
24. *Pap. Edwin Smith,* p. 14; see also p. 47.
25. It has the same style as the non-medical didactic literature of the period.
26. Thus, e.g. in cases 10, 14, 23, 25, 26, 28, 47 but not in cases 34-6.
27. Case 3, gloss D.
27a. A 'father of two tongues' in Arabic obviously is a liar but a 'mother of the brain' is not necessarily a meninx; the latter term would require an explanation.
28. *Pap. Ebers,* 99-102. This shows how necessary it is to rearrange the Egyptian medical literature.
29. P. XIIIf. and again p. 9.
30. P. XIV and again p. 11.
31. See Breasted's account in *Pap. Edwin Smith,* pp. 22ff.
32. *Papyros Ebers. Das Hermetische Buch über die Arzneimittel der alten Aegypter in hieratischer Schrift.* Herausgegeben, mit Inhaltsangabe und Einleitung versehen von Georg Ebers. Mit hieroglyphisch-lateinischem Glossar von Ludwig Stern. Leipzig, 1875, 2 vols. The original papyrus is in the Library of the University of Leipzig.
33. H. Brugsch, Ueber die medizinischen Kenntnisse der alten Aegypter und über ein alt-ägyptisches medicinisches Manuscript im Königl. Museum zu Berlin, *Allgem. Monatsschr. für Wiss. u. Lit.,* 1853, pp. 44-56; H. Brugsch, *Notice raisonnée d'un traité médical datant du XIVe siècle avant notre ère et contenu dans un papyrus hiératique du Musée Royal . . . de Berlin.* Leipzig, 1863. 20 pp.

34. S. Birch, 'Medical Papyrus with the Name of Cheops,' *Zschr. ägypt. Sprache,* 1871, 9:61-4.
35. *Papyros Ebers. Das älteste Buch über Heilkunde.* Aus dem Aegyptischen zum erstenmal vollständig übersetzt von H. Joachim. Berlin, 1890.
36. Listed in Miron Goldstein, *Internationale Bibliographie der altägyptischen Medizin,* 1850-1930, Berlin, 1933.
37. In 1913 W. Wreszinski published a hieroglyphic transcription of the Papyrus, *Die Medizin der alten Aegypter, Bd. 3: Der Papyrus Ebers.* 1. Teil, Umschrift, Leipzig, 1913. A translation and commentary were announced but were never published; the English translation by Cyril P. Bryan (London, 1930) was not made from the Egyptian but from the German version of Joachim.
38. *The Papyrus Ebers, the Greatest Egyptian Medical Document,* translated by B. Ebbell. Copenhagen, 1937. Our quotations are from this version. Wreszinski in his transcription numbered the recipes and cases of disease from 1 to 877 and some writers refer to these numbers. Since Wreszinski's transcription is not accompanied by a translation and most of our readers will not use it, our references are to the pages of the manuscript which are also indicated in Ebbell's translation. In some important cases the number of the line is given in addition to the page number but as a rule the latter will be enough to enable the reader to find a passage without difficulty.
39. A. Erman and H. Grapow, *Wörterbuch der ägyptischen Sprache,* Leipzig, 1926-31;–*Die Belegstellen,* Heft 1, Bd. 2, Heft 1-7, Leipzig, 1935-9.
40. The columns of the manuscript are numbered 1-110 but actually there are only 108 because the scribe jumped from page 27 to 30, leaving out the numbers 28 and 29. The original pagination has been preserved, however, in all editions and translations.
41. Grapow thinks that the compendium was not complete because it does not end with an Explicit and the name of the scribe, such as we have them in *Pap. Berlin,* 191. This may be, but a compilation such as we have in this papyrus was never 'complete' because one could always add to it. However, it is not a fragment. See H. Grapow, 'Bemerkungen zum Papyrus Ebers als Handschrift,' *Zschr. ägypt. Sprache,* 1935, 71:160-4.
42. *Pap. Ebers,* 93, 6.
43. Ibid. 99, 1.
44. Ibid. 103, 19.
45. Grapow I, p. 25ff.

45a. Fragments of this treatise also occur in Pap. Carlsberg no. VIII; see Erik Iversen, Papyrus Carlsberg no. VIII . . . *Det Kgl. Danske Videnskabernes Selskab,* Hist.-fil. Meddelelser XXVI, 5, Copenhagen, 1939, p. 4.

46. E.g. 109.
47. Three cases in the book on women's diseases (*Ebers* 96,16-97,7) are reminiscent of *Pap. med. Kahun* since they are written in the same style.
48. The first treatise has the title *The Physician's Secret: Knowledge of the Heart's Movements and Knowledge of the Heart* and runs from 99,1-99, 12 and 100,2-14.

49. *Pap. Ebers,* 103,1-18=*Pap. Berlin,* 163.
50. So Breasted in *Pap. Edwin Smith,* pp. 4ff. *et passim,* who also makes the unjustified statement that in the papyri other than Edwin Smith disease was treated as 'entirely due to demoniacal intrusions.'
51. *Pap. Ebers,* 97,15-98,22.
52. See Ibid. 1-2, 69, 108.
53. See Ebbell's note, *Pap. Ebers,* 108.
54. Vol. I, pp. 9-11 of his edition of the papyrus.
55. Clemens Alexandrinus, *Stromateis,* lib. VI, cap. 35-7.
56. The others were on anatomy, pathology, surgical instruments, ophthalmology, and gynecology.
57. See W. Scott, *Hermetica,* Oxford, 1924.
58. See Wreszinski, *Pap. Berlin,* pp. xif.
59. It was first published with introduction, glossary, and plates by G. Reisner, *The Hearst Medical Papyrus* (University of California Publications, Egyptian Archaeology, vol. 1), Leipzig, 1905; a new edition with transcription, German translation and commentary was published by W. Wreszinski, 'Der Londoner medizinische Papyrus und der Papyrus Hearst': *Die Medizin der alten Aegypter,* vol. II, pp. 1-133, Leipzig, 1912. Our references are to this edition. An English translation with linguistic and medical commentary by H. L. F. Lutz, S. V. Larkey, and C. D. Leake has been in preparation for some time.
60. See the very convenient concordance of Grapow, I, 72-5.
61. *Pap. Hearst* 173-4 = *Pap. Ebers* 78.
62. *Pap. Hearst,* 212-16.
63. Ibid. 94-124.
64. I myself had such a collection of tested recipes for a long time. The only difference was that having loose-leaf books today I could arrange them alphabetically under the disease for which they were used. All the ancient physician who wrote on a roll of papyrus could do was to add new recipes at the end if there was space left or to write on the back side. Another possibility was to add a leaf of papyrus to the roll. After such a book had been copied several times, there was little order left.
65. It was first reproduced on plates by H. Brugsch in the second volume of his *Recueil de monuments égyptiens,* Leipzig, 1863, plates 85-107, pp. 101-20; hence it is often quoted as *Papyrus Brugsch maior,* the adjective being used to differentiate it from Berlin Papyrus 3027, the one that contains the incantations for mother and child and that is sometimes quoted as *Papyrus Brugsch minor,* although it was neither acquired nor published by Brugsch. W. Wreszinski published Papyrus 3038 in facsimile, with transcription, translation, commentary, and glossary: 'Der grosse medizinische Papyrus des Berliner Museums (Pap. Berl. 3038),' *Die Medizin der alten Aegypter,* vol. I, Leipzig, 1909. Our quotations refer to this edition.
66. *Pap. Berlin,* 154, 161.
67. Ibid. 153, 157, 158.
68. See again the concordance in Grapow I, 72-5.

69. *Pap. Berlin,* 66-76.
70. Ibid. 195-9.
71. Ibid. p. xiv, 'Es sind Vorschriften, die auf dem absurdesten Aberglauben beruhen, die sich aber vielleicht gerade deswegen bis fast zum heutigen Tage erhalten haben.'

71a. *Pap. Berlin,* 163 = *Pap. Ebers* 103, 1-18.

72. Translation by J. Breasted in *Pap. Edwin Smith,* p. 5. The name of the physician occurs once more toward the end of the treatise, 163h.
73. *Hieratic Papyri in the British Museum, Chester Beatty Gift,* London, 1935. Of this collection no. VI is the medical papyrus [Pap. 10,686 of the British Museum].
74. Frans Jonckheere, *Le Papyrus médical Chester Beatty* (La Médecine égyptienne, no. 2), Brussels, 1947. Quoted in the following as *Pap. med. Chester Beatty.* References are to the numbers of recipes given by Jonckheere.
75. No. 12.
76. *Chester Beatty* 26 = *Ebers* 33.
77. See his chapter *Neuordnung der medizinischen Texte,* II, 126-32.
78. I knew a famous gynecologist who prayed on his knees prior to every operation he performed. A physician in Geneva, Switzerland, P. Tournier, makes constant use of religious forces in his practice and his books are widely read, see, e.g. *Médecine de la personne,* Neuchâtel and Paris, 1940; *Désharmonie de la vie moderne,* 1947.
79. Gardiner in *Encyc. Rel. Ethics,* VIII, p. 268, refers to a Greek alchemical treatise that defines the difference between the physician and the magician. According to this treatise the physician is one who acts ἀπὸ βιβλίων . . . μηχανικῶς, 'mechanically and by books,' while the other is a ἱερεύς, a priest who acts 'through his own religious feeling,' διὰ τῆς ἰδίας δεισιδαιμονίας.
80. Herodotus, II, 84. About specialization see W. Spiegelberg, 'Zu dem Spezialistentum in der ägyptischen Medizin,' *Zschr. ägypt. Sprache,* 1917, 53:111; J. G. De Lint, 'Egyptische Specialisten,' *Bijdragen tot de Geschiedenis der Geneeskunde,* 1934, 14:48-52.
81. See Breasted, *Pap. Edwin Smith,* p. xiv; also H. Junker, 'Die Stele des Hofarztes Irj,' *Zschr. ägypt. Sprache,* 1928, 63:70.
82. Junker, loc. cit. pp. 53-70.
83. Another such 'Guardian of the Anus' at the time of the Old Kingdom was Hawi, see J. E. Quibell, *Excavations at Saqqara,* 1905-6, vol. I, pl. XIV. Jonckheere, *Pap. Chester Beatty,* p. 76, refers to a statuette from the XIIth Dynasty representing a man looking at the anus of a woman who is crouching on knees and elbows. The statuette was considered erotic but may very well represent an inspection of the anus by just such a specialist, as Jonckheere very correctly pointed out. The ἰατροκλύστης of a document of the 2nd century B.C. is probably the descendant of the Guardian of the Anus, see Wilcken, *Urkunden der Ptolemäerzeit,* I, 148.7.
84. B. W. Weinberger summ[illegible]zed the literature on Egyptian dentists and dentistry in two papers, 'I[illegible] Dentistry Evolve from the Barbers, Black-

smiths or from Medicine?' *Bull. Hist. Med.*, 1940, 8:965ff.; 'Further evidence that dentistry was practiced in ancient Egypt, Phoenicia and Greece,' ibid. 1946, 20:188ff.

85. He was also 'one understanding the internal fluids,' a gastro-intestinal specialist if there ever was one. See Saqqara I, pl. XIV, Junker, loc. cit.
86. Junker, loc. cit. pp. 69f.
87. F. Jonckheere, 'Coup d'oeil sur la médecine égyptienne; l'intérêt des documents non médicaux,' *Chronique d'Egypte*, 1945, 20:24-32.
88. Sources for the various titles in Junker, loc. cit. p. 64ff.
89. Jonckheere, loc. cit. p. 25. We shall have to wait for more material before definite conclusions may be reached on this point.
90. Junker, loc. cit. p. 65.
91. Jonckheere, loc. cit. p. 25.
92. See R. Fournier, *La Médecine égyptienne des origines à l'école d'Alexandrie*, Bordeaux, 1933.
93. The letter is preserved in the Leyden Papyrus 371. See Jonckheere, loc. cit. p. 31.
94. The love-sick boy in the poem quoted above (p. 291, note 2), says that neither master-physician nor magician could cure him, which hints at the fact that in certain cases both were consulted.
95. Diodorus, I, 82.3.
96. *Pap. Hearst*, 214.
97. *Pap. Ebers*. 1.
98. Ibid.
99. Adolf Fonahn, 'Der altägyptische Arzt IWTI,' *Arch. Gesch. Med.*, 1909, 2:375-8.
100. Further sources in Junker, loc. cit. p. 66. See also *Pap. Berlin*, 163a, where Neterhotep is designated as 'scribe of sacred writings, chief of the excellent physicians.'
101. H. Schaefer, 'Die Wiedereinrichtung einer Aerzteschule in Saïs unter König Darius I,' *Zschr. ägypt. Sprache*, 1899, 37:72-4; the English translation is by Breasted, *Pap. Edwin Smith*, pp. 17f.
102. Xenophon, *Cyropaedia;* the passages are collected in E. Vidal, 'Les idées des Assyriens et des Egyptiens sur la vie et la mort, la santé et la maladie, 3000 ans avant Jésus-Christ,' *Société de Géographie d'Alger, Bulletin*, 1912, 7:569-96.
103. *Odyssey*, IV, 231f.
104. See Jonckheere, loc. cit. p. 29.
105. Ibid.
106. *Pap. Ebers*, 99.
107. *Pap. Edwin Smith*, 1, gloss A.
108. Ebbell in *Pap. Ebers*, p. 14.
109. Jonckheere, loc. cit. p. 26.
110. W. A. Jayne, *The Healing Gods of Ancient Civilizations*, New Haven, 1925, pp. 76-7.
111. See F. Jonckheere, *Autour de l'autopsie d'une momie*, Bruxelles, 1942.

112. The dresser is mentioned twice in *Pap. Edwin Smith* in glosses of case 9 and of case 19. See in this connection Grapow, I, 94.
113. Thus on an ostracon of the British Museum. See Jonckheere, *Chronique d'Egypte*, 1945, 20:32.
114. Ἰατρικὰ ἐρωτήματα, edited and translated into French by Ch. Daremberg and E. Ruelle, *Oeuvres de Rufus d'Ephèse*, Paris, 1879, pp. 195ff. The treatise characteristically begins with the sentence, ἐρωτήματα χρὴ τὸν νοσοῦντα ἐρωτᾶν, 'one must ask the patient questions.'
115. *Pap. Edwin Smith*, 20. Another question about odor from a woman's genitalia may be found in *Pap. med. Kahun*, 2.
116. *Pap. Ebers*, 36.
117. Ibid.
118. Ibid. 41.
119. Ibid. 42.
120. Ibid. 37.
121. E.g. *Pap. Edwin Smith*, 7.
122. Ibid. 3.20, *Pap. Ebers*, 57.
123. About eye symptoms see *Pap. Ebers*, 55ff.
124. *Pap. Edwin Smith*, 8.
125. Ibid. 7.
126. Ibid. 25.
127. Ibid. 31.
128. *Pap. Ebers*, 39.
129. Ibid. 40.
130. *Pap. Edwin Smith*, 7.
131. *Pap. Ebers*, 36.
132. Ibid. 104.
133. Ibid. 37.
134. Ibid. 39.
135. *Pap. Edwin Smith*, 7, the term is explained in gloss G.
136. *Pap. Edwin Smith*, 1-8 *et passim.*
137. Ibid. 4.
138. Ibid. 5.
139. Ibid. 6.
140. Ibid. 13, 17, 37.
141. Ibid. 7.
142. Ibid. 46.
143. *Pap. Ebers*, 107.
144. Ibid. 40.
145. Ibid. 104.
146. See *Pap. Edwin Smith*, 31 and 33, where in both cases the patient as a result of a dislocated or crushed vertebra of the neck is 'unconscious of his two arms and his two legs.'
147. *Pap. Ebers*, 37.
148. *Pap. Edwin Smith*, 39.
149. *Pap. Ebers*, 38.
150. *Pap. Edwin Smith*, 7.

151. *Pap. Ebers,* 99 = *Pap. Edwin Smith,* 1, gloss A.
152. *Pap. Edwin Smith,* p. xvi.
153. Ibid. 1, gloss A.
154. They had water clocks and shadow clocks, and a portable shadow clock from the 13th century B.C. has been found but it would not have been suitable for measuring the pulse. See E. J. Pilcher, *Palestine Exploration Fund,* 1923, 55:85-8; Breasted, *Pap. Edwin Smith,* p. 106.
155. *Pap. Edwin Smith,* 30.
156. Ibid. 32.
157. Ibid. e.g. 3, 4, 5, 7, 8, 10.
158. Ibid. 7.
159. Ibid.
160. Ibid. 48.
161. Ibid. 8.
162. On diagnosis in general see R. Koch, *Die ärztliche Diagnose, Beitrag zur Kenntnis des ärztlichen Denkens,* Wiesbaden, 2nd ed., 1920.
163. By physician I also mean the surgeon.
164. Such as, e.g. the cases 7, 8, 31, but many others also.
165. Particularly in the sections on diseases of the cardia, 36ff. and in the surgical section at the end. Good descriptions of disease syndromes are sometimes also found in the non-medical literature. There could not be a better picture of a snakebite than in the myth of Re being bitten by a snake at the command of Isis (*Turin Pap.* pl. 133, the translation is by T. Eric Peet): 'Re wails, I was stung by a snake which I saw not. It is not fire, it is not water; yet I am colder than water and hotter than fire. My whole body sweats, and I tremble. My eye is not firm, and I cannot see, for water rains down my face as in the heat of summer.'
166. *Pap. Ebers,* 37.
167. Karl Sudhoff examined all passages which might refer to cancer and came to the conclusion that it was impossible to tell from the extant literature whether the Egyptians knew what we consider cancer. See Karl Sudhoff, Krebsgeschwülste in altägyptischen Papyri, *Monatsschr. f. Krebsbekämpfung,* 1933, pp. 171-4.
168. *Pap. Edwin Smith,* 31.
169. E.g. *Pap. Ebers,* 24ff.
170. Ibid. 53f.
171. *Pap. Berlin,* 29-34.
172. *Pap. Ebers,* 107.
173. Ibid. 104f.
174. Ibid. 49.
175. Ibid. 47.
176. Ibid. 91.
177. Ibid.
178. Ibid. 90.
179. Ibid. 37.
180. Ibid. 106.
181. Ibid. 56f.

182. Namely Ebers: 28, Berlin: 12, Hearst: 9, London: 1. See Frans Jonckheere, 'Une maladie égyptienne; l'hématurie parasitaire,' *La médecine Egyptienne,* no. 1, Brussels, 1944. Jonckheere translated the 50 passages and discussed them critically. For a long time it was believed that the *aaa*-disease was the hookworm disease, the 'Egyptian chlorosis,' until E. Pfister (*Arch. Gesch. Med.,* 1913, 6:12-20) demonstrated that it was rather the Bilharzia disease. Ebbell (*Zschr. ägypt. Sprache,* 1927, 62:16) showed convincingly that *aaa* did not designate the disease as a whole but its most apparent symptom, hematuria. This also explains why the phallus is used as determinative of the word.
183. M. A. Ruffer, *Studies in the Paleopathology of Egypt,* Chicago, 1921, pp. 18-19.
184. See B. Ebbell's study, *Altägyptische Bezeichnungen für Krankheiten und Symptome,* Skrifter utgitt av Det Norske Videnskaps-Akademi i Oslo. II. Hist.-Filos. Klasse, 1938, no. 3, 65 pp., a study that supplements Ebbell's previous articles in *Zschr. ägypt. Sprache* and is devoted primarily to terms that are not translated in Erman-Grapow's *Wörterbuch.* The identification of many such terms is extraordinarily difficult and one must be very cautious in using modern terminology. The worms are discussed, p. 34. Numerous recipes against worms are given in *Pap. Berlin,* 1-12, 19-28, *Pap. Ebers,* 16ff. *et al.*
185. *Pap. Ebers,* 39.
186. Ibid. 40.
187. Ibid. 37.
188. Ibid. 39.
189. Ibid. 2ff.
190. Ibid. 47f.
191. Ibid. 95; see also *Pap. Berlin,* 13-18.
192. *Pap. Ebers,* 95-6.
193. See note 184.
194. F. Reinhard, 'Gynäkologie und Geburtshilfe der altägyptischen Papyri,' *Arch. Gesch. Med.,* 1916, 9:315-44; 1917, 10:124-61.
195. Georg Ebers, 'Papyrus Ebers. Die Maasse und das Kapitel über die Augenkrankheiten,' *Abh. phil.-hist. Classe Sächs. Gesell. Wiss.,* 1889, 9:133-336. The section on diseases of the eyes begins p. 199.
196. J. Hirschberg, 'Geschichte der Augenheilkunde': Graefe-Saemisch, *Handbuch der Augenheilkunde,* vol. 12, Leipzig, 1899, pp. 6-27; A. C. Krause, 'Ancient Egyptian Ophthalmology,' *Bull. Inst. Hist. Med.,* 1933, 1:258-76; Max Meyerhof, 'Eye Diseases in Ancient Egypt,' *Ciba Symposia,* 1940, 1:305-10.
197. See Ebbell's discussion in *Alt-ägyptische Bezeichnungen für Krankheiten und Symptome,* Oslo, 1938, p. 50.
198. See Max Meyerhof, 'Brief eines erblindeten Altägypters,' *Mitt. Gesch. Med. Naturwiss.,* 1918, 17:167.
199. See Sir D'Arcy Power, 'Some Early Surgical Cases. I. The Edwin Smith Papyrus,' *Brit. J. Surgery,* 1933-4, 21:1-4, 385-7.

200. Quite apart from the cosmetic and household recipes of Papyrus Ebers many others are simply laxatives or cough remedies.
201. *Pap. Berlin,* 161.
202. *Odyssey,* IV, 229-30.
203. B. Ebbell, 'Die ägyptischen Drogennamen,' *Zschr. ägypt. Sprache,* 1929, 64:48-54.
204. E.g. 25 and 54.
205. See Dinkler, 'La Science pharmaceutique chez les anciens égyptiens,' *Bull. Inst. Eg.,* 1898, fasc. 1, pp. 77-90; F. von Oefele, 'Die Receptierung der alten Aegypter', *Wiener klin. Wschr.,* 1894, 7:870-71.
206. *Pap. Ebers,* 2.
207. Ibid. 56.
208. Ibid. 89.
209. Chauncey D. Leake, 'Ancient Egyptian Therapeutics,' *Ciba Symposia,* 1940, 1:311-22.
210. See F. L. Griffith, 'Notes on Egyptian Weights and Measures,' *Proc. Soc. Bibl. Archaeol.,* 1892-3, 14:403-50; O. Neugebauer, 'Ueber den Scheffel und seine Teile,' *Zschr. ägypt. Sprache,* 1930, 65:42-8.
211. Such indications may be found on almost every page of *Pap. Ebers, Hearst* or *Berlin;* hence references are given here only in the case of special techniques or procedures, or when entire recipes are quoted.
212. *Pap. Ebers,* 4.
213. Ibid. 24.
214. Ibid. 6.
215. Ibid. 32.
216. Pliny, *Nat. hist.,* VIII, 27 (41). About rectal medication see particularly F. Jonckheere's translation and analysis of *Pap. med. Chester Beatty.*
217. *Pap. Hearst,* 7.
218. *Pap. Ebers,* 56.
219. *Pap. Berlin,* 60.
220. *Pap. Ebers,* 54, also *Pap. Berlin,* 46.
221. *Pap. Ebers,* 4.
222. Ibid. 23.
223. Ibid. 24.
224. Ibid. 35.
225. Ibid. 18.
226. Ibid. 61.
227. Ibid.
228. *Pap. Hearst,* 31, 150.
229. *Pap. Berlin,* 140.
230. E.g. *Pap. Ebers,* 27, 61.
231. Ibid. 23.
232. See Jonckheere's discussion, loc. cit. p. 70ff.
233. About plants see Franz Woenig, *Die Pflanzen im alten Aegypten, ihre Heimat, Geschichte, Kultur und ihre mannigfache Verwendung im sozialen Leben, in Kultus, Sitten, Gebräuchen, Medizin, Kunst,* Leipzig, 1886; F. Netolitzky, *Preuves d'aliments et de médicaments dans les*

cadavres séchés de Naga-ed-Der (Mitteil. Deut. Inst. ägypt. Altertumskunde in Kairo), 1. Ergänzungsband, 1943, 33 pp., 22 figs.

234. See B. Ebbell, 'Die ägyptischen aromatischen Harze der Tempelinschrift von Edfu,' *Acta Orientalia*, 17:89-111; P. Coremans, 'Notes de laboratoire: analyse d'une gomme-résine égyptienne,' *Chronique d'Egypte*, 1941, 16: 101-103; R. O. Steuer, 'Stacte in Egyptian antiquity,' *J. Am. Orient. Soc.*, 1943, 63:279-84.
235. *Pap. Ebers*, 47.
236. W. R. Dawson, 'Studies in Medical History: (a) The origin of the herbal. (b) Castor-oil in antiquity,' *Aegyptus*, 1929, 10:47-72. About herbals in Graeco-Roman times see Charles Singer, 'The Herbal in Antiquity and Its Transmission to Later Ages,' *J. Hellenic Stud.*, 1927, 17:1-52.
237. *Pap. Ebers*, 16.
238. Ibid. 67.
239. N. Georgiadès, 'Contribution à l'étude de l'opium égyptien,' *Bull. Inst. Egyptien*, 1917, ser. 5, 11:361-400.
240. The new translation of Pap. Hearst will undoubtedly contain valuable information on the subject as one of the collaborators, Chauncey D. Leake, is a pharmacologist. The following books may profitably be consulted about the action of drugs used in the past: G. Dragendorff, *Die Heilpflanzen der verschiedenen Völker und Zeiten, ihre Anwendung, wesentlichen Bestandtheile und Geschichte*, Stuttgart, 1898; R. Kobert, *Historische Studien aus dem Pharmakologischen Institute der Kaiserl. Universität Dorpat*, Halle a.S., 1889-96, 5 vols.; A. Tschirch, *Handbuch der Pharmakognosie*, Leipzig, 1917-25, 3 vols., 2nd ed., 1930ff.
241. K. Heyser, 'Die Alliumarten im Gebrauch der abendländischen Medizin,' *Kyklos*, 1928, 1:64-102; E. Hirschfeld, 'Scilla,' *Kyklos*, 1929, 2:163-78; H. E. Sigerist, 'Ambroise Paré's Onion Treatment of Burns,' *Bull. Hist. Med.*, 1944, 15:143-9; B. Tokin a.o., 'Phytoncides or Plant Bactericides,' *Amer. Rev. Soviet Med.*, 1944, 1:236-50.
242. *Pap. Ebers*, 30.
243. Ibid. 95.
244. Ibid. 57.
245. Ibid. 74.
246. Ibid. 75; *Pap. Hearst*, 41.
247. *Pap. Ebers*, 52.
248. See O. von Hovorka and A. Kronfeld, *Vergleichende Volksmedizin*, Stuttgart, 1909, 2 vols.
249. *Pap. Ebers*, 65ff.
250. *Ciba Symposia*, 1940, 1:320.
251. *Pap. Ebers*, 13, 27.
252. Ibid. 46.
253. Ibid. 80.
254. H. Thédenat, *Note sur un étui à collyre égyptien conservé au Musée du Louvre* (Mém. Soc. nat. Antiquaires de France), 1881, vol. 41, 27 pp.
255. *Pap. Edwin Smith*, p. 11.
256. *Pap. Hearst*, 10-14.

257. See Chauncey D. Leake, *Ciba Symposia,* 1940, 1:318.
258. *Pap. Ebers,* 70.
259. About the material used see B. Ebbell, *Die alt-ägyptische Chirurgie,* Oslo, 1939, p. 10.
260. An exception is *Pap. Ebers* 91, 12-19, concerning a wound of the ear.
261. Ibid. 70.
262. Ibid. 71.
263. *Pap. Edwin Smith,* 2, gloss B; 10, gloss A.
264. See his discussion of the term in *Pap. Edwin Smith,* p. 229f.
265. Ebbell, loc. cit. p. 10f.
266. *Pap. Ebers,* 107.
267. Ibid. 107-8.
268. Ebbell, loc. cit. p. 123ff.
269. *Pap. Ebers,* 106, 108.
270. Such as, e.g. Khons' swelling, *Pap. Ebers,* 108.
271. Breasted did not pay sufficient attention to the very important surgical section of *Pap. Ebers* and based his conclusions almost entirely on *Pap. Edwin Smith.*
272. *Pap. Edwin Smith,* 39.
273. Th. Meyer-Steineg had Egyptian surgical instruments in his collection at the University of Jena, some of which (two lancets and three knives) he reproduced without commentary in Meyer-Steineg and Sudhoff, *Geschichte der Medizin im Ueberblick mit Abbildungen,* Jena, 2nd ed., 1922, p. 29. My impression is that the instruments are Hellenistic.
274. See Meyer-Steineg and Sudhoff, loc. cit. p. 31, and E. Holländer, *Plastik und Medizin,* Stuttgart, 1912, p. 464ff.
275. *Pap. Ebers,* 89, to which must be added the three recipes (72) 'to expel destruction by eating ulcer on the gums.'
276. *Pap. Hearst,* 8-9.
277. E. A. Hooton, *Oral surgery in Egypt during the Old Empire,* Harvard African Studies I, Cambridge, Mass., 1917.
278. H. Junker, *Giza I. Die Mastabas der IV. Dynastie auf dem Westfriedhof,* Vienna, 1929, vol. 3, p. 256f., pl. 50A.
279. E. Renan, *Mission de Phénicie et la campagne de Sidon,* Paris, 1864, p. 472.
280. Clawson, 'A Phoenician Dental Appliance of the 5th Century B.C.,' *Am. Dent. Soc. Europe Tr.,* 1933, pp. 142-60; also 'Phoenician dental art,' *Berytus,* 1934, 1:23-32.
281. About dentistry in ancient Egypt see V. Guerini, *A History of Dentistry,* Philadelphia and New York, 1909; K. Sudhoff, *Geschichte der Zahnheilkunde,* Leipzig, 2nd ed., 1926; and particularly the publications of B. W. Weinberger, 'Did Dentistry Evolve from the Barbers, Blacksmiths or from Medicine?' *Bull. Hist. Med.,* 1940, 8:965-1011; 'Further Evidence that Dentistry Was Practised in Ancient Egypt, Phoenicia and Greece,' *ibid.* 1946, 20:188-95; 'The Dental Art in Ancient Egypt,' *J. Am. Dent. Ass.,* 1947, 34:170-84.

282. Diodorus, I, 49, 3: ἑξῆς δ' ὑπάρχειν τὴν ἱερὰν βιβλιοθήκην, ἐφ' ἧς ἐπιγέγραφθαι ψυχῆς ἰατρεῖον.

283. The Egyptian word *mtw* or *metu* means vessel, muscle, nerve, tendon; in other words the Egyptians did not differentiate these organs, just as the Greek word νεῦρον for a long time designated both nerve and tendon. There can be no doubt, however, that in these two treatises the *mtw* were vessels since they carried air, liquids, and excrements. See H. Grapow, *Ueber die anatomischen Kenntnisse der altägyptischen Aerzte,* Leipzig, 1935.

284. A. Piankoff, *Le 'cœur' dans les textes égyptiens depuis l'Ancien jusqu'à la fin du Nouvel Empire,* Paris, 1930; see also W. Spiegelberg, 'Das Herz als zweites Wesen des Menschen,' *Zschr. ägypt. Sprache,* 1931, 66:35-7.

285. *Pap. Ebers,* 99, 1-12 and 100, 2-14.

286. *Pap. Edwin Smith,* 1, 6-8.

287. *Pap. Ebers,* 103, 1-18.

288. *Pap. Berlin,* 163-64a. This version has a longer introduction and more recipes.

289. R. O. Steuer, '*Whdw,* Aetiological Principle of Pyaemia in Ancient Egyptian Medicine,' *Bull. Hist. Med.,* Suppl. 10, Baltimore, 1948.

290. Ebbell in the introduction to his translations of *Pap. Ebers* (p. 21ff.) points out that the *metu* discussed in the two treatises designate different vessels, the ones being arteries through which 'the heart speaks,' the others possibly veins, a view that is not shared by other Egyptologists. Personally, I believe that the term *metu* has the same meaning in both treatises, designating vessels, pipes through which everything moves that is in motion in the body, carrying 'the internal fluids' as well as the air. Since both treatises are highly speculative it is probably futile to try to identify the *metu* with any anatomical part we know.

291. The text in *Pap. Ebers* ends here while *Pap. Berlin,* 163 h now has a series of prescriptions beginning 'What is done against it according to the art of the famous physician Neterhotep.'

292. *Pap. Ebers,* 99.

293. Ibid. 100.

294. Ibid.

295. Ibid.

296. *Pap. Hearst,* 94-122, also 228-32, 237-8, 249; see also *Pap. Berlin,* 51, 122, 174-8; *Pap. med. Chester Beatty,* 2, 18. It must be kept in mind that in these recipes *mtw* need not always mean vessels but also muscles, nerves, or tendons.

297. Not less than 24 prescriptions 'to quiet the metu' are found in the texts.

298. The Egyptian language had two terms for brain, a general one meaning viscera at large and designating the brain when it appeared as 'viscera of the head' as is the case in Papyrus Edwin Smith; and another more specific term found in Papyrus Ebers and Hearst. See E. Iversen in *J. Egypt. Archaeol.,* 1947, 33:47-51.

299. See the Oxford English Dictionary or Webster's Dictionary.

300. Grapow, *Ueber die anatomischen Kenntnisse,* etc., p. 18.

301. *Pap. Ebers,* 57.
302. H. Ranke, *Orient. Lit. Ztg,* 1924, 27:558ff.; H. Grapow, loc. cit. p. 5.
303. Georg Ebers, *Die Körperteile, ihre Bedeutung und Namen im Altägyptischen* (Abh. Bayr. Ak. Wiss. I Cl.), 1897, vol. 21, 96 pp.; B. Ebbell, 'Aegyptische anatomische Namen,' *Acta Orient.,* 15:293-310; W. R. Dawson, 'Three Anatomical Terms,' *Zschr. ägypt. Sprache,* 1927, 62:20-23; J. G. de Lint, 'Beitrag zur Kenntnis der anatomischen Namen im alten Aegypten,' *Arch. Gesch. Med.,* 1932, 25:382-90.
304. *Pap. Edwin Smith,* 6.
305. Ibid. 22, gloss A.
306. Ibid.
307. *Mother and Child,* U.
308. Literature in Grapow, loc. cit. p. 23.
309. Clemens Alex., *Stromata,* 634.
310. A. S. Yahuda, 'Medical and Anatomical Terms in the Pentateuch in the Light of Egyptian Medical Papyri,' *J. Hist. Med.,* 1947, 2:549-74; see also his *The Language of the Pentateuch in Its Relation to Egyptian,* Oxford, 1932.
311. Herodotus, III, 129.
312. Ibid.
313. *Pap. Edwin Smith,* 25.
314. Hippocrates, edited by Littré, IV, 144.
315. Apollonius von Kitium, ed. Hermann Schöne, Leipzig, 1896, pl. 14.
316. *Pap. Edwin Smith,* p. 17.
317. See the excellent study of Erik Iversen, *Papyrus Carlsberg No. VIII,* with some remarks on the Egyptian origin of some popular birth prognoses (Det Kgl. Danske Videnskabernes Selskab. Hist. fil. Meddelelser XXVI, 5), Copenhagen, 1939, which presents new material and in which the earlier literature to the subject is also discussed critically.
318. G. Zoëga, *Catalogus codicum Copticorum manuscriptorum qui in Museo Borgiano Velitris adservantur,* Rome, 1810, pp. 626-30.
319. M. U. Bouriant, 'Fragment d'un livre de médecine en copte thébain,' *Acad. Insc. Belles Lettres, C R des Séances,* 1888, ser. 4, 15:374-9.
320. E. Chassinat, *Un papyrus médical copte* (Mém. Inst. Franç. Archéol. Orient, vol. 32), Cairo, 1921, 396 pp. and 20 plates.

IV. MESOPOTAMIA

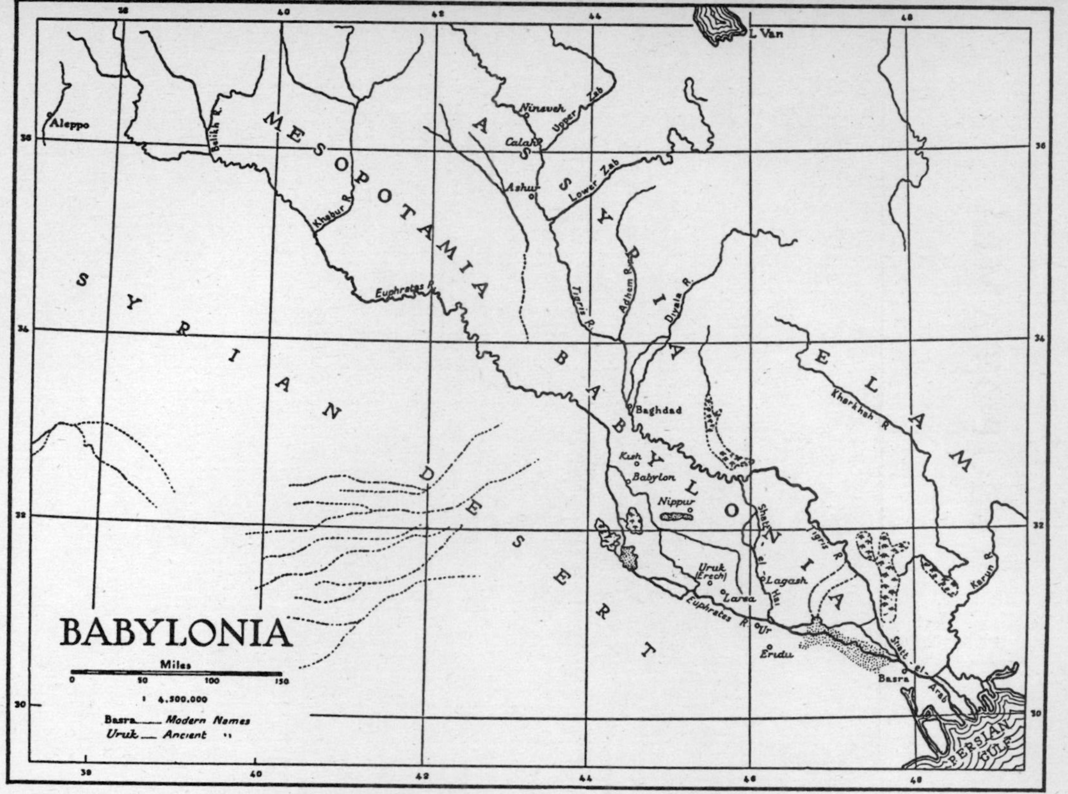

From *A History of the Ancient World* by M. Rostovtzeff. Used by permission of the Clarendon Press, Oxford.

*

1. The Setting

GEOGRAPHY

The rampant flood which no man can oppose,
Which shakes the heavens and causes earth to tremble,
In an appalling blanket folds mother and child,
Beats down the canebrake's full luxuriant greenery,
And drowns the harvest in its time of ripeness.

Rising waters, grievous to eyes of man,
All-powerful flood, which forces the embankments
And mows mighty *mesu*-trees,
Frenzied storm, tearing all things in massed confusion
With it in hurtling speed.[1]

This sounds very different from the Hymn to the Nile, as different as the geography of the two countries was. The Nile could be capricious also, could fail to rise, or rise too much. It had to be watched carefully but on the whole the river was a stabilizing element in the life of the country. It rose and receded at the expected time and the inundation could be controlled to a very large extent through the system of basins, dykes, sluices, and canals that was erected at an early stage. The weather, moreover, was very steady. South of Memphis one could be sure to see Re rising every morning, and even in the Delta a cloudy sky was not a frequent sight. This steadiness of the weather was also a stabilizing factor.

Mesopotamia in spite of many parallel features was a very different country.[2] As the Greek name indicates, it was the 'land between the rivers,' between Euphrates in the west and Tigris in the east. Both rivers came from the mountains of Armenia and flowed to the Persian Gulf, the Tigris on a shorter course while the Euphrates was much longer, much more tortuous, and carried more water. Today the two rivers join near Basrah and flow as one large stream, the Shatt el-Arab, leisurely to the sea, covering a distance of about a hundred miles. But this is recent alluvial land and in antiquity the sea reached much further north so that the rivers never joined but entered the sea separately. This explains why the ruins of the great Sumerian cities, Ur, Eridu, Lagash, are far inland today while they were close to the sea at the time they were built.

Like Egypt, Mesopotamia is a 'gift of rivers' because without them most of the land would be desert. As the rainfall south of the 34th parallel is not sufficient to allow crops, irrigation is necessary and of course possible because the rivers always carry water plentifully. They also flood the land when the snow melts in the mountains of Armenia; the Tigris first, the Euphrates somewhat later, beginning in March and reaching the maximum in May, but unlike that of the Nile their flood is violent and destructive unless it is checked by canals. Hence canals had to be built here also. They were constructed to connect the two rivers and drain water from the Euphrates into the Tigris. They irrigated the land, and the larger ones served at the same time as highways of traffic. Herodotus was impressed by the system of canals he found and pointed out that, unlike what he saw in Egypt, the fields were not irrigated by the rivers directly but rather through manual labor, with pumps.[8] In other words, when the rivers rose in the spring they filled the canals with their surplus water, which then was drained and pumped into the fields.

Just as the rivers of Mesopotamia lack the steadiness of the Nile, so is the climate different from that of Egypt. In the south the summer temperature is usually over 110° and may rise as high as 126° while it may drop to freezing point in winter. All over the country scorching hot days are followed by cold nights. Violent storms are not rare, with torrential rains in the north, or dust storms carrying sand from the desert into the houses through every fissure. It is an enervating climate, the violence of which is strongly reflected in the literature of Babylonia.

Boundaries and divisions of the country were also determined by the rivers. Where they break through the mountains, entering the plain and beginning to take a parallel course, they are about 110 miles apart. Flowing southward they gradually come closer to one another, and in the region of Bagdad the land between the rivers has narrowed down to about 20 miles; it was probably even less in antiquity because the rivers have shifted their beds repeatedly. The land then widens again, ending up with the estuaries of the rivers on the Persian Gulf. The distance from the Armenian mountains to the sea amounts to about 800 miles.

This course of the rivers naturally divided the country into two parts, Lower and Upper Mesopotamia. As in Egypt, culture moved in the direction from south to north. It was in Lower Mesopotamia that the Sumerians developed their high civilization and they were followed by the Babylonians. The agricultural backbone of their economy was the cultivation of the date palm, which thrived in the hot and moist atmosphere of the region, where the fruit was ripened by the hot wind that blew from the south in September. The date provided the people with a rich staple food. When you fly in an airplane at low altitude over Mesopotamia today, the luxuriant plantations of palm trees, lined up as regularly as though on a chess board, still present an impressive sight. It was recognized very early that the date palm was heterosexual and that artificial fertilization increased the crops. In the palace of Ashur-nasir-pal at Calah (Nimrûd) were large-sized reliefs showing the 'sacred tree,' the stylized form of the date palm, with the king on each side assisted by a winged being performing some religious rite connected with the ceremony of fertilizing the tree.[4] At the time of Herodotus, Babylonia had rich crops of cereals, wheat, barley, millet, and sesame,[5] just as Iraq has today.

Upper Mesopotamia, the region north of today's Bagdad, where the kingdoms of Akkad and later of Assyria developed, was different in many ways. Its southern part had agricultural land also, but pastures were in the north, grazing land where mountaineers and nomads kept their flocks. And the northern mountains were rich in minerals, containing gold, silver, lead, iron, and copper. Not far from the ancient Nineveh are the much-coveted oil fields of Mosul, a source of wealth, some day perhaps of ruin, for Iraq.

Mesopotamia like Egypt had natural borders, the sea in the south, the Syrian desert in the west, the mountains of Armenia in the north, and the Zagros mountains and the boulders of the Pushti Ku in the east, 60 to 100 miles from the Tigris. Yet the country was much more open and much more vulnerable than Egypt. Egypt had nothing to fear from the south, west, or north and was attacked from the east almost exclusively. Mesopotamia, on the other hand, was a fertile stretch of land surrounded on three sides by desert nomads and mountain peoples who greedily looked at the country between the rivers, just as Celtic and Germanic tribes looked at the fertile plains of Italy in the beginning of our era. And just as the Alps, a most formidable barrier, had passes, so the mountains bordering on Mesopotamia had passes also, through which many invaders found their way to the plains. And every thousand years Semitic tribes from arid Arabia pushed north in quest of better pastures.

Since Mesopotamia was more open than Egypt its culture spread farther. Not only did it strongly influence the immediate neighbors in Palestine, Syria, Asia Minor, and Persia but there were early contacts with India and possibly even China. Large as the Asiatic continent was, it had caravan trails that crossed the deserts and the mountain ranges and connected the most distant parts with one another. And the caravan brought not only goods from foreign lands but fairy tales, legends, technical knowledge, recipes, drugs, surgical operations. The caravan was a means of communication and of cultural exchange the significance of which cannot be estimated too highly.

What diseases may we expect in such a landscape?[6] In Egypt we were able to consult direct sources, the innumerable bones and the mummies that the dry sand had preserved. The soil of Mesopotamia is humid and the number of skeletons that have survived from early antiquity is very limited. Hence we do not have a paleopathology of Mesopotamia as we have of Egypt. Nor do we have the many wall paintings that adorned Egyptian tombs with scenes of everyday life. Most of our knowledge of the early incidence of disease is derived, therefore, from a study of the literature, medical and other, and we shall see later that it is not easy to make diagnoses from the available texts. But then we may also draw certain conclusions from the general geography of the country and from diseases prevailing today.

We may safely assume that Mesopotamia had in common with Egypt certain water-carried diseases, various forms of dysentery with all their complications. Typhoid fever is frequent today. Flies have always been a plague throughout the Near East. They infected the food, sat on the eyelids of sleeping children and spread diseases of the eyes. The marsh land in the estuaries of the rivers was a breeding place for mosquitoes and Lower Mesopotamia probably had more malaria than Egypt. Leprosy occurred in remote antiquity and the custom of segregating lepers, so familiar to us from Leviticus, originated in Mesopotamia. The medical texts preserved make it evident that diseases of the respiratory tract, particularly acute and chronic bronchitis and pneumonia, were frequent, more so than in Egypt, and this is not astonishing when we remember the climate of the country, with its violent changes of temperature, its cold nights following scorching days. Mesopotamia, moreover, located between East and West, was on the highway of acute epidemic diseases and must have been visited from remote antiquity by a variety of plagues that took their course from East to West.

We shall study the diseases of the country in more detail when we come to the discussion of its medical literature, but before we do this we must try to locate Mesopotamian culture in time.

CHRONOLOGY

The civilization of Mesopotamia is at the same time closer to us and more distant than that of Egypt. It is closer because the Old Testament tells us a great deal about it. We hear of the tower of Babel, of Nineveh that was to be destroyed. Abram came from Ur of the Chaldees, and since the middle of the nineteenth century, when Mesopotamian sites were excavated and cuneiform tablets deciphered, it has become evident how deeply influenced the Hebrews had been—like all ancient peoples of the Near East—by Babylonian civilization. It was found that the Akkadian language, the language of Babylonia and Assyria, belonged to the Semitic family like Hebrew, and old myths familiar to us from early childhood, the story of the creation of the world in seven days, the story of the deluge, and many others, appeared in the literature of Babylonia.[7] We shall see later that through Judaism, Christianity, and Islam ancient Mesopotamian institutions have survived to the present day in the West and in the East, and there can be no doubt that Greek civilization assimilated more Babylonian than Egyptian elements.

On the other hand, the archaeological remains are not so well preserved as those of Egypt. Huge buildings were erected in Mesopotamia too, but their material was clay bricks which did not resist the ravages of time, and the soil did not preserve the infinity of objects such as were found in Egypt, objects that make it possible to visualize the people's everyday life so easily. Nevertheless we can see in our museums reliefs, statues, delicately carved seals, the exquisite works of goldsmiths, enough to show us that Mesopotamia had also created great artistic values.[8]

The history of Mesopotamia is much more complicated than that of Egypt because many peoples, tribes large and small, were involved, and the following pages, needed to locate Mesopotamian civilization in time, cannot do more than give a sketchy outline of the main periods.

Recent excavations have shown that the land between the rivers, like the whole of Western Asia, was inhabited for many centuries before the invention of writing during the stone and early copper age, by people who knew the art of making pottery although they did not yet possess the potter's wheel. When Mesopotamia entered the historical period at about the same time as Egypt, toward the end of the fourth millennium B.C., the country was populated by the Sumerians in the south, by still semi-nomadic Semitic tribes in the north. It was the Sumerians who first developed Mesopotamian civilization, who built the first canals and irrigated the land.[9] A brachycephalic race, very different from the dolichocephalic Semites, they had probably come from the north and had settled in the estuary of the rivers. They spoke an agglutinative language and the script they invented consisted first, like that of the Egyptians and Chinese, of ideograms, of pictures. But it developed into a phonetic stage, with a sign for every syllable without however reaching the stage of the Egyptian or Hebrew scripts which possessed signs for every consonant. The writing material was not papyrus and ink, as in Egypt, but soft clay into which the cuneiform signs were drawn with a stylus made usually of a hard reed with a wedge-shaped end. After such a clay tablet had been covered with writing it was dried in the sun or baked in an oven and became so hard that tens of thousands have survived to the present day.[10] The individual tablet was not large and a book consisted of a series of numbered tablets, each one marked with the title of the book and frequently having as 'catch word' the first line of the following tablet. And just as our library books are stamped with the name of the library, we may find on cuneiform tablets the indication that they belonged to the palace of a certain king.

Just as many Egyptian papyri are fragments, many cuneiform tablets have been found broken or have been damaged in the process of excavation, particularly in the early days when archaeological methods were not so highly developed as they are now. The Assyriologist, therefore, is very often confronted with the difficult task of finding 'joins,' that is, of putting fragments together like the pieces of a jigsaw puzzle.

Texts of particular importance were often written on stone, and in our museums we can see monumental inscriptions relating the deeds of a king, like the stele of Ashur-nasir-pal in the British Museum or the block of black diorite in the Louvre on which the Code of Hammurabi is written.

The first period of Mesopotamian history, the *Classical Sumerian Age,* includes the centuries from about 3000 to 2400 B.C. It was the formative period of a great culture. The village with its huts of reed and mud inhabited by patriarchal families had become a walled city and every city was a state in itself. It was the domain of a god who resided in the center of the city, in the temple, and to whom everything belonged, the temple, the city, and the land around it. He was served by minor gods and by humans: free farmers, who tilled the soil with their slaves, traded with their neighbors, and one of whom was the god's steward, his chief priest, and the people's king.[11] The ruler's function was to worship his god, to keep the canals in order, and to lead his people in the case of conflicts with other city states. He was aided in his tasks by officials who were priests and scribes.

There were many such local gods and we have lists of them indicating their family relations, possessions, and attributes. But some gods stood above all others: Anu, Lord of the Heavens; Enlil, Lord of the Storm; and just as there was a national state and universal authority among the gods, thus it happened that one of the city states on earth subjugated others, gained leadership, and in this way created a national state. This was the case when the kings of Ur, a city on the Euphrates close to the sea, conquered the neighboring city states, and several dynasties of Ur ruled over a Sumerian empire, until Ur in its turn was conquered by the rival city of Lagash. The excavations at Ur have been extraordinarily revealing. They show that the ruler was buried with his entire household, wives and servants. And they also brought to light the exquisite creations of lapidaries and goldsmiths.

The Sumerians developed a culture that lasted for thousands of years, elements of which are still in existence today. Their cuneiform script was taken over by the Semites in the north and other peoples, and was used for the writing of a number of different languages. They began a new month with every new moon, adding an extra month to the year from time to time. The calendar of the oriental Jews and of the Mohammedans is still based on the moon year. Their numeral unit was 60 and we still divide the hour into 60 minutes, the circle into 360 degrees. We shall see later what influence their religious concepts exerted far beyond Western Asia and also how medicine and the sciences were developed within the framework of their theology.

While the city states of Sumer flourished in the first half of the third millennium, northern Mesopotamia, Akkad, was inhabited by semi-nomadic Semitic tribes. The camel was not domesticated yet, and the nomads had herds of asses. They gradually settled on the land and traffic developed between North and South, peaceful commercial relations and also armed conflicts. Around 2400 B.C. Sargon of Akkad defeated the Sumerians. A mighty ruler, he created a vast empire reaching from the Mediterranean to the Persian Gulf and to the mountains of Elam, an empire that was consolidated and enlarged still further by one of his descendants, Naram-Sin, 'the beloved of the moon-god.' Sargon's was the first Semitic empire. Its language became the dominating spoken language of Mesopotamia and in increasing measure also its literary language. Sumerian never disappeared, but in the course of time became the sacred and classical language, as Latin and Greek are to us today. Semitic energy and inventiveness were blended with Sumerian culture and the result was a new and very forceful civilization. Sumerian art and literature had become rigid in many ways, but the Semitic influx revitalized and modernized them. The Akkadians took over not only the Sumerians' system of writing but also their calendar, their weights and measures, and many elements of their religion, science, and medicine.

The period from about 2400 to 2000 B.C., from Sargon to the fall of the Third Dynasty of Ur, is usually called the *Sumero-Akkadian Age*. The tools and weapons were still made of copper because the manufacturing of bronze was not invented before about 2000 B.C. It was a period of flourishing trade with the neighboring countries, with silver as the chief medium of exchange. The empire Sargon had built did not last for more than a century. The subjugated peoples revolted. Sumer and Akkad were separated again and a strong revival of Sumerian culture took place, of which Gudea, viceroy of Lagash, was the chief exponent. He was later remembered as a holy man who fought evil and injustice wherever he found them, and rebuilt temples. The Third Dynasty of Ur, founded by Ur-Engur, pursued a policy of reconciliation. North and South were united again, until around 2025 Mesopotamia was invaded from the east by the people of Elam, who took possession of the Sumerian cities, and from the west by the Amorites, who invaded Akkad and conquered Babylon, at that time still a small and insignificant town.

The Amorites ruled in Babylon and made it a city of such importance that it gave its name to the land it controlled and to the civilization for which it stood. Its local god Marduk was identified with Enlil and was worshiped as far as Babylonian government reached. At his side was Ishtar, the goddess of love. The greatest Amorite king ever to reside in Babylon, who made it the prospering capital of a great empire, was Hammurabi.[12] He fought a thirty years' war with Elam, defeated Larsa, Eshunna, and Mari in the south and west, Assur in the north, and ruled supreme in the very center of Mesopotamia. While art had somewhat declined, the sciences and learning were highly cultivated and flourished at his court. He attracted scholars from far and wide. The classical literature of the past, the great epics and mythological tales, the hymns and prayers, the divination texts, the astrological and medical books were collected, issued in new editions and sometimes in translations. The translating of books was never a problem in ancient Egypt, which had one national language. It evolved, to be sure, and commentaries and glosses might be required for the interpretation of ancient texts. Mesopotamian civilization, however, was from the very beginning bilingual, since Sumerian and the Semitic Akkadian were totally different languages. The Semitic prevailed in Babylonia as well as Assyria but it had different dialects; Sumerian continued to be read, as we just mentioned, and from about 1000 B.C. on, Indo-European peoples entered the scene and began to play a decisive part. Books and documents, therefore, were translated and dictionaries were written for the purpose.

The great city that Hammurabi built is no more. It was destroyed and the Babylon that the Greek travelers admired was not his but Nebuchadnezzar's city. One lasting monument, however, remains to the glory of Hammurabi, greater than any town could be, his Code of Laws, *The Judgments of Righteousness which Hammurabi, the great King set up*. It is the oldest code that has come down to us and its elements are much older and go back to Sumerian times. Hammurabi, however, collected these laws, codified them, and made his Code the law of the land as far as his administration reached. In an absolute monarchy where so much power is vested in the king and in the officials who in the provinces rule in his stead, where there is so much room for arbitrariness, a Code of Laws that states in plain words the rights and duties of the individual, regulates family and property relations and the entire social life of the community, such a Code is a great element of security to the individual as well as to the state. From this Code and from other Babylonian documents we gather that the strong sense of justice expressed in the Old Testament was not peculiar to the Hebrews, but was quite universal in Mesopotamia. It was an inflexible justice, which punished infractions of the law without pity; but it was justice, and not only human but divine justice. The diorite shaft in the Louvre represents Hammurabi standing in front of Shamash the sun god from whom he receives the laws; [13] the monument itself was placed in the temple of Marduk at Babylon.

The Code of Hammurabi tells us a great deal about social life in Babylonia in the second millennium B.C. and we shall refer to it frequently in the following chapter and also later when discussing the position of physician and patient in society.

The period of Hammurabi was one not only of great political and cultural achievements but also of greatly increased trade and economic prosperity. The Babylonians had the uncanny gift of blending business with religion. The temples were centers not only of worship but also of finance, like our present stock exchanges. Indeed, not only the king and his noblemen were wealthy and carried on highly profitable trade but—and even more so—the gods owned riches and endeavored to increase them. Through their habitations, the temples, they owned land and people, and whoever needed money for business could borrow it from the gods at 20 per cent interest.

The Golden Age of Babylonia like that of Egypt did not last very long. The Hittites, breaking through from the north, raided the capital, and the Kassites, wild mountain people who had infiltrated the country in a steady stream, overpowered it, just as the Hyksos probably at about the same time conquered Egypt. And just as the Hyksos strove to become Egyptians, the Kassites were assimilated by the higher culture of Babylonia. They brought new blood but no creative power, and civilization stagnated in Babylonia for about a thousand years, until the short flowering of the Chaldean empire. And in the meantime the cultural centers had shifted to the north.

Assyria was the northeastern bastion of Mesopotamia. A Semitic settlement in the upper valley of the Tigris, it took its name from its tribal god Assur, whose city was built on the western bank of the river. When the local city state grew and gradually became a national state, Assur like Marduk of Babylon was identified with Enlil.

The Assyrians were merchants and pursued an aggressive commercial policy. As early as 1900 B.C., if not earlier, they had a colony at Kanish far up in the north in Asia Minor, the later Cappadocia; we are well informed about it from several thousand clay tablets found there, business documents and letters written in Old Assyrian. In their quest for commercial expansion, for the silver of Cilicia and for access to the Mediterrannean Sea, their interests clashed with those of other nations, the Hittites in the north, the very warlike kingdom of Mitanni on the upper Euphrates, the Arameans in Syria, the Phoenician settlements on the coast, and Babylonia in the south. Assyria became a military state and fought wars with its neighbors ruthlessly, for centuries. Its army with its horse-drawn war chariots was dreaded all over the Near East and although the Hittites were the first to use iron, the Assyrian army was the first to be completely equipped with iron weapons after 1000 B.C. Iron arrow points, swords, and spears were far superior to those made of bronze, and an army that was the first to use improved weapons had a great advantage over its enemies. The Assyrians were also feared for the machines with which they rammed the walls of enemy cities.

Babylon was in Kassite hands and when the Hittite empire fell and Egypt collapsed in the twelfth century, Assyria remained the most powerful state in the Near East. Nineveh, built further up the Tigris on its eastern bank, became the new and beautiful capital of a great empire that flourished from about 750 to 612 B.C. We are well informed about this period, because the documents preserved are numerous. Strong personalities give it color, Tiglath-pileser III (745-727), who subjugated the West and consolidated the empire, Sargon II (722-705), empire-builder, who founded for himself a new capital Dur-Sharrukin, felt a great responsibility for the preservation of Mesopotamian culture and collected books. His son and successor, Sennacherib (705-681), spent much of his life fighting rebellions, sacked Babylonia, was a skilful administrator. Keenly interested in engineering problems he restored Nineveh, using limestone for foundations, alabaster for wall reliefs. He improved the irrigation system, built an aqueduct that brought water from the eastern hills to the city, and he is also remembered for having introduced the cotton plant from India, a plant that for thousands of years was to play a very important part in the economy of the entire Near East.

Egypt was independent of Assyrian rule and as long as this was the case it was a menace in that it constantly incited rebellions in the peripheral provinces. The subjugation of Egypt was the main task of Esarhaddon's reign (681-668), a task in which he only partly succeeded because he died before it was fully accomplished. Still, he was able to add to his titles that of 'King of the Kings of Egypt.' His son and successor, Ashurbanipal (668-626), was not only a great king but also a great scholar, well versed in the classical literature and in the arts and sciences. The excavation of his library at Nineveh was a revelation. Twenty-two thousand clay tablets were found there and brought to the British Museum. We shall see later that we owe to this library most of our knowledge of ancient Mesopotamian medicine. Ashurbanipal's reign was brilliant, Nineveh with its temples, palaces, and gardens more beautiful than ever. Codified Assyrian laws, independent from those of Hammurabi, based on Old Assyrian legal traditions regulated the life of the empire.

And yet under the brilliant surface the empire contained the germs of its downfall. Even today with all our modern means of quick transportation and with the most deadly war weapons, it is impossible to hold an empire if the subjugated nations want independence and are willing to fight for it. This was even more the case in antiquity, when means of communication were relatively slow and vassal states far from the center were always inclined to revolt. Rome was able to hold its empire as long as it brought peace and prosperity to the conquered nations, respected their culture, and was able to fight its wars with its own people. Assyria exacted heavy levies from its vassals. The suppression of frequent rebellions required large armies, which deprived the home economy of manpower and finally forced Assyria to fight its wars with foreign troops that could not be relied upon. Internal dissension, open civil war between the sons of Ashurbanipal, accelerated the process of disintegration, and when the Chaldeans of Babylon joined forces with the Indo-European Medes and attacked Assyria from all sides with armies equipped with the same weapons and using the same tactics as their adversary, Assyria broke down. Nineveh was captured and thoroughly destroyed in 612.

This was the end of a great empire, but once more, although for less than a century, was a Semitic state to flourish in ancient Mesopotamia. It was the so-called New Babylonian Empire of the Chaldeans.

The Chaldeans were a Semitic tribe which in the beginning of the first millennium B.C. lived in the region northeast of the Persian Gulf from where it gradually penetrated into Babylonia. One of its chieftains, Nabopolassar, taking advantage of the disorders that followed the death of Ashurbanipal, assumed the kingship of Babylonia and with the help of Cyaxares and his Medes broke the Assyrian power as we just saw. Nabopolassar himself, and still more his son Nebuchadnezzar, continued the conquest of the Near East, which once more was united under a strong central power. In 586 B.C. Jerusalem was destroyed and many Hebrews were taken as captives to Babylonia.

Nebuchadnezzar (604-561) was not only an empire builder but also a builder of cities. During his long reign he spared no effort to make his capital Babylon the greatest and most beautiful city of the ancient world. Strongly fortified, with monumental gates, it centered around the temple of Marduk with its high tower and the royal palace with its 'Hanging Gardens,' which the Greeks counted among the seven wonders of the world. Nebuchadnezzar remembered the Golden Age of Babylonia, the time of Hammurabi, and his endeavor was to re-create it. The literary documents are written in a style reminiscent of the early days. But a Renaissance is never really a rebirth. The past can never be restored. Just as our Renaissance in the West drew profound inspiration from the arts and letters of Greece and Rome, but actually was deeply influenced by the Middle Ages, in the same way the empire of the Chaldeans was inspired by the classical culture of early Babylonia but continued where the Assyrians had left off. There is an astounding continuity in the history of Mesopotamian civilization for over three thousand years. Sumer was the cradle in which certain social and economic patterns, religious ideas, literary motives, artistic styles first took shape, and in subsequent centuries whoever happened to be in power in this area of the world, Semitic or non-Semitic peoples, desert or mountain tribes, assimilated the culture they found and carried on with it, developing certain of its aspects one step further. Or perhaps, it is not astounding, because we find a similar continuity and assimilating power of culture in Egypt, India, China, and in our own Western world. Thousands of years have passed since the Homeric poems, the dialogues of Plato, the Hippocratic writings, the Acropolis were created, but they are still with us, still exerting a profound influence on our life whether we are aware of it or not.

The New Babylonian Empire was short-lived, an afterglow of the old culture, an Indian summer. New forces were at work in the Eastern Mediterranean world, physical and spiritual, which proved to be irresistible. When Nebuchadnezzar died in 561 B.C., the Greeks had colonized the coasts and islands of the Mediterranean and a new poetry was bursting forth. At the same time the Persians were coming to the fore, ready to push west and south with formidable armies. Nebuchadnezzar's successors were weaklings and internal dissension undermined the empire still further. Cyrus the Great united and disciplined the Persian tribes, defeated the Medes, conquered Sardes, defeating Croesus of Lydia. Secure in the north he now turned east and south and the Chaldeans could see the writing on the wall. Nabonidus, Babylonia's last king, surrendered and Cyrus entered the city of Babylon in 539 or, according to other calculations, in 538. This was the end, and for two hundred years, until the arrival of Alexander of Macedonia, Babylonia was a Persian satrapy. From the second century B.C. on Aramaean was the spoken language of the entire region, a language that had an alphabet and did not need written signs for every syllable. But until the first century B.C. Babylonian scholars were able to write in cuneiform script and could read old Sumerian texts.

A civilization never dies entirely. Empires break up, buildings crumble, but the dying lion that the chisel of an anonymous Assyrian sculptor created on the walls of the royal palace of Nineveh is still with us. We still read the Epic of Gilgamesh, the hero who destroyed monsters and rebelled against the existing order by seeking immortality. A civilization also lives through the contributions it has made to its successors. The Christian and the Mohammedan world through the medium of the Old Testament received and kept alive many ancient Mesopotamian institutions and ideas, the seven-day week and the weekly day of rest, the way of naming the days after the planets, religious and legal concepts, literary motives, and indirectly even, as we shall discuss later, methods of combating diseases.

A civilization continues to live also through the advances it has made in science and technology, although the contributions themselves in these fields are easily forgotten. In the British Museum we stand in front of the sculptures that once adorned the palace of Ashur-nasir-pal at Calah. We see them with our eyes, as Assyrians did 2700 years ago, and we need no interpreter to become aware of their majestic beauty. But who outside of a few specialists knows of and can appreciate the great contributions made by the Assyrians and particularly the Chaldeans to astronomy? What they discovered and formulated became part of the accumulated knowledge upon which the progress of science rests. The results of their discoveries were taken over by the Greeks, who continued research where their predecessors had left off.

This book is obviously not the place to discuss the history of astronomy in Mesopotamia,[14] but a few words should be said about it, because if we look for science, in our sense of the word, in the ancient Orient it is here that we find it and not in medicine.

All over the ancient world the Chaldeans had the reputation of being stargazers. High towers had been built in many places from which people in the clear nights observed the firmament and the motion of the stars. Why did people look at the stars and write down what they saw? Why were they so keenly interested in what happened in the skies? For two reasons: In all ancient civilizations, as among many primitive peoples today, divination played a very important part, and in Babylonia perhaps more than anywhere else, it was generally accepted that the gods revealed their intentions in signs. These omens, spontaneous or provoked, were not only indicative of events but were believed to cause them. The priest's function was to teach the people what they should do in order to keep the gods benevolent, or in order to placate them had they been provoked. To that end he had to interpret the signs, and celestial happenings were particularly important omens. Thus the priests observed the stars, the moon, the five planets then known—Jupiter, Mercury, Saturn, Mars, Venus—the constellations of the zodiac through which the planets took their course. From the eighth century B.C. on they sent regular reports to the court from various points of observation so that evil might be averted through propitiative rites.

This was not astronomy, to be sure, but astrology. The course and interplay of heavenly bodies were studied not for scientific but for religious purposes, but they were studied nevertheless and important observations were made. We may well imagine that in the beginning it must have been particularly the seemingly abnormal happenings such as eclipses or comets that attracted attention and called for interpretation. In the Western world not so long ago comets were believed to be a certain sign of the wrath of God and were held responsible for the outbreak of epidemics. In the course of time the ancient astrologers must have found that there were no abnormal happenings in the sky, that the stars all moved according to eternal laws, and that their motions could be predicted with certainty. Astrology, however, never died but took on different forms, probably in Hellenistic times, and possibly on Egyptian soil, with the theory of the horoscope. Its idea was that the constellation of the planets at a given moment determined events; at the moment of an individual's birth it determined his constitution, character, and fate. Astrology was to play a very important part in late medieval and early Renaissance medicine and we shall, therefore, have more to say about it later.

Astrology was not the origin of astronomy since it had a totally different purpose and very different methods, but it probably sharpened the eye of the observer of celestial phenomena, just as hepatoscopy, divination from the liver of sacrificial animals, although not anatomy, taught priests to observe minute anatomical details. Neugebauer correctly pointed out that the origin of astronomy in Mesopotamia as in other ancient civilizations was rather the very practical need of having a workable calendar which might be used satisfactorily by the farmers as well as by those who were in charge of the cult. Measurement of time, determination of the seasons, lunar festivals, these were, according to Neugebauer, 'the problems which shaped astronomical development for many centuries.'[15] And in the course of these developments the Babylonians attained results that far surpassed those ever reached by the Egyptians and anticipated Greek science. Their methods of computing the ephemerids of the moon and of the planets were truly scientific and make it evident that they also had reached a high level of mathematical knowledge.[16]

NOTES

1. Quoted from H. and H. A. Frankfort, John A. Wilson, Thorkild Jacobsen, William A. Irwin, *The Intellectual Adventure of Ancient Man,* Chicago, 1946, p. 127, a most inspiring book in which Mrs. Frankfort's English versions of Babylonian poetry are of extraordinary beauty. This and other quotations from this book by permission of The University of Chicago Press.
2. About the general geography and history of Mesopotamia see *The Cambridge Ancient History,* vols. I-III, Cambridge, 1923-5; Eduard Meyer, *Geschichte des Altertums,* Stuttgart, 1925-34, 7 parts in 4 vols.; L. J. Delaporte, *Mesopotamia,* New York, 1925; G. Contenau, *La Civilisation d'Assur et de Babylone,* Paris, 1937.
3. Herodotus, I, 193.
4. See e.g. E. A. Wallis Budge, *Assyrian Sculptures in the British Museum,* London, 1914, plate XI. For a different interpretation see Contenau, *Civilisation,* p. 193.
5. Herodotus, loc. cit.
6. See G. Contenau, *La Médecine en Assyrie et en Babylonie,* Paris, 1938, pp. 1-4.
7. See, e.g. A. Heidel, *The Babylonian Genesis,* Chicago, 1942; *The Gilgamesh Epic and Old Testament Parallels,* Chicago, 1946.
8. See S. Harcourt-Smith, *Babylonian Art,* New York, 1928.
9. C. L. Woolley, *The Sumerians,* Oxford, 1928; *Ur of the Chaldees: A Record of Seven Years of Excavation,* London, 1929; H. Frankfort, *Archaeology and the Sumerian Problem,* Chicago, 1932.
10. B. Meissner, *Die Keilschrift,* Berlin, 2nd ed., 1922.
11. H. Frankfort, *Kingship and the Gods,* Chicago, 1948.

12. There is no consensus about the time at which he ruled except that it is generally accepted that he held his throne for 43 years. R. Campbell Thompson in *The Cambridge Ancient History,* vol. I, p. 487, assumes that he ruled 2123-2081 B.C., while Breasted (*Ancient Times, a History of the Early World,* 2nd ed., Boston, 1935, p. 169) gives the date as 1948-1905 and Albright as c.1728-1686 (*From the Stone Age to Christianity,* 2nd ed., Baltimore, 1946, p. 364). About the chronology of Mesopotamia see Arno Poebel, *J. Near Eastern Studies,* 1942, 1:247-306; 1943, 2:56-90.
13. See the very interesting thesis of H. Frankfort (*Kingship and the Gods,* Chicago, 1948, p. 157), according to which 'the regularity of the sun's movements suggested . . . the thought of inflexible justice and an ubiquitous judge.' In Egypt 'justice was part of an established order created by Re.'
14. The basic collections of texts are: R. Campbell Thompson, *The Reports of the Magicians and Astrologers of Nineveh and Babylon,* London, 1900, 2 vols.; Ch. Virolleaud, *L'Astrologie chaldéenne,* Paris, 1908-12, 4 vols. The basic studies on astronomy are Franz Xaver Kugler, S.J., *Sternkunde und Sterndienst in Babel. Assyriologische, astronomische und astralmythologische Untersuchungen,* Münster i.W., 1907-24, 2 vols. (with many texts); see also Carl Bezold, *Astronomie, Himmelsschau und Astrallehre bei den Babyloniern,* SB. Heidelberger Ak. Wiss., Phil.-hist. Kl., 1911, and particularly the numerous studies of O. Neugebauer, today undoubtedly the outstanding authority in the field, who at the present time is preparing a collection of astronomical cuneiform texts. His article, 'The History of Ancient Astronomy, Problems and Methods,' *J. Near Eastern Studies,* 1945, 4:1-38, gives an excellent survey of the field with a good bibliography.
15. Loc. cit. p. 14.
16. About Babylonian mathematics see O. Neugebauer, *Mathematische Keilschrifttexte* [Quellen u. Stud. Gesch. Math. Astron. Phys.], Berlin, 1935 8, 3 vols.; *Vorlesungen über Geschichte der antiken mathematischen Wissenschaften,* vol. 1: *Vorgriechische Mathematik,* Berlin, 1934; F. Thureau-Dangin, *Textes mathématiques babyloniens,* Leiden, 1938.

*

2. Social Environment

The social and economic structure of Mesopotamian society obviously underwent changes in the course of 3000 years but, just as in Egypt, certain elements of it remained unchanged through the ages or were modified only slightly. The geography was the same, which means that Mesopotamia at all times was a country the prosperity of which depended on irrigation. The clay of the soil provided always the same building material and stuff for the manufacturing of an infinity of objects from jars to furniture and coffins. The economy of the country remained a slave economy throughout the course of Babylonian history. In this brief chapter, which is necessary in order to have at least a sketchy picture of the social environment in which the life of the people in whose health and illness we are interested unfolded, we shall consider primarily the conditions that prevailed during the Golden Age of Hammurabi. His Code of Laws is an excellent source and we possess, moreover, a wealth of other documents from that period. We shall, however, also compare certain conditions with those in the Sumero-Akkadian period and also with those in the Assyrian and Chaldean empires.[1]

We mentioned in the previous chapter that the Sumerian city-states consisted of freemen who with their slaves as laborers produced the food and goods society required, and that one of these freemen was king-priest of the group. It may well be that these city-states were originally primitive democracies and that a king was elected only in periods of emergency, but kingship became hereditary and with the unification of the country and growing centralization of power the local king-priests became provincial governors.

Conquest by foreign races led to a further stratification of society and at the time of Hammurabi it consisted of three classes. The upper class, *amelu*, or patricians, to use a term familiar from Roman history, were landed proprietors and holders of high offices at the court, in the administration, in the army, and in the temples. Together with the crown and the temples they were the chief owners of the means of production, had wealth and power, enjoyed many privileges, and also had greater responsibilities. Damage done to a patrician was punished more severely than if it were done to the member of a lower class[2] but on the other hand a patrician who committed an offense met with a harsher punishment than the member of a lower class committing the same offense.[3]

The next class, which held a position between patricians and slaves, were the *mushkinu* or to use a Roman term again plebeians. They were laborers mostly, or small merchants, small officeholders, school teachers, beggars. They worked on the land as farm laborers or share croppers. They were permitted to own property and to hold slaves but most of them were poor and dependent on the patricians.

The slaves, *ardu,* were a large and very important class because they were the chief laborers in agriculture and industry and hence produced the wealth of the country. Their labor gave the patricians, the priests, and the court the leisure to engage in cultural activities. Slaves were either the children of slaves, or free people who had been sold by their parents because of general poverty or to pay off a debt, or they were prisoners of war. Victorious wars were a tremendous source of labor power. Thus we hear that when Sargon II in the eighth century B.C. conquered Urzana he captured 20,960 prisoners.[4] Lost wars on the other hand were a great drain on the countries' labor power. Not only were thousands of slaves lost who had been drafted into the army but entire cities were depopulated.

There was no stigma attached to slavery, for the good reason that everybody might become a slave in time of war. A slave could marry a free woman and in such a case his children were free.[5] A slave girl very often was her master's concubine and she herself and her children became free after the master's death.[6] Slaves could be liberated by their owners or could purchase their liberty. Otherwise they were the personal property of their masters. They were marked and the male slave's head was shaved. They worked in the fields, in the garden, in the house, and were craftsmen. The owner of slaves would sometimes rent them out for farm labor during the harvest and if such a slave died or became sick compensation had to be paid for him. Babylonian slaves, like Egyptian serfs, were subject to levy for forced labor. If the government needed large numbers of workmen for repairing canals or building new ones or for city construction, or if it needed soldiers for the army, it could draw upon the slave reserves of the country.

Since slaves were objects of property the various codes protected the owners against losses. Very interesting from a medical point of view is article 278 of the Code of Hammurabi, according to which the sale of a slave, male or female, was annulled if the *bennu* disease befell him or her within one month. In Assyrian sales contracts of the seventh century B.C. the term was extended to one hundred days and a second disease, *sibtu,* was included as a cause for making a sale void.[7] There has been much speculation about the nature of these diseases, and I think that Karl Sudhoff's explanation is the most convincing.[8] On the basis of careful philological and medical interpretation of the passages involved, he came to the conclusion that *bennu* was a spastic disease, possibly epilepsy, and *sibtu* a contagious disease, possibly leprosy. As a parallel he pointed to Greek contracts from Hellenistic Egypt in which these very diseases (ἱερὰ νόϐος and ἐπαφή) were mentioned as reasons for returning a slave.[9]

The land was owned by the Crown, the temples, and private individuals; slaves, hired farm laborers, or share croppers tilled the soil. The Code of Hammurabi, however, mentions another type of landholding, namely land bestowed upon soldiers as fiefs. In times of peace the soldier lived on his farm and he could count on a secure income from it, but in times of war he had to serve in the army. Such land could not be sold but was passed on to the son, who with the farm assumed his father's military obligation.[10]

In Assyria a middle class developed that held a position between patricians and plebeians, a class that included the free craftsmen and professional people, *ummane,*[11] in other words, potters, blacksmiths, painters, and also scribes, architects, and bankers. At the same time we find a strict guild organization similar in many ways to that of the Islamic world in the Middle Ages. The various trades had certain sections of town assigned to them just as in the Arabic *sūq* of today we still can see the leather workers in one street, the potters in another, and similarly streets for every single trade. The Assyrian craftsmen's organization had a semi-military character, with chiefs of various grades who were responsible for the work of the members of the guild as well as for the collection of taxes and the fulfilment of other obligations.

The social unit here as in Egypt was the family.[12] We do not know at what age people married in Hammurabi's days, but they were in all probability young, since the newly wed frequently went to live with the parents of the husband. No marriage was valid without legal contract.[13] The suitor brought a gift of silver to the father of the prospective bride and he in turn gave his daughter a dowry. The Code is very explicit about what is to be done with bridal gift and dowry in case of breach of promise, divorce, or similar occurrences.[14] Most men had only one wife, but those who could afford it could marry more than one, or have concubines. This happened particularly when the first wife had no children, in which case she also could be repudiated. If, however, a man took a second wife because his first wife had become sick, he was not allowed to divorce the sick wife but was obliged to keep her in the house and support her as long as she lived,[15] unless she preferred to leave, in which case the dowry was to be returned to her.[16]

The Code gives detailed instructions about divorce which was easy for the man, not so easy but nevertheless possible for the wife.[17] Adultery if established beyond doubt was punished by drowning, but if the husband pardoned his wife, her partner could count on being pardoned by the king.[18] A woman suspected of adultery could be forced to submit to an ordeal.[19] The position of woman in society was relatively high. Women were priestesses and could engage in trade and in various professional activities. In many legal matters they had equal rights with men.

We do not know very much about childbirth but it seems likely that women gave birth to their children as in Egypt, squatting on bricks or on a parturition chair or then lying on the bed.[20] And here as in Egypt they were aided by one or several midwives and protected against evil spirits with amulets, prayers, and magic rites. Nergal, the god of pestilence, and Labartu, the demon, had to be propitiated; evil spirits, the ghosts of 'a woman that hath died in travail, or a woman that hath died with a babe at the breast, or a weeping woman that has died with a babe at the breast' [21] were to be kept off. Ishtar was invoked or Shamash the sun god.

> May this woman give birth happily! May she give birth, may she stay alive and may the child in her fare well! May she walk in health before thy divinity! May she give birth happily and worship thee! [22]

Children could be adopted by married couples, after which they had all the rights and duties of children born in the house. Or a craftsman adopted a boy and taught him his trade, or a temple woman adopted a little girl. The Code of Hammurabi has detailed regulations about adopted children.[23]

On the other hand, here as almost everywhere in antiquity there was no objection to the destruction of newborn children. People who were too poor to raise a large family or those priestesses who were not allowed to have children threw the newly born into the well or exposed him in the desert. Or the mother did what happened to Moses, 'took for him an ark of bulrushes, and daubed it with slime and with pitch, and put the child therein, and she laid it in the flags by the river's brink.'[24]

Children were nursed here, as in the entire ancient Orient, for the first three years, by their mothers if they had enough milk or by a wet nurse if the parents could afford her. She was remunerated in money or in kind and the Code again was very strict in order to prevent abuses. If a child given into the care of a nurse died and the nurse was convicted of having substituted another child in his stead, her breasts were cut off.[25]

Boys were not circumcized. The custom was apparently not of Semitic but of African origin and the Hebrews took it over from the Egyptians.

As the climate of Mesopotamia was very different from that of Egypt the costume was very different also.[26] Egyptian dresses were usually made of linen, but the cold nights of Mesopotamia required a woolen cloak in antiquity as they do at the present time. But linen was used also in Mesopotamia, particularly for under garments, and the Babylonians, moreover, had fabrics made of cotton. At the time of Herodotus the Babylonian costume consisted of a long linen shirt; over this the men wore a coat made of cloth and a short white cloak. Their long hair was tied with a ribbon; they had a signet ring on their finger and carried a cane with a carved ornamented head.[27] This rather elaborate costume was the result of a long development. In the early days of Sumer, people living in the hot estuaries of the rivers probably wore very little and a reminiscence of this primitive nudity survived in certain cults. The laborer at work probably never wore more than a string belt or a short girdle. In the Sumero-Akkadian period the chief costume of men and women consisted of a rectangular piece of cloth draped in folds over the left shoulder, somewhat like a Roman toga. A heavy bonnet completed the costume. This is how King Gudea is represented in various statues.[28] He is, moreover, shaved, although the fashion later required men to have long beards. The Kassites introduced a new garment, a robe with short sleeves, which has remained the basic costume of the Near East to the present day and is the dalmatic of the Catholic Church. It was worn with a belt around the middle; the material used changed in the course of time and also according to the social status of the individual. The robe was frequently embroidered, an art in which the Assyrians were masters. A kind of scarf or shawl was wrapped over the robe not so much for decoration as for protection against the cold. The bonnet was replaced by a cap. The woman's dress was very much the same except that it was more lavishly decorated and women wore more jewelry. Bright were the festive colors, while those of mourning were dark; like the Hebrews, the Babylonians rent their clothes and girded themselves with sackcloth when mourning the dead.

The custom of women being veiled in public, so characteristic of the Islamic world, can be traced back to Assyria. The old Assyrian laws codified around 1100 B.C. contain very stringent regulations on the subject. Married women, widows, daughters of freemen, 'a bondswoman who with her mistress goes on the highway,' and even the married temple courtesan were veiled, while wearing the veil was strictly forbidden to unmarried temple courtesans, all prostitutes, and slaves. The Assyrian Laws state: [29]

> He who sees a veiled harlot, shall arrest her; he shall produce free men as witnesses and bring her to the entrance of the residency. Her jewelry shall not be taken from her but the man who has arrested her shall take her clothing; she shall be beaten 50 stripes with rods, and pitch shall be poured on her head.

If a slave is caught veiled, her ears are cut off. On the other hand, a man who sees a veiled prostitute or slave and does not report her, receives fifty lashes, 'his ears shall be pierced, and a cud shall be passed through them and be tied behind him; and in addition he shall do labor for the king for one full month.'[30]

Here as in Egypt and all over the East, ointments, cosmetics, and perfumes were used profusely, but we have no evidence that the Babylonians were as clean as the Egyptians. Purity was an important concept with them also, but it was a spiritual concept and their purity rites were primarily symbolic. We shall see later that aspersion with water played an important part in their magic ritual, but unlike the precepts in Leviticus it had hardly any hygienic significance. The Babylonians washed their hands before meals, as all people do who eat with their fingers, and poured water over their hands after meals. But they probably washed head and body only on festive occasions. Only very rich people had bath tubs and used a mixture of oil and potash with the bathing water. All kinds of taboos were attached to the canals, and, as the welfare of the country depended largely on them, it was considered a sin to urinate into them.

The diet was chiefly vegetarian.[31] Bread, made mostly of barley and baked into flat loaves, was the staple food, but other cereals—spelt, wheat, and sesame—were used also. A mush made of flour, milk, and honey was a popular dish. The country was rich in vegetables. In the royal garden of Merodach-Baladan, sixty different kinds were cultivated, including such staple vegetables as onions, leek, garlic, beans, turnip, radish, cucumber, colocynth, lettuce, dill, and others.[32] The date provided a high caloric food rich in sugar. It could be eaten fresh and dried, baked into cakes, made into a kind of honey, and used in a great variety of ways. Even the stones were not lost but were burned to make charcoal. The vine and apple trees grew in the northern part of Mesopotamia, fig trees probably everywhere. A fruit and vegetable garden is the pride of every household in an arid country and when we see with what loving care such a garden is nursed today we realize it certainly was the same in the past. Water is everything in these countries.

Where it is available the vegetation is luxuriant and where there is no water, there is desert.

The country was probably not so rich in cattle and other domestic animals as was Egypt, nor had it the wealth of wild birds that bred along the Nile. The sheeps' wool, moreover, was needed for textiles. Meat except in the house of the very rich appeared on the table only on festive occasions; here as in Egypt fish was the chief source of animal protein. In the house of the lower classes the food was served heaped in a large bowl; the whole family squatted or sat with crossed legs around it and everyone helped himself from it with his fingers in a way we may still observe in the Near East. The rich had tables and ate sitting on chairs or, in the late Assyrian period, reclining on couches as the Greeks did.

Drinking water came from the rivers and canals and there can be no doubt that it was contaminated very often and that intestinal diseases were frequent. In some houses the water was kept cool in jars suspended in drafty places. Milk was a food rather than a drink. Among the fermented beverages, beer was by far the most popular. It was the *kvas* type of beer similar to that of Egypt. Palm wine was made from the sweet juice gathered from the shoots of the date palm and also from the fruits. But wine was also made from grapes and some was imported from Syria, where a famous brand was produced. All these wines were very sweet and rather strong. Banquets at which wine was served liberally became noisy affairs. The 'bodies' of the guests 'became joyful, they shouted much, their heart was exalted' or the drinker's 'liver was loosened and he became gay.'[33] On the way home he felt unsteady on his legs and sometimes the drunkenness was such that the doctor's advice was sought. A recipe has been preserved which gives a striking description of alcoholic intoxication:[34]

> If a man has taken strong wine and his head is affected and he forgets his words and his speech becomes confused, his mind wanders and his eyes have a set expression; to cure him take licorice . . . beans, oleander . . .[35] to be compounded with oil and wine before the approach of the goddess Gula[36] and in the morning before sunrise and before anyone has kissed him let him take it, and he will recover.

Food taboos did exist although it seems that they were not so strict as those of the Mosaic Code. Man was pledged 'not to eat what the god and the goddess loath.'[37] The pig was considered unclean and a source of illness but pork was eaten by some, nevertheless, except on certain days. Other foods such as roast meat, fish, and onions were not to be eaten on certain days, and we shall have to say more about the highly developed hemerology of the Babylonians. Lack of food not only in periods of famine but voluntary abstinence as a sign of mourning was considered a cause of illness. In a Late Assyrian letter the king is urged not to mourn for Shamash longer than half a day and to have a second meal that day. The writer then continues, saying that 'fasting, abstinence from food and drink afflict the mind, illness follows.'[38]

Housing[39] was not very different in Mesopotamia from what it was in Egypt, although architectural styles varied. The reed hut was probably the earliest dwelling here also, and the clay brick became the chief building material. The country was very poor in stone and timber; in the south stone is nonexistent. Assyria had some quarries from which stone could be cut, but bricks were much cheaper and had the additional advantage that they kept the heat out more effectively. Clay, which was available in unlimited quantities, was pressed into molds and the bricks thus obtained were dried in the sun. They could be hardened still further by being baked in an oven; or bits of straw or reed were mixed with the clay, adding to the solidity of the brick.

Houses were, as a rule, built around a courtyard, here as in Egypt. They had no windows. Light and air entered through the doorways, one opening into the street and others leading to the courtyard. Flat roofs were very popular then as today because the family could retire there after sunset to enjoy the coolness of the night. Flat roofs, however, required timber, but the trunks of palm trees covered with clay were good enough for that purpose. Only the very rich could afford to purchase cedar wood imported from Mount Lebanon. But even palm trees were not cheap in addition to the fact that they were not too solid, and this is probably the reason why houses were roofed with brick vaults at an early time.

What the proportion between flat and vaulted roofs was in different periods is impossible to tell, because the roof is the first part of the house that collapses; but it is very likely that not only granaries and storerooms were vaulted. From the point of view of hygiene both types of roof have advantages and disadvantages. Vaults give more air to a room, particularly when they have an opening on the top as those have that are seen on relief pictures.[40] On the other hand they do not provide terraces on which people can sleep, as flat roofs do. Of course, it was possible to combine the advantages of both by having some rooms vaulted and others not, and judging from pictures we find that this was actually done.

The mansions of the rich and the royal palaces had not only one courtyard but several, in other words they were combinations of houses. There is no doubt that the block house was developed in Mesopotamia as it was in Egypt, although Herodotus probably exaggerated when he said that all houses in Babylon were three to four floors high.[41] We also know from excavations that not all streets were straight. The better houses had bathrooms with asphalt floors and toilets with water that flushed the night soil into the street. Palaces and other large houses had regular sewers, vaulted brick conduits that collected rain water, bath water, night soil, and other refuse and drained it out of the house. We never hear of any organized disposal of sewage, but it is obvious that the farmer used whatever he could get hold of as manure, unless he needed the animal dung and at times even human dung for fuel. Charcoal was a luxury and the kitchen stove was at best heated with dried desert plants.

The architect who built a house in the days of Hammurabi was remunerated according to a tariff and assumed a liability for his work.[42] I mention this because we shall have to discuss later the surgeon's liability in more detail and we shall see that the pattern was the same. If a house was not built solidly and it collapsed and killed the owner, the architect was to be killed. If the owner's son was killed, the architect's son had to pay with his life. A slave had to be replaced as did other damaged property, draconic laws which followed the principles of the *lex talionis,* eye for eye, tooth for tooth.

It brings to mind present-day practices during the housing shortage when we hear that he who bought a house, in addition to paying the purchase price, had to make gifts to the seller and the witnesses.[43]

The common man's furniture was simple enough, consisting of a bed or two, a few chairs, a table, a few chests for storing clothes and whatever possessions the family had. At the court, however, and in the houses of the nobility, from Sumerian days to the time of the Chaldeans, furniture and utensils were much more elaborate and reflected the achievements of the arts and crafts of the period. We have no tomb, however, preserved from Mesopotamia comparable to that of Tutenkhamon; from what remains we have, it seems that the Mesopotamians did not cultivate the art of living as the Egyptians did, and had not their easy-going ways. Their climate was more trying, their religion more somber, their art more rigid.

Life consisted generally of hard work, but there was also time for rest and recreation. Dancing and singing were universal. Music was played with a variety of instruments and the tunes were perhaps not so different from those that we hear in Bagdad on a summer night. Games were played, precursors of chess. Friends met for a banquet and drinking bout to celebrate some event or went for a sailing party on the river. The rich were passionate hunters here as everywhere. And religion, the cult of the gods, provided holidays, festivals, strong emotions. When the gods feasted in heaven commemorating an event of their life and career, the humans, rich and poor, were invited to partake of their rejoicing. Farmers came from the country, prayed, sacrificed, followed the processions, and the temple prostitutes had a profitable day.

Every ancient civilization had a certain hemerology. Some days in the calendar were considered lucky, others unlucky. Unlucky days were not holidays in themselves, but since no business must be transacted on such days, and nothing important undertaken, they became more or less holidays. The great significance of Babylonia in this respect was that the 7th, 14th, 21st, and 28th days of the month, which were considered unlucky, occurred at a regular interval.[44] They were probably the precursors of the Jewish Sabbath, of the weekly day of rest, which was taken over by both Christianity and Islam.[45] The Greeks and Romans had just as many holidays in the course of the year, but at irregular intervals. The institution of a weekly day of rest was extraordinarily important as a measure of physical as well as mental hygiene in that it set a definite elementary rhythm to man's life, instituting a day of rest and recreation after every six days of labor. And regularity, rhythm, is an essential factor of health.

We may end this brief chapter by reporting what an Assyrian considered the good life. In a letter found in the library of Ashurbanipal, the king's servant Adad-shum-usur petitioned his lord Esarhaddon to give his son a position at the court. In the first part of the letter he pictures how excellent conditions are, but in spite of all his soul is distressed and his mind depressed because his son is not yet in the presence of the king his lord and because he has nobody at the court to intercede for him. The letter begins: [46]

Ashur the king of the gods has mentioned the name of the king my lord for the rule of Assyria. Shamash and Adad by their true revelation have established the rule of the king my lord over all countries, a favorable rule, righteous days, years of justice, heavy rains, full streams, good prices. The gods are propitious, religion thrives, temples are richly furnished. The great gods of heaven and earth are exalted in the reign of the king my lord. Old men dance, young men play music, women and maidens gladly perform the task of womanhood, procreation is common, sons and daughters are brought forth, childbirth is exceeding satisfactory. The one whose sins condemn him to death, the king my lord lets live. Those who were captive during many years, you have delivered. Those who were ill many days, recover. The hungry are satisfied, the lean become fat, the naked are covered with garments.

NOTES

1. For a general survey of ancient Mesopotamian culture see M. Jastrow, *The Civilization of Babylonia and Assyria,* Philadelphia, 1915; B. Meissner, *Babylonien und Assyrien,* Heidelberg, 1920-24, 2 vols. [cited as Meissner]; L. Delaporte, *La Mésopotamie et les civilisations babylonienne et assyrienne,* Paris, 1924; G. Furlani, *La Civiltà babilonese e assira,* Rome, 1929;

G. Contenau, *La Civilisation d'Assur et de Babylone,* Paris, 1937 [cited as Contenau, *Civilisation*].

2. E.g. *Code,* 207-8 or 209-14.
3. E.g. *Code,* 116.
4. D. D. Luckenbill, *Ancient Records of Assyria and Babylonia,* Chicago, 1927, vol. II, p. 30; Contenau, *Civilisation,* p. 249.
5. *Code,* 175.
6. *Code,* 170ff.
7. S. Schiffer, Beihefte, *Orient. Lit. Zeit.,* I, Berlin, 1907, pp. 2-12.
8. Karl Sudhoff, 'Die Krankheiten *bennu* und *sibtu* der babylonisch-assyrischen Rechtsurkunden,' *Arch. Gesch. Med.,* 1911, 4:353-69.
9. Such contracts are collected in Karl Sudhoff, *Aerztliches aus griechischen Papyrus-Urkunden,* Leipzig, 1909, p. 142ff.
10. See *Code,* 26ff.
11. See Sidney Smith in *Cambridge Anc. Hist.,* vol. III, p. 96ff.
12. About family and family life see R. C. Thompson in *Cambridge Anc. Hist.,* vol. I, p. 522ff., and Meissner, vol. I, p. 389ff.
13. *Code,* 128.
14. Ibid. 138ff., 159.
15. Ibid. 148.
16. Ibid. 149.
17. Ibid. 137ff.
18. Ibid. 129.
19. Ibid. 132.
20. Sources are listed in Meissner, vol. I, p. 390.
21. R. Campbell Thompson, *The Devils and Evil Spirits of Babylonia,* London, vol. I, 1903, p. 41. This and the other numerous quotations from this book by permission of Luzac and Co. Ltd., London.
22. *Beitr. Assyr.,* x, 1, no. 1, 25ff.; Meissner, vol. I, p. 390
23. *Code,* 185ff.
24. *Exodus,* 2, 3; compare with this *Cuneiform Texts . . . in the Brit. Mus.,* XIII, 42, 6ff.; Meissner, vol. I, p. 392.
25. *Code,* 194. About wet nurses in general see V. Scheil, 'Les Nourrices en Babylonie,' *Rev. Assyr.,* 1914, 11:175-82.
26. About clothing see Meissner, vol. I, p. 407ff.; Contenau, *Civilisation,* p. 237.
27. Herodotus, I, 195.
28. See, e.g. *Rev. Assyr.,* 1907, vol. 6, plate I.
29. G. R. Driver and J. C. Miles, *The Assyrian Laws,* Oxford, 1935, pp. 408-9.
30. Ibid. p. 409.
31. About food see Meissner, vol. I, p. 413ff.; Contenau, *Médecine,* p. 28f.
32. R. C. Thompson in *Cambridge Anc. Hist.,* vol. I, p. 500.
33. P. Dhorme, *Textes religieux assyro-babyloniens,* Paris, 1907, p. 41.
34. F. Küchler, *Beiträge zur Kenntnis der Assyrisch-Babylonischen Medizin,* Leipzig, 1904, pp. 32-3 (English translation by M. Jastrow in 'The Medicine of the Babylonians and Assyrians,' *Proc. Roy. Soc. Med.,* Sect. Hist. Med., 1914, p. 152.
35. The text lists eleven drugs, most of which are unidentified.

36. Which means as much as 'in the evening before the stars rise.'
37. For this and the following see Meissner, vol. II, p. 137f.
38. R. H. Pfeiffer, *State Letters of Assyria* [Am. Orient. Ser. 6], New Haven, 1935, p. 186.
39. About housing see Meissner, vol. I, p. 274ff.; Contenau, *Civilisation*, p. 142; and archaeological monographs about excavated cities such as R. Koldewey, *Das wiedererstehende Babylon*, Leipzig, 4th ed., 1925; E. Unger, *Babylon nach der Beschreibung der Babylonier*, Berlin, 1931; H. R. Hall and C. L. Woolley, *Ur Excavations*, London, 1927; G. Loud, *Khorsabad*, Chicago, 1936, and many others.
40. Such a picture may be found in Contenau, *Civilisation*, p. 147.
41. Herodotus, I, 180.
42. *Code*, 228-33.
43. Sources in Meissner, vol. I, p. 367.
44. Another ill-starred day was the 49th (seven times seven), counting from the first of the preceding month.
45. For a discussion of this matter see K. Sudhoff, 'Hygienische Gedanken und ihre Manifestationen in der Weltgeschichte,' *Deutsche Revue*, 1911, 4:40-50, reprinted in *Skizzen*, Leipzig, 1921, p. 143ff.
46. R. H. Pfeiffer, *State Letters of Assyria*, New Haven, 1935, p. 118f.

*

3. Principles and Sources of Mesopotamian Medicine

If we wish to understand Mesopotamian medicine we must keep in mind that religion dominated and permeated all aspects of the civilizations that flourished in that area, from the early days of Sumer to the very end of the New Babylonian empire. At the time when the pre-Socratic philosophers were investigating nature in Greece and a new rational medicine was developed in schools flourishing on islands and along the coasts of the Mediterranean, Babylonian medicine was still religious in its general outlook. This does not mean that physicians had not accumulated a certain store of empirically gained observations and treatments, but we shall see that they were fitted into the traditional religious system. The beginning of a separation between magico-religious and empirico-rational medicine that we found in Egypt never took place in Mesopotamia, and we have no texts comparable in any way to Papyrus Edwin Smith or to certain sections of Papyrus Ebers. There is no doubt that new excavations will bring forth new texts and surprises may possibly occur. We know that surgery was practiced in Babylonia and that operations were performed even on the eye. At the moment, we have no surgical book, but some day a series of tablets may be found listing surgical cases and operations. As a whole, however, I do not expect great surprises. We possess many texts from different periods and they all reflect very much the same spirit. They are actually extraordinarily monotonous.

Babylonian religion [1] was primarily of Sumerian origin, although obviously it also contained Semitic elements. The cosmic deities of the Sumerians, the Lords of Heavens, Storm, Earth, and Water, Anu, Enlil, Nintu, Enki, were taken over by the Semites. Their names might change or local deities, Marduk, Ashur, and others were identified with them, but their authority remained through the millennia. They ruled supreme in heaven and on earth, together with the other deities that constituted the rich Mesopotamian pantheon.

After having created from chaos heaven and earth, the rivers Tigris and Euphrates, the canals and ditches, the gods created man. Like a potter they made him of clay but mixed with flesh and blood of a god who had been killed for the purpose. This is why god is in man. And this process of creation is renewed whenever a child is born.[2]

The gods created man for their service, to carry the yoke and labor for them, to build habitations (that is, temples) for them, to till the soil, reap crops, breed animals to be sacrificed to them. Service of the gods was man's duty and the purpose of his life. The temple was the palace of the god where he resided, had his furniture, his cart, his boat, his servants and musicians, his concubines, like any earthly ruler. But not only the priests were his servants, all of mankind was, and the king was his chief steward. He who served the gods well lived happily on earth, and he who neglected them or transgressed their commandments was punished. Sickness sent by gods directly or through the medium of demons was the chief form of punishment, for the individual's own sin, for that of his parents or his clan.[3] But sickness could also befall man because he had not been cautious and the evil spirits had taken hold of him, although he had not committed any offense. Sin, sickness, and possession by demons, however, were so intimately connected that the terms became almost synonymous.[4]

These views are very familiar to us because we encountered them in Egypt and among primitive peoples, and we know how man reacted to disease wherever he held such views. Religion and magic provided the means to influence gods and events, to avert evil and restore health. Leading a pure life, observation of taboos, prayer, sacrifice, and the whole gamut of magic instruments and procedures from amulets to solemn incantations, were the methods employed, and the interpretation of omens revealed the intentions of the gods. We shall discuss this in detail later and shall illustrate it with texts.

In the theocratic societies of ancient Mesopotamia medicine remained religious, or we may better say, magico-religious. It taught the people how to avoid illness, how to restore health, and thus to postpone death, by propitiating or reconciling the gods. Life after death was conceived as dreary and colorless, and we saw how Gilgamesh rebelled against fate and sought the immortality that was granted only to gods.

The law was divorced from religion. Hammurabi on the famous diorite stone was pictured standing in front of Shamash and promulgated his Code in the name of his god, but even before his time a distinction was made between priestly and civil jurisdiction and gradually the administration of the law was taken away from the priests entirely and placed in the hands of civil judges and secular courts.[5] Such a divorce from religion never took place in medicine and the various categories of healers were always made up of members of the clergy.

Babylonian magic was an integral part of religion.[6] Magic usually is, in most ancient civilizations. Whether the reciting of a prayer is a religious or a magic performance depends on what you expect from it, and it is sometimes difficult to tell where a prayer ends and an incantation begins. Magic was the means to exert a certain control over the transcendental world and obviously was used not only for medical purposes but whenever man was in distress or wanted to have a wish fulfilled, when he needed rain for the fields to have rich crops, and even for such trivial matters as the desire not to be molested by dogs.[7]

Magic was a perfectly legitimate science, man's chief means of protection, and without the possession of some magic formulae and objects a family would have felt utterly helpless. But there was also illegitimate black magic by which a man could harm his fellow man, and the accusation of such magic was a serious matter for which the Code of Hammurabi prescribed trial by ordeal.[8] The individual under suspicion had to jump into the river, and if the river took hold of him and he drowned, his guilt was evident and the accuser could take his house. On the other hand, if he floated and thus was proved to be guiltless the accuser was killed and his house given to the victim.

While everybody had some knowledge of magic, just as everyone knew prayers and was familiar with certain rites, yet the higher, the specialized knowledge and practice of magic was in the hands of priests, diviners, exorcists, and physicians, who had studied the ancient texts, had been trained in temples and initiated into a science of which much was kept secret.[9] Mesopotamian magic is particularly important not only because we possess a wealth of texts that make it possible to study the subject in great detail, but also because much of it survived in the West and in the East through Jewish, Syriac, and Mandaic channels.[10]

In studying the history of ancient Mesopotamian medicine, we must always remember that in all civilizations of this area religion, magic, science, and learning were one, an inseparable whole, and it is as such that we must approach it.

It was relatively easy to get hold of the literary sources of Egyptian medicine. The number of papyri preserved is limited; they can be dated with fair accuracy and most of them have been edited and translated competently. They have been known for some time and much work has been devoted to their philological and medical interpretation. They present enough unsolved linguistic problems, to be sure, and we saw that we had to draw on non-medical texts also in order to get a better integrated picture of Egyptian medicine. But still it is possible to have all medical papyri on one table at the same time, which makes it easy to compare passages and in general to work with these texts.

The situation is infinitely more complicated with the literary sources of Mesopotamian medicine.[11] The first difficulty is one of definition. When is a text to be considered medical and when not? We have a large number of tablets that list symptoms of disease and indicate pharmacological treatments, very much in the style of some of the Egyptian papyri. They represent one aspect of Mesopotamia's religious medicine, texts that contain a vast amount of empirically gained observations and treatments and impress us as being largely rational in our sense of the word. They obviously are medical books, written by and for priest-physicians.

But then we know that disease was believed to be caused primarily by demons, ghosts, and a great variety of evil spirits. We know that divination was the chief method of making a diagnosis, a prognosis, and of averting an impending evil. We know that prayers, incantations, and other magic rites were the treatments most frequently employed. We possess very many tablets describing the demons, their ways and evil doings. The literature on hepatoscopy alone is very considerable and we have many texts listing and interpreting other omens. Prayers and incantations are found among the earliest literature preserved and the number of texts we possess is very large indeed.

Should we discard this entire literature as non-medical and leave it to the historian of religion and magic? Of course not. Any text that deals with health and disease is of the greatest interest to us. This magical and religious literature is obviously not concerned with disease alone. Demons had more than one way of plaguing man; omens were consulted to foretell and sometimes forestall all kinds of events, and people prayed to their gods or performed magic rites not only to have their health restored; but there is no doubt that disease took a very important place in this literature, which thus becomes one of our chief sources of medical thought and practices in Mesopotamia.

As early as 1894 K. Tallqvist published the important Maqlû texts,[12] a series of incantations and rites, mostly of imitative magic using fire to destroy the evil. Two years later H. Zimmern published the Shurpu series,[13] a collection of similar texts, and in the following years he edited a number of other documents dealing with magic.[14] In 1902 David W. Myhrman published the very important Labartu texts,[15] incantations and rites directed against one of the chief causes of illness, the female demon Labartu. R. Campbell Thompson's two volumes, *The Devils and Evil Spirits of Babylonia,*[16] giving transliterations and a translation of three major series of magic texts,[17] contain not only great literary documents but very important sources of medical history. Many more such texts have been published since then [18] and there can be no doubt that future excavations will bring forth new tablets.

The dating of texts presents another and very serious difficulty. The majority of our medical books and documents come from the library of Ashurbanipal; since he lived in the seventh century B.C. we have a *terminus ante quem.* We know that these books cannot have been written later, but many were copies of older books, of texts that may well go back to the third millennium B.C. The fact that most of them are written in Sumerian does not mean that they are of Sumerian origin, since Sumerian was the language of learning which physicians used just as Roman doctors wrote medical books in Greek, and Western European doctors in Latin until the early nineteenth century. The Sumerian language, of course, evolved, just as medieval or eighteenth-century scientific Latin is different from that of Cicero. Study of the language and style does give a lead in regard to the age of a text but is not a certain criterion because an old text may not have been copied literally but rather written in the scholastic jargon of the copyist's day; or writers were purists at times, and tried to express themselves in the language and style of the remote past. The humanists' Latin in the Renaissance was much closer to the language of Cicero than that of their medieval precursors or later successors.

Apart from language and style we know that a book is older than its Assyrian copy when parallel texts have been found on tablets excavated in older sites, and as a matter of fact, we have a considerable number of such tablets. The German excavation of Ashur, in a site some centuries older than Ashurbanipal's time, brought forth many important medical texts. The earliest Sumerian incantations that we have, about 40 short texts written on small tablets, can be traced to the IIIrd Dynasty of Ur.[19] Old Babylonian texts have been found at Nippur. They are longer, written on larger tablets in several columns, sometimes six or even eight.[20] At the time of Hammurabi interlinear Akkadian translations were added to the original Sumerian text.

While it is possible to date a number of texts with fair accuracy there are still very many of which we do not know more than the *terminus ante quem* and about the origin of which we can only speculate. Falkenstein's and Kunstmann's [21] studies were interesting attempts to bring some order into the early incantation texts by analyzing their literary genre and the different types. There was literature on the sick man and his treatment from the third millennium on, here as in Egypt, and every century added to the store of knowledge. But it is not possible yet to write a consecutive history of early Mesopotamian medicine. We may at best distinguish between old and young elements and may point out that the physicians of Ashurbanipal's time had books describing symptoms and drugs available, which so far could not be traced to the second or third millennium. We must, however, keep in mind that very old texts, very old incantations, and lists of omens were still used when the Persians conquered the land and even later. The oral tradition, moreover, played in all ancient civilizations a part that cannot be estimated highly enough. People knew very much more than was written in books.

The editor and translator of cuneiform texts faces many difficulties. The first arises from the fact that tablets are frequently broken, particularly those excavated in the early days. When we look at the plates of R. Campbell Thompson's *Assyrian Medical Texts from the Originals in the British Museum,*[22] we soon find that hardly one of the tablets with which he had to deal was not damaged. Sometimes the fragments are large and contain much text, other times they are very small. The editor, therefore, after having read the texts must look for joins, for fragments that belong together. But these fragments do not fit like those of a jigsaw puzzle that have been neatly cut with a fine saw; the edges instead have frequently crumbled off and words are missing. Fortunately we possess a number of medical texts not in one but in several copies and it is often possible to fill in gaps from such duplicates.

The editor of such a text, after having collected the fragments, first copies the text in cuneiform script, then transliterates it into Latin characters, and finally translates it into a modern language.

We mentioned the enormous difficulties encountered in the identification of Egyptian technical terms, particularly of drugs. Here the task while difficult enough is easier in so far as Akkadian, Babylonian, and Assyrian were Semitic languages into which Sumerian texts were frequently translated. Coptic, the late development of ancient Egyptian, is a language with a very limited vocabulary, while Hebrew, Syriac, and Arabic are very rich languages with a considerable medical literature, with technical terms and many plant names, which obviously are very helpful in our attempts to identify medical matters in the old literature of Mesopotamia.

Work on the medical texts proper centered in the beginning around the Kouyunjik Collection of the British Museum, that is, the tablets from the library of Ashurbanipal. A. H. Sayce was probably the first to attempt a translation of such texts, in 1885.[23] The medical terminology was little known at that time and in 1904 Friedrich Küchler published, translated, and discussed the same texts and a number of others in a very important monograph[24] which actually opened up the field. From then until 1921 shorter or longer medical texts were made known incidentally,[25] and in 1921 and 1922 E. Ebeling published a larger number of tablets from the British Museum.[26] He had edited the religious texts found by the Germans at Ashur,[27] many of which dealt with health and disease, and he planned to publish a volume with all cuneiform medical texts available at that time. He was apparently not aware that a British Assyriologist had been engaged in the same task for a very long time, namely R. Campbell Thompson, who in 1923 published on 107 plates the text of 660 cuneiform medical tablets, thus practically exhausting the medical holdings of the Kouyunjik Collection.[28] Before a satisfactory translation could be attempted, it was necessary to identify as many drugs as possible. Thompson did this in his *Assyrian Herbal*,[29] a monograph on about 250 Assyrian vegetable drugs based on a thorough examination of all known medical texts and of more than 120 fragments of cuneiform plant lists. These lists include chiefly plants with medicinal value and are particularly important because they frequently give synonyms and equivalents or brief descriptions of plants. At the same time Thompson also engaged in studies on Assyrian chemistry,[30] and then he set out transliterating, translating, and interpreting his medical texts. He did it in a series of papers of varying length, widely scattered in journals.[31] Of course, it would be more convenient to have the entire medical literature of Mesopotamia collected in several volumes, with the texts arranged chronologically and according to subjects. On the other hand, many translations are still tentative, much editorial work remains to be done, new joins and new tablets will undoubtedly be found, so that it may be too early to think of a Corpus of Mesopotamian medicine. Whoever undertakes such a task will lean heavily on R. Campbell Thompson's findings. Rarely has a field of research been covered so broadly and so thoroughly by one man.

It remains for us to discuss briefly the style of the medical literature and since we shall devote much space to the magic and religious texts, we shall write here primarily about the medical literature proper. The Babylonians were more systematic than the Egyptians. They codified their laws at an early date. They listed carefully their astronomical observation, their astrological findings, and what the various methods of divination taught them. And in the same way their medical books were collections of cases arranged systematically under a certain heading.[32] The principle of classification was either etiological, symptomatic, or clinical. A famous book included cases listed under the heading, 'If the hand of a ghost seizes on a man,'[33] another 'If a woman gives birth to a child with . . .'[34] Or the cases were arranged according to the sick organ, 'If a man is affected in the lungs,'[35] 'If a man's eyes hurt,'[36] or according to the dominating symptom such as jaundice.[37] Collections of prognoses were also made such as the series 'When you approach a sick man,' or 'When the incantation priest goes to the house of a sick man.'[38] These were not purely magic divination texts because the view was held that the symptoms of disease, the deviations from the norm the physician perceived on the patient's body, or in its functions, or in its ejections, were omens also, signs that indicated and caused the sick man's fate, signs that had to be interpreted correctly and had to be counteracted by treatment. Such an attitude toward the symptoms made it possible to include numerous rational elements in a system of otherwise religious medicine.[39]

When the cases were too numerous to be recorded on one tablet, a second tablet was filled with text, or as many as were necessary. They were numbered, and for greater safety each tablet had as a 'catch-word' the beginning of the next tablet. Together they formed a book the title of which consisted of the initial words, just as one of the most famous Salernitan books was and still is known as *Circa instans,* and the papal encyclicals are named in the same way.

Babylonian like the other books were not only copied but edited; elaborate compilations were made from various texts. Medical books like those dealing with technical matters are perhaps the least static of all. Magic and religious texts cannot be changed easily because their wording is all-important and slight changes might affect the action of a spell or charm in the people's mind. Medical texts, on the other hand, underwent constant changes, here as in Egypt. In Babylon and in Nineveh, just as later in Alexandria, scholars undertook the great task of collecting, editing, classifying, and rearranging the literature that had come down to them, just as before them the oral traditions had been collected and written down. Much of this editorial work was done during the first Babylonian Dynasty at the time of Hammurabi. Again, the Kassites in their endeavor to assimilate Babylonian learning made inventories of libraries and archives, copied and abstracted books. The text of a *Treatise on the Lucky Days* was established on the basis of seven tablets, from copies of Sippar, Nippur, Babylon, Ur, Larsa, Uruk, and Eridu. After having made abstracts, and having made a selection, the scholars presented it to Nazimarullash, King of the Universe.'[40]

The reconstruction of the final versions of such compendiums from tablets and fragments found in various places, and the analysis of the constituent parts are now one of the major tasks of modern editors. R. Labat in an admirable study[40] restored the order of the *Book of Prognoses* and showed that it had an unusually elaborate structure in that it did not consist of one series alone, but had four other prognostic series worked into the major text, and that the tablets had two numbers each, one referring to the series as a whole and one to the sub-series. Labat was able to identify 27 tablets as belonging to this book, one which is unusually important also because it shows a systematic arrangement that we are not accustomed to find in such books. The title of the whole series is 'When the incantation priest goes to the house of a sick man,' and so is the title of the first sub-series. The text discusses the significance of omens observed on the way to the sick, around the house, or in the sick room. Then follows a long sub-series consisting of 12 tablets and entitled 'When you approach a sick man.' It contains prognoses arrived at from the observation of skull, head, hair, temples, forehead, eyes and their parts, nose, nostrils, tongue, mouth, voice, ear, face, throat, arms, forearms, palms, loins, back, epigastrium, abdomen, entrails, lower abdomen, intestines, thighs, buttocks, feces, penis, urine, testicles, knees, and feet. In other words, we have here in a prognostic text a systematic arrangement *a capite ad calcem* as we have it in a surgical text, in Papyrus Edwin Smith.

The next sub-series comprising 10 tablets is entitled, 'If the first day when he is sick the sight of the blow . . .' and discusses the prognostic evaluation of the patient's condition or behavior from the first to the sixth day of his illness and thereafter, the symptoms observed in the beginning, during the course, and after the illness, those that occur in the morning, in the evening, at night, the patient's desires and the symptomatology of a number of diseases. The last and perhaps incomplete sub-series was probably entitled, 'If the hand of the sick is taken' and listed symptoms caused by various demons.

This was a very elaborate textbook indeed, the result of a long development. We shall quote a few passages from it in a later chapter. It does not include treatments since it is a purely prognostic book, but it lists symptoms because it is impossible to make prognoses from nothing. Prognoses also occur in other, not specialized, medical texts as part of the general discussion of a case.[41]

The style encountered in this literature is very similar to that of Egypt for the good reason that it is the logical order to present a case. First the symptoms must be listed. To the patient they are the disease, the subject of his complaint, that which impels him to consult a doctor. The symptoms determine the physician's actions and so he must know them. Sometimes only the dominating symptom is given, 'a man is sick of a cough,'[42] or 'a man's mouth and nostrils hold fetor.'[43] Sometimes we have very elaborate and detailed descriptions,

> If a man's head hurts him, his mouth pricks him, his eyes trouble him, his ears sing, his throat chokes him, his neck-muscles hurt him . . . his fundament, his breast, his shoulders and his loins hurt him, his fingers are cramped, his stomach is inflamed, his bowels are hot . . . his hands, his feet and his knees ache . . .[44]

On the basis of the symptoms observed the physician could make a diagnosis which might be magical or rational and very frequently was etiological: the disease is 'the hand of a ghost or the hatred of a goddess'[45] or it is 'choking of the passage.'[46] Or various possibilities are indicated. In the case just quoted of a man who had pains in the head and other limbs, the patient might be 'sick of retention, either restriction of constipation or restriction of breath . . . or is sick of kidney trouble or of bile or of jaundice . . . or is sick from a curse, or is sick of ulcers [?], or of rheumatism, or of the hand of a ghost . . . or is sick of the demon, "Raiser of the Head for Evil."' In the majority of cases no diagnosis is given because it is implicit in the symptomatology. When a man suffers of a cough or of a headache no diagnosis is needed because the symptom is the disease.

In a complete description of a case symptomatology and diagnosis will be followed by a prognosis indicating that the sick man will recover, or will die, or will linger and die.[47] The favorable prognosis more frequently follows instructions for the treatment and thus assumes the character of a recommendation, or it introduces the treatment with the words: 'For his recovery thou shalt . . .'[48] Very many cases do not include a prognosis. The art of foretelling the future of a patient was divination, a highly specialized art that was in the hands of a special category of priests. It had its own literature and we have just mentioned one of its outstanding books.

Instructions for the treatment conclude the discussion of a case. It may be magical or consist in the application of drugs. It may be a mere reference to a certain incantation that must be performed and the text of which could be found in special collections. Or we have the full text of the spell and detailed instructions on how to perform the ritual.

In very many cases listed in the medical texts proper a series of treatments follows immediately the mention of the symptoms, or even of the single symptom which serves as heading of the tablet. Thus,[49] 'if a man is full of itch, fennel and . . . together thou shalt bray, mix in oil, anoint and he shall recover.'

If ditto, ricinus, sumach, thou shalt bray, in . . . wash, the rind of . . .

If ditto, with oil of fishes' insides (?) thou shalt anoint . . .

If ditto, scab of the housewall thou shalt rub, and anoint (?) . . .

Storax, fennel, ricinus, these three drugs for itch . . . , root of barhuš, root of tamarisk, cummin . . . thou shalt apply.

In other words, these particular tablets contained collections of recipes and nothing else, and had thus the same character as certain sections of Papyrus Ebers and of other Egyptian medical papyri. As a matter of fact, the medical literature of Egypt and that of Mesopotamia were very similar in style although they differed a great deal in content and concepts. Archaic civilizations always have common features even when there is no direct intercourse between them. It is the time element that makes it. Man needs a certain time to develop certain techniques, ideas, philosophies. Not only were the civilizations of Egypt and Mesopotamia contemporary but also those of neighboring countries between which there was constant intercourse. It is no wonder that they learned much from one another and that they exchanged people, technical knowledge, and ideas, sometimes peacefully and sometimes violently in periods of war.

And now we should like to know what the content has been of Mesopotamia's medical literature, taking it in the broadest sense of the word, including magic and religious texts in so far as they have any relation to health and disease. But first we must have a brief look at the sick man and his healers in their mutual relationship.

NOTES

1. The literature on religion in Mesopotamia is very considerable. Some of the basic general books to consult on the subject are: M. Jastrow, *Die Religion Babyloniens und Assyriens,* Giessen, 1907-12; A. Ungnad, *Die Religion der Babylonier und Assyrer,* Jena, 1921, a collection of texts in translation; S. N. Kramer, *Sumerian Mythology: A Study of Spiritual and Literary Achievements in the Third Millennium B.C.,* Philadelphia, 1944; E. Dhorme, *Les Religions de Babylonie et d'Assyrie,* Paris, 1945.
2. A. Heidel, *The Babylonian Genesis,* Chicago, 1942.
3. The concept of disease being a punishment for sin must be Semitic because it does not occur in the early Sumerian incantations as A. Falkenstein has shown, *Die Haupttypen der Sumerischen Beschwörung,* Leipzig, 1931, p. 56.
4. See L. W. King in *Encycl. Rel. Ethics,* New York, vol. VIII, p. 253.
5. *Cambridge Anc. Hist.,* vol. I, p. 511.
6. The most recent monographic discussion is G. Contenau, *La Magie chez les Assyriens et les Babyloniens,* Paris, 1947. See also the literature on Babylonian religion.
7. E. Ebeling, 'Babylonische Beschwörung gegen Belästigung durch Hunde,' *Mitt. Vorderasiat. Gesell.,* 1916, pp. 17-21. To have a dog urinate against you may have been considered more than a nuisance, namely an evil spell or an evil omen.
8. *Code,* 2.
9. Contenau, *Magie,* p. 54ff.
10. *Encycl. Rel. Ethics,* vol. VIII, p. 255.
11. The most recent monograph on Mesopotamian medicine is G. Contenau, *La Médecine en Assyrie et Babylonie,* Paris, 1938, an excellent book, to which we owe a great deal (to be cited as Contenau, *Médecine*). It has the most exhaustive bibliography ever published on the subject. A physician and one of France's most distinguished Assyriologists, Curator of Oriental Antiquities at the Louvre and Professor at the Ecole du Louvre for many years, Contenau was better qualified than anybody else to write such a book. B. Meissner, *Babylonien und Assyrien,* Heidelberg, vol. II, 1925, has a long chapter on medicine, pp. 283-323, which may be consulted profitably.

A very good earlier survey is M. Jastrow, 'The Medicine of the Babylonians and Assyrians,' *Proc. Roy. Soc. Med.*, Sect. Hist. Med., 1913, pp. 109-76. See also W. R. Dawson, *The Beginnings, Egypt and Assyria* [Clio medica., vol. I], New York, 1930.

12. K. Tallqvist, *Die assyrische Beschwörungsserie Maqlû*, Leipzig, 1894.
13. H. Zimmern, *Die Beschwörungstafeln Shurpu*, Leipzig, 1896.
14. Such as *Ritualtafeln für den Wahrsager, Beschwörer und Sänger*, Leipzig, 1901.
15. David W. Myhrman, 'Die Labartu-Texte. Babylonische Beschwörungsformeln nebst Zauberverfahren gegen die Dämonin Labartu,' *Zschr. Assyr.*, 1902, 16:141-200.
16. R. Campbell Thompson, *The Devils and Evil Spirits of Babylonia, Being Babylonian and Assyrian Incantations against the Demons, Ghouls, Vampires, Hobgoblins, Ghosts, and Kindred Evil Spirits, Which Attack Mankind*, Luzac's Semitic Text and Translation Series, vols. XIV-XV, London, 2 vols., 1903-4.
17. Utukki Limnûti (Evil spirits), Ašakki Marsûti (Fever sickness), and Ti'i (Headache).
18. They will be listed in subsequent chapters.
19. They are listed and discussed in A. Falkenstein, *Die Haupttypen der Sumerischen Beschwörung*, Leipzig, 1931.
20. Ibid. p. 8ff.
21. Walter G. Kunstmann, *Die Babylonische Gebetsbeschwörung*, Leipzig, 1932.
22. London, 1923.
23. A. H. Sayce, 'An Ancient Babylonian Work on Medicine,' *Zschr. f. Keilschriftforschung*, 1885, 2:1-14, 205-16. About literature to 1902 see von Oefele, *Keilschriftmedicin, Einleitendes zur Medicin der Kouyunjik Colloction*, Breslau, 1902 [Abh. z. Gesch. d. Med., Heft 3]. See also his *Materialien zur Bearbeitung babylonischer Medizin*, Berlin, 1902 [Mit. Vorderasiat. Ges., vol. VII, no. 6]; 'Zwei medizinische Keilschrifttexte,' *Mitt. Gesch. Med. Naturwiss.*, 1904, 3:217-24.
24. Friedrich Küchler, *Beiträge zur Kenntnis der assyrisch-babylonischen Medizin*, Leipzig, 1904 [Assyr. Bibliothek, vol. 18]. (To be cited as Küchler.) Küchler was aided by von Oefele, who studied the same texts at about the same time; see his *Keilschriftmedizin in Parallelen*, Leipzig, 1904 [Der alte Orient, vol. 4, no. 2].
25. Such as the texts published by V. Scheil: 'Un Document médical assyrien,' *Rev. Assyr.*, 1916, 13:35-42; 'Fragment de tablette médicale,' *Rev. Assyr.*, 1917, 14:87-9; 'Tablette de pronostics médicaux,' ibid. 121-31; 'Quelques Remèdes pour les yeux,' *Rev. Assyr.*, 1918, 15:75-80; H. F. Lutz, 'A Contribution to the Knowledge of Assyro-Babylonian Medicine,' *Am. J. Semit. Lang. Lit.*, 1919-20, 36:67-83; M. Jastrow, 'The Medicine of the Babylonians and Assyrians,' *Proc. Roy. Soc. Med.*, Sect. Hist. Med., 1914, 7:109-76; 'Babylonian-Assyrian Medicine,' *Annals Med. Hist.*, 1917, 1:231-57; M. S. Langdon, *The Babylonian Expedition of the University of Penn-*

sylvania, 1914, vol. xxxi: The Constantinople Medical Text, No. 179, pp. 51-75.

26. E. Ebeling, 'Keilschrifttafeln medizinischen Inhalts,' *Arch. Gesch. Med.*, 1921, 13:1-42, 129-44; 1922, 14:26-47, 65-78; *Keilschrifttexte medizinischen Inhalts*, Berlin, 1922, Heft i, ii.
27. E. Ebeling, *Keilschrifttexte aus Assur religiösen Inhalts*, Leipzig, 1915ff.
28. R. Campbell Thompson, *Assyrian Medical Texts from the Originals in the British Museum*, London, 1923.
29. R. Campbell Thompson, *The Assyrian Herbal*, London, 1924.
30. R. Campbell Thompson, *On the Chemistry of Ancient Assyrians*, London, 1925. Later publications on the subject were: 'An Assyrian Chemist's Vademecum,' *J. Roy. Asiat. Soc.*, 1934, pp. 771-85, and *A Dictionary of Assyrian Chemistry and Geology*, London, 1936.
31. R. Campbell Thompson, 'Assyrian Medical Texts,' *Proc. Roy. Soc. Med.*, 1924, 17:1-34; 1926, 19:29-78; 'Assyrian Prescriptions for Diseases of the Head,' *Am. J. Sem. Lang. Lit.*, 1907-8, 24:1-6, 323-53; 'Assyrian Prescriptions for Ears,' *J. Roy. Asiat. Soc.*, 1931, pp. 1-25; 'Assyrian Prescriptions for Diseases of the Chest and Lungs,' *Rev. Assyr.*, 1934, 31:1-29; 'Assyrian Prescriptions for Diseases of the Stomach,' *Rev. Assyr.*, 1929, 26:47-92; 'Assyrian Prescriptions for Diseases of the Urine . . . ,' *Babyloniaca*, 1934, 14:57-151; 'Assyrian Prescriptions for Diseases of the Feet,' *J. Roy. Asiat. Soc.*, 1937, pp. 265-86, 413-32; 'Assyrian Prescriptions for Treating Bruises or Swellings,' *Am. J. Semit. Lang. Lit.*, 1930, 47:1-25; 'Assyrian Prescriptions for Ulcers,' *J. Soc. Orient. Research*, 1931, 15:53; 'Assyrian Medical Prescriptions against Šimmatu "Poison,"' *Rev. Assyr.*, 1930, 27:127-35; 'A Babylonian Explanatory Text,' *J. Roy. Asiat. Soc.*, 1924, pp. 452-7; 'Assyrian Prescriptions for the "Hand of a Ghost,"' *J. Roy. Asiat. Soc.*, 1929, pp. 801-23; 'Assyrian Prescriptions for Stone in the Kidneys, for the "Middle" and for Pneumonia,' *Arch. Orientforsch.*, 1936-7, 11:336-40.
32. F. von Oefele, 'Babylonian Titles of Medical Textbooks,' *J. Am. Orient. Soc.*, 1917, 37:250-56.
33. Thompson, *J. Roy. Asiat. Soc. Gr. Brit. Ireland*, 1929, pp. 801-7.
34. See F. von Oefele, loc. cit. note 32.
35. Thompson, *Rev. Assyr.*, 1934, 31:19.
36. Thompson, *Proc. Roy. Soc. Med.*, Sect. Med. Hist., 1926, 19:35.
37. Küchler, p. 51ff.
38. F. W. Geers, 'A Babylonian Omen Text,' *Am. J. Semit. Lang. Lit.*, 1926-7, 43:22-41; see also R. Labat, note 40.
39. See Hermann Schneider's interesting discussion in *Kultur und Denken der Babylonier und Juden*, Leipzig, 1910, p. 548ff.
40. R. Labat, 'Un Traité médical akkadien, essai de reconstitution de la série enûma ana bît marsi âšipu illiku.' *Rev. Assyr.*, 1945-6, 40:27-45.
41. See O. Temkin's discussion of Babylonian literature in 'Beiträge zur archaischen Medizin,' *Kyklos*, 1930, 3:117ff.
42. Thompson, *Rev. Assyr.*, 1934, 31:7.
43. Thompson, *Proc. Roy. Soc. Med.*, Sect. Hist. Med., 1926, 19:67.
44. Ibid. 56.

45. Thompson, *Am. J. Semit. Lang. Lit.*, 1907, 24:352.
46. Thompson, *Babyloniaca,* 1934, 14:121.
47. See Temkin, *Kyklos,* 1930, 3:117ff.
48. This is the case particularly in the tablets on 'Diseases of the Chest and Lungs,' see Thompson, *Rev. Assyr.*, 1934, 31:1-29.
49. Thompson, *Proc. Roy. Soc. Med.*, Sect. Med. Hist., 1926, 19:50.

*

4. Patient and Physician

Herodotus tells us that the Babylonians made no use of physicians, that they brought their sick to the market place and that the passers-by looked at them, asked them about their complaints, and if they had had the same disease or knew of someone who had suffered from a similar ailment, advised them what remedies to use.[1]

Herodotus' statement about Egyptian physicians, about the many specialists, is fully confirmed by Egyptian literature and also by archaeological findings. In Babylonia, however, he must have been grossly misinformed. Perhaps he meant that the Babylonians had not the kind of physicians he had encountered in Egypt, that great variety of specialists. There can be no doubt that patients were occasionally placed in front of the houses or even on the market place and that the neighbors gave their opinion about them. This still happens with poor people all over the East. But we have an infinity of documents to prove that all ancient civilizations of Mesopotamia had physicians, and not only one category but several. Patients, therefore, were not left to the mercy of their families or of neighbors but received expert treatment according to standards prevailing at the time.

Health was considered a great good. 'May Shamash and Marduk give thee health' was a formula frequently used in Babylonian letters of Hammurabi's time.[2] And in Assyria the letter writer addressed the king with 'May Ninib and Gula give to the king my lord happiness and health.'[3] Hence, disease was a great curse and the position of the sick man in society was aggravated particularly by the view that illness was a punishment for sin. This at least was the case as soon as the Semitic influence became strong.

Here we encounter a view which, transmitted through Judaism to the West, was to play an extremely important part to our very days. The sick man was a sinner. He had stolen, killed, committed perjury or adultery, had spit into a river, drunk from an impure vessel, done whatever the society of which he was a member considered sinful, and as a result his god or guardian spirit had abandoned him, whereupon he fell an easy prey to the demons.[4] He was sick and suffered, and deserved it. His suffering made his sin apparent to all. He was branded with the odium of sinfulness and this obviously gave the sick man an isolated position in society. Not only was the course of his daily life different from that of his fellow men but he was in disgrace. In order to be reintegrated into society and to be at peace with the transcendental world he had to submit to all kinds of magic and religious rites, which constituted the treatment of his illness and which we shall have to discuss in detail.

This concept that disease was a punishment for sin was dominant in the Old Testament. God had revealed his law. He who obeyed it piously lived in happiness but he who transgressed it was punished, and illness and suffering at large were the chief punishments. This was a thought of pitiless logic and simplicity. Christianity endeavored to overcome it by glorifying suffering but never quite succeeded. Throughout the Middle Ages and even later, epidemics were frequently considered visitations inflicted by God upon mankind. On a higher level the old retributive view of disease is frequently encountered today in the outraged feelings of patients who consider their sufferings as undeserved.

Today, in civilized countries the individual is held responsible for his own actions only, not for those of his relatives or clan.[5] In Mesopotamia, where the family was very closely knit, the view was generally accepted that an individual might suffer not only for his own sins but for those of his parents or clan. This view is very familiar to us from the Old Testament. Even in our days infants suffering from congenital syphilis are sometimes considered the innocent victims of their parents' sin, and there was a time when the term *lues insontium,* 'syphilis of the innocents,' was applied to them.

Albright has very correctly pointed out that the Babylonians had a deeper feeling for problems of divine justice and of suffering than the Egyptians,[6] and therefore the righteous man suffering innocently presented a problem that disturbed them a great deal. It was treated in poems several times, counterparts to the Book of Job. The hero was aware of having led a virtuous life. He had done everything that might be expected not only of an honest but also of a pious man: [7]

I only heeded prayer and supplication,
my very thought was supplication, sacrifice habitual to me.
The days when gods were worshiped were my heart's delight,
those when I followed (the procession) of the goddess were
  my gain and profit.
Adoration of the king was joy to me,
music for him a source of pleasure.
And I instructed my estate to observe the ritual of the gods,
I taught my people to revere the name of the goddess.

Yet in spite of all his good deeds, sickness and other evils had befallen him:

Alu-disease covers my body like a garment;
sleep in a net enmeshes me;
my eyes stare but see not,
weakness has seized my body.

The diviners consulted could not interpret the omens and the incantation priests had no cure. His god did not succor him, did not stretch out a helping hand, and his goddess had no pity for him, did not walk at his side. His enemy rejoiced.

Why this undeserved misery? This was a problem indeed which could be explained only by assuming that the ways of the gods were mysterious and beyond human comprehension:

What to one's heart seems bad, is good before one's god.
Who may comprehend the mind of gods in heaven's depth?
The thoughts of a god are like deep waters, who could fathom them?
How could mankind, beclouded, comprehend the ways of gods?

This was not a satisfactory explanation to a people that expected and felt entitled to strict justice.[8] Hence, it is no wonder that such voices of rebellion were heard more than once, perhaps for the last time and most impressively in a statement of aging Ashurbanipal, who had a premonition of the disintegration of his great empire:

> The rules for making offerings to the dead and libations to the ghosts of the kings my ancestors, which had not been practised, I reintroduced. I did well unto god and man, to dead and living. Why have sickness, ill-health, misery and misfortune befallen me? I cannot away with the strife in my country and the dissensions in my family. Disturbing scandals oppress me alway. Misery of mind and flesh bow me down; with cries of woe I bring my days to an end.[9]

The fact that righteous people suffered without being aware of any sin committed led to resignation, to the assumption that god's ways were not comprehensible; but it may at a certain time also have shaken the belief in the purely spiritual origin of disease and may have driven man to search for other causes of illness.

In Babylonia we also find the first codified expression of the idea that an individual is entitled to compensation for the loss of health caused to him by another individual. This view was generally accepted in all ancient civilizations and the most primitive reparation for an injury was provided by the *ius talionis*, 'eye for eye, tooth for tooth, hand for hand, foot for foot.'[10] Retaliation satisfied the desire for vengeance. It did not replace the lost organ nor did it compensate materially for it, but in the Code of Hammurabi as well as in the Mosaic Code it was the customary sanction among social equals. If, however, the victim was socially inferior, compensation in money took place. Thus the Code of Hammurabi prescribed:[11]

> Art. 196. If a man has destroyed the eye of a patrician, his own eye shall be destroyed.
>
> Art. 197. If he has broken the bone of a patrician, his bone shall be broken.
>
> Art. 198. If he has destroyed the eye of a plebeian, or broken a bone of a plebeian, he shall pay one mina of silver.

Art. 199. If he has destroyed the eye of a man's slave, or broken a bone of a man's slave, he shall pay half his value.

Art 200. If a man has knocked out the teeth of a man of the same rank, his own teeth shall be knocked out.

Art. 201. If he has knocked out the teeth of a plebeian, he shall pay one-third of a mina of silver.

In the Mosaic Code the man who injured his slave compensated by letting him free, an interesting regulation: [12]

And if a man smite the eye of his servant, or the eye of his maid, that it perish; he shall let him go free for his eye's sake.

And if he smite out his servant's tooth, or his maidservant's tooth; he shall let him go free for his tooth's sake.

The Assyrian laws had stringent regulations concerning injury to the genital organs and injury that caused miscarriage to a pregnant woman. Paragraph 8 of the Middle Assyrian Laws read: [13]

If a woman has crushed a man's testicle in an affray, one of her fingers shall be cut off; and if although a physician has bound it up, the second testicle is affected with it and becómes inflamed or if she has crushed the second testicle in the affray, both her [nipples?] [14] shall be torn off.

A public penalty is imposed on a man who 'has struck a lady by birth and has caused her to cast the fruit of her womb.' The punishment was a fine consisting of the payment of a considerable amount of lead, fifty blows with rods, and one month of forced labor for the king.[15] Injuries causing miscarriage in women of lower birth were a different matter.[16] The penalty was private not public and consisted in talion or monetary compensation. Miscarriage through injury, like voluntary abortion, deprived the husband of offspring, and he was entitled to protection against such a loss. The punishment for abortion was very harsh: 'If a woman has cast the fruit of her womb by her own act and charge and proof have been brought against her, she shall be impaled and shall not be buried.' [17]

These laws were much stricter than those of the Babylonian Code, which merely foresaw monetary fines for the perpetrator of an injury causing miscarriage; the amount of the fine was determined by the social status of the victim. Only in the case of death of a patrician woman resulting from such an injury was retaliation applied and the daughter of the offender killed.[18] Mild also were the regulations for the compensation of an injury inflicted unintentionally. Among persons of equal rank the offender only paid for the doctor. And even in case of death of the victim the penalty was a mere fine.[19]

By far the most humane of the ancient Oriental Codes was that of the Hittites, of which we have a version of probably the thirteenth century B.C.[20] The brutal beatings, mutilations, and executions so frequently mentioned in the Assyrian Laws are not found in this document. Penalties were as a rule monetary compensations, and the amount to be paid varied according to social rank. Breaking of a freeman's hand or foot cost 20 shekels of silver but only half that amount if the victim was a slave.[21] A very reasonable regulation prescribed that if a man had injured another individual and rendered him unable to work, he must bring another man into the house to work for him, pay the doctor's bill, and a compensation of 6 shekels of silver when the patient recovered.[22] The tariff of fines had been reduced considerably. For a head wound one had to pay formerly 6 shekels of silver, 3 to the victim and 3 to the palace but 'now,' the Code says, 'the king has abolished the amount for the palace.'[23] The penalties for causing miscarriage in a woman were much milder than in the Assyrian Laws, and a very sensible differentiation was made according to the age of the embryo. If it happened to a free woman in the 10th month the compensation was 10 shekels of silver, but only 5 if it was in the 6th month, and it was 5 if the victim was a slave woman in the 10th month.[24] Even manslaughter and murder were not punished by death but compensation was given 'in kind.' A man who killed a slave unintentionally must replace him by giving another slave in his stead, but in the case of murder he had to give two slaves. For murder of a free man the compensation was four slaves, and two for manslaughter.[25] The same Code already mentions compensation in money for manslaughter as being customary in certain regions.[26] Strangely enough there was a death penalty for sexual intercourse with cattle, a practice that must have been fairly frequent with a pastoral people. The law may have come from Semitic influence, since we find it also in Leviticus.[27] But here again Hittite law was more humane, for the king could pardon the culprit.[28] There is a new spirit in the Code of the Hittites. Their civilization was dominated by Babylonia to be sure, but they were different people who had come from the North and they were members of the great Indo-European family.

Compensation laws are in no way peculiar to the ancient Orient. We find them in the Twelve Tables of Rome, in the *Lex Salica,* in the Anglo-Saxon Codes, and there is a steady development from there to our modern workmen's compensation laws.

The sick man always has a special position in society because illness suddenly disturbs his daily routine, throws him brutally out of gear, and makes him helpless, a burden to his fellow men. But illness also gives privileges. It excuses the sick from many duties ordinarily expected from individuals in good health, even from the duty of reporting to his king. We find this expressed very graphically in the state letters of Assyria. Esarhaddon, who kept close track of his officials, inquired about one Iratti and was informed about him in a letter written by another official.

> Concerning Iratti, of whom the king my lord wrote, I have worked with him, I have travelled about with him. Since he has not presented himself, the king should be informed that he is ill. Hereafter may the king my lord not blame us on his account. He has received two or three wounds [?] and knows no peace of mind.[29]

Another letter, written by a disease-stricken official to the same ruler, explained:

> Concerning what the king wrote, 'Why did you not come to Ashshur?' I am ill: I do not even go to the market place (?). Were I to go, I should die by the way . . . may I not be deprived of the protection of the king my lord. May he appoint at my side an exorcist and a physician . . . may they perform the ceremonies on my behalf. . .[30]

Another official asked for a physician to be sent: 'Now the handmaid of the king, Bau-gamelat, is seriously ill, she does not eat a morsel. Now may the king my lord give instructions; may a physician come to see her.'[31]

This brings us to a discussion of the physician and other healing personnel in Babylonia and Assyria. In Egypt we encountered specialists for the diseases of every part of the body. Physician, magician, and priest of Sekhmet were the chief groups of healers mentioned in Papyrus Ebers. Here in Mesopotamia we have three major types of priests dealing with sick people. One was the *bârû,* the seer, a priest specialized in divination. He knew omens and how to interpret them. He made diagnosis and prognosis and it was assumed that the patient's fate depended largely on his findings. Sick people were obviously not his only concern, since heavenly signs were consulted on every opportunity, but they held an important place in his day's work. The next and probably most important member of the medical corps was the *âshipu,* the exorcist or incantation priest. His task was to perform the rites required for driving out an evil spirit from the body of a patient and for reconciling him with his god. Like the diviner he was not concerned with sick people exclusively. Expiation rites had to be performed on many occasions and disease was not the only consequence of sin. But there is no doubt that exorcising evil spirits was one of his major functions. The third group of healing priests, finally, was represented by the *âsû,* the physician in the stricter sense of the word, the priest who devoted all his activities to the sick and who also, in addition to charms, knew drugs and was able to perform operations. *Azu* in Sumerian means one who knows water and *iazu,* another designation for the physician, one who knows oil.[32] We shall see later that water and oil played a very important part in divination practices and there can be no doubt that the *azu,* or *âsû* as he was called in the Semitic languages, was a diviner originally.

As priests, the physicians belonged to the most educated class of society; they were well versed in the art of reading and writing, familiar with the old traditions, and trained in their special field. Their education took place in schools connected with the major temples of the country. Physicians who were attached to the palace at the time of the Assyrian empire had to take an oath of office, and we have an interesting letter to the subject written by a priest: "To the king my lord, your servant Ishtar-shum-eresh: May Nabu and Marduk bless the king my lord. The scribes, the seers, the magicians, the physicians, the bird gazers, the courtiers, residing in the city, took the oath [of office] on the 16th of Nisan. Accordingly, tomorrow they may swear allegiance [to the king].'[33] And the same priest reported to his king: 'The 20th, the 22nd, the 25th, are auspicious [days] for the taking of the oaths. When the king my lord gives the order, they can take [the oaths].'[34]

Was medicine like other sacred knowledge kept as a secret not to be divulged to the profane? This is highly probable, certainly for the earlier periods. Many religious texts end with some formula such as: 'May he who knows instruct him who knows. And may he who knows not, not read this.' And 'he who does not keep the secret will not remain in health.—His days will be shortened.'[35]

Physicians worshiped particularly Ninib and Gula, who were considered great healing deities. Ninib, Enlil's son, was invoked by physician and patient alike. Gula, his consort, was the great female physician who resuscitated the dead by touching them with her pure hands.[36] She was the goddess of potions and poisons and the dog was her emblem. Ashurnasirpal erected a shrine for her. Ninazu, 'Lord of Physicians,' was another important healing deity and the emblem of his son Ningishzida was a double-headed snake. We shall see later that in Mesopotamia as in Egypt most gods had healing functions, particularly the great cosmic deities of Sumer and among them Ea, Lord of Water, first of all. Physicians worshiped him as their ancestor.

Physicians like other priests were attached to the court of the king and probably also to the courts of high officials such as governors of provinces. Their number cannot have been very large because in the state letters of Assyria we find constant requests for physicians to be sent from the court to somebody who had fallen ill. Physicians had ranks here as in Egypt. A physician-in-chief, a *rabî asê*, is mentioned in a fragment from Nineveh.[37] Other physicians were available to the population, that is, to those who could pay for them. The Code of Hammurabi included a fee schedule for physicians—or rather for surgeons, although the word used is *azu*, and it seems that there was no special term to designate the surgeon. It is interesting, however, that the Code was concerned with the activities of physicians only in so far as they were manual. This is the earliest physicians' tariff of which we know. The fee was determined by success and type of the operation and by the social status of the patient. For the successful treatment of a serious wound or for a successful operation on the eye, the fee was 10 shekels of silver if the patient was a patrician, 5 if he was a plebeian, and for a slave the owner paid in such a case 2 shekels. For the successful treatment of a broken bone or for the successful (surgical) treatment of an internal organ, the fee was 5, 3, or 2 shekels respectively. If, however, an operation ended fatally or if an eye operation resulted in loss of the eye, the physician's hands were cut off. If the slave of a plebeian died in the course of an operation, the physician was to give slave for slave, and he had to pay half the slave's price if his eye was lost.[38] These were Draconic regulations and it is hard to understand how any physician had the courage to perform an operation when he constantly ran the risk of losing his hands at the first unsuccessful performance. We know from other civilizations that laws frequently remained on paper and were never applied because they were not applicable. They were formulated as a matter of policy and as a warning against abuse but would have defeated their own purpose had they been applied literally. This was in all probability the case here also. But these paragraphs are extremely interesting, nevertheless, because they represent a first attempt of society to protect itself by way of legislation against misuse of the physician's power, a power granted to him by society and without which the physician cannot fulfil his function. The physician's liability for his actions was in every respect very similar to that of the architect[39] or of the shipbuilder.[40]

Physicians did not work on the 7th, 14th, 19th, 21st, and 28th days of the month, days considered unlucky,[41] and here as in other ancient civilizations it would have been unethical for them to attend to a hopeless case. 'If a man suffers of a ahhazu, his head, his face, his whole body and even the root of his tongue are affected; to such a sick the physician shall not put his hand, such a man will die, not recover.'[42]

Babylonia like Egypt had veterinarians and the Code of Hammurabi prescribed their fee and liability. For a successful operation performed on an ox, a cow, or a donkey the veterinary surgeon was entitled to one-sixth of a shekel of silver, but if the animal died he had to pay the owner one-quarter of its value.[43]

The Code also mentions the *gallabu,* the barber who may be considered as an auxiliary to the physician in that he also performed minor surgery. One of his functions was the branding of slaves, and since such marks were indelible, owners of slaves and the barber himself had to be protected against abuses.[44] According to Contenau, the barber also performed dental operations.[45] This is quite possible. At any rate we know that teeth were extracted in Assyria. A late but very interesting letter addressed to Esarhaddon said: [46]

> Replying to what the king my lord wrote me, 'send me your true diagnosis.' I have given my diagnosis to the king my lord in one word: 'Inflammation!' He whose head, hands and feet are inflamed, owes his state to his teeth: his teeth should be extracted. On this account his insides are inflamed. The pain will presently subside, the condition will be most satisfactory.

I think it would be futile to consider this document an anticipation of the modern theory of focal infection and the part played in it by oral sepsis. It is rather the result of a simple speculation. The elementary observation that when a tooth ached, the head, that is the cheek, was frequently swollen and sometimes very conspicuously so, must have led to the conclusion that other swellings were due to the same cause. Extraction of the sick tooth removed the pain and the swelling of the cheek. It did not affect the swelling of hands and feet but few treatments were effective anyway.[47]

The barber may have pulled teeth but the physician attended to them also, as we know from a letter of Arad-Nana who wrote to his king: 'concerning the condition of the tooth of which the king wrote me, I have helped it to heal, its condition is notably better.' [48]

The wet nurses may be considered another group of auxiliary medical personnel. We mentioned them and the laws concerning them in another connection so we need not repeat the material here.

We know the names of relatively many Babylonian and Assyrian physicians. They had seals like other persons of importance, and a number of these very attractive seals are preserved. They wrote letters to the King their Lord, some of which we still have. We also know that like their Egyptian colleagues the doctors of Mesopotamia were in demand at foreign courts.

Thus the seal of the physician Ur-Lugal-edin-na, who lived at the time of Gudea's son, is preserved at the Louvre,[49] which also possesses the seal of the Assyrian physician Makkur-Marduk, who succeeded his father Sin-Asharid in the profession.[50] At foreign courts Babylonian physicians competed with those of Egypt. Around 1300 B.C. the Egyptian physician Pareamakhu was in demand at several Anatolian courts and at about the same time the Babylonian doctor Raba-sha-Marduk was at the Hittite court.[51] Around 1280 B.C. the king of Babylon sent a physician and an exorcist to the Hittite monarch Hattusil.[52]

By far the most picturesque account of medical life in Mesopotamia is to be found in the state letters of Assyria. They are late documents, to be sure, most of them written in the seventh century B.C. but there are good reasons to assume that conditions were not so very different from what they had been before. Particularly attractive are the letters of two physicians of Esarhaddon,[53] Arad-Nana and Adad-shum-usur. They contain consilia, the physician's opinion on a malady of the king or of a member of his court with advice for treatment, or reports on the condition of a patient to whom the physician had been dispatched. Some are long, some are short, and almost all of them reveal that characteristic blend of religious, magical, and empirical elements. We cannot conclude this chapter better than by quoting passages from some of these letters. They begin with a standard formula such as: 'To the king my lord, your servant Arad-Nana: Very hearty greetings to the king my lord. May Ninurta and Gula give to the king my lord happiness and health.' Then follows the advice. The king suffered from a disease which apparently affected his hands and perhaps other joints, some kind of arthritis or gout. He had written to his physician about it, who advised: [54] 'The king should be anointed while he rests, on account of the wind. He should have incantations performed over pure water, in the basin in which he regularly washes his hands;

he should not pour (this water) away. Quickly the gout (?) will leave . . .'

The king once complained that his forbears had had better attention when they had been sick, an accusation which Arad-Nana refused to accept: [55] 'If the king says, "He is here," he should write me, I shall come.' This and similar passages show that Arad-Nana apparently did not live in the royal palace but perhaps in a temple. If he had belonged to the immediate entourage of the king he would have been near him all the time, in the capital as well as on journeys, and there would have been no need for writing letters. The same epistle refers to drugs sent by the physician to his lord:

> The herbs which I have sent to the king are for (use on) two (different) occasions. They are called 'BU' herb and 'PA.TI' herb. They are dissimilar. One is like a sprout, the other is for the thread on the cavity (?) (of the liver). The liver will be considerably benefited. At once, the king my lord will say, 'For what else are they good?' They are good for an incantation of deliverance, they are helpful to a woman with birth pangs.

It would be impossible to find a better illustration for the magic character of certain herbs.

Esarhaddon was impatient.[56] He repeatedly said to his physician: 'Why do you not recognize the nature of this illness of mine, Why do you not bring about its cure?' Whereupon Arad-Nana 'sealed and sent a letter':

> Let them read it to the king, let them explain it to the king my lord. If it is agreeable in the sight of the king my lord, let a magician perform an exorcism (?) (and) a ceremony against (it). Let the king take this bath: immediately his fever will leave the king my lord. That anointing with oils should be done two or three times for the king my lord, as the king knows (?). If the king so wills, let him do it tomorrow. That disease is in the pus. They should bring licorice to the king. Exactly as they have done twice already, they should massage (him) vigorously. I intend to come and give instructions. At once the perspiration of the king will come. I am sending to the king my lord a concoction (?) of those things; let him apply it to the flesh of his neck. May the king anoint himself on the appointed day with the liniment which I am sending.

Esarhaddon, however, consulted not only his *âsû*, his physician, but also his *âshipu*, his exorcist. He complained to Marduk-shakin-shum:[57] 'My arms (and) legs are limp, and I cannot open my eyes. I am smeared (with liniments) and abed with fever, it burns my very bones,' whereupon the priest answered: 'at (the root) of this there is no sin. Ashur, Shamash, Bel, (and) Nabu will bring about the recovery. His illness will leave, (his condition) is truly most satisfactory. Let them serve (?) whatever is good, let him eat (it).'

The king had the health of the crown prince much at heart and physicians had to send him reports about him. Thus Arad-Nana wrote:[58] 'All is well with the crown prince. The rites which we prepared for (him), we have performed at intervals of an hour and forty minutes all through the day: he walks, he is well, he gains strength, but he stays (indoors).' And another physician Adad-shum-usur reported:[59] 'Concerning the medicine about which the king my lord wrote (me), it is perfectly safe. As the king my lord has commanded, in all haste we shall give it to those slaves to drink. Afterwards the crown prince may drink (it). But I, what am I saying! I am an old man without his senses! The king's commands shall be fulfilled even as are those of a god.'

The interesting statement that drugs were tested on slaves before they were given to members of the royal family reminds us of the fact that 2400 years later, in A.D. 1722 the inoculation of smallpox was tested on seven criminals and six orphans before it was practiced on the children of the Princess of Wales.

Magic played an important part in the treatments discussed in these letters, but sometimes they consisted of simple and effective manual procedures, as were employed in the case of a patient who had a nosebleed, about whom Arad-Nana wrote:[60]

> The rab mugi reported to me as follows: 'Yesterday, toward evening, there was profuse bleeding.' Those bandages are applied inexpertly; they are placed upon the cartilages of the nose, bandaging the cartilage. On account of the bleeding, (the dressing) should be placed inside the nostrils; the breathing will be hindered, but the flow of blood will cease. If agreeable to the king, I shall come there tomorrow (and) teach (them how to do it). For the present may I hear good news.

And over and over again physicians and other officials reaffirmed their loyalty to the king their lord and their readiness to comply with his orders unhesitatingly, as Arad-Nana did when he said:[61]

As to what the king wrote me, 'Your business is to hasten when the face of Ashur-mukin-palea becomes pale,'—I am at his side, I have kept my eyes on his face. I have come to reassure the king my lord. Now let the king my lord reckon a full month, (after that time), I stake my life on his being able to do any kind of work.

The great charm in these letters is that they were not written for publication and hence give a spontaneous picture of medical life as it unfolded at the Assyrian court.

NOTES

1. Herodotus, I, 197.
2. See *Cambridge Anc. Hist.*, vol. I, p. 547.
3. R. H. Pheiffer, *State Letters of Assyria*, New Haven, 1935, no. 287, p. 200.
4. Contenau, *Civilisation*, p. 109. L.-R. Le Port, *Les Causes Morales du mal physique dans la médecine assyro-babylonienne*, Thèse, Montpellier, 1925.
5. We have had enough examples to the contrary in recent years, but *Sippenhaft* and execution of entire families in Hitler Germany were reversals into primitive savagery or possibly a revival of old Semitic concepts.
6. W. F. Albright, *From the Stone Age to Christianity*, Baltimore, 1946, p. 149.
7. The following quotations are from Frankfort *et al.*, *The Intellectual Adventure of Ancient Man*, Chicago, 1946, pp. 213ff. About the poem see also Ch.-F. Jean, *La Littérature des Babyloniens et des Assyriens*, Paris, 1924, pp. 195-8; A. Ungnad, *Die Religionen der Babylonier und Assyrer*, Jena, 1921, pp. 227-30.
8. One version of the poem has a happy end in that the sufferer is restored to his previous condition.
9. *Cambridge Anc. Hist.*, vol. III, p. 127.
10. Exodus, 21, 24.
11. *The Hammurabi Code and the Sinaitic Legislation*, by Chilperic Edwards, London, 1921, p. 38.
12. Exodus, 21, 26-7.
13. *The Assyrian Laws*, by G. R. Driver and John C. Miles, Oxford, 1935.
14. The word is missing in the text but must have meant an organ that occurs in pairs such as hands (Tallqvist) or breasts (Scheil) or nipples (Driver and Miles).
15. *The Assyrian Laws* § 21.

16. Ibid. §§ 50-52. See the discussion of these somewhat confused paragraphs by Driver and Miles, p. 108ff.
17. Ibid. § 53.
18. *Code of Hammurabi,* 209-14.
19. Ibid. 206-8.
20. Heinrich Zimmern, *Hethitische Gesetze aus dem Staatsarchiv von Boghazköi,* Leipzig, 1922.
21. Ibid. 11-12.
22. Ibid. 10.
23. Ibid. 9.
24. Ibid. 17-18. (The months were moon months.)
25. Ibid. 1-4.
26. Ibid. 5.
27. *Leviticus,* 20, 15.
28. *Hethitische Gesetze,* II, 73.
29. R. H. Pfeiffer, *State Letters of Assyria,* no. 282, p. 196.
30. Ibid. no. 283, p. 197.
31. Ibid. no. 281, p. 196.
32. See Meissner, *Babylonien and Assyrien,* Heidelberg, vol. 2, 1925, p. 284; R. Dumon, 'La Profession de médecin d'après les textes assyro-babyloniens,' *J. Asiat.,* 1897, 9:318-26.
33. Pfeiffer, *State Letters* . . . no. 211, p. 154.
34. Ibid. no. 341, p. 232.
35. See Meissner, loc. cit. vol. II, p. 139f.
36. Ibid. vol. II, p. 31.
37. R. Labat, *Rev. Assyr.,* 1945-6, 40:34.
38. *Code,* 215-23.
39. Ibid. 228ff.
40. Ibid. 234ff.
41. Meissner, loc. cit. vol. II, p. 286.
42. Küchler, p. 63.
43. *Code,* 224-5.
44. Ibid. 226-7.
45. Contenau, *Médecine,* p. 33.
46. Pfeiffer, *State Letters* . . . no. 284, p. 198.
47. One must be very careful in the interpretation of such documents, since they may be translated very differently. Thus G. G. Cameron translated the crucial passages of this letter in the following way: 'The truth to the king my lord I shall speak: the burning of his head, his hands, his feet (wherewith) he burns (is) on account of his teeth. His teeth (are) coming out; on account of (that) he burned. In his chamber he lay down. (But) now (he is) very well . . .' See G. B. Denton, 'A New Interpretation of a Well-known Assyrian Letter,' *J. Near East. Stud.,* 1943, 2:314-15. See the discussion by B. W. Weinberger in *An Introduction to the History of Dentistry,* St. Louis, 1948, vol. I, pp. 32-6.
48. Pfeiffer, no. 291, p. 203.
49. S. Langdon, *Rev. Assyr.,* 1920, 17:51.

50. Contenau, *Médecine,* p. 42.
51. W. F. Albright, loc. cit. p. 159.
52. A. Leix, *Ciba Symposia,* 1940, 2:672.
53. The chief editions and translations of the epistolary literature of Mesopotamia are: R. F. Harper, *Assyrian and Babylonian Letters Belonging to the K. Collection in the British Museum,* Parts 1-4, Chicago, 1892-1914; and L. Waterman, *Royal Correspondence of the Assyrian Empire,* Ann Arbor, vols. 1-3, 1930-31, vol. 4, 1936. A very attractive selection is that of R. H. Pfeiffer, *State Letters of Assyria,* New Haven, 1935, from which all our quotations have been taken by permission of Professor Pfeiffer.
54. Pfeiffer, no. 287, p. 200.
55. Ibid. no. 288, p. 201.
56. Ibid. no. 286, p. 199.
57. Ibid. no. 285, p. 198.
58. Ibid. no. 290, p. 202.
59. Ibid. no. 294, p. 204.
60. Ibid. no. 290, p. 202.
61. Ibid. no. 291, p. 203.

*

5. Content of Mesopotamian Medicine

We must now consult the texts and try to visualize how the Mesopotamians conceived disease to be, how it appeared to them, and what they did to ward it off and to restore health. We shall find many views that we have encountered in Egyptian medicine and many that are very familiar to us from primitive medicine. This will allow us to be very brief in discussing principal matters and to place all emphasis on the particularly Babylonian or Assyrian aspects of the problems. We can do it the better since the literature that has come down to us is extraordinarily rich and colorful. Many concepts, views, methods met with among primitive tribes today, ascertained in field work through observation and interviews, occurred in ancient Mesopotamia also but on a much higher plane, and they were expressed in an extremely forceful literature of great poetic beauty.

CAUSE OF DISEASE

We mentioned before that spirit intrusion was considered the chief cause and the very essence of disease, and we must now study who these spirits were, by what mechanisms they took hold of man, and what means of protection he possessed against them.

Like the Egyptian, and even more so, the Babylonian lived in a world that was haunted by evil spirits. They were everywhere, in the dark corners of the house, in the attic, in ruins, and on waste lands; they roamed the streets of the city at night, hid behind rocks and trees on the open land ready to attack you when you passed by; they rode howling with the stormwind. There was not a place on earth where you could feel safe. Yet, it would be a great mistake to assume that the life of the Babylonian was one of perpetual terror, far from it. If you led a righteous life, worshiping the gods, keeping the ghosts of your ancestors in the Underworld by feeding them with regular offerings, if you respected taboos and possessed the necessary amulets and charms, there was no reason why you should be afraid of spirits. They were kept in check and had no power over you, although it happened here and there that they attacked a man without apparent reason.

By way of comparison, we may say that today we know that we live in a world which is haunted by bacteria. They are in our homes, in the food we eat, in the air we breathe, in the dust of our cities; and if we climb a high mountain where the air is pure and the soil is covered with virginal snow, we still cannot escape bacteria because we carry them with us, having millions of them in our intestinal tract. And yet we are not afraid of them. If we live hygienically, keep fit, and possess not amulets and charms but the necessary immunizations, they have no power over us even though they get the better of us sometimes without apparent reason.

In Mesopotamia evil spirits took hold of a man for three major reasons. One was lack of caution, or simply fate. This seems to have been the dominating view in Sumer, where disease was not yet considered a punishment for sin.[1] One of the chief types of the

Sumerian incantation was the so-called prophylactic type, the purpose of which was to keep the demons away from man: [2]

Man may enter the house—thou shalt not enter it.
Man may approach the house—thou shalt not approach it!
If something enters, thou shalt not enter.
With an entering man thou shalt not enter!
With an outgoing man thou shalt not enter.

Or the demon is threatened that he will find neither food nor drink: [3]

Until thou art removed, until thou departest
From the man, the son of his god,
Thou shalt have no food to eat,
Thou shalt have no water to drink,
Thou shalt not stretch forth thy hand
Unto the table of thy father Enlil, thy creator.
Neither sea water, nor sweet water,
Nor bad water, nor Tigris water,
Nor Euphrates water, nor pond water,
Nor river water shalt thou drink.
If thou wouldst fly up to heaven
Thou shalt have no wings,
If thou wouldst lurk in ambush on earth
Thou shalt secure no resting place.
Unto the man, the son of his god,
Come not nigh,
Get thee hence!

These were protective incantations used to keep off the spirits as were also a variety of amulets, notably those representing the demons, of which type a number are preserved in our museums.[4]

Man's destiny was in the hands of the gods. A Babylonian frightened by evil omens addressed Ea, Shamash, and Marduk in a prayer that said: [5]

To appoint fates and to fashion destinies is in your hand;
Ye are they who decree the fates of life; Ye are they who fashion the destinies of life.

Ye are they who ordain the decree of life . . .
I upon whom evil prodigies and signs have come,
Am afraid, melancholy and cast into gloom.
On account of the evil omen of an eclipse of the moon, on account of the evil omen of an eclipse of the sun.

Since omens not only indicated impending evil but actually brought it, great caution and skill were required to counteract them, and the gods were implored to 'blot out unlucky prodigies and signs, shivering dreams, evil and not good,' and to 'perform expiations for prodigies and signs, how many soever there be.' [6]

Lack of caution opened the door to the demons, but sin did it still more, and this became the dominating cause of spirit intrusion. What actions were considered sinful? The views obviously changed in the course of time. Every society has a set of taboos which may not be violated without sanction. We saw that in certain primitive tribes illness inflicted by the deity directly or through demons was the only form of social sanction. In the civilizations that flourished in Mesopotamia, the state in its codes of laws defined what was right and wrong, and civil courts punished the transgressor. But many commandments and prohibitions had a purely moral character, were not included in the codes, and yet were very important for the normal functioning of society. If you incited the father against the son, the son against the father, the mother against the daughter, and the daughter against the mother, friend against friend; if you brought discord into a united family, said yes for no, had a straight mouth but a crooked heart [7]—these were all offenses that were not punished in civil courts but by the gods, who withdrew their protection from you, whereupon the evil spirit took hold of you. There obviously was some overlapping between the moral and the legal codes. Murder, theft, adultery, fraud were sins as well as offenses punished under the law, but the moral code was a most formidable social means of coercion since it constantly kept people in line by threatening them with the wrath of the gods and torture by evil spirits. Lists of sins have been preserved [8] and we shall come back to them in a moment when we discuss the concept of contagion.

'May the protecting genius and the guardian spirit be continually on the house' an Assyrian prayed,[9] but when he sinned, the guardian spirit abandoned him. Sometimes he was not aware of having sinned or was assailed for somebody else's sin and prayed:

Loosen my disgrace, the guilt of my wickedness; remove my disease; drive away my sickness; a sin I know (or) know not I have committed; on account of a sin of my father (or) my grandfather, a sin of my mother (or) my grandmother, on account of a sin of an elder brother (or) an elder sister, on account of a sin of my family, of my kinsfolk (or) of my clan . . . the wrath of god and goddess have pressed upon me.[10]

Lack of caution and sin were not the only ways of falling a victim to the evil spirits. A man could also become sick as a result of sorcery, of black magic, and we mentioned before how severely punished the sorcerer was. Black magic was always coexistent with white magic because it seemed obvious that if it was possible to remove a spell, it was also possible to cast one. We do not know very much about methods of black magic, because these are secret and illegitimate matters not recorded in books, but we may safely assume that sorcerer and witch used potions and philters, sent bad dreams, used methods of sympathetic magic, and recited incantations that gave them power over the spirits through which they harmed their victims. Their action was one more mechanism through which the individual was laid open to the assault of demons; but as the sorcerer interfered with the divine order, and this to an evil end, he was punishable by law, and the incantation priest fought him just as he did the demons. The series Maqlû, mentioned before, deals primarily with the combating of witchcraft.

As in Mediterranean countries, we find here also the belief in the evil eye as a source of witchcraft, although it may not have been quite as outspoken as in Egypt. We also hear of the evil mouth, the evil tongue, the evil finger that may bewitch an individual. A tablet of the British Museum in Sumerian and Assyrian has the following exorcism:

O witch, whosoever thou art, whose heart conceiveth my misfortune, whose tongue uttereth spells against me, whose lips poison me, and in whose footsteps death standeth, I ban thy mouth, I ban thy tongue, I ban thy glittering eyes, I ban thy swift feet, I ban thy toiling knees, I ban thy laden hands, I bind thy hands behind. And may the Moon-god (Sin) destroy thy body, and may he cast thee into the Lake of Water and Fire.[11]

It is obvious that black magic was used not only to destroy an enemy but also for less nefarious purposes, to win a girl's love, and in other similar matters.

We have to discuss one more cause of disease, a very important one, and one which through the medium of Judaism was to play a great part in Western medicine: namely, contagion. The idea was that the sick who was possessed by evil spirits was taboo for the duration of his illness. He was unclean, and this impurity was contagious. He who touched him, slept on his bed, sat on his chair, ate out of his plate, or drank from his cup became impure also and open to the invasion of spirits.[12] There were many ways of becoming impure. Disease was one, and probably the chief one, but there were other more trivial ones:

While he walked in the street,
While he made his way through the broad places,
While he walked along the streets and ways,
He trod in some libation that had been poured forth, or
He put his foot in some unclean water,
Or cast his eye on the water of unwashen hands,
Or came in contact with a woman of unclean hands,
Or glanced at a maid with unwashen hands,
Or his hand touched a bewitched woman,
Or he came in contact with a man of unclean hands,
Or saw one with unwashen hands,
Or his hand touched one of unclean body.[13]

The concept of contagion was purely spiritual, not in any way medical, but it had hygienic consequences. You did not touch the sick unnecessarily, for fear of being contaminated. And whoever had become impure had to undergo an atonement ritual, had to perform purification rites, which again were spiritual in concept but had hygienic implications. These ideas are familiar to us from Leviticus. The Greeks never had a clear concept of the contagiousness of disease, but the Jews did, and had developed methods of segregating sick people whose impurity was particularly severe, such as lepers. Their views on the subject were in all probability of Babylonian origin.[14] And when in the Middle Ages the church decided to fight leprosy, against which physicians were helpless, it applied the precepts of Leviticus,[15] and these became the basic methods of our modern measures applied in the combating of communicable diseases. The original concept of the contagiousness of disease conditions, however, can be traced back to Babylonia.

And now we must look more closely at the evil spirits. Basically they are not so very different from those of Egypt or other archaic civilizations, but they are more picturesque, have more personality, and many have names. The literature about them and their doings is very considerable. R. Campbell Thompson, who did the pioneering work in this field also,[16] distinguishes three classes of spirits.

The first consists of the ghosts of the dead, which, instead of being in the dreary Underworld, roam on earth in search of a body. They are the ghosts of people who remained unburied: 'He that lieth in a ditch . . . He that no grave covereth . . . He that lies uncovered, whose head is uncovered with dust, the king's son that lieth in the desert, or in the ruins, the hero whom they have slain with the sword.'[17] We mentioned before that what kept the ghosts in the Underworld was the offerings and libations presented to them by the family of the dead. But when he had no family or the sacrifices were neglected, the ghost returned to the upper world. An incantation said:

> Whether thou art a ghost unburied,
> Or a ghost that none careth for,
> Or a ghost with none to make offerings to it,
> Or a ghost that hath none to pour libations to it,
> Or a ghost that hath no posterity.[18]

And finally here as everywhere else it was believed that the ghosts of those dead who had not fulfilled their task on earth were restless: the ghosts of children, of brides and of women who died in childbirth; or the ghosts of people who died in abnormal circumstances, who 'died of hunger in prison' or 'died of thirst in prison'; or 'he whom the bank of a river hath made to perish, he that hath died in the desert or marshes, he that a storm has overwhelmed in the desert.' [19]

The second class consisted of spirits born from the union of a demon and a human. Such was Alû, a spirit horrible to look at, hiding in caverns and ruins but always ready to pounce on a victim, born from the intercourse of man and a spirit such as Lilîtu or Ardat lilî.

The third group was made up of devils, of spirits which were of the same nature as the gods but whose function it was to perform evil deeds. Most of them were of Sumerian origin but some were Semitic such as in a general way Ilu limnu, the evil god, more specifically Lilû the male, or Lilîtu the female night spirit, or Ardat lilî, the restless ghost of a woman. We are familiar with Lilith, the screech owl of the Old Testament [20] who according to later traditions bore children to Adam, devils and spirits.

The evil spirits frequently appeared in groups. Such a group of six was a combination of Utukku, the ghost of a dead, Alû the spirit just mentioned, Ekimmu another ghost, of Semitic origin, Gallu, a devil, sexless, who sometimes appeared roaming the streets in the form of a bull, Ilu just mentioned, and Rabisu, the lurking demon who set the hair on the victim's body on end. Or the demons appear in triads, such as the Semitic Lilû, Lilîtu, and Ardat lilî, or the Sumerian Labartu, Labasu, Ahhazu. Labartu was a very important spirit, daughter of Anu, who lived in the mountains or in the cane brakes of marshes and whose specialty was to attack children. She was the sister of the seven evil demons just as Narûdu was the sister of the seven benevolent spirits.[21] Labasu was a ghoul, Ahhazu, the seizer, but there is some uncertainty about their exact meaning. Pazuzu was a storm demon,[22] and other spirits were identified with specific diseases. Nergal, god of pestilence, sun at noontime when it kills,[23] had fourteen attendants who infested mankind with fever diseases. Ashakku also caused fever and consumptive diseases; [24] Tiʾu, headaches and similar ailments; [25] Namtaru, diseases of the throat; [26] Sualu, such of the chest. And in addition to these well-defined devils, there were legions of anonymous spirits, the Evil Seven and many others who pounced on the wanderer. A few texts will best illustrate the ways of the demons and the methods by which they attacked mankind. We are well informed about them because the incantation priest exorcising a patient frequently began the ceremony by describing the spirits. Being uncertain with which he was dealing, he addressed many of them, hoping to hit the right one. A very forceful incantation of great beauty began: [27]

Cold and rain that minish all things . . .
They are the evil Spirits in the creation of Anu spawned.
Plague Gods, the beloved sons of Bel,
The offspring of Ninkigal.
Rending in pieces on high,
Bringing destruction below,
They are the Children of the Underworld.
Loudly roaring on high,
Gibbering below,
They are the bitter venom of the gods.
The great storms directed from heaven—those are they,
The owl, that hoots over a city—that is they,
They are the children born of Earth,
That in the creation of Anu were spawned.
The highest walls, the thickest walls,
Like a flood they pass.
From house to house they break through,
No door can shut them out,
No bolt can turn them back,
Through the door like a snake they glide,
Through the hinge like the wind they blow;
Estranging the wife from the embrace of a husband,
Snatching the child from the loins of a man,
Sending the man forth from his home.
They are the burning pain
That bindeth itself upon the back of a man.
The god of the man is a shepherd
Who seeketh pasture for the man,
Whose god unto food leadeth him.
Whether thou be a hag-demon,

Or a ghoul,
Or a robber-sprite
Or a harlot (that hath died) whose body is sick,
Or a woman (that hath died) in travail,
Or a weeping woman (that hath died) with a babe at the breast,
Or an evil man (that hath died),
Or an evil spirit,
Or one that haunteth the neighbourhood . . .

The text continues in the same vein, and we see the priest feeling his way to reach the spirit responsible for the patient's illness, and after having listed sufficient possibilities, he exorcises the fever invoking an entire pantheon.

The Evil Seven are pictured in an incantation of the same series: [28]

Seven are they, seven are they,
In the Ocean Deep seven are they,
Battening in Heaven seven are they,
In the Ocean Deep as their home they were reared,
Nor male nor female are they,
They are the roaring windblast,
No wife have they, no son do they beget;
Knowing neither mercy nor pity,
They hearken not unto prayer or supplication.
They are horses reared among the hills;
The Evil Ones of Ea,
Throne-bearers to the gods are they.
They stand in the highway to befoul the path,
Evil are they, evil are they,
Twice seven are they!

In another text the Seven are described as being the South Wind, a dragon with mouth agape, a grim leopard that carried off children, a terrible serpent, a furious beast, a rampant . . . an evil windstorm. 'These seven are the Messengers of Anu, the king bearing gloom from city to city.' [29]

Another incantation from another series was used in the treatment of a patient assailed by seven demons but not the anonymous spirits of the previous texts:

Fever (Ashakku) unto the man, against his head hath drawn nigh,
Disease (Namtaru) unto the man, against his life, hath drawn nigh,
An evil Spirit (Utukku) against his neck hath drawn nigh,
An evil Demon (Alu) against his breast hath drawn nigh,
An evil Ghost (Ekimmu) against his belly hath drawn nigh,
An evil Devil (Gallu) against his hand hath drawn nigh,
An evil God (Ilu) against his foot hath drawn nigh,
These seven together have seized upon him,
His body like a consuming fire they devour.[30]

This was undoubtedly a case of a severe fever disease and the spirit intrusion was particularly serious. Other exorcisms were addressed to an individual demon. One of Thompson's series dealt with Tĭ'u, the evil spirit of headache, and the following description shows him roaming over the desert and attacking the victim: [31]

Headache roameth over the desert, blowing like the wind,
Flashing like lightning, it is loosed above and below;
It cutteth off him who feareth not his god like a reed,
Like a stalk of henna it slitteth his thews.
It wasteth the flesh of him who hath no protecting goddess,
Flashing like a heavenly star, it cometh like the dew;
It standeth hostile against the wayfarer, scorching him like the day,
This man it hath struck and
Like one with heart disease he staggereth,
Like one bereft of reason he is broken,
Like that which has been cast into the fire he is shrivelled,
Like a wild ass . . . his eyes are full of cloud,
On himself he feedeth, bound in death;
Headache whose course like the dread windstorm none knoweth,
None knoweth its full time or its bond.

This is a description of great force and beauty and the patient is pictured as one who has been attacked by a very serious illness, meningitis, encephalitis, or something similar. Examples could be multiplied indefinitely but there is no need of doing so since the texts are easily available to those who are interested in this particular literature. There is just one more incantation that we must quote in this connection because of its unusual interest. The demon in this text is the Worm who gnaws at the teeth of man, thus causing toothache, and the incantation includes the story of the creation. The text was discovered and first published by Thompson:[32]

After Anu made the heavens,
The heavens made the earth,
The earth made the rivers,
The rivers made the canals,
The canals made the marsh,
The marsh made the Worm.
The Worm came weeping unto Shamash,
(Came) unto Ea, her tears flowing:
'What wilt thou give me for my food?
What wilt thou give me to destroy?'
'I will give thee dried figs (and) apricots.'
'Forsooth, what are these dried figs to me, or apricots?
Set me amid the teeth, and let me dwell in the gums,
That I may destroy the blood of the teeth,
And of the gums chew their marrow.
So shall I hold the latch of the door.'

It was an incantation for people suffering from toothaches, and the Worm was exorcised with the words: 'Since thou hast said this, O Worm, may Ea smite thee with his mighty fist!' The whole text was repeated three times, whereupon a salve was applied to the sick tooth.

On the statuettes preserved, the Babylonian demons look fierce and remind us of the masks of present primitive tribes. The storm demon Pazuzu was partly human, partly wild beast, and partly bird with huge wings.[33] Labartu on a relief from Susa is pictured with an animal face, holding a snake in one hand and a weapon in the other. Together with her are her brothers, the Evil Seven.[34] Other demons are pictured with bulging eyes which spell the victim, others with two faces which do not fit together,[35] and still others with horns and animal feet. The Christian devil was a reminiscence of these Mesopotamian demons, and the medieval and Renaissance painters pictured him very much in the same spirit as the Assyrian artists.

These statuettes, made of terra cotta and sometimes of bronze, were used as amulets. You knew the demon, knew what he looked like, you had him in hand by possessing his effigy, and this protected you against him. The bronze Pazuzu of the Louvre Museum has a ring on top which shows that it must have been worn attached to the belt or to a necklace.

It was a strange world, this world of evil spirits lurking in every corner, always ready to assail you. But with some caution man could live in it merrily and with not more concern than we have when we cross an avenue of one of our large cities, where we are constantly threatened by much more destructive forces.

DIVINATION

A man had fallen ill. As a result of sin or for some other reason an evil spirit had taken hold of him. He suffered, was impure, had dropped out of society, and was in disharmony with the world at large. His obvious desire was to return to his previous condition, to be reintegrated into the society of his fellow men, and to be again at peace with the transcendental world. The task of the healer was to help him in this endeavor and to perform the necessary rites. And since treatment was strictly etiological, the first task was to diagnose the sin that had been committed—if any—the demon who was plaguing the patient, and, furthermore, to find out what intentions the gods had with the sick, whether his illness was harmless or fatal and whether he would be sick for a short or a long time.

Divination, the interpretation of omens, was the chief method employed to answer these questions or, in other words, to make diagnosis and prognosis. It was in addition considered the most important preventive measure. And since practically all phenomena and all happenings might be signs revealing the intentions of the gods, divination was a highly developed branch of learning which called for a specialized category of priests, for the *bârû*, the diviner.[36]

Absurd as most systems of divination appear to us today, they nevertheless go back to certain elementary observations. The mistake was that causal relations were assumed to exist where this was not the case, and that systems were built on the basis of such assumptions. I see birds flying to my left and at that very moment

I stumble and break a foot. Living in the twentieth century after Christ, I consider this a mere coincidence, and as I think in terms of science I should accept a causal relation between the two events only—and then only hypothetically—if the same accident happened under the same circumstances more than once and not only to me but also to others. Man of the pre-scientific age reasoned differently and believed in the causal relation between two events without further controls. If he broke his foot when he saw birds flying on his left, it seemed obvious to him that the birds, revealing the intentions of the gods, had announced and brought bad luck. The next step for him was to deduce that if birds to the left meant bad luck, birds to the right must mean good luck, and such a conclusion was the beginning of a system. Only careful statistical data would have revealed the fallacy of such a system, but this would have been a scientific approach inconceivable at that time.

Yet we must be careful in judging omens and I think that an example from our own days will make clear what I mean. At all times it was believed that the behavior of certain animals, today particularly of cats, had the significance of omens. A black cat crossing my path means bad luck; a cat washing her ears with her paw announces a letter; a cat sleeping in a distorted position on its ear announces rain. Many people believe in these signs, which at closer examination appear to belong to very different categories. There is no evidence whatever that the color of a cat has any influence on our life, nor is there any connection between her washing an ear and the mail. But when my cat sleeps on her ear, I invariably find that the barometer has dropped. Cats, in other words, react to sudden drops of atmospheric pressure, and their behavior in such a case is not an omen in the magical sense but a scientific phenomenon.

There is another point that we must keep in mind, namely that the most abstruse omens do exert an influence on people as soon as they believe in them. If somebody is convinced that a black cat crossing his path brings bad luck, he will feel uncertain and will be inclined to make mistakes. The general who in the past went to battle knowing that the stars were against him had good chances of losing it, because he was bound to feel that it was a vain undertaking to fight against destiny, when he thought that the odds were against him and all in favor of his adversary.

In discussing primitive medicine, we saw that omens may be divided into two major groups, of which one includes the infinite variety of spontaneous signs while the other consists of signs sought by the diviner. There is no limit to the number of spontaneous omens; practically everything could be indicative of divine intentions, the behavior of animals, plants, rivers, the physiognomy of people, their dreams, animal and human births that occurred at a given moment, and, of course, the stars and all heavenly phenomena. The diviner whose task it was to interpret these omens had to be a very keen observer of his environment, able to perceive the slightest phenomena and the most minute deviations from the norm. And he had to be learned in order to interpret what he saw.

Omens were sought through various methods, among which the most important was the examination of the liver of sacrificed animals. From Babylonia hepatoscopy spread all over the Eastern section of the Mediterranean. But this was an expensive method since a sheep had to be slaughtered each time. A cheaper oracle probably used in the case of poor people consisted in having a drop of oil poured on water and watching what happened. Or a flame was lit and from its flickering conclusions were drawn. Divination was an endless field and we cannot possibly discuss it in any detail or in all its aspects. All we can do in this brief chapter is illustrate with a few texts the chief methods of divination used in connection with the sick man.

Different as these methods all were, they had one point in common, namely that the oracles were simple. The gods did not reveal themselves in intricate sentences. Their omens stated in simple terms that a sick man would live or die, that there would be rain or a drought, that a battle would be won or lost. The diviners invoked Shamash the sun god, whose light penetrates everywhere and makes everything apparent, or Adad, who revealed himself in thunderstorms.[37]

Studying now some spontaneous omens, we must recall the prognostic book which begins with the series 'When an incantation priest goes to the house of a sick man' and which lists mostly animal omens seen on the way to the patient or in the sick room. Any animal encountered may indicate and determine the patient's fate, a pig, a wolf, a serpent, or a bird:

If a man go to the house of a sick man (and) a falcon goes along at his right, that sick man will get well.
If the falcon goes along on his left side, that sick man will die.
If in the morning in the rear of a sick man's house a falcon proceeds from an inclosure at the right to an inclosure at the left, that sick man will speedily recover.
If in the morning in the rear of a sick man's house a falcon proceeds from an inclosure at the left to an inclosure at the right, his sickness will be protracted.
If in the morning in the rear of a sick man's house a falcon flies away, that sick man will die.[38]

Or the animal may be an insect:

If a scorpion falls upon a sick man, after the 10th day he will die.
If a scorpion drops itself on the sick man, his sickness will be long.
If a scorpion stands at the head of a sick man's bed, his sickness will quickly leave him.
If a scorpion stands on the wall before a sick man, his sickness will leave him.
If a scorpion enters a sick man's lap, that sick man will live.[39]

The right side brought good luck and the left side bad luck, and this remained so for ages throughout the Mediterranean world, so much so that the Latin word for left, *sinister,* assumed a sinister meaning. Animal omens obviously had significance not only for sick people but on every occasion. Sometimes the origin of an omen is not easily apparent. If a dog extinguished a fire in somebody's house, it meant that a command would be issued to this house.[40] But if a dog stood in your way, it meant that you would encounter some obstacle,[41] and this was a simple case of sympathetic magic. Sometimes rational considerations seemed to be at the bottom of omens. If sheep howled pitifully in their fold, it meant that the fold would be destroyed. And when sheep ate one another's vermin a famine was impending among the cattle.[42] A vague attempt to correlate natural occurrences with the incidence of illness may be found in omens taken from the observation of a river. When the water rose in the month of Nisan and the river had the color of blood, it announced death in the country. And when the river seemed stagnant like a pond, diseases of the chest were to be expected. Fevers resulted in other cases. But then we read that when the river carried yellow plants, jaundice occurred in the country.[43] These omens are certainly not more than a vague foreboding of epidemiological ideas.

Birth omens were another important group of signs.[44] Abnormal human and animal births were striking and believed to be very portentous. Monstrous births at all times captured human imagination,[45] and children born with one eye or two heads, or Siamese twins may have given rise to the belief in Cyclopes and other fabulous beings. But abnormal births do not occur frequently and these unusual happenings were assumed to be omens foretelling the fate of the king, the royal family, or the state:

> If an ewe gives birth to three fully developed (lambs), the dynasty will meet with opposition, approach of an usurper, the country will be destroyed.
>
> If an ewe gives birth to five, destruction will ravage the country, the owner of the house will die, his state will be destroyed.[46]

There was no limit set to the diviners who systematized this knowledge. They had no hesitation to have an ewe give birth not only to five lambs but also to six, seven, eight, nine and even ten lambs. Giving birth to nine meant the 'end of the dynasty,' and 'if an ewe gives birth to ten, a weakling will acquire universal sovereignty.'[47] Imagination ran wild when an ewe was supposed to have given birth to five, 'one with the head of a bull, one with a lion-head, one with a jackal-head, one with a dog-head and one with the head of a lamb.'[48] Jastrow pointed out that this merely meant that the heads resembled those of such animals[49] but I do not think that we must look for rational explanation in every case, just as we need not try to explain how a woman gave birth to as many as eight children simultaneously.[50] We do not attempt to interpret the illustration of Muscio's *Gynaecia,* in which eleven infants are pictured in one uterus.[51] And if a bitch or sow was listed as having a litter of thirty, we need not think that this was more than a speculative assumption; the number might just as well have been sixty or a hundred and twenty. Abnormal births were not common events and hence were reported. Thus the Assyrian butcher Uddanu informed the astrologer Nergalêtir that his sow had given birth to a pig with eight legs and two tails, whereupon the astrologer put the pig in salt, carried it home, and recorded the event.[52]

Birth omens were not as important medically as others and constituted a method of divination used for events of greater consequence than the individual lot of an average patient. But like hepatoscopy they sharpened the eye of the diviner and greatly enriched anatomical terminology, since terms had to be coined to designate in great detail the various parts of the body and deviations from their normal appearance.[53] Jastrow laid great stress on the texts that mention a woman giving birth to a lion, dog, pig, ox, ass, lamb, or other animals[54] and, pointing out that this merely meant a resemblance of the infant with such animals, he developed the thesis that this was the beginning of the 'science' of physiognomy,[55] which flourished in Greece and thereafter in the Western world from G. B. Porta[56] to Lavater.[57] In all these physiognomic studies, comparison with animal parts played a certain role and physiognomy assumed the character of an omen 'science' in so far as it was believed that the external features of an individual reflected his character and general psychosomatic constitution.

In Babylonia as in most other archaic civilizations people believed in the reality of dreams and also in the power they exerted as revelations of divine intentions. Some dreams were easy to understand, were mere wish fulfilments, or reflected everyday occurrences. But the meaning of others was dark and had to be interpreted by the priests. They could tell you that you must expect illness if you dreamed that you twisted your nose, that you pulled your teeth, pressed your cheeks, or lacerated your tongue.[58]

If a man in his dream

goes down into the earth, he will die and will not be buried in the earth. If he goes down into the earth and sees dead people, his days will be short.

If the same, and dead people are seen, the evil Utukku will seize him.
If the same, and he embraces a dead, he will die of the setu disease.[59]

Dreams, of course, not only announced ill health and death but also good luck, realization of desires, booty, profits, success, and other pleasant happenings.[60] In all epics from that of Gilgamesh to the Homeric hymns and later poems, the gods spoke to the heroes in prophetic dreams, exhorting, warning them, or simply announcing what would happen to them.

Of all the spontaneous omens the most forceful ones were probably those that could be read in the heavens, from the general constellation, from the relation between fixed stars and planets, from eclipses, comets, and similar occurrences.[61] We mentioned astrology before and saw that divination was its chief purpose. Its literature had the same character as that concerning other omens, that is, it listed happenings as they had been observed and added the events to be expected in each case. One text goes as far back as the Old Babylonian period; [62] various collections were compiled during the Kassite period, and judicial astrology reached its climax at the time of the Late Assyrian empire. The chief collection of texts preserved is named after its opening words, *Enuma Anu Enlil* (As Anu and Enlil).[63] It is divided into four parts dealing with omens derived from the observation of moon, sun, planets and other stars, and meteorology. This was a large collection, which consisted of at least 70 tablets at the time of Ashurbanipal and kept growing steadily. Another source of judicial astrology is to be found in the reports and letters sent regularly to the court by astrologers stationed in strategic points of observation all over the country.

Astrology even more than the interpretation of birth omens required a complicated machinery, not only highly specialized diviners, but also observation towers in different parts of the empire and a fast messenger service. Hence the stars were not consulted to determine the outcome of the illness of a poor farmer or craftsman. Like the birth omens and even more so, heavenly signs were read and interpreted in matters concerning the nation, the chances of a campaign, the welfare of the king, his family, and court. A few examples will illustrate this [64]

If one sees the moon on the first day of the month, there will be quiet and peace in the land.

If an eclipse takes place in the month Nisan at the time of the first night-watch, there will be destruction; brother will kill brother.

If the sun is darkened on the first Nisan, the king of Babylon will die.

If Mercury is visible for one month, there will be rain and floods.

If Venus has disappeared in the morning from the first to the thirtieth day in the month Nisan, there will be mourning in the country.

If it rains eight days in the month Nisan, it means wealth of the people.

If it rains eight days in the month Siwan, the king will die.

If it rains eight days in the month Adar, it means a good crop and luxuriant vegetation.

We see that this kind of judicial astrology had little relation to medicine. Jastrow pointed out that astrology was 'resorted to for the purpose of determining the course and outcome of a disease, according to the day of the month on which it began, or according to phenomena observed in the moon or the planets at the time that the disease was raging.'[65] We have some texts that illustrate this point, but we must keep in mind that the theory of the horoscope made its appearance at the very end of Babylonian history, that it developed in Egypt, in Hellenistic times. There was no astrological medicine of any consequence in early Mesopotamia. Such a system developed much later through the combination of elements of Ptolemy's astronomy and Galen's medical system. Then, in the Middle Ages and Renaissance it played a very important part and we shall discuss it in detail in a later volume of this book.

Omens were not only spontaneous signs but also had to be sought by special methods; among these hepatoscopy, the examination of the liver of sacrificial animals, was by far the most important and the most highly developed.[66] It was an old method and texts can be traced back to the time of Sargon I and Naram-Sin.[67] The literature was very extensive and texts were written on tablets in the usual way, but here perhaps more than anywhere else the need was felt for illustrations; in fact not only do we have tablets with illustrations, that is with designs, of the anomalies of the liver,[68] but we have texts written on clay models of the liver.[69]

The underlying theory was that when the god consulted accepted the sacrifice of an animal, a sheep as a rule, he identified himself with the spirit of the animal so that his intentions were reflected in its organs and particularly in the liver, which was considered the seat of the soul and the center of life.[70] The consultation of the liver oracle was a highly ceremonial affair.[71] It took place in front of the statue of the god. The question was formulated in writing and the tablet was deposited at the feet of the god. Prayers, purifications, libations, preceded the sacrifice. Then the sheep was slaughtered; the abdominal cavity was opened and the diviner examined liver and intestines *in situ;* he cut out the liver and inspected the place it had taken in the cavity, the 'palace of the liver' as it was called. And finally he put the organ in front of him in such a way that the side with the gall bladder was facing him. Now his chief work began: he inspected the surface of the liver, inch by inch, the left, the right, the square lobe, the lobus caudatus, processus capillaris and processus pyramidalis, the gall bladder and its ducts, the blood vessels connected with the liver, lymph glands, the entire surface anatomy of the organ. He looked for malformations, for the design of the superficial veins; whatever he saw had a definite meaning that had been established centuries before and was recorded in the scriptures that he had studied in order to be a *bârû*. What he observed on every single part of the liver he wrote down, and the sum total was the god's answer to the suppliant's question. If all signs were favorable or unfavorable you knew what you had to do. If of twelve signs ten were favorable and two unfavorable you had good chances to succeed with whatever your project happened to be. Texts were arranged according to parts of the liver: [72]

If the path (possibly the ligamentum falciforme) is double and there is a drawing between both parts, my army will meet disaster.

If the path is double and a 'weapon' is between both parts looking downward, my army will rise and kill the enemy.

If the finger (processus pyramidalis) is like the ear of a lion, the king will be unmatched.

If the finger is like the tongue of an ox, the king's intimate friends will rise against him.

If the gall bladder is perforated on top, it means good luck to the king.

If the gall bladder is perforated below to the left, it means disaster to the enemy's army.

These few examples show that this elaborate oracle was consulted primarily in affairs of the state, but liver omens were sought also in matters of health and disease if the patient was sufficiently prominent: [73]

If the shanû [74] is double as well as the nîru [74] and if they are strongly designed the sick man will die.

If idem and if there is a lump of flesh at the bottom of the na,[74] . . . curse will befall the sick and he will die.

If idem, and if the ductus hepaticus falls to the right the sick will live but will not accomplish his desire.

If the bladder is long the king will live a long time.

If the processus pyramidalis is normal, he who brings the sacrifice will be in good health and he will live a long time.

The clay livers that have come down to us are very interesting. The one in the British Museum may be as old as the time of Hammurabi; it represents a normal sheep's liver and was in all probability used for the instruction of students. From Babylonia hepatoscopy spread all over the Near East and as far as Italy. Thirty-two clay models representing abnormal livers were found at Tell Hariri, the site of the capital of the Mâri empire which was destroyed by Hammurabi.[75] Other such models were excavated at Boghaz Keui, the Hittite capital,[76] and in Palestine. And finally there is a famous Etruscan bronze model of the liver found at Piacenza around 1877. It reflects a different system of hepatoscopy and the question of its origin is still controversial.[77]

The diviner who examined the liver also inspected other organs, such as the kidneys; in organs that occur in pairs, the usual distinction was made between right and left. Thus destruction of the right kidney meant death of the queen and, in the case of war, destruction of the army, but if the left kidney was affected it indicated that the enemy's queen would die and the enemy's army would perish.[78]

The intestines as they present themselves when you open the abdominal cavity were investigated also and conclusions were drawn from their general arrangement and design.[79] Various pictures of them have been preserved.

The diviner obviously was a keen observer since his primary task consisted in perceiving the slightest variations on the surface of the organs under examination. He was completely familiar with their surface anatomy and had names for every part.[80] But neither the liver nor the kidneys were cut open and the priest was probably not in the least interested in their internal structure. His approach to animal organs was in no way scientific but was purely religious and magical.

The interpretation of birth omens, judicial astrology, and hepatoscopy were complicated and expensive methods of divination that required an elaborate ceremonial. Simpler methods were needed for the everyday purposes of the common man. The observation of animals and other objects of nature was a method such as we have seen. Another popular and inexpensive method consisted in dropping oil into a cup filled with water and watching what happened:

If I drop oil on water, and the oil sinks and rises again . . . it means bad luck for a sick man.

If a ring forms from the oil in Eastern direction and remains thus it means: for a campaign that I shall undertake it and shall make plenty of booty; for a sick it means that he will recover.

If two rings develop from the oil, one large, the other small, the wife of the man will give birth to a boy; for a sick it means that he will recover.

If the oil disperses and covers the cup, the sick will die; the army will be destroyed.

If the oil bubble moves in Eastern direction, the sick will die.[81]

Two textbooks dealing with this kind of divination existed at the time of Hammurabi.[82] Another inexpensive method consisted in observing a flickering flame: [83]

If the flame of a light is dark, the sick will die within three days.

If the flame of a light is greenish, the lord and the lady of the house will meet disaster.

If the flame of a torch is bright, the house will thrive.

And finally the very symptoms of an individual's illness were considered omens; as we mentioned before, such a view opened the door to a rational approach to the phenomena of disease. But the symptoms were omens also in another sense, in that they predicted the individual's fate not only in so far as his health was concerned but in general:

If a pustule develops on his lower lip to the right, he will experience misery.

If a pustule develops on his lower lip to the left, he will pile up money and goods.[84]

I think that one reason for the fallacy of divination is to be sought in the fact that whenever a diviner observed an omen, he counteracted it with some magic rite, so that no one knew what might have occurred if the omen had been left to exert its nefarious influence.

TREATMENT

And now the treatment. It was etiological, was meant to remove the cause of illness and thus to readjust the sick man to his environment and to the world at large. To this end the patient atoned for his sin or that of his people and placated his gods. Witchcraft had to be destroyed and demons were expelled with incantations. Since we encountered the same views in Egypt and also to a certain extent among primitive peoples of our own time, we need not repeat what we have said and our task will consist rather in stressing the Mesopotamian aspects of expiation rites, and in illustrating them with a few texts. We may do it the better as the literature available is both rich and forceful.

When a man had sinned and was ailing as a result of it he sometimes addressed himself to his god directly, with prayer and sacrifice. Such a prayer from the library of Ashurbanipal, but addressed to an old Sumerian deity, read: [85]

O! Ninlil, lady of the gods, I have turned unto thee.
To spare and to show favour thou knowest. Thy mantle I have taken hold of.
A heavy sin (?) I carry, I know not to bear it.

Because of (my) transgression known and unknown I have become weak.
Because of the evil I have done and have not done I perish, O! lady,
(Because) of the sin which since the time of my youth I have carried
And which the apostle of god has known or not known I suffer greatly
Daily (?), O! my lady, may my evil be expelled.
May thy good breath blow and the darkness be brightened.
From trouble and calamity that distress take thou my hand,
May not my offender prosper who exults over me.
May I live, may I prosper and the greatness of thy great divinity ever shall I cherish.

Prayers sometimes began with exuberant praising of the god invoked. Thus, addressing himself to Nergal, god of pestilence, the suppliant said:[86]

Mighty Lord, thou exalted, first-born of Nunamnir,
First among the Anunnaki, Lord of the Battle,
Offspring of Kutushar, the great Queen,
Nergal, thou mightiest god, favorite of Ninmenna!
Thou art radiant in the bright Heavens, high is thy abode,
Great art thou in the Underworld, knowest no rival,
With Ea in the gods' assembly thy counsel is supreme,
With Sin in the Heavens thou seest all.
Thy father Enlil gave thee all, the black-headed ones, all that breatheth,
The cattle in the fields, he entrusted it all into thy hands.

After having thus praised the god, the suppliant formulated his complaints and endeavored to propitiate Nergal, ending his prayer with the words:

Absolve my guilt, cancel my sin!
May the wrath of thy divine heart be appeased,
May the angered god and the angered goddess again be at peace with me!
Thy might I will proclaim and I will sing thy praise.

In other cases prayer was combined with an elaborate ritual. A fragmentary tablet in the British Museum gives a graphic picture of such an expiation ritual.[87] A prayer in which the sick man expressed all his anguish was to be recited three times and furthermore:

His arms behind him thou shalt turn (?), and as long as his sickness [lasts] before the stars water and . . . beer libate and do not kneel. On the roof . . . he shall sleep, and in the morning ten shekels of šadānu-stone thou shalt . . . With water wash thyself and anoint thyself with oil . . . Before Shamash a censer of cypress thou shalt place, and this šadānu-stone thou shalt remove. Before Shamash thou shalt put (give) it. Over it he shalt speak as follows: O Kagina-stone, šadānu, darling of Shamash, the far-famed judge, like my father, my begetter, [forgive] my wrongdoings . . .

Here, in other words, we have a combination of prayer, sacrifice, religious and magic rites. Sacrifice played an important part in all these rituals. Words were not enough to appease the angered deity, who expected offerings in addition, incense, libations of milk, beer, wine and solid food, bread, fruit, and, when the patient could afford it, the meat of animals. But sacrifice had a deeper magic meaning in that the animal slaughtered was offered to the god as a substitute for the sick man:

The kid is a substitute for mankind,
He hath given the kid for his life,
He hath given the head of the kid for the head of the man,
He hath given the neck of the kid for the neck of the man,
He hath given the breast of the kid for the breast of the man.[88]

The kid or a suckling pig or some other virgin animal was sacrificed to appease the irate god and thereby to save the life of the patient. This was sympathetic magic pure and simple and similar magic was used when a patient had been bewitched. Both the Maqlû and the Shurpu series deal to a large extent with the destruction of witchcraft through fire. A good example of imitative magic is given in the following text, which was recited while images of wizard and witch were burned:[89]

Scorching Fire, warlike son of Heaven,
Thou the fiercest of thy brethren,
Who like Moon and Sun decidest lawsuits—
Judge thou my case, hand down the verdict.
Burn the man and woman who bewitched me;
Burn, O Fire, the man and woman who bewitched me;

Scorch, O Fire, the man and woman who bewitched me;
Burn them, O Fire;
Scorch them, O Fire;
Take hold of them, O Fire;
Consume them, O Fire;
Destroy them, O Fire.

This was an incantation in which the oral rite was combined with a manual one, in this case one of imitative magic. Incantation, indeed, was by far the most frequent and the oldest method of treatment. A demon had taken hold of a man and the *âshipu,* the exorcist, endeavored to drive the evil spirit out by chanting the right words and performing the necessary rites. Following Falkenstein's classification of the Sumerian incantations,[90] we may divide this literature into four major groups, each of which is characterized by a certain style.

Many incantations begin with having the priest step forward and say who he is and what magic power he possesses. He then says what he is doing, prays for protection against the demons, exhorts them not to do any harm, and brings the ceremony to a climax when addressing himself directly to the demons he pronounces the fateful words: 'By Heaven be thou exorcised, by Earth be thou exorcised.' This pattern is followed more or less closely in many of the texts preserved, such as the following: [91]

The man of Ea am I,
The man of Damkina am I,
The messenger of Marduk am I,
My spell is the spell of Ea,
My incantation is the incantation of Marduk,
The Ban of Ea is in my hand,
The tamarisk, the powerful weapon of Anu,
In my hand I hold;
The date spathe, mighty in decision,
In my hand I hold.
Unto my body may they not draw nigh,
Before me may they wreak no evil,
Nor follow behind me.
On the threshold where I stand, let them not set themselves;

Where I stand, there stand thou not!
Where I sit, there sit thou not!
Where I walk, there walk thou not!
Where I enter, there enter thou not!
By Heaven be thou exorcised! By Earth be thou exorcised!

The reference to Marduk makes evident that we are dealing with a Babylonian text and tamarisk and date spathe appear as powerful apotropaic weapons. An elaborate ritual is described in the following incantation of which I quote only the introduction:[92]

The Sorcerer-priest that maketh clear the ordinances of Eridu am I,
The Herald that goeth before Ea am I,
Of Marduk, sage magician (and) eldest son of Ea,
The Herald am I,
The Exorciser of Eridu, most cunning in magic am I;
O thou evil demon, turn thee to get hence,
O thou that dwelleth in ruins, get thee to thy ruins,
For the great lord Ea hath sent me;
He hath prepared his spell for my mouth
With a censer for those Seven, for clear decision,
He hath filled my hand.
A raven, the bird that helpeth the gods,
In my right hand I hold;
A hawk, to flutter in thine evil face,
In my left hand I thrust forward;
With the sombre garb of awe I clothe thee,
In sombre dress I robe thee,
A glorious dress for a pure body.
Fleabane (?) on the lintel of the door I have hung,
St. John's wort (?), caper (?), and wheatears
On the latch I have hung;
With a halter as a roving ass
Thy body I restrain;
O evil Spirit, get thee hence,
Depart, O evil Demon!

This text gives a most vivid description of how such a ceremony was performed. The priest had been called to the patient's house. Plants of magic significance were hung on the lintel of the door and on the latch. The sick man was dressed in somber garb and since he was delirious or raving he was tied to the bed. Then the priest stepped up to him, dressed in dark clothes, swinging a censer, holding a raven in one hand, a hawk in the other. He came as the herald of Ea and of his son Marduk, endowed with the divine power embodied in the magic words of pure spells and he exorcised the demons by Heaven and Earth.

Another group of incantations follows a slightly different pattern. The priest begins by describing the life and evil doings of the demons in general, then refers to a special attack on a man, the patient under treatment. We next hear of Marduk reporting to his father Ea, asking for advice and receiving instructions for a sometimes very complicated ritual which has the power to drive out the demons. The incantation ends with a prayerlike wish that the evil spirits may spare the patient and that good spirits may take their place. We have quoted so many texts describing the ways of the demons that we shall not repeat them here but will rather give a few examples of Ea's instructions to Marduk, that is, of magic ritual:

> Go, my son (Marduk),
> Take a white kid of Tammuz,
> Lay it down facing the sick man and
> Take out its heart and
> Place it in the hand of that man;
> Perform the Incantation of Eridu,
> The kid whose heart thou hast taken out
> Is li'i-food with which thou shalt make an 'atonement' for the man,
> Bring forth a censer (and) a torch,
> Scatter it in the street,
> Bind a bandage on that man,
> Perform the Incantation of Eridu,
> Invoke the great gods
> That the evil Spirit, the evil Demon, evil Ghost,
> Hag-demon, Ghoul,
> Fever, or heavy sickness
> Which is in the body of the man,
> May be removed and go forth from the house!
> May a kindly Spirit, a kindly Genius be present! [98]

A figure of clay of the sick man was made in the following ritual: [94]

Go, my son (Marduk),
Pull off a piece of clay from the deep,
Fashion a figure of his bodily form (therefrom) and
Place it on the loins of the sick man by night,
At dawn make the 'atonement' for his body,
Perform the Incantation of Eridu,
Turn his face to the west,
That the evil Plague-demon which hath seized upon him
May vanish away from him.

And still more outspoken was the rite of sympathetic magic in this ritual: [95]

Fashion a figure of him in dough,
Put water upon the man and
Pour forth the water of the Incantation;
Bring forth a censer (and) a torch,
As the water trickleth away from his body
So may the pestilence in his body trickle away.
Return these waters into a cup and
Pour them forth in the broad places,
That the evil influence which hath brought low (his) strength
May be carried away into the broad places,
That the spittle which hath been spat
May be poured forth like the water,
That the magic which mingleth with the spat-forth spittle
May be turned back,
By the magic of the Word of Ea,
The chanting lips which have uttered the ban,—
May their bond be loosened!
That this man may be pure, be clean!
Into the kindly hands of his god may he be commended.

Among these texts are beautiful prayers of the incantation priests to the gods for assistance in their difficult task, such as the following: [96]

O Ea, King of the Deep, to see . . .
I, the magician, am thy slave.

March thou on my right hand,
Be present on my left;
Add thy pure spell unto mine,
Add thy pure voice unto mine,
Vouchsafe (to me) pure words,
Make fortunate the utterances of my mouth,
Ordain that my decisions be happy,
Let me be blessed where'er I tread,
Let the man whom I (now) touch be blessed.
Before me may lucky thoughts be spoken,
After me may a lucky finger be pointed.
Oh, that thou wert my guardian Genius,
And my guardian Spirit!
O god that blesseth, Marduk,
Let me be blessed, where'er my path may be!
Thy power shall god and man proclaim;
This man shall do thy service,
And I too, the magician, thy slave.

In this case the priest performed the elementary rite of touching the patient with his hand. He did even more in the following case: [97]

When I draw near unto the sick man,
When I examine the muscles of the sick man,
When I compose his limbs,
When I sprinkle the water of Ea on the sick man,
When I subdue the sick man,
When I bring low the strength of the sick man,
When I recite an incantation over the sick man,
When I perform the Incantation of Eridu,
May a kindly Spirit, a kindly Guardian, be present at my side.

The manual rites used in driving out spirits were manifold but not very different from those discussed in previous sections of this volume. A demon was transferred through magic formulae into a pot of water, which was then broken so that the water was spilled.[98] Or he was driven into a little boat, which then sailed away; or was tied into magic knots, or an onion was peeled and one peel after the other was thrown into the fire while the priest recited the appropriate incantation.[99] Or gold or precious stones were used here as in Egypt by those who could afford them. In a ritual against Labartu the house was cleaned, a picture of the demon was made of clay from the house and placed at the head of the patient. A brazier into which a sword was thrust was also placed at the head of the sick man and kept there blazing for three days. At the end of the third day the picture of the demon was carried out of the house, destroyed with the sword, buried in a corner of the wall, and surrounded with flour and water. And when you returned to the house you were not to look back.[100]

A third group of incantations was primarily prophylactic. Again the life of the evil spirits was described in vivid colors and the magic formulae were to keep them away from man. We have given examples of such texts before and need not repeat them.

Just as in Egypt incantations were used to consecrate objects of the ritual, we also find in Babylonia a group of similar texts which were recited over plants and other drugs to give them their magic power.

The more pronounced the Semitic element became in Mesopotamian civilization, the more outspoken the concept of sin as cause of disease was and the more we encounter the prayer-type of incantation.[101] The old Sumerian spells remained popular, demons were driven out through the same oral and manual rites for thousands of years, but the purer the concept of the deity became the more the sick man addressed himself to his god directly in prayers, hesitatingly in Mesopotamia but unreservedly in Judaism and Christianity.

Throughout the course of its history Mesopotamian medicine maintained its religious and magic character, but at the same time it was able to include many elements, observations, treatments, techniques that we consider rational and these we must briefly discuss now.

NOTES

1. See Falkenstein, *Die Haupttypen der Sumerischen Beschwörung*, Leipzig, 1931, p. 56.
2. Ibid. p. 35ff. The text quoted is p. 41.

3. Ibid. p. 42; R. Campbell Thompson, *The Devils and Evil Spirits of Babylonia,* London, 1903-4, cited as Thompson, *Devils,* vol. i, pp. 60-63.
4. See, e.g. C. Frank, 'Köpfe babylonischer Dämonen,' *Rev. Assyr.,* 1910, 7:21-32; W. G. Schileico, 'Tête d'un démon assyrien à l'Ermitage Impérial de Saint-Pétersbourg,' *Rev. Assyr.,* 1914, 11:57-9; V. Scheil, 'Labartu et autre amulette,' *Rev. Assyr.,* 1929, 26:10-11.
5. C. J. Mullo-Weir, 'A Prayer to Ea, Shamash, and Marduk,' *J. Roy. Asiat. Soc. Gr. Brit. Ireland,* 1929, pp. 285-8.
6. Ibid.
7. H. Zimmern, *Die Beschwörungstafeln Shurpu,* Leipzig, 1896, tablet ii.
8. J. Morgenstern, 'The Doctrine of Sin in the Babylonian Religion,' *Mitt. Vorderasiat. Gesell.,* 1905, 10:3ff.; S. Langdon, 'Sin,' *Encycl. Rel. Ethics,* vol. xi, pp. 531-3; Ch. F. Jean, *Le Péché chez les Babyloniens et les Assyriens* [Monografie del Collegio Alberoni, no. 3], Piacenza, 1925; G. Furlani, 'Sulle liste babilonesi e assire di peccati,' *Rendiconti R. Accad. Naz. Lincei, Cl. Sc. morali, stor., filol.,* 1930, ser. 6, vol. 6, pp. 118-46.
9. C. J. Mullo-Weir, 'Fragments of Two Assyrian Prayers,' *J. Roy. Asiat. Soc. Gr. Brit. Ireland,* 1929, p. 762.
10. Ibid.
11. E. A. Wallis Budge, 'A Guide to the Babylonian and Assyrian Antiquities,' British Museum, 1908, p. 71.
12. Zimmern, Shurpu II, 100.
13. Thompson, *Devils,* vol. ii, p. 136ff.
14. See Thompson's discussion in *Devils,* vol. ii, p. 4ff.
15. Leviticus, 13.
16. Thompson, *Devils.*
17. Ibid. vol. i, p. xxxi.
18. Ibid. vol. i, p. 41.
19. Ibid. vol. i, p. xxxi.
20. Isaiah, 34, 14.
21. Meissner, vol. ii, p. 203.
22. Ibid. vol. ii, p. 204.
23. Contenau, *Civilisation,* p. 91.
24. Meissner, vol. ii, p. 201.
25. M. Bartels in an early study, *Zsch. Assyr.,* 1893, 8:179-84, tried to identify Tî'u with erysipelas. It is always a mistake to make such close identifications since they usually project modern concepts into the past.
26. Meissner, vol. ii, p. 200.
27. Thompson, *Devils,* vol. i, p. 51ff.
28. Ibid. vol. i, p. 77ff.
29. Ibid. vol. i, p. 89ff.
30. Ibid. vol. ii, p. 29.
31. Ibid. vol. ii, p. 65ff.
32. Cuneiform Texts, part xvii, pl. 50, again, with translation, in *Devils,* vol. ii, p. 160ff.; and a revised translation in *Proc. Roy. Soc. Med.,* Sect. Hist. Med., 1926, 19:59-60; see also B. Meissner, *Mitt. Vorderasiat. Gesell.,* ix, 3, p. 40ff.

33. A very good bronze copy is in the Louvre.
34. V. Scheil, 'Labartu et autre amulette,' *Rev. Assyr.*, 1929, 26:10-11.
35. See the very ingenious interpretation of Contenau in *Médecine,* p. 88ff. He pointed out that the Babylonian word for the human face occurred in the dual form, meaning that the face consists of two halves joined in the most perfect way while in the case of demons the two faces do not make one whole.
36. The literature about Mesopotamian divination is very considerable. One of the most recent and comprehensive monographs is: G. Contenau, *La Divination chez les Assyriens et les Babyloniens,* Paris, 1940, with good bibliography (quoted in the following as Contenau, *Divination*). Pioneer work in the field was done by A. Boissier who published numerous texts and whose *Documents assyriens relatifs aux présages,* Paris, 1894-9, 3 vols., and *Choix de textes relatifs à la divination assyro-babylonienne,* Geneva, 1905, 2 vols., are a mine of information. Important also is Ch. Fossey, *Textes assyriens et babyloniens relatifs à la divination,* Paris, 1905. The classical book on ancient divination, A. Bouché-Leclercq, *Histoire de la divination dans l'antiquité,* Paris, 1879-80, 4 vols., may still be consulted profitably for Greek and Roman parallels.
37. Contenau, *Divination,* pp. 29f.
38. F. W. Geers, 'A Babylonian Omen Text,' *Am. J. Sem. Lang. Lit.*, 1926/27, 43:29.
39. Ibid. p. 33.
40. J. Hunger, *Babylonische Tieromina nebst griechisch-römischen Parallelen* [Mitt. Vorderasiat. Ges. xiv, 3], Berlin, 1909.
41. Ibid.
42. A. Ungnad, *Die Religion der Babylonier und Assyrer,* Jena, 1921, p. 323.
43. A. Boissier, *Choix de textes,* vol. ii, p. 235ff.; Contenau, *Médecine,* p. 104.
44. Ch. Fossey, 'Présages tirés des naissances,' *Babyloniaca,* 1912-1913, 5:1-256; M. Jastrow, *Babylonian-Assyrian Birth-omens and Their Cultural Significance,* Giessen, 1914; L. Dennefeld, *Babylonisch-assyrische Geburts-Omina, zugleich ein Beitrag zur Geschichte der Medizin* [Assyriol. Bibl., vol. 22], Leipzig, 1914; A. Ungnad, 'Das Alter der Geburtsomina,' *Orient. Lit. Zeit.*, 1917, 20:139-40; E. F. Weidner, 'Kommentare zu den Geburtsominatexten,' *Am. J. Sem. Lang. Lit.*, 1921-22, 38:187-206.
45. See Eugen Holländer, *Wundergeburt und Wundergestalt in Einblattdrucken des fünfzehnten bis achtzehnten Jahrhunderts,* Stuttgart, 1921; A. Sonderegger, *Missgeburten und Wundergestalten in Einblattdrucken und Handzeichnungen des 16. Jahrhunderts,* Zürich, 1927.
46. Jastrow, loc. cit. p. 17ff.
47. Ibid. p. 18.
48. Ibid.
49. Ibid. note 1.
50. Ibid. p. 31.
51. In *Codex Bruxellensis* 3714, Saec. ix. Reproduction in K. Sudhoff, *Ein Beitrag zur Geschichte der Anatomie in Mittelalter,* Leipzig, 1908, plate 23, fig. 13.

52. R. C. Thompson, *The Reports of the Magicians of Nineveh,* London, 1900, vol. I, p. 107, no. 277; Contenau, *Médecine,* p. 130.
53. H. Holma, *Die Namen der Körperteile im Assyrisch-Babylonischen* [Ann. Acad. Sci. Fennicae, ser. B, vol. 7, no. 1], Helsinki-Leipzig, 1911.
54. Jastrow, loc. cit. p. 40.
55. About physiognomic omens see A. Boissier, 'Iatromantique, physiognomie et palmomantique babyloniennes,' *Rev. Asiat.,* 1911, 8:33-9; F. R. Kraus, *Die physiognomischen Omina der Babylonier,* Leipzig, 1935.
56. G. B. Porta, *De humana physiognomia,* Sorrento, 1586.
57. J. K. Lavater, *Physiognomische Fragmente,* Leipzig, 1775-8, 4 vols.
58. H. F. Lutz, 'An Omen Text Referring to the Action of a Dreamer,' *Am. J. Sem. Lang. Lit.,* 1919, 35:145-57.
59. Contenau, *Médecine,* p. 126.
60. Contenau, *Divination,* p. 157ff.
61. See Contenau, *Divination,* p. 299ff.; O. Neugebauer, *J. Near Eastern Stud.,* 1945, 4:14ff.; Ch. Virolleaud, 'Présages tirés des eclipses de soleil et de l'obscurcissement du Soleil ou du ciel par les nuages,' *Zsch. Assyr.,* 1902, 16:201-39; V. Scheil, 'Présages tirés de Vénus,' *Rev. Ass.,* 1917, 14:142-5.
62. V. Šileiko, 'Mcndlaufprognosen aus der Zeit der ersten babylonischen Dynastie,' *C. R. Ac. Sc. URSS,* 1927, B. p. 125-8.
63. Ch. Virolleaud, *L'Astrologie chaldéenne,* Paris, 1908-12; E. F. Weidner, 'Die astrologische Serie Enûma Anu Enlil,' *Arch. Orientforsch.,* 1942, 14:172-95.
64. From Ungnad, *Religion,* p. 316ff.
65. M. Jastrow, *Proc. R. Soc. Med.,* Sect. Hist. Med., 1914, 7:124.
66. C. Bezold, *Einige Bemerkungen zur babylonischen Leberschau* [Religionsgeschichtliche Versuche und Vorarbeiten], Giessen, 1905, pp. 240-52; M. Jastrow, 'Notes on Omen Texts,' *Am. J. Sem. Lang. Lit.,* 1907, 23:97-115; M. Jastrow, 'Hepatoscopy and Astrology among the Babylonians and Assyrians,' *Proc. Am. Phil. Soc.,* vol. 49, pp. 646-76; A. Ungnad, 'Ein Leberschau–Text aus der Zeit Ammisadugas,' *Babyloniaca,* 1908, 2:257-74; E. F. Weidner, 'Zur babylonischen Eingeweideschau,' *Mitt. Vorderasiat. Ges.,* 1916, 21:191-8; E. F. Weidner, 'Zahlenspielereien in akkadischen Leberschautexten,' *Orient. Lit. Zeit.,* 1917, 20:257-66; L. Dennefeld, *Die babylonische Wahrsagekunst,* Strasbourg, 1919; V. Scheil, 'Nouveaux Présages tirés du foie,' *Rev. Assyr.,* 1930, 27:141-54; H. Dillon, *Assyro-Babylonian Liver-Divination,* Rome, 1932; J. Nougayrol, 'Textes hépatoscopiques d'époque ancienne conservés au Musée du Louvre,' *Rev. Assyr.,* 1941, 38:67-88; 1945-6, 40:56-98.
67. A. Boissier, 'Les Présages de Sargon et de Naram-Sin. Extraits des livres des haruspices,' *Rev. Sémit.,* 1902, 10:275-80; V. Scheil, 'Oracles au sujet de Sargon l'Ancien,' *Rev. Assyr.,* 1929, 26:9-10.
68. Contenau, *Divination,* p. 242.
69. E. A. Wallis Budge, *A Guide to the Babylonian and Assyrian Antiquities,* British Museum, 1908, no. 148, p. 174.
70. A. Merx, *Le Rôle du foie dans la littérature des peuples sémitiques* [Florilegium Melchior de Vogüe], Paris, 1909, pp. 427-44; M. Jastrow,

'The Liver as the Seat of the Soul,' *Studies in the History of Religions Presented to C. H. Toy*, New York, 1912, pp. 143-68.

71. See Contenau, *Divination*, p. 257ff.
72. Ungnad, *Religion*, p. 312ff.
73. From Boissier, *Choix de textes*, vol. I, pp. 65, 69ff.; see Contenau, *Médecine*, p. 117f.
74. Parts of the liver which are not identified with certainty.
75. M. Rutten, 'Trente-deux Modèles de foies en argile inscrits provenant de Tell-Hariri [Mâri],' *Rev. Assyr.*, 1938, 35:36-70.
76. E. F. Weidner, Staatl. Mus. Berlin. *Keilschrifturkunden aus Boghazköi*, Heft IV, pp. 71-5.
77. V. Poggi, 'Di un bronzo piacentino,' *Atti. Mem. Stor. Patr. Emilia*, 1879, 4:1-26; A. Körte, 'Die Bronzeleber von Piacenza,' *Mitt. Deut. Arch. Inst.*, Röm. Abt., 1905, 20:348-79; C. Thulin, *Die Götter des Martianus Capella und die Bronzeleber von Piacenza*, 1906; W. von Bartels, *Die Etruskische Bronzeleber von Piacenza in ihrer symbolischen Bedeutung*, Berlin, 1910; G. Furlani, 'L'epatoscopia babilonese et l'epatoscopia etrusca,' *Atti del Primo Congresso Internaz. Etrusco*, Firenze, 1929, pp. 122-66; G. Furlani, Mantica Hittita e Mantica Etrusca, *Studi Etruschi*, 1936, 10:1-12.
78. L. W. King, 'Heart and Reins' in relation to Babylonian liver divination, *J. Manchester Orient. Soc.*, 1911, pp. 95-8.
79. B. Meissner, 'Omina zur Erkenntnis der Eingeweide des Opfertieres,' *Arch. Orientforsch.*, 1934, 9:118-22.
80. See M. Jastrow, 'Divination through the Liver and the Beginnings of Anatomy,' *Trans. Coll. Phys. Philadelphia*, 1908, 29:117-38; M. Jastrow, 'The Signs and Names for the Liver in Babylonian,' *Zsch. Assyr.*, 1906, 20:105-29.
81. Ungnad, *Religion*, p. 314.
82. J. Hunger, *Becherwahrsagung, bei den Babyloniern*, Leipzig, 1903.
83. Ungnad, *Religion*, p. 316; A. Boissier, *Choix de textes*, 1905, vol. I, p. 170ff.
84. Ch. Virolleaud, *Babyloniaca*, vol. I, p. 91ff.; Contenau, *Divination*, p. 213.
85. M. Sidersky, 'Assyrian Prayers,' *J. Roy. Asiat. Soc.*, 1929, p. 781f.
86. Ungnad, *Religion*, p. 223.
87. C. J. Mullo-Weir, 'Fragment of an Expiation-Ritual against Sickness,' *J. Roy. Asiat. Soc.*, 1929, pp. 281-4.
88. Thompson, *Devils*, vol. II, p. xxxii.
89. *Maqlû*, Tablet II, 104-15; translation by H. A. Frankfort in Frankfort *et al.*, *The Intellectual Adventure of Ancient Man*, Chicago, 1946, p. 134.
90. A. Falkenstein, *Die Haupttypen der Sumerischen Beschwörung*, Leipzig, 1931.
91. Thompson, *Devils*, vol. I, p. 23ff.
92. Ibid. vol. I, p. 133ff.
93. Ibid. vol. II, p. 32ff.
94. Ibid. vol. II, p. 100ff.
95. Ibid. vol. II, p. 108ff.
96. Ibid. vol. I, p. 26ff.

97. Ibid. vol. I, p. 18ff.
98. *Encycl. Rel. Ethics,* vol. VIII, p. 255.
99. See Jastrow, *Proc. Roy. Soc. Med.,* Sect. Hist. Med., 1913, p. 115f.
100. D. W. Myhrman, 'Die Labartu-Texte,' *Zschr. Assyr.,* 1902, 16:161.
101. See W. G. Kunstmann, *Die Babylonische Gebetsbeschwörung,* Leipzig, 1932.

*

6. Rational Elements in Mesopotamian Medicine

When we analyzed the Book of Prognoses, we mentioned that when the priest-physician was called to a patient, he observed not only phenomena of the sick man's environment but also of his body and general behavior. They too were signs, omens that must be interpreted and that revealed the patient's condition and impending fate. The physician, in other words, observed what we call symptoms of disease and listed them in books arranged according to the organ affected. Scanty as his anatomical knowledge was, he obviously was able to determine roughly the seat of a pain, of an inflammation, or of an itch. Thus we have series of tablets dealing with diseases of the head and its parts, of the lungs, of stomach and intestines, of the feet and other organs. We do not know whether these series, or at least some of them, were meant to be parts of an encyclopedia of medicine arranged *a capite ad calcem* but this is possible.

We have discussed the general character and style of this medical literature proper in a previous chapter. Our task here shall be to give an idea of the rational elements included in the religious system of Mesopotamian medicine by analyzing some tablets and quoting some typical passages.

Beginning with the head [1] we find prescriptions to be applied when a man has a pain in the head, when 'his head is bent with pain gripping his temples,' when the head throbs, or burns, when it 'burns and his head is bent, his head being as on fire, and the hair stands up,' or 'a man's brain contains fire and myalgia afflicts the temples and smites the eyes, his eyes are afflicted with dimness, cloudiness, a disturbed appearance, with the veins bloodshot, shedding tears.' This is a graphic description of a violent headache which may result from very different conditions so that it would be unwise to attempt a diagnosis. Or we read that the head has an itch, or a scab, that it smells unpleasantly, or contains water. The latter remark must not be interpreted as meaning hydrocephalus, because the physician had certainly not opened such a skull. The water, if there was any, was probably sweat, particularly when, as in the recipe immediately following, the forehead is mentioned as containing water. Or the patient simply felt as if he had water in the head.

In Mesopotamia just as in Egypt people of rank did not like to see their hair turn gray and the remedies they applied,[2] gall of a black ox, gall of a scorpion, gall of a pig, the head of a black raven, the head of a stork combined with opium, some other drugs and various oils, were in a way similar to those used in Egypt. It was a serious matter also when a woman's hair grew weak and thin, and in such a case charms and amulets were indicated.[3]

Pain in the brow was a localized headache, which was treated with various drugs, but a stronger remedy was needed 'when his brow pains a man and he vomits and is sick, his eyes being inflamed, it is the hand of a ghost; then reduce to ashes human bones and bray them; anoint him with them in cedar oil and he will recover.'[4] Not only the hand of a ghost but also 'the hatred of a goddess against his life' was responsible for a man's right temple hurting him and his right eye being swollen and letting tears flow.[5] The remedy, nevertheless, consisted of a mixture of drugs, and all through this literature we find this constant combination of magic, religious, and empirical elements.

The hand of a ghost seizing a man also caused diseases of the ears, and a series of tablets was devoted to them.[6] The 'ears sing,' and the patient was advised to put his fingers in his ears and to say: 'Wherever thou be, may Ea restrain thee,' whereupon drugs were introduced into the ears either directly or with wool or through fumigation. Otitis media was described: 'fire extends into the interior of his ear and it dulls the hearing,' the interior swells, pus exudes with offensive fetor, and the condition is very painful. The treatment consisted in the application of various drugs, in fumigations, and on the fourth day the interior was to be cleansed and alum was blown into the ear through a tube.[7]

Diseases of the eyes must have been as frequent in Mesopotamia as in Egypt, and we have a number of texts concerning them.[8] The eyes are sick, affected, failing, dim; they hurt, are inflamed, secrete matter, tears flow; or they are dry, will not open, are full of blood, full of yellow rheum, full of flesh growing, a film is in the eyes, they do not see, or can see nothing by day but can see everything by night, the object of vision is indistinct or it is multiplied. Jaundice of the eye is considered a symptom of a serious condition: 'When a man suffers from jaundice of the eye and his disease rises into the interior of his eyes, the water of the interior of his eyes is green like copper . . . his interior parts being raised return food and drink, the disease desiccates this man's entire body: he will die.'[9] The Babylonians and Assyrians must have known as much about diseases of the eyes as the Egyptians did, and their treatments were not so very different. Vegetable, animal, and mineral drugs were applied, charms were spoken, and operations must have been performed at an early date since reference to such an operation is made in the Code of Hammurabi.

Of other diseases affecting parts of the head, we may mention those of the mouth:[10] fetor, dry saliva, unhealthy saliva or such that flows too freely, 'if a man's saliva comes when he is talking and he ejects his spittle into a man's face, his teeth ache, his mouth hurting (?) him, the eructation of . . .'[11] 'If the saliva in a man's mouth does not cease to flow, that man has been bewitched';[12] the cure, however, is not to be sought in charms but rather in giving a potion of mustard, oak galls, licorice root, and liquidambar; in another recipe tamarisk-(galls), galbanum, fir-turpentine, pine-turpentine, are brayed together to make a potion—drugs which have astringent and disinfecting qualities. Another, rather serious condition is encountered when a man's mouth hurts him and is twisted to the right or left so that he cannot speak [13]—some form of paralysis against which the recommended drugs hardly had any effect.

A series of tablets has the title 'If a man's teeth ache.' [14] The sick tooth was treated with charms or with drugs or with both. The drugs were astringents like alum, or gums, or vinegar, flour, frogs, oil, root of mandrake, and various other vegetable and animal products. The drugs were applied to the tooth directly or with wool. When the teeth were loose and decay had set in, the gums were massaged with various drugs 'until blood comes forth.' When a man's teeth had become yellow, the physician was advised to bray together '"salt of Akkad," ammi, Lolium, pine-turpentine, (with these) with thy finger [thou shalt rub his teeth] . . . cleanse his mouth and nostrils . . . wash his mouth with honey, oil (and) kurunnu-beer . . . with a feather thou shalt make him vomit, and (then) thou shalt bray lupins (and) turmeric together, [let him drink (them)] in oil and kurunnu-beer, [and he shall recover].' In other cases the mouth was cleansed with the forefinger, around which a strip of linen had been wound.[15]

Diseases of the respiratory organs must have been frequent in Mesopotamia and we have many texts dealing with them. The outstanding symptoms, cough, sputum, dyspnea, and chest pain, are described graphically. A man 'coughs dry, ejecting no saliva,' [16] or the 'lungs cough up pus and the inward parts,' [17] or 'a man is affected in his lungs and they vomit exceedingly.' [18] Hemorrhage may be meant although it is not certain, in a passage that reads: 'if black, evil (?) blood comes from the "mouth" of the left lung of a man . . .' [19] A pain in the chest, or in chest and loins, or in chest, epigastrium, and loins is mentioned in many of these texts and undoubtedly describes the pleural and bronchopulmonary pain. Dyspnea is probably referred to in several passages which say: 'if a man's lungs pant with his work,' [20] although the translation is not certain. 'When the breath of a man's mouth is difficult,' [21] is probably also a reference to dyspnea.

'A man is affected in his lung passage' [22] or 'suffers from the "pipe of the lungs,"' [23] means that the patient has a disease of the bronchi or upper respiratory organs. An Assyrian tablet published by Labat and Tournay gives a good description of bronchitis:

If the patient suffers from hissing cough, if his wind-pipe is full of murmurs, if he coughs, if he has coughing fits, if he has phlegm: bray together roses and mustard, in purified oil drop it on his tongue, fill, moreover, a tube with it and blow it into his nostrils. Thereafter he shall drink several times beer of the first quality; thus he will recover.[24]

Another text, referring probably to pneumonia, lists as symptoms fever, chest pain, coughing and much sputum, loss of flesh, and 'the leg is heavy to him.'[25]

In the tablets dealing with diseases of the chest, we have a number of diagnoses although they do not go beyond naming the organ affected. 'If a man's breast hurts him, his epigastrium burns him, his stomach [is inflamed (swollen)] . . . that man has lung-trouble.'[26] More interesting is the fact that magic as well as rational causes were made responsible for the same kind of disease. 'If a man's breast and loins hurt him, he vomiting, that man sorcery has attacked . . .'[27] But then we find similar symptoms develop after a sudden chill:[28] 'If a man, having fallen into water and being taken out, his pain extends either to his side or to his . . . as his breath goes in and out . . .' The treatment recommended in this case was very sensible. The chest was fomented with water in which fennel had been boiled, after which balsamic poultices were applied. This remained the treatment of pleurisy and pneumonia for several thousand years.

Stomach and intestines were the seat of many diseases and we have Assyrian instructions on what should be done 'if a man's stomach holds fire,[29] if his epigastrium 'blows the fire of his stomach' or 'brings up the fire of the stomach,' if a man's epigastrium is 'overloaded with heat' or, 'to remove fire of the stomach.' Anus trouble is to be expected 'if a man eats bread, drinks beer and is constricted, ejecting his saliva, (his stomach) being "fettered," his bowels cry out (?).' But sorcery is involved, 'if a man's stomach is inflamed, his epigastrium burning . . . food and beer being bound, that man has eaten or drunk some sorcery.' Texts describe how the interiors hurt, grip you, devour you, rise, cut you,[30] how the stomach is distended, puffed up, full of acid, with a pain in its pit, with heartburn, vomiting bile when the individual eats. A recipe is for 'when a man's interiors regurgitate and his interior parts are inflamed, when his interiors make noises, return food and water.' [31] The conditions described are colic, constipation, diarrhea, vomiting, lack of appetite and its contrary, a voracious appetite. Jaundice was a very important symptom complex. 'If a man's body is yellow, his face is yellow . . . jaundice is the name of the disease.' [32] Prescriptions were given for the cases when the bile 'gripped' a man [33] and jaundice filled his eye.

Numerous are also the diseases of the genito-urinary organs mentioned in Assyrian tablets.

If a man in his sleep or in his walking has seminal discharge and he does not know that he went to his wife and his penis and his 'cloth' are full of seminal fluid, thou shalt mix in oil 'clay of the dust of the mountain-stone' and horned alkaḷi. Thou shalt smear a plaster on the point of the man's 'tongue.' Thou shalt pour it on the man's sore. And in oil and wine thou shalt mix it. He shall drink it and he will recover.[34]

While there is no evidence of syphilis it seems very likely that gonorrhea did occur, at least we have several passages that point to purulent discharges from the urethra, such as:

If a man's urine is like the urine of an ass, that man is sick of gonorrhea; if a man's urine is like beer-yeast, that man is sick of gonorrhea; if a man's urine is like wine-yeast, that man is sick of gonorrhea; if a man's urine is like gummy paint (varnish), that man is sick of gonorrhea.[35]

Discharge of blood or of pus and blood is mentioned in other passages: 'If a man discharges blood from his penis like a woman' [36] or, 'If from a man's penis blood and pus come forth on him, like the seizure of a jackal . . .' [37] Spermatorrhea, retention of urine, incontinence of urine, impotence are other troubles discussed in these texts, which also include prescriptions relative to sexual intercourse and general love charms.

The occurrence of renal calculus is evidenced by several texts and it seems that a distinction was made between hard and soluble stones.[38] Thus a prescription read: 'Whether it be hard or soluble stone, or gonorrhea, or strangury, or anus-trouble, or urine coming drop by drop . . .' [39] The drugs prescribed, black saltpeter, shell of ostrich-egg, pine-turpentine,[40] may not be expected to have had any effect.

Other prescriptions were for diseases of the legs and feet: [41] 'If the flesh of a man's legs has been strained so that he cannot walk,' or 'if the feet are bent and cannot straighten themselves; if a man's feet hold "poison" . . . his feet being out of control; if sickness comes out on a man's leg and it grows like a pustule.' Treatments were largely pharmacological and drugs were prescribed for internal as well as external use.

Another series dealt with symptoms localized in the tendons of the lower extremity, notably the *Kabartu* and *Sagalla* diseases,[42] which perhaps included such ailments as rheumatism, arthritis, and sciatica. These are chronic diseases against which we even today have few effective treatments, and it is no wonder that the Babylonians combated them primarily with incantations.

Examples could be multiplied indefinitely, but I think that the texts quoted are sufficient to make it evident that Babylonian and Assyrian physicians observed and described a great many symptoms of disease and, like their Egyptian colleagues, were able to correlate symptoms and saw that some usually occur in combination. Their concept of disease was not ontological like ours. The chief symptom was the disease, or the organ affected gave it the name. The causation of disease was magical or religious, to be sure, but such a view did not exclude the assumption that natural causes, such as heat, cold, food, poison, or the bite of animals also played a part in the genesis of illness. If you were sick because a scorpion had stung you,[43] this was a natural enough cause, but it still remained to be explained why the scorpion had bitten you and not someone else.

The purpose of diagnosis, as we saw, was not only to ascertain the cause of an illness, the sin committed or the demon involved, but also to ascertain character and seat of the disease. And we also found that a prognosis was made not only from external omens but from the interpretation of symptoms of disease.[44] The prognosis was not only favorable or unfavorable but sometimes more detailed: 'If the kabartu-illness is violent, the ban has "gripped" him; he will quiet down but will die later.' [45] The prognosis was sometimes combined with a verdict such as the advice to the physician not to handle a hopeless case.[46] We also have indications with regard to the course of a disease and the time that it may be expected to last or has lasted. Thus a disease is a 'swollen joint lasting two years,'[47] and 'if the tendons of his leg devour him suddenly, he cannot stand and walk, this is a Sa.Gal-disease of two years.'[48] A patient of the Liptu-series[49] who is cold in the daytime, hot at night, 'will be sick seven days and will recover.' Diseases have their time and course, and the physician must know when the moment has come for him to act: 'If a man's feet are full of diseases, these diseases have a term, the day of the diseases has been fulfilled . . .' then, before sunrise the physician will perform the incantation.[50]

Incantations frequently consisted of both an oral and a manual rite. While pronouncing the magic words, the priest performed symbolic gestures such as touching the patient with his hand, or he gave him objects charged with magic power, a string with magic knots, precious stones to be worn around the neck, or drugs compounded into a potion. The words gave the drugs their power to heal, and the medical literature proper is full of such combination treatments, much more so than the Egyptian literature. But then in Mesopotamia, too, we find many prescriptions of drugs without any indication of magic words. This does not necessarily mean that nothing was said while the drugs were given, because the words may have been taken for granted. Even in our days some patients recite a *Pater Noster* or *Ave Maria* or make the sign of the cross when they take medicine, and such rites do not appear in our textbooks. Yet there can be no doubt that pharmacological treatments were applied in Mesopotamia independently at times. Two trends came together, magic and empirical. People took drugs as manual rites of a spell, but at all times they had also known and used herbs and other drugs apart from medicine, as house remedies that gave relief and did not require any explanation.

The materia medica of Mesopotamia as investigated and identified by R. Campbell Thompson[51] includes about 250 medicinal plants, 120 mineral substances, and 180 animal and other—mostly unidentified—drugs. This does not include the various vehicles, wines, beers, fats, oils, honey, wax, and milks. Systematic as the Babylonians were, they listed their drugs not only for lexicographic reasons—although it was important enough to know the Babylonian equivalent of a Sumerian plant name—but also with a medical end in view.[52] Thus we have tablets written in three columns of which the first lists the drugs, the second the diseases for which each is to be used, and the third indicates in which form the drug must be applied, e.g.: 'root of licorice—a cough remedy—bray and drink it with oil and beer'; or 'root of sunflower—a remedy for toothache—put it on the tooth.'[53] Other texts enumerated the drugs indicated for diseases of a single organ, the eye, the mouth, or the anus. 'For sickness of the mouth' and 'to be placed upon the mouth' were such drugs as male pestilence root, green kulkullanu, turnip, khalulaia, root of sun plant, and others.[54] Still shorter texts merely listed drugs and the diseases against which they served without any further instructions.

The physician who decided upon a pharmacological treatment thus had a variety of books available for ready consultation; from mere lists of drugs and diseases to regular textbooks with symptomatology, diagnosis, prognosis, and more detailed instructions in regard to the treatment of a certain case of sickness.

The Mesopotamian materia medica was very similar to that of Egypt. Among vegetable drugs we find: fruits, such as grape, apple, pomegranate, fig; common vegetables, like garlic, onion, leek, bean, lupin, lettuce, cucumber, and pumpkin; cereals, like barley, wheat, millet, or spelt; spices and condiments were used a great deal, fennel, saffron, thyme, mustard, caraway seed, chicory, turmeric, or flowers like rose and anemone. Just as in Egypt, a great variety of resins and gums were ingredients of prescriptions; among these were myrrh, storax, ambra, opopanax, asafetida, galbanum, gum of fir and pine, and turpentine from these two trees. The country's trees and shrubs, date palm, cedar, cypress, pine, tamarisk, laurel, juniper, myrtle, box and others, provided many drugs prepared from their roots, wood, leaves, fruit, or from substances exuded. Among the more effective vegetable drugs were hellebore, hyoscyamus, mandrake, opium,[55] and hemp.[56]

When we come to animal drugs, we find all the elements of the

Dreckapotheke represented—urine, feces, hair, ground bones of animals and man. The use of fat, blood, liver, meat, and other parts of various animals could have had a rational foundation, and the borderline between dietetic and pharmacological treatment was by no means sharp. It is very likely, however, that most prescriptions of this kind had a magic origin and were intended to appease or to disgust the demon, or to gain power over him.[57] In the course of time magical and empirical elements became so interwoven that the original intention was no longer clear and a drug was given on traditional grounds.

The number of animals from which organs were used was very large. As a matter of fact, it had no limits, since parts of every animal might become ingredients of a recipe. This is not the case with plants, because some are venomous and kill whoever eats them, while the fat or meat even of a poisonous snake may be consumed without any harm.

The animals whose parts were prescribed more frequently were the domestic animals: cattle, sheep, goat, pig, donkey, dog; among wild animals: lion, wolf, fox, gazelle, the mouse and the frog, a yellow and a green frog. Birds were also frequently used for medicinal purposes: chicken, pigeon, raven, stork, swan, owl, falcon, vulture, and others.

Much more important was the use of mineral substances, of which Babylonians and Assyrians had considerable knowledge that they applied in a highly developed technology.[58] Mineral drugs occur frequently in recipes for diseases of the eyes, and here as in Egypt sulphur was used in the treatment of skin diseases. Among the chemical elements and compounds encountered in Assyrian prescriptions, we find white and black sulphur, sulphate of iron, arsenic, yellow sulphide of arsenic, arsenic trisulphide, black saltpeter, antimony, iron oxide, magnetic iron ore, sulphide of iron, pyrites, copper dust, verdigris, mercury, alum, bitumen, naphtha, calcined lime and a variety of not identified stones.

The materia medica consisted primarily of the natural products of the homeland but drugs were also imported, here as in Egypt. Thus the drug 'dadanu'[59] was used in four varieties, one native

Assyrian, two imported from Canaan and one from the peninsula of Sinai or the African coast.[60]

The first task in studying such texts is philological and consists in attempting to identify the drugs. R. Campbell Thompson did the pioneering work on this subject, and by investigating all the material available and the present flora of Mesopotamia succeeded in making many identifications. Some are conjectural, to be sure, and others will be changed on the basis of new materials, but it will always be remembered that Thompson did the spade work in this very difficult field. The next task will be medical and we shall have to decide which drugs appeared in recipes for magic reasons and which had an empirico-rational foundation, which were effective and which not. Here as in Egypt—and in our own time—drugs must have been prescribed occasionally merely because the patient expected something to be done.

The recipes not only list drugs, but give sometimes detailed instructions on how to compound and apply them. They were brayed in a mortar, as a rule, and if liquid were strained. Infusions were made in wine or in strong vinegar. Grape wine and date wine, sweetened wine, and wine that was 'neither purified nor clarified' were frequently used as vehicles, as were also various kinds of milk. Curd was a vehicle particularly for drugs used in the treatment of diseases of the eyes. Thus a recipe for a man whose 'eyes are sick and full of blood . . . blood and tears coming forth from the eyes, a film closing over the pupils . . .' read:

> . . . thou shalt beat leaves of tamarisk, steep them in strong vinegar, leave them out under the stars; in the morning thou shalt squeeze them in a helmet: white alum, storax, 'Akkadian salt,' fat, cornflour, nigella, 'gum of copper,' separately thou shalt bray: thou shalt take equal part of them, put them together; pour them into the helmet in which thou hast squeezed the tamarisk; in curd and šuniš-mineral thou shalt knead it, and open his eyelids with a finger and put it in his eyes. While his eyes contain dimness, his eyes thou shalt smear, and for nine days thou shalt do this.[61]

I have quoted this text as an example of an elaborate recipe that gives a graphic picture of how an eye remedy was compounded and applied. Other compositions were rubbed into the eye with a bronze blade.[62] Potions were frequently drunk through a tube, and tubes were also used to blow medicaments into nose, ear, urethra, and anus. Salves and ointments prepared with a great variety of fats were rubbed into the skin in an operation that amounted to some kind of massage. Or the salve was smeared on a piece of cloth or leather which then was placed on the sore part and attached with a bandage.

Fumigation was a very popular method of treating various organs with drugs. Thus the ears were fumigated with 'seed of juniper, seed of laurel, liquidambar, male and female, horse hair, glue (?), by means of fire.'[63] Diseases of chest and lungs seemed to respond particularly well to such treatments:

> . . . if a man is affected in the lungs, thou shalt spread powder of tar over a thornfire, let the smoke enter his anus . . . his mouth and nostrils, it shall make him cough(?): thou shalt bathe him with water of Vitex: thou shalt anoint the whole of his body with curd: thou shalt bray linseed either in milk (?) . . . , bind on him for three days, and let his tongue hold honey and refined oil . . .[64]

This is a good example of a combined treatment including fumigation, medicated bath, anointment, poultice, and internal medication. Fumigation of a different kind was one with 'pig-dung, dog-dung, jackal-dung, fox-dung, gazelle-dung, ammi (?), salicornia-alkali, hart's horn, sulphur, bitumen, human bone, glue, (?), in fire,[65] which was practiced when a ghost had seized a man. The acrid smoke which must have developed from such a mixture was obviously directed at the ghost.

Like their Egyptian colleagues, the Assyrian doctors possessed an apparatus for inhalations. A decoction of various drugs was placed into a pot, which was sealed with wheaten dough after a reed-tube had been inserted into it. The pot was placed on fire and then: 'thou shalt put it [the tube] into his mouth, let him draw the steam up by the reed-tube into his mouth . . . it shall strike his lungs: for nine days thou shalt do this.'[66] Suppositories and enemas were given for rectal medication; in the local treatment of urinary diseases, drugs were injected or blown into the urethra through a copper or bronze tube.

The prescriptions also contain instructions in regard to the time when a remedy was to be made and when it was to be taken. Potions were frequently prepared in the evening and were kept open during the night 'under the stars,' whereupon patients had to drink them in the morning 'on an empty stomach.' [67] 'In the morning without a meal let him drink' [68] or, 'in the morning before the sun rises, before he puts foot to the ground he shall drink.' [69] Or a potion was to be taken in the evening, 'he shall drink it at the approach of the star.' [70]

It is striking that unlike the Egyptian prescriptions those of Assyria rarely contain indications about weights and measures. They do sometimes. Thus we may find that various drugs must be compounded in 'equal parts,' or 'equal portions.' [71] In some cases, we hear what the weight was to be: '10 shekels of fir-turpentine, 10 shekels of roses, 10 shekels of galbanum, mustard, salicornia-alkali, these six drugs as local regulator (?) of the bile he shall drink.' [72] As a rule, however, we have no indications, and this is particularly strange since some highly toxic drugs were used, such as mandrake, opium, hemp or hyoscyamus. It may be that there was a certain convention in regard to the amount that was to be taken, so that it need not be prescribed explicitly in each case, and the physician must have known that there was a maximal dose for some drugs.

Here as in Egypt, we have no special treatises on diets. It was not until the Greek period that the regulation of a patient's diet became one of the chief methods of treatment, but it is obvious that attention was always paid to a sick man's mode of living, and to what he ate and drank. A prescription for 'a man sick of a cough' read: 'Ground lolium, pounded roses, as mixture thou shalt mix, let him eat it in oil and honey; let him drink soup of pig's meat; when he goes to stool thou shalt light a fire before him, he shall direct it to his anus, and shall recover.' [73] In this prescription we have a combination of pharmacological, dietetic, and physical treatments. Another recipe including dietetic considerations read: 'If a man has a pain inside, food and drink coming back to his mouth, bandage his head and breast. Boil . . . let him eat it with honey, lamb fat and butter. Let him refrain from eating onions, white onions and kidnu for three days, and not wash himself with water and he will recover.' [74]

Physical means were also employed in the treatment of patients. We already mentioned the application of heat, the use of medicated baths and massage. In order to make a sick man vomit, the physician tickled his throat with a feather.[75] Cramps were treated with hot or cold water and various manipulations as described in the following instructions: [76]

> If a man has cramps, let that man sit down with his feet under him, pour boiled . . . and cassia juice over his head and he will recover.
>
> If *ditto*, let him kneel and pour cold water on his head.
>
> If *ditto*, place his head downwards and his feet [under him?], manipulate his back with the thumb, saying 'be good,' manipulate his arms fourteen times, manipulate his head fourteen times, rolling him on the ground . . .

We know that surgery was practiced at an early date in Mesopotamia, since the Code of Hammurabi dealt with the surgeon's liability. It is also perfectly obvious that the armies had surgeons who knew how to treat wounds. Patients must have been bled here as everywhere else in antiquity, either through phlebotomy or cupping.[77] Yet since we do not possess a single surgical text we know nothing about Babylonian and Assyrian surgery. This in itself is not astonishing because surgery is not learned from books, as we mentioned in the case of Egypt. Yet we would expect to have texts dealing with the treatment of wounds, abscesses, tumors, and other surgical diseases. It is very possible that further excavations will bring such texts to light.

A system of medicine that was dominated by magic and religion, and the purpose of which was to rehabilitate an individual and to reconcile him with the transcendental world, obviously included psychotherapy. The soul-searching of a patient who was convinced that he suffered because he had sinned had a liberating effect; and the rites performed and the words spoken by the incantation priest had a profound suggestive power. Mesopotamian medicine was psychosomatic in all its aspects.

Unlike Egypt, Mesopotamia never developed a rational theory of life in health and disease, and we have nothing comparable to the Egyptian theory of the *metu.* The gods created man, gave life to every individual born, and they also sent illness. Disease had a seat, to be sure; it affected the body as a whole or a certain organ, but the localization was vague as also was the Babylonian's anatomical knowledge, which here, as in all archaic civilizations, was derived from observations on animals—in the kitchen and on the sacrificial altar—and from chance observations on wounded people.

The only literature dealing with parts of the body consisted of lists of names in Sumerian and Akkadian.[78] Occasionally organs were related to a specific god, as in Egypt,[79] but there is no doubt that the Babylonians did not dissect bodies, and there is no reason why they should have done so. Their approach to the problems of disease was not a realistic anatomical one but was spiritual. This also explains why they did not speculate about what we should call the physiological functions of the organs, but rather considered them the seat of emotions and of mental functions in general. Thus the heart was believed to be the seat of the intellect, the liver of affectivity, the stomach of cunning, the uterus of compassion, ears and eyes of attention.[80] Similar views survived the centuries and millennia, and are still reflected in our language, when we speak of someone being kind-hearted, choleric, or bright-eyed.

Disease was sent by the gods and caused by evil spirits or witchcraft, but we saw that natural causes such as exposure to cold or alcoholic intoxication were occasionally made responsible for illness. We also find primitive attempts to explain the mechanism of a disease rationally. A man is sick because his 'body is full of uncleanness.'[81] In another case a 'man is sick of a painful swelling and the muscle of his heel is full of "wind,"'[82] or 'a man is sick of a painful swelling and his feet are full of blood.'[83] We also remember the letter of Nabu-nasir in which he made sick teeth responsible for burning of head, hands, and feet.[84] The texts are vague and do not state explicitly that uncleanness, wind, or blood are the immediate cause of the patient's illness. We are not justified to declare on the basis of these and similar passages that the Assyrians had a humoral or pneumatic theory of disease.[85] They never developed pathological theories of this type, but they certainly knew that humors, air, uncleanness, played a part in the genesis of diseases, and had observed that a sick organ affected other parts of the body.

*

Epilogue

The great civilizations of Egypt and Mesopotamia were contemporaneous and developed in neighboring territories. Traffic between the countries was lively from remote antiquity on. Goods were exchanged in friendly intercourse and nations clashed in armed conflicts at times. It is no wonder that the two civilizations had a great deal in common. They developed from the stone age to the copper, bronze, and iron ages at about the same time. Their economy, their form of government, their religion, their art and literature, their mode of living were similar in many ways, and their medicine consisted basically of the same magic, religious, and empirical elements. But the geography of the two countries was different, and so were the carriers of their culture. Hence, we find significant differences in religious concepts, in the administration of justice, in artistic styles, and in general customs. In medicine, while the elements were the same, yet the emphasis was different. Egypt, so far as our present knowledge goes, developed the empirical and rational side more highly and earlier than Mesopotamia, where magic and religious practices maintained their dominating influence to the very end.

Both countries lost their independence in the course of the first millennium B.C., but many elements of their culture survived them and were taken over and assimilated by the peoples who succeeded them. This was particularly the case with technical knowledge. Literature is bound to the language of a people, art is the most subtle expression, the rare flower of its culture, and cannot be transplanted to another people, at least not without undergoing profound changes. But technical knowledge, means and methods, cross borderlines in space and time. The accumulated experience of centuries in mathematics, astronomy, astrology, engineering, agriculture, and medicine are passed on, become the starting point of new developments, or at least act as stimulus and ferment. Theories are not so easily propagated since they are deeply rooted in the general philosophy of a society, an expression of the attitude of man toward his fellow man, toward nature and the world at large. A young people may adopt a theory from an old civilization on which it borders or to which it succeeds, but merely as a loan. Sooner or later it will create its own systems to explain the world, to explain the phenomena of life in health and disease. But facts, observations, treatments, drugs, and operations that have stood the test of time are taken over and incorporated into the body of a society's own experiences.

Both Egypt and Mesopotamia, and the latter perhaps in a higher degree, influenced their neighbors, the peoples of Syria, Asia Minor, and of the islands of the Eastern Mediterranean. The empires of the Hittites, of Mitanni and many others perished, but the Hebrew people survived all vicissitudes of their history and were to play a particularly important part as transmitters of Oriental knowledge to the Christian West as well as to the Islamic East. Deeply influenced by Mesopotamian civilization, they were also in close touch with Egypt. They had no medical literature proper, but the books of the Old Testament reflected medical views and passed them on to the medieval world in the West and in the East. We shall discuss Biblical medicine when it begins to exert its influence as a link between the Ancient Orient and the Middle Ages.

The conquest of Babylonia and Egypt by the Persians in the sixth century B.C. marked the final eclipse of the Ancient Orient and the decisive victory of the Indo-European peoples. They were to lead the destinies of the Near East until the advent of Islam, and those of Europe and India to the present day. As long as Mesopotamian civilization was creative and strong, it assimilated foreign conquerors without difficulty, but even in the sixth century before Christ, when it had long completed its course, it was strong enough to imprint its stamp upon the Persians, who wrote their triumphant inscriptions in cuneiform script and borrowed and adapted elements of Mesopotamian art. They also used the Aramaic alphabet from which the Middle Persian Pehlevi alphabet was derived, and wrote their diplomatic correspondence with the West in Aramaic, which was becoming the international language of the Near East.

From a provincial town Babylon once more, for a very short while, became a world capital when Alexander the Great established his residence there in 331 B.C., but his sudden death eight years later prevented the city from becoming the glorious center of a great Graeco-Asiatic empire. Babylonians and Greeks had met long before the time of Alexander. Through the intermediary of Crete and Phoenicia, Mesopotamia like Egypt influenced Greece at an early date. In the cities of Asia Minor a constant interchange, not only of goods but also of ideas, took place and we shall see how the pre-Socratic philosophers borrowed from their Eastern neighbors. The physicians did also and learned from Egypt and Mesopotamia more than the mere use of certain drugs.

Another channel through which Mesopotamian medical lore was transmitted to the Middle Ages was the Syriac medical literature, which flourished in the schools of the Nestorians on Mesopotamian soil. Consisting for the most part of translations from the Greek, it nevertheless included many early Oriental elements.[86]

These, however, were mere reminiscences. When Babylon fell to the Persians, a new medicine was dawning, created by the Western branch of the Indo-European family, the Greeks, and by its Eastern branch, the Indians. The discussion of this new medicine as it developed in East and West will be the subject of our next volume.

NOTES

1. About diseases of the head see Thompson's translations in *Amer. J. Sem. Lang.*, 1907-8, 24:1-6, 323-53; *Proc. Roy. Soc. Med.*, Sect. Hist. Med., 1924, 17:2-22; op. cit. 1926, 19:55-7.
2. Thompson, *Proc. Roy. Soc. Med.*, Sect. Med. Hist., 1924, 17:12.
3. Ibid. p. 10f.
4. Thompson, *Am. J. Sem. Lang.*, 1907-8, 24:350.

5. Ibid.
6. Thompson, 'Assyrian Prescriptions for Diseases of the Ears,' *J. Roy. Asiat. Soc.*, 1931, pp. 1-25.
7. Ibid. pp. 8-10.
8. Thompson, 'Assyrian Medical Texts,' *Proc. Roy. Soc. Med.*, Sect. Hist. Med., 1924, 17: 22-34; op. cit. 1926, 19:30-55; V. Scheil, 'Quelques Remèdes pour les yeux,' *Rev. Assyr.*, 1918, 15:75-80; Arlington C. Krause, 'Assyro-Babylonian Ophthalmology,' *Ann. Med. Hist.*, 1934, N.S. 6:42-55.
9. F. Küchler, *Beiträge zur Kenntnis der assyrisch-babylonischen Medizin*, Leipzig, 1904, p. 55.
10. Thompson, *Proc. Roy. Soc. Med.*, Sect. Hist. Med., 1926, 19:69-78.
11. Ibid. p. 73.
12. Ibid. p. 77.
13. Ibid. p. 71f.
14. Ibid. pp. 57-62. See B. W. Weinberger's discussion in his *An Introduction to the History of Dentistry*, St. Louis, 1948, vol. I, p. 36ff.
15. Thompson, loc. cit. p. 70
16. Thompson, 'Assyrian Prescriptions for Diseases of the Chest and Lungs,' *Rev. Assyr.*, 1934, 31:8.
17. Ibid. p. 17.
18. Ibid. p. 19.
19. E. Ebeling, 'Keilschrifttafeln medizinischen Inhalts,' *Arch. Gesch. Med.*, 1921, 13:16.
20. Thompson, loc. cit. p. 20.
21. Ibid. p. 21.
22. Ibid. p. 22.
23. Ebeling, loc. cit. p. 14.
24. R. Labat and Jacques Tournay, 'Un Texte médical inédit,' *Rev. Assyr.*, 1945-6, 40:115.
25. Ebeling, loc. cit. p. 17.
26. Thompson, loc. cit. p. 2f. and many similar passages here as well as in Ebeling.
27. Thompson, loc. cit. p. 10.
28. Thompson, 'Assyrian Prescriptions for Stone in the Kidneys, for the "Middle," and for Pneumonia,' *Arch. Orientforschung*, 1936-7, 11:336-40.
29. See Thompson, 'Assyrian Medical Prescriptions for Diseases of the Stomach,' *Rev. Assyr.*, 1929, 26:47-92.
30. Küchler, p. 1ff.
31. Ibid. p. 27.
32. Küchler, p. 55.
33. Ibid. p. 51ff.
34. H. F. Lutz, 'A Contribution to the Knowledge of Assyro-Babylonian Medicine,' *Am. J. Sem. Lang. Lit.*, 1919-20, 36:74.
35. Thompson, 'Assyrian Prescriptions for Diseases of the Urine, etc.,' *Babyloniaca*, 1934, 14:108-9.
36. Lutz, loc. cit. p. 74.
37. Thompson, loc. cit. p. 96.

38. Ibid. p. 111ff.
39. E. Ebeling, *Keilschrifttexte aus Assur religiösen Inhalts*, II, no. 73, obv. 1ff., 18ff.
40. Thompson, *Arch. Orientforschung*, 1936-7, 11:338.
41. Thompson, 'Assyrian Prescriptions for Diseases of the Feet,' *J. Roy. Asiat. Soc.*, 1937, pp. 265-86, 413-32.
42. E. Ebeling, 'Keilschrifttexte medizinischen Inhalts,' *Arch. Gesch. Med.*, 1921, 13:129-44; op. cit. 1923, 14:26-47.
43. Ch. Fossey, 'Textes inédits ou incomplètement publiés: Recettes contre les piqûres,' *Zschr. Assyr.*, 1905-6, 19:175-81; R. C. Thompson, 'Assyrian Medical Prescriptions against Shimmatu "poison,"' *Rev. Assyr.*, 1930, 27:127-36.
44. See O. Temkin's discussion in *Kyklos*, 1930, 3:126ff.
45. Ebeling, *Arch. Gesch. Med.*, 1923, 14:34.
46. E.g. in Küchler, p. 63.
47. Thompson, 'An Assyrian Incantation against Rheumatism,' *Proc. Soc. Bibl. Archaeol.*, 1908, 30:68.
48. Ebeling, loc. cit. 1921, 13:132.
49. A series dealing with the prognostic evaluation of a pustule or abscess, published by Ch. Virolleaud, 'Pronostics sur l'issue de diverses maladies,' *Babyloniaca*, 1907, p. 96ff. See Contenau, *Médecine*, p. 174ff.
50. Ebeling, loc. cit. 1923, 14:35.
51. R. Campbell Thompson, *The Assyrian Herbal*, London, 1924.
52. Such lists are published in *Cuneiform Texts from Babylonian Tablets, etc. in the British Museum*, vol. XIV; some of them have been reproduced and translated by M. Jastrow, 'The Medicine of the Babylonians and Assyrians,' *Proc. Roy. Soc. Med.*, Sect. Hist. Med., 1914, 7:152ff.; others by V. Scheil, 'Un Document médical assyrien,' *Rev. Assyr.*, 1916, 13:35-42.
53. Meissner, vol. II, p. 295.
54. Jastrow, loc. cit. p. 157.
55. Haupt, *Zschr. Assyr.*, vol. 30, pp. 60-66; Justin Zehnder, 'Le Pavot et son usage chez les assyriens,' *Soc. Helvét. Sc. Nat.*, Lausanne, 1928, Sect. de Pharmacie.
56. W. F. Albright, 'Assyr. *martakal* "Haschisch" und amurtinnu "Sidra,"' *Zsch. Assyr.*, 1926, 37:140.
57. See the discussion of M. Jastrow, loc. cit. p. 158ff.
58. See Thompson, *On the chemistry of ancient Assyrians*, London, 1925; 'An Assyrian Chemist's Vademecum,' *J. Roy. Asiat. Soc.*, 1934, pp. 771-85; 'On some Assyrian minerals,' ibid. 1933, pp. 885-95; *A Dictionary of Assyrian Chemistry and Geology*, London, 1936.
59. According to Jastrow, loc. cit. p. 154, a thorn, while Thompson, *Herbal*, p. 77, believes it to be gum arabic.
60. *Cuneiform Texts in the Brit. Mus.*, XIV, pl. 21, col. 5, lines 18-22, Jastrow, loc. cit. p. 154.
61. Thompson, *Proc. Roy. Soc. Med.*, Sect. Hist. Med., 1924, 17:28-9.
62. Ibid. pp. 25, 27.
63. Thompson, *J. Roy. Asiat. Soc.*, 1931, p. 4.

64. Thompson, *Rev. Assyr.*, 1934, 31:18.
65. Thompson, *J. Roy. Asiat. Soc.*, 1929, p. 802.
66. Thompson, *Rev. Assyr.*, 1934, 31:19.
67. Labat and Tournay, *Rev. Assyr.*, 1945-6, 40:115.
68. Thompson, *Proc. Roy. Soc. Med.*, Sect. Hist. Med., 1924, 17:21.
69. Thompson, *Babyloniaca*, 1934, 14:126.
70. Lutz, *Am. J. Sem. Lang.*, 1919-20, 36:72ff.
71. Thompson, loc. cit. p. 108.
72. Labat and Tournay, loc. cit. p. 115. Other example Thompson, loc. cit. p. 106.
73. Thompson, *Rev. Assyr.*, 1934, 31:6.
74. M. Jastrow, 'Babylonian-Assyrian Medicine,' *Ann. Med. Hist.*, 1918, 1:241.
75. Thompson, loc. cit. p. 17 *et passim.*
76. Jastrow, loc. cit. p. 241.
77. It was formerly believed that the seal of the physician Ur-Lugal-edinna preserved at the Louvre included the picture of two cupping vessels and of another instrument for bleeding, a kind of lancet (see R. Zehnpfund, 'Zukakîpu, das Schröpfinstrument der Babylonier,' *Beitr. z. Assyr.*, 1902, 4:220-26). Meissner (vol. II, p. 285) thought that the vessels were recipients for salves and the lancets surgical needles, while Contenau (*Médecine*, pp. 41-2) believes that the vessels or vases are symbols of the god of vegetation and that the instruments that look like lancets or needles are whips such as are commonly used by shepherds.
78. H. Holma, 'Die Namen der Körperteile im Assyrisch-Babylonischen,' *Ann. Acad. Scient. Fennicae*, ser. B, vol. 8, 1. Helsinki, 1911.
79. Ibid. XIV. *Cuneiform Texts in the Brit. Mus.*, XXIV, 45, 51ff.; Meissner, vol. II, p. 293.
80. P. Dhorme, *L'Emploi métaphorique des noms des parties du corps en hébreu et en akkadien*, Paris, 1923; Meissner, vol. II, p. 293.
81. Thompson, *J. Soc. Orient. Research*, 1931, 15:54.
82. Thompson, *J. Roy. Asiat. Soc.*, 1937, p. 284.
83. Ibid.
84. R. H. Pfeiffer, *State Letters of Assyria*, New Haven, 1935, p. 198.
85. See A. Leix, *Ciba Symposia*, 1940, 2:681.
86. Such a book was published by E. A. Wallis Budge, *Syrian Anatomy, Pathology and Therapeutics, or 'The Book of Medicines,'* London, 1913, 2 vols., a book which includes an abstract from Galen's περὶ πεπονθότων τόπων, Hellenistic astrological medicine and a popular Syrian medical book with 'native prescriptions'; see M. Jastrow, *Ann. Med. Hist.*, 1918, 1:255-6.

APPENDIX I

*

Histories of Medicine

Medical history was written at all times. The author of the Hippocratic treatise on *Ancient Medicine* speculated about the origins of the craft.[1] The writer or writers who compiled the *Anonymus Londinensis* collected physicians' and philosophers' views on the etiology of diseases and on physiology.[2] Celsus felt impelled to begin the medical section of his Encyclopaedia with a historical sketch,[3] and Soranus, in the second century of the Christian era, wrote biographies of physicians.

The tradition was not lost in the Middle Ages. Even in early medieval manuscripts we find a short text outlining the history of medicine,[4] and in the East Ibn abī Uṣaibi'a's story of the physicians [5] remained unsurpassed for many centuries. Renaissance writers such as Polydore Vergil,[6] and particularly Symphorien Champier,[7] wrote outlines of medical history. New editions were published of the Greek and Arabic classics, not for historical reasons but as textbooks. Ancient medicine was alive until the nineteenth century and whatever medical historiography there was, was pragmatic as a matter of course. K. Sprengel significantly called his great book *Versuch einer pragmatischen Geschichte der Arzneykunde*,[8] a book that in Sudhoff's opinion—which I fully share—was unsurpassed for over a century.

The attitude toward the past of medicine changed in the course of the nineteenth century, and the writing of medical history followed the trends of general historiography. It cannot be the purpose of this brief appendix to analyze these trends [9] or to give a bibliography of the numerous histories of medicine written in every country during the century. The following select list intends rather to acquaint the reader with (1.) general histories of medicine, (2.) histories of medical disciplines, (3.) histories of medicine of single countries, and (4.) histories of diseases, which today may be consulted profitably. Books dealing with special periods or special problems have been or will be referred to in footnotes as our work proceeds.

1. GENERAL HISTORIES OF MEDICINE

We must distinguish between books written by one man and those written by a group of historians. The latter have the advantage that every chapter is written by a specialist, but on the other hand, the serious disadvantage that they do not present an integrated picture of developments. It usually happens, moreover, that the individual contributions are very uneven in quality. The two chief books of this type are:

Handbuch der Geschichte der Medizin, initiated by Th. Puschmann, edited by M. Neuburger and J. Pagel, Jena, 1902-5, 3 vols. Very unbalanced and uneven, antiquated in many ways but still useful for the enormous amount of material it contains.

Histoire générale de la médecine, de la pharmacie, de l'art dentaire et de l'art vétérinaire, ed. by Laignel-Lavastine and B. Guégan, Paris, 1936-49, 3 vols. Beautifully presented with superb illustrations; text very unbalanced with some very competent and some rather poor contributions.

Of the books written by individual historians, the following may be mentioned:

Heinrich Haeser, *Lehrbuch der Geschichte der Medicin und der epidemischen Krankheiten,* Jena, 3rd ed., 1875-82, 3 vols. Still a very useful book, chiefly for the literature it gives and for the excellent summaries of medical achievements in certain periods.

E. T. W. Withington, *Medical History from the Earliest Times,* London, 1894. Short and witty.

Max Neuburger, *Geschichte der Medizin,* Stuttgart, 1906-11, vol. 1 and vol. 2, part I. English edition, London, 1910-25. Includes antiquity and the Middle Ages. The most philosophic history of medicine.

Sir William Osler, *The Evolution of Modern Medicine,* New Haven, 1921. Interesting as it shows how a great clinician looked at the history of his science.

Karl Sudhoff, *Kurzes Handbuch der Geschichte der Medizin* [=3rd and 4th ed. of Julius Leopold Pagel, *Einführung in die Geschichte der Medizin*], Berlin, 1922. An authoritative account with comprehensive bibliographic references; primarily a history of medical science and medical literature.

Th. Meyer-Steineg and Karl Sudhoff, *Geschichte der Medizin im Überblick mit Abbildungen,* Jena, 3rd ed., 1928. A good short presentation.

Charles Singer, *A Short History of Medicine,* Oxford, 1928. Concise, didactic, an excellent introductory book.

Fielding H. Garrison, *Introduction to the History of Medicine,* Philadelphia and London, 4th ed., 1929. Somewhat unbalanced in that one half of the book is devoted to the 19th and 20th centuries, but valuable for its wealth of biographical and bibliographical data.

Henry E. Sigerist, *Einführung in die Medizin,* Leipzig, 1931. (*Man and Medicine,* New York and London, 1932; also French, Swedish, Dutch, Italian, Chinese.) A cross-section through modern medicine, developed historically.

Henry E. Sigerist, *Grosse Ärzte,* Munich, 2nd ed. [1933]. (*Great Doctors,* London and New York, 1933; also Spanish.) A short biographic history of medicine.

L. Aschoff and P. Diepgen, *Kurze Übersichtstabellen zur Geschichte der Medizin,* Munich, 3rd ed., 1936. Convenient for quick orientation.

Victor Robinson, *The Story of Medicine,* New York, 2nd ed., 1943. A good general survey, competently written with a strong personal touch.

D. Guthrie, *A History of Medicine,* London, 1945. Short, rather conventional survey.

Richard H. Shryock, *The Development of Modern Medicine,* New York, 1947. The history of medicine seen by a social historian and giving a brilliant 'interpretation of the social and scientific factors involved.'

Cecilia C. Mettler, *History of Medicine,* Philadelphia, 1947. Not a history of medicine but a series of essays on the history of the various medical disciplines, rather disconnected and not very critical.

A. Pazzini, *Storia della medicina,* Milan, 1947, 2 vols. Competent and well written.

Arturo Castiglioni, *Storia della medicina,* Milan, new (3rd) ed., 1948, 2 vols. (2nd English ed., New York, 1947, in one vol.; also French, Spanish, Portuguese, German.) The best one- or two-volume presentation of the subject available at the moment.

2. HISTORIES OF MEDICAL DISCIPLINES AND ALLIED SUBJECTS

There are monographs available on the history of most medical sciences and specialties but many of these books are out of date. Some of the volumes of the very attractive series *Clio Medica* have been included, but one must keep in mind that they are very short and some of them very sketchy. The chief books to be consulted profitably as a first approach are:

ANATOMY: Ch. Singer, *The Evolution of Anatomy*, London and New York, 1925; G. W. Corner, *Anatomy* (Clio Medica), New York, 1930; J. L. Choulant, *Geschichte und Bibliographie der anatomischen Abbildungen*, Leipzig, 1852 (English edition by M. Frank, Chicago, 1920); F. J. Cole, *A History of Comparative Anatomy from Aristotle to the Eighteenth Century*, London, 1944.

BACTERIOLOGY: W. Bulloch, *The History of Bacteriology*, London and New York, 1938; W. Ford, *Bacteriology* (Clio Medica), 1939.

BIOLOGY: E. Rádl, *Geschichte der biologischen Theorien seit dem Ende des 17. Jahrhunderts*, Leipzig, 1905-9, 2 parts (part I reissued 1913) (English edition by E. J. Hartfield, London and New York, 1930); E. Nordenskiöld, *Die Geschichte der Biologie*, Jena, 1926. Ch. Singer, *A Short History of Biology*, London, 1931 (American edition: *A History of Biology*, New York, 1950.)

BOTANY: Ernst Meyer, *Geschichte der Botanik*, Königsberg, 1854-7, 4 vols.; J. Sachs, *Geschichte der Botanik vom 16. Jahrhundert bis* 1860, Munich, 1875; J. R. Green, *A History of Botany*, 1860-1900, Oxford, 1909; R. J. Harvey-Gibson, *Outlines of the History of Botany*, London, 1919.

CHEMISTRY: H. Kopp, *Geschichte der Chemie*, Braunschweig, 1843-7, 4 vols.; H. Kopp, *Die Entwicklung der Chemie in der neueren Zeit*, Munich, 1873; J. Ch. Hoefer, *Histoire de la chimie*, Paris, 1867, 2 vols.; C. Graebe, *Geschichte der organischen Chemie*, Berlin, 1920, continued by P. Walden, *Geschichte der organischen Chemie seit* 1880, Berlin, 1941; F. Lieben, *Geschichte der physiologischen Chemie*, Leipzig and Vienna, 1935; H. E. Fierz-David, *Die Entwicklungsgeschichte der Chemie*, Basle, 1945

DENTISTRY: B. W. Weinberger, *An Introduction to the History of Dentistry*, St. Louis, 1948, 2 vols. (vol. II is devoted to America); B. W. Weinberger, *Orthodontics, an Historical Review of Its Origin and Evolution, including an Extensive Bibliography*, St. Louis, 1926, 2 pts.; V. Guerini, *A History of Dentistry from the Most Ancient Times until the End of the* 18*th Century*, Philadelphia and New York, 1909; K. Sudhoff, *Geschichte der Zahnheilkunde*, Leipzig, 2nd ed., 1926; H. L. Strömgren, *Die Zahnheilkunde im achtzehnten Jahrhundert*, Copenhagen, 1935; H. L. Strömgren, *Die Zahnheilkunde im neun-*

zehnten Jahrhundert, Copenhagen, 1945; C. Proskauer, *Iconographia odontologica,* Berlin, 1926.

DERMATOLOGY: P. Richter, 'Geschichte der Dermatologie,' *Handbuch der Haut- und Geschlechtskrankheiten,* vol. 14, Berlin, 1928; W. A. Pusey, *The History of Dermatology,* Springfield, Ill., 1933.

EDUCATION: Th. Puschmann, *Geschichte des medizinischen Unterrichts von den ältesten Zeiten bis zur Gegenwart,* Leipzig, 1889.

EMBRYOLOGY: J. Needham, *A History of Embryology,* Cambridge, 1934; A. W. Meyer, *The Rise of Embryology,* San Francisco and London, 1939; B. Bloch, *Die geschichtlichen Grundlagen der Embryologie bis auf Harvey* (Nova Acta Kais. Leop. Karol. Deut. Ak. Naturf., vol. 82, no. 3), Halle, 1904.

GYNECOLOGY: I. Fischer, 'Geschichte der Gynäkologie,' *Biologie u. Pathologie des Weibes,* vol. I, pp. 1-202, Berlin and Vienna, 1924; P. Diepgen, *Geschichte der Frauenheilkunde,* I. 'Die Frauenheilkunde der Alten Welt,' *Handbuch der Gynäkologie,* edited by W. Stoeckel, 3rd ed., vol. 12, part I, Munich, 1937; E. W. Jameson, *Gynecology and Obstetrics* (Clio Medica), New York, 1936.

HYGIENE AND PUBLIC HEALTH: Sir George Newman, *The Rise of Preventive Medicine,* Oxford, 1932. Sir Arthur Newsholme, *The Evolution of Preventive Medicine,* Baltimore, 1927; A. Newsholme, *The Story of Modern Preventive Medicine, a Continuation,* Baltimore, 1929; Ch.-E. A. Winslow, *The Conquest of Epidemic Diseases, a Chapter in the History of Ideas,* Princeton, 1943; P. Trisca, *Aperçu sur l'histoire de la médecine préventive,* Paris, 1923; A. Castiglioni, 'Storia dell'igiene,' *Trattato italiano d'igiene,* Turin, 1926; A. Fischer, *Geschichte des deutschen Gesundheitswesens,* Berlin, 1933, 2 vols. (limited to Germany but with many sidelights on other countries); Th. Weyl and M. Weinberg, 'Zur Geschichte der sozialen Hygiene,' *Handbuch der Hygiene,* edited by Th. Weyl, 4th supp. vol., Jena, 1904; A. Gottstein, *Geschichte der Hygiene im 19. Jahrhundert,* Berlin, 1901.

MEDICINE: J. Petersen, *Hauptmomente in der geschichtlichen Entwicklung der medicinischen Therapie,* Copenhagen, 1877; *Hauptmomente in der älteren Geschichte der medicinischen Klinik,* Copenhagen, 1889; K. H. Faber, *Nosography: the Evolution of Clinical Medicine in Modern Times,* New York, 2nd ed., 1930; H. Rolleston, *Internal Medicine* (Clio Medica), New York, 1930.

MILITARY MEDICINE: F. H. Garrison, *Notes on the History of Military Medicine,* Washington, 1922; A. Cabanès, *Chirurgiens et blessés à travers l'histoire,* Paris, 1918; S. Saitta, *Il servizio sanitario di guerra attraverso i secoli,* Catania, 1924.

NEUROLOGY: J. Soury, *Le Système nerveux central; structure et fonction; histoire critique des théories et des doctrines,* Paris, 1899; F. H. Garrison, 'History of Neurology,' *Textbook of Nervous Diseases,* edited by Ch. L. Dana, New York, 10th ed., 1925.

NURSING: L. R. Seymer, *A General History of Nursing,* London, 1949; V. Robinson, *White Caps: The Story of Nursing,* Philadelphia, 1946; M. A. Nutting and L. L. Dock, *A History of Nursing,* New York, 1907-12, 4 vols.; L. L. Dock and I. M. Stewart, *A Short History of Nursing,* New York, 4th ed., 1938.

OBSTETRICS: E. C. J. von Siebold, *Versuch einer Geschichte der Geburtshülfe,* Tübingen, 2nd ed., 1901-2, 2 vols. (reprinted from 1st ed., Berlin, 1839-45); H. Fasbender, *Geschichte der Geburtshülfe,* Jena, 1906; H. Thoms, *Classical Contributions to Obstetrics and Gynecology,* Springfield and Baltimore, 1935.

OPHTHALMOLOGY: J. Hirschberg, 'Geschichte der Augenheilkunde,' *Handbuch der gesamten Augenheilkunde,* edited by Graefe-Saemisch, Leipzig, 1899-1918, 4 vols. in 10 pts.; B. Chance, *Ophthalmology* (Clio Medica), New York, 1939.

ORTHOPEDICS: E. M. Bick, *History and Source Book of Orthopaedic Surgery,* New York, 1933; S. Mencke, *Zur Geschichte der Orthopädie,* Munich, 1930; R. B. Osgood, *The Evolution of Orthopaedic Surgery,* St. Louis, 1925.

OTO-RHINO-LARYNGOLOGY: A. Politzer, *Geschichte der Ohrenheilkunde,* Stuttgart, 1907-13, 2 vols.; K. Kassel, *Geschichte der Nasenheilkunde von ihren Anfängen bis zum* 18. *Jahrhundert,* Würzburg, 1914 (continued in articles in *Zschr. Laryng. Rhinol. Grenzgeb.,* 1914-22, vols. 7-11); C. Chauveau, *Histoire des maladies du pharynx,* Paris, 1901-6, 5 vols.; J. Wright, *History of Laryngology and Rhinology,* Philadelphia, 2nd ed., 1914.

PEDIATRICS: J. von Bokay, *Die Geschichte der Kinderheilkunde,* Berlin, 1922; F. H. Garrison, 'History of Pediatrics,' *Pediatrics,* edited by I. A. Abt, vol. I, Philadelphia, 1923; J. Ruhräh, *Pediatrics of the Past,* New York, 1925; G. F. Still, *The History of Paediatrics,* London, 1931.

PATHOLOGY: E. R. Long, *A History of Pathology,* Baltimore, 1928; E. R. Long, *Selected Readings in Pathology,* Springfield, Ill., 1929; E. B. Krumbhaar, *Pathology* (Clio Medica), New York, 1937; H. Ribbert, *Die Lehre vom Wesen der Krankheit in ihrer geschichtlichen Entwick-*

lung, Bonn, 1899; E. Goldschmid, *Entwicklung und Bibliographie der pathologisch-anatomischen Abbildung*, Leipzig, 1925.

PHARMACY AND PHARMACOLOGY: G. Dragendorff, *Die Heilpflanzen der verschiedenen Völker und Zeiten*, Stuttgart, 1898; A. Tschirsch, *Handbuch der Pharmakognosie*, Leipzig, 2nd ed., 1933ff.; H. Schelenz, *Geschichte der Pharmazie*, Berlin, 1904; E. Kremers and G. Urdang, *History of Pharmacy*, Philadelphia, 1940; H. Peters, *Aus pharmazeutischer Vorzeit*, Berlin, 1888-91, 2 vols. (Transl. in part by W. Netter as *Pictorial History of Ancient Pharmacy*, Chicago, 1889); J. Berendes, *Das Apothekenwesen: seine Entstehung und geschichtliche Entwicklung bis zum XX. Jahrhundert*, Stuttgart, 1907; A. Benedicenti, *Malati, medici e farmacisti attraverso i secoli*, Milan, 2nd ed., 1946.

PHYSIOLOGY: M. Foster, *Lectures on the History of Physiology during the Sixteenth, Seventeenth and Eighteenth Centuries*, Cambridge, 1901; J. F. Fulton, *Physiology* (Clio Medica), New York, 1931; *Selected Readings in the History of Physiology*, Baltimore, 1930; K. J. Franklin, *A Short History of Physiology*, 2nd ed. London, 1949.

PSYCHIATRY: G. Zilboorg and G. H. Henry, *A History of Medical Psychology*, New York, 1941; O. Beyerholm, *Psykiatriens historie*, Copenhagen, 1937; H. Lähr, *Die Literatur der Psychiatrie, Neurologie und Psychologie von* 1459-1799, Berlin, 1900.

SCIENCE: G. Sarton, *Introduction to the History of Science*, Baltimore, 1927-48, 3 vols. in 5; Ch. Singer, *A Short History of Science, to the Nineteenth Century*, Oxford, 1941; W. C. Dampier, *A History of Science and Its Relation with Philosophy and Religion*, Cambridge, 3rd ed., 1942; W. T. Sedgwick and H. W. Tyler, *A History of Science*, New York and London, 1917; P. Brunet and A. Mieli, *Histoire des sciences*, Paris, vol. I, 1935; F. Sherwood Taylor, *A Short History of Science and Scientific Thought*, New York, 1950.

SOCIAL MEDICINE: R. Sand, *Vers la médecine sociale*, Paris and Liège, 1948; P. Diepgen, *Geschichte der sozialen Medizin*, Leipzig, 1934.

SURGERY: J. F. Malgaigne, *Histoire de la chirurgie en occident depuis le VIe jusqu'au XVIe siècle*, Paris, 1840; J. S. Billings, 'The History and Literature of Surgery,' *A System of Surgery*, edited by F. S. Dennis, Philadelphia, 1895; E. J. Gurlt, *Geschichte der Chirurgie und ihrer Ausübung*, Berlin, 1898, 3 vols.; W. von Brunn, *Kurze Geschichte der Chirurgie*, Berlin, 1928; Sir D'Arcy Power, *A Short History of Surgery*, London, 1933; E. Zeis, *Die Literatur und Geschichte der plastischen Chirurgie*, Leipzig, 1863; H. Graham, *The Story of Surgery*, New York, 1939.

TROPICAL MEDICINE: H. Harold Scott, *A History of Tropical Medicine*, London, 1939, 2 vols.

UROLOGY: C. Vieillard, *L'Urologie et les médecins urologues dans la médecine ancienne*, Paris, 1903; E. Desnos, 'Histoire de l'urologie,' *Encyclopédie française d'urologie*, edited by A. Pousson and E. Desnos, vol. I, Paris, 1914.

VETERINARY MEDICINE: C. P. Leyman, *History of Veterinary Medicine*, Cambridge, 1898; F. Smith, *The Early History of Veterinary Literature*, London, 1919-30, 3 vols.

3. MEDICAL HISTORIES BY COUNTRIES

Medicine is international and it is very difficult to write its history when you have to limit yourself to the area of a given country. Vesalius was born in Brussels, studied in France, did his decisive work in Italy, printed his great book in Switzerland, was in Spain and the Netherlands with the imperial court, and died on a Greek island. He belongs to Europe and to the world. His personality would have to be re-evoked in more than one national history. Albrecht von Haller was born in Switzerland, where he spent the greater part of his life, but his crucial years were those when he worked at Göttingen, which at the time owed allegiance to the king of England. Another problem is presented by the fact that cultural centers shifted a great deal. The importance of Greece in antiquity was very different from its importance during the Middle Ages or the seventeenth and eighteenth centuries.

These difficulties are probably responsible for the fact that there are not very many good national histories of medicine and that those of a number of countries are antiquated and out of print. Yet I think that every country should have its national medical history written, and that such a book should be in the hands of every doctor of the country, because he should be aware of his national heritage, of the historical moment at which he happens to be living, and of the tasks that lie ahead of him. Such a book must be free from any nationalism. A good national historian, as a matter of fact, is always humble, because he is well aware not only of achievements but also of failures and shortcomings and of goals still to be reached. Such a book will picture a nation's particular health problems, which obviously are different in Norway from those in India. It will discuss the development of social, economic, and political conditions that prevailed in the course of time and affected man's life. It will picture what was done to maintain and restore health, who the physicians were, under what conditions and in what institutions they worked, and what contribution they made to world medical science.

Such a book presupposes preliminary studies and, indeed, there is a rich literature on medicine in various countries at a given period, or on certain aspects of medicine in a certain country. Such books we shall of course quote but not in this short bibliography. Our purpose here is to list some general national medical histories, some of which are very good while others are not quite satisfactory.

ARGENTINA: E. Canton, *Historia de la medicina en el Rio de la Plata,* Madrid, 1928, 4 vols.; J. R. Beltran, *Historia del Protomedicato de Buenos Aires,* Buenos Aires, 1937.

AUSTRIA: M. Neuburger, *Die Entwicklung der Medizin in Oesterreich,* Vienna and Leipzig, 1918 (many other publications of the same author deal with special periods of Austrian medicine); L. Schönbauer, *Das medizinische Wien,* Vienna, 2nd ed., 1947.

BELGIUM: C. Broeckx, *Essai sur l'histoire de la médecine belge avant le XIXe siècle,* Brussels, 1838. E. Renaux, A. Dalcq and J. Govaerts, *Aperçu de l'histoire de la médecine en Belgique,* Brussels, 1947.

CANADA: J. J. Heagerty, *Four Centuries of Medical History in Canada,* Toronto, 1928, 2 vols.; W. B. Howell, *Medicine in Canada* (Clio Medica), New York, 1933.

CHINA: K. C. Wong and Wu Lien-Teh, *History of Chinese Medicine,* Shanghai, 2nd ed., 1936; W. Morse, *Chinese Medicine* (Clio Medica), New York, 1934; E. H. Hume, *The Chinese Way in Medicine,* Baltimore, 1940.

DENMARK: V. Ingerslev, *Danmarks laeger og laegevaesen fra de aeldste tider undtil aar 1800,* Copenhagen, 1873, 2 vols.

FRANCE: J. Guiart, *Histoire de la médecine française,* Paris, 1947; Laignel-Lavastine and R. Molinery, *French Medicine* (Clio Medica), New York, 1934.

GERMANY: H. Rohlfs, *Geschichte der deutschen Medicin: Die medicinischen Classiker Deutschlands,* Leipzig, 1875-85, 4 vols.; A. Hirsch, *Geschichte der Medizinischen Wissenschaften in Deutschland,* Munich and Leipzig, 1893; G. Sticker, *Die Entwicklung der ärztlichen Kunst in Deutschland,* Munich, 1927.

GREAT BRITAIN: Sir D'Arcy Power, *Medicine in the British Isles* (Clio Medica), New York, 1930; J. D. Comrie, *History of Scottish Medicine,* London, 2nd ed., 1932.

GUATEMALA: C. Martínez Durán, *Las ciencias médicas en Guatemala,* Guatemala, 1941.

ITALY: S. de Renzi, *Storia della medicina italiana,* Naples, 1845-8, 5 vols.; A. Castiglioni, *Italian Medicine* (Clio Medica), New York, 1932.

JAPAN: Y. Fujikawa, *Geschichte der Medizin in Japan,* Tokyo, 1911 (Engl. ed. in Clio Medica, New York, 1934).

LATIN AMERICA: A. A. Moll, *Aesculapius in Latin America,* Philadelphia, 1944.

MEXICO: F. A. Flores, *Historia de la medicina en México,* Mexico, 1886-8; F. Ocaranza, *Historia de la medicina en México,* Mexico, 1934; I. Chavez, *México en la cultura medica,* Mexico, 1947.

NETHERLANDS: J. Banga, *Geschiedenis van de geneeskunde en van hare beoefenaaren in Nederland,* Leeuwarden, 1868, 2 vols.

NORWAY: Fr. Grön, J. Kobro, and I. Reichborn-Kjennerud, *Medisinens historie i Norge,* Oslo, 1936.

PORTUGAL: M. Lemos, *Historia da medicina em Portugal,* Lisbon, 1891, 2 vols.; L. De Pina, *Histoire de la médecine portugaise,* Porto, 1935.

RUMANIA: Ionescu-Gomoiu, *Istoria medicinei si a invatamantului medical in Romania,* Bucharest, 1936.

RUSSIA: W. M. Richter, *Geschichte der Medicin in Russland,* Moscow, 1813-17, 3 vols.; W. H. Gantt, *Russian Medicine* (Clio Medica), New York, 1937; D. M. Rossiski, *Bibliograficheski ukazatel russkoi literatury po historii meditsiny s 1789 do 1928 g.,* Moscow, 1928.

SPAIN: A. H. Morejon, *Historia bibliográfica de la medicina española,* Madrid, 1842-52; E. Garcia del Real, *Historia de la medicina en España,* Madrid, 1921.

SWEDEN: J. F. Sacklén, *Sveriges läkare-historia ifran Konung Gustav I :s till närvarande tid,* Nyköping, 1822-35, 4 vols., continued by A. H. Wistrand, A. J. Bruzelius, and C. Edling, Stockholm, 1853-76.

UNITED STATES OF AMERICA: F. R. Packard, *History of Medicine in the United States,* New York, 2nd ed., 1931, 2 vols.; J. G. Mumford, *A Narrative of Medicine in America,* Philadelphia, 1903; H. E. Sigerist, *Amerika und die Medizin,* Leipzig, 1933 (*American Medicine,* New York, 1934).

URUGUAY: R. Schiaffino, *Historia de la medicina en Uruguay,* Montevideo, 1927-37, 2 vols.

4. HISTORIES OF DISEASES

In our chapter, 'Disease in Time and Space,' we indicated much literature on the subject which will not be repeated here. The following brief list is made up of monographs on a few major diseases. A comprehensive critical bibliography of the history of diseases, including articles in journals, would be highly desirable but would probably fill a whole volume. So far the best source still is the *Index Catalogue of the Surgeon-General's Library*. A recent publication which covers the history of fourteen diseases is, A. Pazzini and A. Baffoni, *Storia delle malattie* (Edizioni Clinica Nuova), Rome, 1949. More modest in scope was *A Short History of Some Common Diseases,* edited by W. R. Bett, London, 1934.

CHLOROSIS: A. Hansen, *Om chlorosens den aegte blegsots optraeden i Europa gennem tiderne,* Kolding, 1928.

CHOLERA: G. Sticker, *Abhandlungen aus der Seuchengeschichte und Seuchenlehre,* vol. 2, *Die Cholera,* Giessen, 1912.

DIPHTHERIA: E. Behring, *Die Geschichte der Diphtherie,* Leipzig, 1893.

EPILEPSY: O. Temkin, *The Falling Sickness: A History of Epilepsy from the Greeks to the Beginnings of Modern Neurology,* Baltimore, 1945.

EXANTHEMATA: J. D. Rolleston, *History of the Acute Exanthemata,* London, 1937.

GOUT: W. Gaidner, *On Gout: Its History, Its Causes and Its Cure,* London, 1849; M. Klibanoff, *Zur Lehre der Gicht in geschichtlicher Beziehung von Hippokrates zu Paracelsus,* Berlin, 1912; C. Frank, *La Goutte: sur quelques points controversés ou mal connus de son histoire,* Paris, 1922.

HEMOPHILIA: G. Sommerlad, *Geschichte der Hämophilie,* Diss., Leipzig, 1927.

HEART DISEASES: Sir Humphry Davy Rolleston, *Cardio-vascular Diseases since Harvey's Discovery,* Cambridge, 1928; F. A. Willius and Th. E. Keys, *Cardiac Classics. A Collection of Classic Works on the Heart and Circulation,* St. Louis, 1941.

INFLUENZA: F. G. Crookshank, *Influenza,* London, 1922.

LEPROSY: D. Zambaco, *La lèpre à travers les siècles,* Paris, 1914.

MOUNTAIN SICKNESS: Paul Bert, *La Pression barométrique, recherches de physiologie expérimentale,* Paris, 1878 (Engl. ed., Columbus, Ohio, 1943); Carlos Monge, *Acclimatization in the Andes,* Baltimore, 1948.

OCCUPATIONAL DISEASES: G. Rosen, *The History of Miners' Diseases,* New York, 1943.

PLAGUE: G. Sticker, *Abhandlungen aus der Seuchengeschichte und Seuchenlehre*, vol. I, *Die Pest*, Giessen, 1908-10, 2 parts.

POLIOMYELITIS: M. Fishbein (editor), L. Hektoen, E. M. Salmonsen, *A Bibliography of Infantile Paralysis*, Philadelphia, 1946.

SCURVY: A. F. Hess, *Scurvy, Past and Present*, Philadelphia, 1920; R. Krebel, *Der Scorbut in geschichtlich-literarischer, pathologischer, prophylactischer und therapeutischer Beziehung*, Leipzig, 1836.

SMALLPOX: E. M. Crookshank, *History and Pathology of Vaccination*, London, 1889, 2 vols.

TUBERCULOSIS: A. Predöhl, *Die Geschichte der Tuberkulose*, Hamburg and Leipzig, 1888; M. Piéry and Roshem, *Histoire de la tuberculose*, Paris, 1931; A. Castiglioni, 'Storia della tuberculosi,' *Trattato della tuberculosi*, edited by L. Devoto, Milan, 1931, vol. I; A. Ilvento, *La tuberculosi attraverso i secoli*, Turin, 1933; G. B. Webb, *Tuberculosis* (Clio Medica), New York, 1936.

TUMORS: J. Wolff, *Die Lehre von der Krebskrankheit von den ältesten Zeiten bis zur Gegenwart*, Jena, 1907-28, 4 vols. (vol. I in 2nd ed., 1929).

TYPHUS: H. Zinsser, *Rats, Lice and History*, Boston, 1935; T. von Györy, *Morbus Hungaricus*, Jena, 1901.

VENEREAL DISEASES: J. K. Proksch, *Die Literatur über die venerischen Krankheiten*, Bonn, 1889-1900, 3 vols.; E. Jeanselme, 'Histoire de la syphilis,' *Traité de la Syphilis*, Paris, 1931, vol. I; G. Sticker, 'Entwurf einer Geschichte der ansteckenden Geschlechtskrankheiten,' *Handbuch der Haut- und Geschlechtskrankheiten*, Berlin, 1931, vol. 23.

NOTES

1. Ed. Littré, I, 573ff.
2. W. H. S. Jones, *The Medical Writings of Anonymus Londinensis*, Cambridge, 1947.
3. Prohoem., 1ff.
4. See, e.g. *Arch. Gesch. Med.*, 1921, 13:148ff.; *Kyklos*, 1930, 3:418ff.
5. Edited by A. Müller, 1884.
6. See *Bull. Hist. Med.*, suppl. 3, 1944, p. 65ff.
7. *De claris medicinae scriptoribus*, Lugduni, 1506, *et al.*
8. The first edition in 5 vols. was published 1792-1803. The 1st part was issued in 4th ed., 1846; parts 2-5 in 3rd ed., 1823-8; a 6th part in 2 vols. was added by B. Eble, 1837-40.

9. A beginning has been made by P. Diepgen and his students, particularly Edith Heischkel. See her excellent summary of these studies, '*Die Geschichte der Medizingeschichtsschreibung*,' *Einführung in die Medizinhistorik*, edited by W. Artelt, Stuttgart, 1949, pp. 202-37. Artelt's book is an excellent introduction to medical historical research. About present problems see G. Rosen, 'Levels of Integration in Medical Historiography,' *J. Hist. Med.*, 1949, 4: 460ff.

APPENDIX II

*

Source Books of Medical History

A recent German publication makes it possible for us to reduce this appendix to a minimum, namely, Walter Artelt, *Einführung in die Medizinhistorik, ihr Wesen, ihre Arbeitsweise und ihre Hilfsmittel,* Stuttgart, 1949. It is the first publication of its kind and contains a wealth of information. Whoever engages in medical historical research must have recourse to this book, and libraries will find it very useful. It has gaps, to be sure, and one may not agree with every statement the author makes, but it is a truly remarkable book that will save time and trouble to many workers in the field.

Considering the fact that Artelt's book is easily available, this appendix will merely supplement it by listing the chief periodicals and the chief collections of medical classics. It will also indicate some biographical and bibliographical reference books which are so important that they cannot be omitted from any such bio-bibliography.

1. PERIODICALS

The first periodicals devoted to medical history were published in the eighteenth century. Their number was very small and even in the nineteenth century the journals founded by some optimistic scholar usually did not last very long. Medical historians published their papers in general medical, historical, or philological journals. Owing to the fact that Rudolf Virchow was very interested in medical history, his *Archiv,* chief organ of the new pathology, published a large number of very important historical papers. Similarly the *Bulletin of the Johns Hopkins Hospital* brought many excellent historical contributions because the first group of Hopkins doctors consisted of men to whom medical history meant a great deal.

In the beginning of our century, medical historical societies were founded in a number of countries and most of them launched periodicals that are still issued today. Another stimulus was the creation of institutes of the history of medicine most of which called for new means of publication. In 1914 G. Sarton was able to analyze 62 journals devoted to the history of science (*Isis*, 1914, 2:132ff.).

Periodicals are perhaps the most important repositories of the results of research, and every institution that engages in studies of medical history should acquire as many of them as possible. In the following list only those journals of the history of the natural sciences have been mentioned that include the history of the medical sciences.

ARGENTINA: The chair of medical history in Buenos Aires issues two periodicals:

Universidad nacional. Facultad de ciencias médicas. Catedra de historia de la medicina. *Publicaciones,* vol. I, Buenos Aires, 1938ff.

Revista argentina de historia de la medicina, vol. I, Buenos Aires, 1942ff.

The Sociedad de Historia de la Medicina de la Plata publishes:

Archivos argentinos de historia de la medicina, vol. I, La Plata, 1944ff.

BELGIUM: The most important periodical of the history of science was launched in Belgium by George Sarton and was published there for many years until it was taken over by the History of Science Society, namely *Isis, Revue consacrée à l'histoire et à l'organisation de la science,* vol. I, 1913ff. Now published as *Isis, An International Review Devoted to the History of Science and Civilization* (vol. 40, 1949).

Osiris, Studies on the History and Philosophy of Science, and on the History of Learning and Culture, vol. 1, Bruges, 1936ff. (subtitle varies).

BRAZIL: *Revista Brasileira de Historia da Medicina,* vol. I, Rio de Janeiro, 1949ff.

CANADA: *Historical Bulletin, Notes and Abstracts Dealing with Medical History,* issued quarterly by The Calgary Associate Clinic, Calgary, vol. 1, Alberta, 1936ff.

CHINA: *The Chinese Journal of Medical History,* published quarterly by The Chinese Medical History Society, vol. 1, Shanghai, 1947ff.

DENMARK: *Medicinsk-Historike Smaaskrifter,* nos. 1-18, Copenhagen, 1912-17.

Centaurus: International Magazine of the History of Science and Medicine, vol. I, Copenhagen, 1950.

ENGLAND: *Proceedings of the Royal Society of Medicine,* Section of the History of Medicine, since 1913.

Studies in the History and Method of Science, edited by Ch. Singer, vols. 1-2, Oxford, 1917-21.

Research studies in medical history. Wellcome Historical Medical Museum, vol. I, 1922ff.

Annals of Science, a quarterly review of the history of science since the Renaissance, vol. 1, London, 1936ff.

FRANCE: *Bulletin de la Société Française d'Histoire de la Médecine,* vol. I, Paris, 1902ff., continued as *Mémoires de la Société Française d'Histoire de la Médecine,* vol. I, Paris, 1945ff.

Thales, published by Institut d'Histoire des Sciences et des Techniques, Université de Paris, vol. I, 1934ff.

Hippocrate, Revue d'humanisme médical, vol. 1, Paris, 1933ff.

Aesculape, Revue . . . illustrée latéro-médicale (became organ of Société Internationale d'Histoire de la Médecine), vols. 1-30, Paris, 1911-40 (vols. 5-12, 1914-22, never published; vol. 13, 1923, also as, new series, vol. 1).

Bulletin de la Société d'Histoire de la Pharmacie, vol. 1, Paris, 1913ff.; continued as *Revue d'histoire de la pharmacie,* vol. 1, 1930ff.

Earlier periodicals were:

La France médicale, revue d'études d'histoire de la médecine, vols. 1-64, Paris, 1854-1921.

La chronique médicale, vol. 1ff., Paris, 1894-1920.

Bulletin de la Société Médico-Historique, Paris, 1909-10.

GERMANY: *Mitteilungen zur Geschichte der Medizin und der Naturwissenschaften,* vols. 1-40, Leipzig, 1902-43, a bibliographic journal published by the German Society of the History of Medicine and Science, extended from vol. 31 on to include the history of technology.

Archiv für Geschichte der Medizin, vols. 1-20, Leipzig, 1907-28; continued as *Sudhoffs Archiv für Geschichte der Medizin,* vols. 21-6, Leipzig, 1929-33, and as *Sudhoffs Archiv für Geschichte der Medizin und der Naturwissenschaften,* vol. 27, Leipzig, 1934ff. It was supplemented by a series of monographs: *Studien zur Geschichte der Medizin,* vol. 1, Leipzig, 1907ff.

The Leipzig Institute of the History of Medicine furthermore published:

Beiträge zur Geschichte der Medizin, vol. 1 (only vol. published), Zurich, 1925.

Kyklos, Jahrbuch des Instituts für Geschichte der Medizin, etc., vols. 1-4, Leipzig, 1928-32.

Arbeiten des Instituts, etc., vols. 1-2, Leipzig, 1930-32.

Vorträge des Instituts, etc., vols. 1-4, Leipzig, 1928-31.

The Berlin Institute of the History of Medicine and Science published:

Quellen und Studien zur Geschichte der Naturwissenschaften und der Medizin, vol. 1, Berlin, 1931ff.

Abhandlungen zur Geschichte der Medizin und der Naturwissenschaften, vol. 1, Berlin, 1934ff.

Further series, all of which were discontinued during the war but may some day be resumed, are:

Jenaer medizin-historische Beiträge, vol. 1, Jena, 1912ff.

Münchener Beiträge zur Geschichte und Literatur der Naturwissenschaften und Medizin, no. 1, Munich, 1926ff.

Acta Paracelsica, no. 1, Munich, 1930ff. (See *Nova acta Paracelsica* under Switzerland).

Arbeiten zur Kenntnis der Geschichte der Medizin im Rheinland und in Westfalen, vols. 1-12, Jena, 1929-33.

Older German periodicals:

Archiv für die Geschichte der Arzneykunde, edited by Th. L. Wittwer, Nurenberg, 1790. (Only one volume published.)

Beiträge zur Geschichte der Arzneiwissenschaft, edited by K. Sprengel, vols. 1-2, Halle, 1794-6.

Historisch-literarisches Jahrbuch für die deutsche Medizin, edited by L. Choulant, vols. 1-3, Leipzig, 1838-40.

Janus, Zeitschrift für Geschichte und Literatur der Medicin, edited by A. W. E. Th. Henschel, vols. 1-3, Breslau, 1846-8. (Reprinted 1931.)

Janus, Central-Magazin für Geschichte und Literärgeschichte der Medicin, ärztliche Biographik, Epidemiographik, medicinische Geographie u. Statistik, vols. 1-2, Gotha, 1851-3. (Reprinted 1931.)

Deutsches Archiv für Geschichte der Medicin und medicinische Geographie, edited by H. Rohlfs, vols. 1-8, Leipzig, 1878-85.

Abhandlungen zur Geschichte der Medizin, edited by H. Magnus, M. Neuburger, K. Sudhoff, nos. 1-18, Breslau, 1902-6.

ITALY: *Atti delle riunioni della Società Italiana di Storia Critica delle Scienze mediche e naturali,* Perugia, Faenza, Venetia, 1907-9, continued as, *Rivista di Storia critica delle scienze mediche e naturali,* vol. 1, Siena (later Florence), 1910-12ff.

Archivio di storia della scienza, vols. 1-8, Rome, 1919/20-27, continued as *Archeion* (which became the organ of the Internat. Committee of the History of Science), vol. 9ff., 1928ff., continued as *Archives internationales d'histoire des sciences,* vol. 1, Paris, 1947/48ff.

Bolletino dell'Istituto Storico Italiano dell'Arte Sanitaria, vols. 1-14, Rome, 1921/22-34, continued as *Atti e memorie, Accademia dell'Arte Sanitaria,* 2nd series, vol. 1, 1935ff. (published as supplement to *Rassegna di clinica, terapia e scienze affini*).

Castalia, Rivista di storia della medicina (from 1947 on the subtitle was *La medicina nella storia e nel arte*), vol. I, Milan, 1945ff. Primarily the organ of the Milanese School directed by N. Latronico who also edits a series of monographs:

Collana di studi di storia della medicina, Milan, vol. 1, 1945ff.

Università di Roma. Istituto di Storia della Medicina:

Lavori, Rome, vol. 1 (1938-9), 1940.

Collezione C: Studi e ricerche storico-mediche, Rome, 1942ff.

NETHERLANDS: *Janus, archives internationales pour l'histoire de la médecine et pour la géographie médicale,* vol. 1, Amsterdam (later Haarlem, then Leiden), 1896-1940.

Bijdragen tot de geschiedenis der geneeskunde, vol. 1, Amsterdam, 1921ff. (published as supplement to *Nederl. Tijdschrift voor Geneeskunde*).

PERU: *Anales de la Sociedad Peruana de Historia de la Medicina,* vol. 1, Lima, 1939ff.

POLAND: *Archiwum historji i filozofji medycyny oraz historji nauk przyrodniczych,* vol. 1, Poznan, 1924ff.

PORTUGAL: *Archivos de historia da medicina portugueza,* vols. 1-6, Porto, 1887-96, N. S. 1910-15.

SPAIN: *Trabajos de la cátedra de historia crítica de la medicina,* vol. 1, Madrid, 1933ff.

SWEDEN: *Lychnos* (organ of the Swedish Society of the History of Science), vol. I, 1937ff.

SWITZERLAND: *Veröffentlichungen der Schweizerischen Gesellschaft für Geschichte der Medizin und der Naturwissenschaften*, vol. 1, Zurich, 1922ff.

Gesnerus, Vierteljahrsschrift für Geschichte der Medizin u. der Naturwissenschaften, vol. 1, Aarau, 1943ff.

Ciba Zeitschrift (Ges. für chemische Industrie in Basel), vol. 1, Basle, 1933ff.

Nova acta Paracelsica, Jahrbuch der schweizerischen Paracelsus-Gesellschaft, Einsiedeln, 1944ff.

Zürcher medizingeschichtliche Abhandlungen, vol. 1, Zurich, 1924ff.

Berner Beiträge zur Geschichte der Medizin und der Naturwissenschaften, vol. 1, Berne, 1944ff.

TURKEY: *Türk tib tarihi, archives d'histoire de la médecine turque*, Istanbul.

Istanbul Universitesi Tib tarihi enstitüsü, *Adet & Sayi*, Istanbul.

UNITED STATES OF AMERICA: *Bulletin of the History of Medicine* (organ of the American Association of the History of Medicine and the Johns Hopkins Institute of the History of Medicine), vol. 1, Baltimore, 1933ff.; vols. 1-6, 1933-8 issued as the Institute's *Bulletin;* vols. 1-2 as supplements to the *Johns Hopkins Hospital Bulletin*, vols. 52-3; index of vols. 1-20 published 1950.

Johns Hopkins University, Institute of the History of Medicine. *Publications:*

1st ser., *Monographs*, vol. 1, 1942ff.

2nd ser., *Texts and Documents*, vol. 1, 1941ff.

3rd ser., *Hideyo Noguchi Lectures*, vol. 1, 1934ff.

4th ser., *Bibliotheca Medica Americana*, vol. 1, 1937ff.

Journal of the History of Medicine and Allied Sciences, vol. 1, New York, 1946ff.

Ciba Symposia (Ciba Pharmaceutical Products, Inc.), vol. 1, Summit, N. J., 1939ff.

Alcmeone, rivista trimestrale di storia della medicine, vol. 1, New York, 1939ff.

Bulletin of the Society of Medical History of Chicago, vol. 1, Chicago, 1911ff. (published irregularly).

Periodicals that have been discontinued:

Medical Life, vols. 1-45, New York, 1894-1938.

Annals of Medical History, vols. 1-10, New York, 1917-28; new series, vols. 1-10, 1929-38; third series, vols. 1-4, 1939-42. Index published by H. Schuman, New York, 1946.

Medical Library and Historical Journal (Association of Medical Librarians), vols. 1-5, Brooklyn, 1903-7; continued as *Aesculapian, A Quarterly Journal of Medical History, Literature and Art*, vol. 1, Brooklyn, 1908-9.

Medical Leaves, Chicago, vols. 1-5, 1937-43.

2. CLASSICS OF MEDICINE

The study of texts is the essential part of the researcher's work and the study of the classics of medicine has, in addition, great educational value.[1] Ancient texts and, as matter of fact, all texts that were not printed under the author's supervision, must be edited. We shall mention—and when necessary discuss—the various editions of ancient and medieval writers in the course of this work. Here we shall merely draw attention to some general collections of medical classics that may be consulted profitably by students and physicians. Such series are extremely welcome because they make important studies easily available.

In America we have an excellent collection:

Medical Classics, edited by Emerson C. Kelly, Baltimore, 1936-41, 5 vols.

The Johns Hopkins Institute of the History of Medicine published a number of classics in its *Bulletin of the History of Medicine* and made them available in reprints; [2] it also published classics in two of its series of publications, already mentioned.

America also has some excellent anthologies of classical medical texts, among them the *Selected Readings* published by Charles C Thomas in Springfield, Ill., and Baltimore, Md. To date they cover physiology, pathology, classical descriptions of disease, obstetrics, and gynecology, and will undoubtedly be extended to other fields. Other recommendable books of this type have been listed in the preceding section of this appendix. A very good general anthology intended primarily for students is:

Logan Clendening, *Source Book of Medical History*, New York, 1942.

In England around the middle of last century the Sydenham Society included in its series of publications a certain number of classics from various periods, in English translation, and so did its successor, the New Sydenham Society. They are listed in the second series of the Index-Catalogue of the Surgeon General's Library. In recent time, Charles Singer launched a series which in four volumes included works of Paré,

Sydenham, Laennec, and Lister,[3] and R. T. Gunther published fourteen volumes of texts and studies dealing with *Early Science in Oxford.*[4]

Germany had two very important series which unfortunately were discontinued long ago. One was an extensive collection of classics of science, while the other was devoted to classics of medicine:

Ostwald's Klassiker der exakten Naturwissenschaften, Leipzig, Engelmann (close to 200 numbers, small booklets in pocketsize).

Klassiker der Medizin, edited by Karl Sudhoff, Leipzig, 1910-23, J. A. Barth.

Incunabula and other early printed books, which have not only historical but artistic value, have frequently been reprinted in facsimile and there is hardly one such series that does not include some medical book. Two series exclusively devoted to the history of medicine and science produced some beautiful books but never got beyond the fifth volume:

Alte Meister der Medizin und Naturkunde, edited by G. Klein, Munich, 1910-12, 5 vols.[5]

Monumenta medica, edited by H. E. Sigerist, Milan and Florence, 1923-8, 5 vols.

Holland has a series of classics that is a model of its kind and should be imitated by other countries:

Opuscula selecta neerlandicorum de arte medica, vol. 1, Amsterdam, 1907ff. (vol. 17 was issued in 1943).

The series is published by the chief medical journal of the country, the *Nederlandsch Tijdschrift voor Geneeskunde,* and contains in large volumes a great number of the country's classical writings in the original language and in translation into English, German, or some other of the more widely understood languages.

Russia undertook to publish classics in the nineteen-thirties:

Klassiki biologii i meditsiny, Moscow and Leningrad, Ogiz, 1935ff. (Some of the volumes came out under the auspices of the All-Union Institute of Experimental Medicine.)

In Spain Pedro Lain Entralgo founded in 1946 a series, *Clasicos de la medicina.*

It would be very desirable if one of our bibliographers could prepare an index of all treatises and papers included in these various collections as some may be easily overlooked.

3. BIOGRAPHICAL AND BIBLIOGRAPHICAL REFERENCE BOOKS

To identify a physician of the past or an old book, to find data on a man's life, or literature on a given subject, may be easy or may be extremely difficult. We may find what we are looking for in a few minutes in one of the current dictionaries that every library has in its reading room, or we may have to embark in painstaking studies in libraries and archives. Yet the number of reference books available that we may consult in such cases is extremely large. In building up a department of medical history, first attention must be given to reference books. They are much more important than rare books. Of course, it is nice to have both, but rare books are read and studied very infrequently while reference books are used all the time. A reference collection must be such that it allows a quick first orientation on any problem of medical history or any question of background. The Johns Hopkins Institute of the History of Medicine has an excellent collection, conveniently located in one room, and it would be tempting to give a catalogue of it; this, however, would be beyond the scope of this appendix and it is hardly necessary, since we have excellent books guiding us to the basic reference materials.

One such book that can be recommended warmly is:

A Handbook of Medical Library Practice, edited by Janet Doe, Chicago, 1943.

Written primarily for librarians, it is of greatest benefit also to all those who use medical libraries and its excellent section on Reference Work by Eileen R. Cunningham includes an annotated list of 603 reference books.

Artelt's *Einführung in die Medizinhistorik*, mentioned before, has a very good section on bibliographies to which we should like to refer the reader.

Every period of medical history has its special bibliographic problems. The Greek, Roman, and medieval texts have been transmitted in manuscripts, and whoever wants to edit such texts must have recourse to the numerous catalogues of manuscripts of our libraries. More bibliographic work has probably been devoted to the incunabula than to any other group of printed books. Catalogues devoted exclusively or primarily to medical manuscripts or incunabula will be discussed later in this work, when we come to the periods in question. All I can do here is give a short select list of a few general reference books that I found particularly useful:

Encyclopedias, modern and old, will be found very helpful and I should like to draw particular attention to one that has rendered me unusually good services for many years:

Grosses vollständiges Universal-Lexicon aller Wissenschafften und Künste, published by Johann Heinrich Zedler, Halle and Leipzig, 1732-54, 64 vols. and 4 suppl.

Most countries have published dictionaries of national biography, all of which include many physicians. The following are some special dictionaries in the order in which they are usually consulted:

Biographisches Lexikon der hervorragenden Ärzte aller Zeiten und Völker, edited by August Hirsch, E. Gurlt, and A. Wernich, 2nd ed. prepared by Wilhelm Haberling, Franz Hübotter, and Hermann Vierordt, Berlin and Vienna, 1929-35, 5 vols. and suppl.

Biographisches Lexikon hervorragender Ärzte des neunzehnten Jahrhunderts, edited by Julius Pagel, Berlin and Vienna, 1901.

I. Fischer, *Biographisches Lexikon der hervorragenden Ärzte der letzten fünfzig Jahre*, Berlin and Vienna, 1932-3, 2 vols.

Hermann Vierordt, *Medizin-geschichtliches Hilfsbuch mit besonderer Berücksichtigung der Entdeckungsgeschichte und der Biographie*, Tübingen, 1916.

Bayle and Thillaye, *Biographie médicale par ordre chronologique d'après Daniel Leclerc, Eloy, etc.*, Paris, 1855, 2 vols.

Dezeimeris, Ollivier and Raige-Delorme, *Dictionnaire historique de la médecine ancienne et moderne*, Paris, 1828-39, 4 vols.

Biographie médicale, edited by A.-J.-L. Jourdan, as part of *Dictionnaire des sciences médicales*, Paris, 1820-5, vols. 1-7.

Benj. Hutchinson, *Biographia medica, or Historical and Critical Memoirs of the Lives and Writings of the Most Eminent Medical Characters, that Have Existed from the Earliest Account of Time to the Present Period*, London, 1799, 2nd ed., London, 1809, 2 vols.

N. F. I. Eloy, *Dictionnaire historique de la médecine ancienne et moderne*, Mons, 2nd ed., 1778, vols. 1-4.

A. C. P. Callisen, *Medicinisches Schriftsteller-Lexicon der jetzt lebenden Ärzte, Wundärzte, Geburtshelfer, Apotheker, und Naturforscher aller gebildeten Völker*, Copenhagen, 1830-45, 33 vols.

Nouvelle biographie générale, Paris, 1853-66, 46 vols.

Biografia universale antica e moderna, Venice, 1822-31, 65 vols.

For the history of the exact sciences the best biographical dictionary still is:

J. C. Poggendorffs *Biographisch-literarisches Handwörterbuch für Mathematik, Astronomie, Physik, Chemie und verwandte Wissenschaftsgebiete,* Leipzig, 1863-1926, 5 vols. in 7.

Dictionaries specializing on certain countries or periods will be mentioned in later volumes of this work.

As to general bibliographic reference books, their number is endless. The most comprehensive is undoubtedly:

Index-Catalogue of the Library of the Surgeon-General's Office, United States Army, published in Washington since 1880. The first three series number 47 volumes, the fourth series is in course of publication since 1936.

The *Index-Catalogue* is particularly valuable as it lists not only books but also journal articles and even chapters of books. It obviously has gaps, since it is not a world bibliography, but the catalogue of a given library, which, although one of the largest, cannot possibly be complete.

For the older literature the *Bibliothecae* of A. von Haller are still perhaps the best sources of information:

Bibliotheca botanica, Zurich, 1771-2, 2 vols. Modern index by J. C. Bay, Berne, 1908.

Bibliotheca anatomica, Zurich, 1774-6, 2 vols.

Bibliotheca medicinae practicae, Basle, 1776-88, 4 vols.

Bibliotheca chirurgica, Berne and Basle, 1774-5, 2 vols.

They superseded:

J. J. Manget, *Bibliotheca scriptorum medicorum veterum et recentiorum,* Geneva, 1731, 4 pts. in 2 vols. (although the book may still be consulted).

Some early and still useful bibliographies are:

L. Choulant, *Handbuch der Bücherkunde für die ältere Medicin,* Leipzig, 2nd ed., 1841; reprinted Munich, 1926.

L. Choulant, *Bibliotheca medico-historica sive Catalogus librorum historicorum de re medica et scientia naturali systematicus,* Leipzig, 1842.

J. Rosenbaum, *Additamenta ad Ludovici Choulanti Bibliothecam medico-historicam,* Halle, 1842 and 1847. Specimen I and II.

A. Pauly, *Bibliographie des sciences médicales, bibliographie—biographie—histoire—épidémies—topographies—endémies,* Paris, 1874.

Rare books may be located in:

J. G. T. Graesse, *Trésor de livres rares et précieux,* Dresden, 1859-1900, 7 vols. in 8.

J. C. Brunet, *Manuel du libraire et de l'amateur de livres*, Berlin, 5th ed., 1922, 6 vols.

An extremely valuable book is:

F. H. Garrison and L. T. Morton, *A Medical Bibliography: A Check-list of Texts Illustrating the History of the Medical Sciences*, London, 1943.

This is an annotated bibliography, which lists the basic books in every field of medicine. It is a selection, of course, but it includes 5506 items and I have never consulted it in vain.

A difficult and so far unsolved problem is how to keep track of current medical historical literature. Before the war, we had two journals that reported on new publications, books as well as papers, the German *Mitteilungen zur Geschichte der Medizin, der Naturwissenschaften und der Technik* and the American *Isis*. The *Mitteilungen* were discontinued during the war, and *Isis*, having to cover the field of the entire history of science and civilization, cannot devote too much space to medicine. The *Quarterly Cumulative Index Medicus*, published by the American Medical Association in Chicago, includes medical history publications but in no way systematically.

It was felt that a solution might be found if every country would publish annually its national bibliography, and that these bibliographies could then be consolidated, possibly by the *International Society of the History of Medicine*, once it begins to function. From 1940 on, the *American Association of the History of Medicine* published annually in its organ, the *Bulletin of the History of Medicine*, the *Bibliography of the History of Medicine of the United States and Canada* (edited by Genevieve Miller).

Switzerland began publishing its national bibliography in *Gesnerus*, vol. 1, 1943/44.

Other national bibliographies, although not issued periodically, are:

J. E. Kroon, *Catalogus van werken en artikelen van Nederlanders op historisch genees-, schei-, wis-, natuurkundig en natuurwetenschappelijk gebied*, 1 Januari 1900 tot 30 September 1923, Leiden, 1923.

Adalberto Pazzini, *Bibliografia di storia della medicina Italiana*, Milan, 1939.

Publishing such bibliographies raises another difficult problem. Many papers and even books are worthless, are simply popular articles written for the entertainment of their authors and a few readers. In other words, should such bibliographies endeavor to be as complete as possible, or should they be critical?

A promising attempt at reviewing critically recent literature in a given field was made very successfully by O. Temkin, 'Recent Publications in Egyptian and Babylonian Medicine,' *Bull. Inst. Hist. Med.*, 1936, 4:247-56, 341-7.

The whole question of bibliography must be discussed nationally and ultimately internationally. It may not be as acute here as it is in other medical fields, but it must be solved nevertheless.

NOTES

1. See H. E. Sigerist, 'Classics of Medicine,' *Bull. Hist. Med.*, 1944, 16:1-12.
2. They are listed in *Bull. Hist. Med.*, 1944, 16:5-6.
3. London, 1921-4.
4. Oxford, 1921-45.
5. Listed in *Index-Catalogue*, third series.

APPENDIX III

*

Museums of Medical History

The study of the antiquities of medicine is very important as it involves valuable primary sources. It is a difficult study because objects are scattered all over the world and because the field is extremely broad. The medical historian obviously is interested not only in old surgical instruments and pharmacy jars but also in the antiquities of housing, clothing, nutrition, in burial rites, and all conditions that affect the people's health. As a result, there is not a museum in the world that does not contain some items of significance to the student of medical history. Large institutions such as the Metropolitan Museum in New York, the British Museum in London, or the Louvre in Paris, all have sections illustrating the daily life of the Egyptians, the Greeks, or the Romans, and are veritable mines of information to us as to all students of antiquity, quite apart from the inscriptions and other medical texts they possess. All museums of cultural anthropology have many objects illustrating primitive medicine. Local historical museums, sometimes very small ones, may contain objects of great importance to medical history. Where excavations are carried out, antiquities are unearthed that illustrate aspects of life that had some bearing on health and disease. This is the case not only with the great sites—Athens, Pompeii, Herculaneum—but also with such small Roman outposts as Vindonissa in Switzerland. It obviously is impossible to mention in these few pages all museums that are of interest to us. The student of medical history should never miss an opportunity to visit museums, because he will never do so without profit. All we can do here is list a few typical collections we have visited or about which we have special information, and outline what the future tasks must be to make antiquities available to medico-historical research.

Most important obviously are the institutions devoted primarily, if not exclusively, to the history of medicine and to the history of science. The outstanding example is:

The Wellcome Historical Medical Museum and Library in London (Museum at 28 Portman Square, W.1., Library at 183 Euston Road, N.W.1.). The collection was built up by the late Sir Henry S. Wellcome.[1] It is by far the richest collection covering the entire field of the history of medicine and the allied sciences, and is not only an educational but a research center of the greatest importance. The Museum contains approximately 200,000 objects, many of which are unique specimens, about 800 pictures, and a large and valuable collection of prints. The Library contains about 220,000 volumes, together with 5000 manuscripts and over 100,000 autographed letters. There are 612 incunabula, which constitute the second largest collection of medical and allied incunabula in existence, and the sixteenth and seventeenth century material is even more important. A brochure was recently published describing the Library. A *Catalogue Raisonné* of the incunabula is being published shortly, and the great catalogue of the entire Library, now in card form, is being prepared for publication. The Museum has for many years organized exhibitions on various occasions, and the catalogues of these provide useful reference material. The latest are the *Catalogue of Books, Manuscripts and Relics Commemorating the Bicentenary of Edward Jenner*, published in 1949, and the *Catalogue of an Exhibition Illustrating Medicine in 1850*, published in 1950, both by the Oxford University Press. The Museum also publishes a series of scholarly monographs by specialists in various subjects.

Other collections devoted primarily to the history of medicine are the following:

The Medico-Historical Museum of Copenhagen (68 Bredegade).[2] Founded in 1907 by C. J. Salomonsen, it became the property of the University in 1918 and is located in the old building of the Surgical Academy.

Medizingeschichtliche Sammlung der Universität Zürich. Initiated in 1915 by G. A. Wehrli, it became the property of the Canton of Zurich in 1932 and is located in the tower of the main building of the University. Particularly rich in the field of folk-medicine.

Museum of Historical and Cultural Medicine of the Cleveland Medical Library Association, Cleveland, Ohio (11,000 Euclid Avenue).[3] Initiated by D. P. Allen and developed by H. Dittrick.

In France several medical schools have created museums:

Musée d'Histoire de la Médecine de la Faculté de Médecine de Paris.

Musée Historique de la Faculté Mixte de Médecine et de Pharmacie de Lyon.[4]

Musée Flaubert et d'Histoire de la Médecine, located in the Hôtel-Dieu of Rouen, 51 rue de Lecat.[5]

Wherever Departments or Institutes of the History of Medicine were created, collections of objects grew up as a matter of course. Some of them are small but they all have the advantage of being handled expertly and of having full use made of them for research. Some such institutions are:

The Johns Hopkins Institute of the History of Medicine, Baltimore, Md. (1900 E. Monument Street).[6]

The Historical Library, Yale Medical Library, New Haven, Conn. (333 Cedar Street). It possesses notably a pharmacy and a weight and measures collection built up and presented by E. C. Streeter.[7]

The Department of Medical History of the Medical School of the University of Kansas, Kansas City.[8]

Istituto di Storia della Medicina dell'Università di Roma, founded in 1937 by A. Pazzini, the most important institute of its kind in Italy.[9]

Rome has another remarkable museum, that of the *Accademia di Storia dell'Arte Sanitaria.*[10]

The *Institute of the History of Medicine* at the Medical Faculty of the *Charles University* in Prague has collections of books and portraits but not of objects. However, the *Medical Museum* in Prague II collects all documents and objects concerning the history of medicine in Bohemia and also possesses a collection of coins and medals related to medical subjects. The *Museum of Pharmacology* in the Purkyně-Institute, moreover, has collections from apothecary's shops of the sixteenth and seventeenth centuries.[11]

Before the war all Polish universities had Institutes of the History of Medicine, all of which had collections.[12] Today the subject is taught in Warszawa, Krakow, Poznán, Wroclaw, Lodź, Lublin, and at the Medical Academy in Gdansk, and the Institutes are being reconstructed.

In Rumania, Bucharest has a *National Institute of the History of Medicine,* founded in 1935 by V. Gomoiu, which in addition to books and documents includes medals and medical and pharmaceutical objects.[13] The University of Cluj has an *Institute of the History of Medicine, Pharmacy and Medical Folklore* with rich collections.[14]

In central Europe the following Institutes possess collections that have survived the war:

Karl Sudhoff-Institut für Geschichte der Medizin und der Naturwissenschaften an der Universität Leipzig (Talstrasse 33).[15]

Institut für Geschichte der Medizin und der Naturwissenschaften an der Universität Berlin (Universitäts-Strasse 3b).

Institut für Geschichte der Medizin an der Universität Jena, founded by Th. Meyer-Steineg, with collections of Graeco-Roman antiquities.

The Institute at the University of Frankfurt a. M. is in the process of reorganization.

Institut für Geschichte der Medizin an der Universität Wien, created by M. Neuburger, located in the Josephinum, with very considerable collections.[16]

The *Genootschap voor Geschiedenis der Geneeskunde Wiskunde en Natuurwetenschappen,* in addition to having a library in Leiden, founded in 1942, in co-operation with the Nederlandsch Tijdschrift voor Geneeskunde, a collection of medals *Scientia Medica et Naturalia in Nummis.*[17]

The *Rijksmuseum voor de Geschiedenis der Natuurwetenschappen,* the Netherland's State Museum of the History of Science, also located at Leiden, includes collections of great importance to the history of medicine.[18]

In China, a *Medical History Museum* was opened in 1938 in Shanghai, organized by the Chinese Medical History Society, which acts as Medical History Section of the Chinese Medical Association.[19]

Museums devoted to the history of science usually contain objects that also concern the history of the medical sciences. Some have been mentioned before; others are:

Museo e Istituto di Storia delle Scienze, in Florence (Piazza dei Giudici 1).[20]

Museo Nazionale della Scienza e della Tecnica, in Milan, located in Monasterio di S. Vittore, founded by government decree of 1947.[21]

National Museum of Science and Industry, in London.

Museum of the History of Science, in Oxford. (In the Old Ashmolean; a *Brief Guide* by F. Sherwood Taylor was published in 1949.)

Deutsches Museum von Meisterwerken der Naturwissenschaft und Technik, in Munich.

The history of pharmacy is well represented in museums. Pharmacy jars are works of art and hence popular collectors' items. Almost all museums of medical history possess antiquities of pharmacy and some like the Wellcome Museum have very considerable holdings. Some special collections in addition to those mentioned before are:

The Squibb Ancient Pharmacy, in New York (58th Street and 5th Avenue).[22]

American Institute of the History of Pharmacy, in Madison, Wisconsin.[23]

Schweizerische Sammlung für Historisches Apothekenwesen, in Basle (Totengässlein 3).[24]

Musée d'Histoire de la Pharmacie, in Paris (4, avenue de l'Observatoire).[25]

Raccolta di Storia della Farmacia, in the Pharmacological Institute of the University of Pavia.[26]

A division of *Germanisches Nationalmuseum,* in Nürnberg.[27]

Pharmaziegeschichtliche Sammlung im Thüringer Museum zu Eisenach.[28]

Historical pharmacies or pharmaceutical utensils are also to be found in ancient hospitals such as, e.g. the Ospedale Maggiore in Milan.

We find, furthermore, that medical museums serving needs of current medicine, anatomy, pathology, or health education occasionally have historical divisions or sections that became historical in the course of time. Italian medical schools have old medical collections some of which were founded centuries ago.[29] Historical items may be found in the following museums:

Royal College of Surgeons, in London (Lincoln's Inn Fields). It contained, among others, John Hunter's famous collection of anatomical preparations, much of which was destroyed by bombs during the Second World War.[30]

Army Medical Museum, in Washington.[31]

Deutsches Hygiene Museum, in Dresden, with good historical material prepared upon the initiative and under the supervision of Karl Sudhoff.

Staatliche Mediko-Historische Sammlung im Kaiserin-Friedrich-Haus für das ärztliche Fortbildungswesen, in Berlin.

This very fragmentary list of museums of medical history gives an idea of the types of institutions that we have today. It seems to me that the following postulates should be fulfilled in order to make the antiquities of medicine readily available to research:

1. Every country should have at least one institution that would collect, classify, and catalogue systematically medical objects of all kinds. To such an institution hospitals, pharmacies, laboratories, physicians, and other medical personnel could turn over whatever items they no longer need (objects, documents, books, etc.). Such an institution could be a university institute or a museum, publicly or privately owned and oper-

ated. Every country's national medical association should feel a strong responsibility for the preservation of its national medical heritage.

2. An inventory should be made of existing medico-historical collections. This could be made nationally first, possibly as a project of the national associations of the history of medicine. The national inventories could then be combined into an international handbook.

3. An index or indices should be made of non-movable antiquities of medicine such as hospitals, aqueducts, statues of physicians, temples of healing deities, et cetera, with photographs and full descriptions. Such indices might be prepared nationally or according to subjects, by one institution specializing on water supplies and sewage systems, another on monuments, while a third may wish to prepare an index of Graeco-Roman antiquities.

NOTES

1. *Handbook to the Wellcome Historical Medical Museum*, London, 1920; new edition, 1927.
2. See W. von Brunn, 'Das medizinische Museum in Kopenhagen,' *Münch. med. Wschr.*, 1934, 81:1436; D. Guthrie, 'The Medico-Historical Museum in Copenhagen,' *Medicine Illustrated*, 1949, 3:134-6.
3. See H. Dittrick, 'Medical History Collections in the United States and Canada,' II, 'Collections in Cleveland, Ohio,' *Bull. Hist. Med.*, 1940, 8:1214-45. The paper describes the holdings of all public and private medico-historical collections in Cleveland and in doing so it sets an example that should be followed by other cities.
4. A catalogue by Jules Guiart in *Annales de l'Université de Lyon*, 3e série, médecine, fasc. II, Paris, Masson, 1941, 272 pp., 16 plates.
5. See Lecaplain, 'Le Musée de l'Ecole de Médecine de Rouen,' *Aesculape*, 1924, pp. 1-6; catalogue by R.-M. Martin, Rouen, 1947; see *Arch. Intern. Hist. Sc.*, 1949, 2:807.
6. See the Annual Reports of the Institute in *Bull. Hist. Med.*
7. See the Annual Reports of the Library.
8. L. Clendening, 'The Library and Museum of the Department of Medical History of the University of Kansas,' *Bull. Hist. Med.*, 1940, 8:742-8, illus.
9. See A. F. La Cava, 'L'Istituto di Storia della Medicina dell'Università di Roma,' *Castalia*, 1947, 3:31-4.
10. See the reports in *Atti e Memorie dell'Accademia dell'Arte Sanitaria.*
11. Information kindly supplied by Prof. Miloslav Matoušek of Prague.
12. See, e.g. (W. Szumowski), *L'Institut d'Histoire de la Médecine de l'Université Jagiellonienne de Cracovie*, a pamphlet published on the occasion of VIIth Internat. Hist. Congress, in 1933; see also notes in *Archiwum Historij i Filozofij Medycyny.*
13. Information kindly supplied by Dr. V. Gomoiu.

14. V. L. Bologa, 'L'Institut d'Histoire de la Médecine et de la Pharmacie de Cluj (Roumanie),' *Archeion,* 1928, 9:517-20; V. L. Bologa, 'Institutul de Istoria Medicinei, Farmaciei si de Folklor Medical din Cluj,' *Boabe de Grau,* June, 1932; see also annual reports in *Clujul Medical.*
15. H. E. Sigerist, 'Forschungsinstitute für Geschichte der Medizin und der Naturwissenschaften,' *Forschungsinstitute, ihre Geschichte Organisation und Ziele,* edited by L. Brauer, Mendelsohn Bartholdy, and A. Meyer, Hamburg, 1930, vol. I, pp. 391-405.
16. T. Oliaro, 'L'Istituto di Storia della Medicina in Vienna,' *Minerva Medica,* 1933, no. 20, 19 May.
17. D. Burger, *Arch. Intern. Hist. Sc.,* 1948, 1:513-16; 1949, 2:936-8.
18. See the annual Reports of the Director published by the Ministry of Education, Arts, and Sciences.
19. K. C. Wong, Report of the Chinese Medical History Society, *Arch. Internat. Hist. Sc.,* 1949, 2:545-51.
20. About its origin see C. Del Lungo, 'Il museo di fisica e di storia naturale di Firenze ed il museo degli strumenti antichi di fisica e di astronomia,' *Arch. Stor. Sc.,* 1919, 1:153-6.
21. See *Castalia,* 1948, 4:46.
22. Catalogue by George Urdang, New York, E. R. Squibb and Sons, 1940.
23. G. Urdang, 'The American Institute of the History of Pharmacy,' *Bull. Hist. Med.,* 1941, 10:690-700.
24. J. A. Häfliger, *Pharmazeutische Altertumskunde und die Schweizerische Sammlung für historisches Apothekenwesen an der Universität Basel,* Zürich, 1931. Pages 27-38: list of 230 European public and private collections possessing objects that concern the history of pharmacy.
25. See *Arch. Internat. Hist. Sc.,* 1949, 2:810, and current notes in *Rev. Hist. Pharm.*
26. P. Mascherpa, 'Una collezione storica della farmacia nella R. Università di Pavia,' *La Chimica,* 1943, no. 8, 34 pp., illus.
27. F. Ferchl, *Deutsche Apotheken-Altertümer* [Bilderbücher des Germanischen Nationalmuseums Heft 4], Nürnberg, 1936.
28. W. Fiek, *Die pharmaziegeschichtliche Sammlung im Thüringer Museum zu Eisenach* [Veröffentl. Ges. Gesch. Pharm.], n.d.
29. A medico-chirurgical museum was founded in Ravenna in the early 18th century; see A. F. La Cava, 'Il più antico museo medico-chirurgico,' *Castalia,* 1945, 1:109-14.
30. A. Keith, *Illustrated Guide to the Museum of the Royal College of Surgeons,* London, 1910. About the destruction see *Bull. Hist. Med.,* 1941, 10:631-2.
31. See C. F. Craig, 'The Army Medical Museum,' *Mil. Surgeon,* 1919, 15:670 87.

APPENDIX IV

*

Literature on Paleopathology Since 1930

The main result of the classical studies of Roy L. Moodie, Marc Armand Ruffer, and L. Pales was the recognition that disease must be as old as life itself and that it occurred at all times in the same basic forms that we see today. Once this was established through the investigation of sufficient and adequate human and animal remains the interest in paleopathology decreased for a while. When the incidence of arthritis had been evidenced for a certain period and region, the examination of hundreds of additional bones might reveal a few more cases of arthritis but nothing new concerning the disease.

New techniques, however, gave a certain impetus to these studies, notably the use of x-rays in the examination of bones and of mummies and, more recently, the application of serological methods.

Roy L. Moodie's book, *Paleopathology, an Introduction to the Study of Ancient Evidences of Disease,* Urbana, Ill., Univ. of Illinois Press, 1923, has at the end (pp. 545-57) a bibliography that includes most publications on the subject to 1922. The book of Léon Pales, *Paléopathologie et pathologie comparative,* Paris, Masson & Cie, 1930, contains a bibliography (pp. 293-348) of 660 titles including those of Moodie's book and additional items published between 1923 and 1930. The student of paleopathology is referred to these excellent bibliographies and in the following we merely list some titles published since 1930.

We shall discuss the paleopathology of America in Volume IV of this work and on this occasion shall give a bibliography of the subject. We have included here some titles dealing with American material mainly on account of their methodological interest.

Abbott, K. H. and Courville, C. B., 'Historical Notes on Meningiomas; Hyperostoses in Prehistoric Skulls,' *Bull. Los Angeles Neurol. Soc.*, 1939, 4:101-13.

Almeida Prado, A. de, 'Evolução em patologia,' *An. Fac. de Med. da Univ. de São Paulo* (pt. 2), 1941, 17:733-73.

——, 'Paleopatologia,' *São Paulo Méd.*, 1944, 1:9-14.

B. M., 'Zeugen prähistorischer Kämpfe,' *Umschau*, 1929, 33:473.

Banerjee, D. N., 'Paleopathology,' *J. Indian Med. Ass.*, 1941, 10:263-7.

Basedow, H., 'Diseases of the Australian Aborigines,' *J. Trop. Med. and Hyg.*, 1932, 35:177-85, 193-8, 209-13, 229-33, 247-50, 273-8.

Baudouin, M., 'Une Lésion inconnue de la rotule chez un préhistorique,' *Paris méd.*, 1935, 96-470-73.

Beltrán, J. R., 'Las enfermedades dentarias en la prehistoria,' *El Noticioso Médico Mundial*, 1938, no. 18, 4 pp.

——, 'Las incognitas de la cirurgía prehistórica,' *Bol. y Trab., Soc. Argent. de Cirujanos*, 1941, 2:715-21.

Bouquet, H., 'Die Krankheiten des Ur-Menschen,' *Deut. Aerzte Ztg.*, 1943, 9: no. 407.

Boyd, W. C. and Boyd, L. G., 'An Attempt to Determine the Blood Group of Mummies,' *Proc. Soc. Exp. Biol.*, 1934, 31:671-2.

——, 'Blood Grouping Tests on 300 Mummies, with Notes on the Precipitin-Test,' *J. Immunology*, 1937, 32:307-19.

——, 'Les Groupes sanguins chez les anciens Egyptiens,' *Chronique d'Egypte*, 1937, 12:41-4.

Candela, P. B., 'Blood Group Reactions in Ancient Human Skeletons,' *Amer. J. Phys. Anthrop.*, 1936, 21:429-32.

——, 'Blood Group Determinations upon Minnesota and New York Skeletal Material,' *Amer. J. Phys. Anthrop.*, 1937, 23:71-8.

Castaldi, L., 'I più antichi documenti medici (paleopatologia),' *Rassegna internaz. di Clin. e Terap.*, 1937, 18:148-58.

Chamberlain, E. B. and Taft, R. B., 'Ancient Arthritis [in Mastodon],' *Radiology*, 1938, 30:761-2.

Congdon, R. T., 'Spondylolisthesis and Vertebral Anomalies in Skeletons of American Aborigines, with Clinical Notes on Spondylolisthesis,' *J. Bone & Joint Surg.*, 1932, 14:511-24.

Courville, C. B. and Abbott, K. H., 'Cranial Injuries of Pre-Columbian Incas with Comments on Their Mechanism, Effects and Lethality,' *Bull. Los Angeles Neurol. Soc.*, 1942, 7:107-30.

Cressman, L. S. and Larsell, O., 'A Case of Probable Osteomyelitis in an Indian Skeleton,' *West. J. Surgery*, 1945, 53:332-5.

Decker, F. H. and Bohrod, M. G., 'Medullary Artifacts in Prehistoric Bones,' *Am. J. Roentgenol.*, 1939, 42:374-5.

Denninger, H. S., '*Osteitis fibrosa* in Skeleton of Prehistoric American Indian,' *Arch. Path.*, 1931, 11:939-47; also *Tr. Chicago Path. Soc.*, 1931, 13:408-18.

———, 'Paleopathological Evidence of Paget's Disease,' *Ann. Med. Hist.*, 1933, 5:73-81.

———, 'Prehistoric Syphilitic Lesions. Example from North America,' *Southwestern Med.*, 1935, 19:202-4.

Desfosses, P., 'Paléontologie et médecine,' *Presse méd.*, 1935, 43:2061.

Dorn, H. F., 'The Increase in Average Length of Life,' *Pub. Health Rep. U. S.*, 1937, 52:1753-77.

Ehrenberg, K., 'Neuere Untersuchungen über Krankheitserscheinungen bei vorzeitlichen Tieren und ihre Ergebnisse,' *Med. Klinik*, 1931, 27:172-4.

Fisher, A. K., 'Additional Paleopathological Evidence of Paget's Disease,' *Ann. Med. Hist.*, 1935, 7:197-8.

Franz, L. and Winkler, W., 'Die Sterblichkeit in der frühen Bronzezeit Niederösterreichs,' *Zschr. f. Rassenk.*, 1936, 4:157-63.

Gieseler, W., 'Bericht über die jungpaläolithischen Skelettreste von Stetten ob Lontal bei Ulm,' *Verh. Ges. Phys. Anthrop.*, 1937, 8:41-8.

Gilmour, J., 'Heads and Tales, or Prehistoric Surgery,' *Univ. Durham Coll. Med. Gaz.*, 1929-30, 30:33-42.

Given, J. C. M., 'Palaeopathology and Evolution,' *Lancet*, 1928, 1:164-6.

Guiart, J., 'Una incursione medica nella preistoria,' *Biol. med.*, 1932, 8:71-92.

Handley, R. S., 'Case of Multiple Thoracic Injuries in Roman Britain,' *Brit. J. Surg.*, 1937, 25:461-4.

Hofschlaeger, R., 'Von den Krankheiten des vorgeschichtlichen Menschen,' *Ciba Zschr.*, 1939, 6:2319-24.

Holden, H. S., 'Some Observations on the Wound Reactions of *Ankyropteris corrugata*,' *J. Linn. Soc. London*, 1931 48:643-55, 1 plate, 16 figs.

Hrdlička, A., 'Seven Prehistoric American Skulls with Complete Absence of External Auditory Meatus,' *Am. J. Phys. Anthrop.*, 1933, 17:355-77.

Janssen, H.-L., 'Wundbehandlung in der Vorzeit,' *Deut. med. Wschr.*, 1933, 59:1098-9.

Jonckheere, Frans: *Autour de l'autopsie d'une momie, Le scribe royal Boutehamon,* Bruxelles, 1942.

Jones, E. W. A. H., 'Studies in Achondroplasia,' *J. Anat.,* 1931-2, 66: 565-77.

Krogman, W. M., 'The Pathologies of Pre- and Protohistoric Man,' *Ciba Symposia,* 1940, 2:432-43.

——, 'The Medical and Surgical Practices of Pre- and Protohistoric Man,' *Ciba Symposia,* 1940, 2:444-52.

——, 'The Skeletal and Dental Pathology of an Early Iranian Site,' *Bull. Hist. Med.,* 1940, 8:28-48.

Krumbhaar, E. B., 'A Pre-Columbian Peruvian Tibia Exhibiting Syphilitic (?) Periostitis. With Recognizable Varieties of Bone Marrow Cells,' *Ann. Med. Hist.,* 1936, 8:232-5.

Lang, F. J., '*Ostitis fibrosa* in ihren genetischen Beziehungen zur Osteomalacie und Rachitis,' *Beitr. z. path. Anat. u. allg. Path.,* 1931, 87: 142-60.

MacKay, C. V., 'Some Pathological Changes in Australian Aboriginal Bones,' *Med. J. Australia;* 1938, 2:537-55.

Martin, C. P., 'Some Variations in the Lower End of the Femur Which Are Especially Prevalent in the Bones of Primitive People,' *J. Anat.,* 1932, 66:371-83.

Michaelis, L., 'Vergleichende mikroskopische Untersuchung an rezenten, historischen und fossilen Knochen,' *Veröffentl. a. d. Kriegs- und Konstitutions-Path.,* no. 24; *Jena,* 1930, vol. 6: no. 1.

Miller, J. L., 'Some Diseases of Ancient Man,' *Ann. Med. Hist.,* 1929, n. ser. 1:394-402.

Mollison, T., 'Zeichen gewaltsamer Verletzungen an den Ofnet-Schädeln,' *Anthrop. Anz.,* 1936, 13:79-88.

——, 'Die Verletzungen am Schädel und den Gliedmassenknochen des Rhodesiafundes,' *Anthrop. Anz.,* 1938, 14:229-34.

Moodie, R. L., 'Studies in Paleopathology, xxiii: Surgery in pre-Columbian Peru,' *Ann. med. Hist.,* 1929, n. ser. 1:698-728.

——, 'California Sabre Tooth; Facial Asymmetry following Loss of Sabre,' *Pacific Dent. Gaz.,* 1929, 37:764-6.

——, 'Unusual Skull from Pre-Columbian Peru,' *Am. J. Surg.,* 1930, 8:903-4.

——, 'Prehistoric Surgery in New Mexico,' *Am. J. Surg.,* 1930, 8:905-8.

——, 'Hypertrophy in Sacrum of Sabre Tooth, Pleistocene of Southern California,' *Am. J. Surg.,* 1930, 8:1313-15.

——, 'Pleistocene Luxations,' *Am. J. Surg.,* 1930, 9:348-62.

Moodie, R. L., 'Studies in Paleopathology, xxviii: The Phenomenon of Sacralization in the Pleistocene Sabre-tooth,' *Am. J. Surg.*, 1930, 10:587-9.

——, 'Suggestion of Rickets in the Pleistocene,' *Am. J. Surg.*, 1930, 10:162-3.

——, *Roentgenologic Studies of Egyptian and Peruvian Mummies.* Field Museum of Natural History, Anthropology, Memoirs, vol. III, Chicago, 1931, 66 pp., 76 plates.

Nikolaev, L. P., 'Kostnye zabolevaniya v doistorichestkom periode,' *Ortoped. i Travmatol.*, 1935, 9:3-10.

Panneton, P., 'Le Premier Malade connu dans l'histoire de l'humanité,' *Union méd. du Canada*, 1944, 73:804-5.

Pardal, R., 'Sobre paleopatología americana; reacción hiperostósica sugestiva de un meningioma subyacente, en un cráneo indígena de Mendoza,' *Prensa méd. argent.*, 1939, 26:1585-92.

——, 'Sobre paleopatología americana; "cribra orbitalia," lesión bilateral del techo de las órbitas en un cráneo indígena del Brasil,' *Prensa méd. argent.*, 1944, 31:167-70.

Popp, H., 'Krankheiten und Chirurgie des Urmenschen,' *Med. Welt*, 1939, 13:127-9.

Ritchie, W. A. and Warren, S. L., 'Occurrence of Multiple Bony Lesions Suggesting Myeloma in Skeleton of Pre-Columbian Indian,' *Am. J. Roentgenol.*, 1932, 28:622-8.

Rivet, L., 'Pathologie et chirurgie préhistoriques,' *Presse méd.*, 1945, 53:402.

Rogers, L., 'History of Craniotomy: an Account of the Methods Which Have Been Practiced and the Instruments Used for Opening the Human Skull during Life,' *Ann. Med. Hist.*, 1930, n. ser., 2:495-514.

Rokhline, D. G., Roubachewa, A., and Maikowa-Stroganowa, 'La Cyphose des adolescents, recherche paléopathologique,' *J. de Radiol. et d'Electrol.*, 1936, 20:246-51.

Rostock, P., 'Unfall- und Kriegschirurgie in Ägypten vor 4500 Jahren,' *Chirurg*, 1938, 10:127-30.

Schultz, A. H., 'Notes on Diseases and Healed Fractures of Wild Apes, and Their Bearing on the Antiquity of Pathological Conditions in Man,' *Bull. Hist. Med.*, 1939, 7:571-82.

Sedwick, H. J., 'Observations on Precolumbian Indian Skulls Unearthed in New York State,' *J. Amer. Dent. Ass.*, 1936, 23:764-73.

Shattuck, G. C., 'Lesions of Syphilis in American Indians,' *Amer. J. Trop. Med.*, 1938, 18:577-86.

Shaw, A. F. B., 'Histological Study of the Mummy of Har-mosě, the Singer of the Eighteenth Dynasty (*c.* 1490 B.C.),' *J. Path. and Bact.*, 1938, 47:115-23.

Shore, L. R., 'Some Examples of Disease of the Vertebral Column Found in Skeletons of Ancient Egypt. A Contribution to Palaeopathology,' *Brit. J. Surg.*, 1936, 24:256-71.

Sjövall, Einar, 'Die Bedeutung der Skelettanalyse bei Grabuntersuchungen,' *K. Fysiograf. Sällskapets Lund Förhandl.*, 1933, 2 (10):1-24.

Snorrason, E. S., 'Rheumatism, Past and Present, in the Light of Paleopathology and Social Pre-history,' *Canad. Med. Ass. J.*, 1942, 46:589-94.

Steppuhn, O. and Utkina-Ljubowzowa, X., 'Proteolytische Zellfermente von ägyptischen Mumien (etwa 3000 jährig) und Mammut (etwa 30,000 bis 100,000 jährig),' *Biochem. Ztsch.*, 1930, 226:237-42.

Sticker, Georg, 'Zur Pathologie der Alemannen,' *Verhandl. Ges. Phys. Anthropol.*, 1935, 7:28-30.

——, 'Zur Pathologie der Alemannen,' *Med. Welt*, 1935, 9:739-41.

Szörényi, Elisabeth, 'Echinanthus scutella Lam., ein pathologischer Seeigel aus dem ungarischen Eozän,' *Palaeobiologica*, 1931, 4:251-6.

Tecoz, H. F., 'Les Maladies de l'homme préhistorique,' *Praxis*, Bern, 1944, 33:174.

Tello, J. C. and Williams, H. U., 'Ancient Syphilitic Skull from Paracas in Peru,' *Ann. Med. Hist.*, 1930, n. ser. 2:515-29.

Terra, H. de., 'The Siwaliks of India and Early Man,' *Early Man*, Internat. Sympos., Acad. Nat. Sc., Philadelphia, 1937, pp. 257-68.

Vallois, H. V., 'Les Maladies de l'homme préhistorique,' *Rev. Scientifique*, 1934, 72:666-78.

——, 'La Durée de la vie chez l'homme fossile,' *C. R. Acad. Sc.*, 1937, 204:60-62; also *Anthrop.*, 1937, 47:499-532.

Wakefield, E. G. and Dellinger, S. C., 'Diseases of Prehistoric Americans of South Central United States,' *Ciba Symposia*, 1940, 2:453-64.

—— and Camp, J. D., 'Study of Osseous Remains of Primitive Race Who Once Inhabited Shelters of Bluffs of Ozark Mountains,' *Am. J. Med. Sc.*, 1937, 193:223-8.

Weidenreich, F., 'Duration of Life of Fossil Man in China and Pathological Lesions Found in His Skeleton,' *Chinese Med. J.*, 1939, 55:34-44.

Wilke, Georg, '*Die Heilkunde in der europäischen Vorzeit*, Leipzig, 1936.

Williams, G. D., Ritchie, W. A., and Titterington, P. F., 'Multiple Bony Lesions Suggesting Myeloma in Pre-Columbian Indian Aged Ten Years,' *Am. J. Roentgenol.*, 1941, 46:351-5.

Williams, H. U., 'The Origin and Antiquity of Syphilis: the Evidence from Diseased Bones. A Review, with Some New Material from America,' *Arch. Pathol.*, 1932, 13:779-814, 931-83.

———, 'The Origin of Syphilis: Evidence from Diseased Bones; a Supplementary Report,' *Arch. Dermat. and Syph.*, 1936, 33:783-7.

Wilson, G. E., 'A Study in American Paleohistology,' *Am. Naturalist*, 1927, 61:555.

Wyman, L. C. and Boyd, W. C., 'Blood Group Determination of Prehistoric American Indians,' *Amer. Anthrop.*, 1937, 39:583-92.

Young, F. B., 'Paleopathology,' *Nebraska Med. J.*, 1931, 16:26-9.

The following titles deal particularly with *Paleodontology*, or the ancient evidence of anomalies and diseases of the teeth:

Adloff, P., 'Ueber die Bedeutung des Gebisses für die Beurteilung der zum Menschen in Beziehung stehenden fossilen Reste,' *Anat. Anz.*, 1933, 75:542-9.

———, 'Ergänzende Bemerkungen zur Beurteilung des Gebisses von Sinanthropus Pekinensis,' *Anat. Anz.*, 1941, 91:160-75.

Bentzen, Raymond C., 'Dental Conditions among the Mimbres People of Southwestern United States Previous to the Year 600 A.D. An Original Study of the Teeth and Jaws from a Series of Skeletons Unearthed by the Jenks Expedition,' *Dental Cosmos*, 1929, 71:1068-73.

Boule, M. and Vallois, H., 'L'Homme fossile d'Asselar (Sahara),' *Rev. Stomatol.*, 1935, 37:608-17.

Branson, C. C., 'Paleontologic Development of Skull and Teeth,' *Internat. J. Orthodontia*, 1931, 17:315-24.

Buschan, G., 'Ueber künstliche und natürliche Veränderungen an den Zähnen, Pflege und Behandlung derselben bei den Natur- and frühgeschichtlichen Völkern,' *Wien med. Wschr.*, 1936, 86:874-9.

Cave, A. J. E., 'Remarks on Certain Neolithic Skulls,' *Proc. Roy. Soc. Med.*, 1938, 31:1373-81.

Chabert, L., 'Quelques Remarques sur l'appareil masticateur des Néanderthaliens,' *J. méd. Bordeaux*, 1938, 115:81-9.

Christophersen, K. M., 'Investigations into Dental Conditions in the Neolithic Period and in the Bronze Age in Denmark,' *Dent. Rec.*, London, 1939, 59:575-85.

———, 'Ueber die Zahnverhältnisse bei einer Volksgruppe der Wikingerzeit; odontologische Untersuchungen aus der Grabstätte bei Trelleborg (Seeland)', *Acta odont. scand.*, 1940, 2:87-108.

Conaway, E. B., 'A Dental Radiographic Study of Two Mummies,' *Radiogr. & Clin. Photogr.*, 1937, 13:21-2.

de la Borbolla, D. F. Rubin, 'Types of Tooth Mutilation Found in Mexico,' *Am. J. Phys. Anthrop.*, 1940, 26:349-65.

Derry, D. E., 'Incidence of Dental Diseases in Ancient Egypt,' *Brit. Med. J.*, 1933, 1:112.

Dreyer, T. F., 'Dental Caries in Prehistoric South Africans,' *Nature*, 1935, 136:302-3.

Fisher, A. K., Kuhm, H. W., and Adami, G. C., 'Dental Pathology of the Prehistoric Indians of Wisconsin,' *Bull. Pub. Museum of City of Milwaukee*, 1931, 10 (3):331-74.

French, E. L., Tefft, H., *et al.*, 'Composition of Precolumbian Teeth; Calcium, Phosphorus, and Carbon Dioxide Determinations on All the Dentin and All the Enamel,' *J. Dent. Res.*, 1939, 18:547-56.

Gregory, W. K., 'New Models Illustrating Evolution of Human Dentition,' *Internat. J. Orthodontia*, 1934, 20:1077-81.

——— and Hellman, M., 'South African Fossil Man-Apes and Origin of Human Dentition,' *J. Am. Dent. Ass.*, 1939, 26:558-64; Abstract: *Nature*, 1939, 143:25-6.

———, 'The Upper Dental Arch of Plesianthropus Transvaalensis Broom and Its Relations to Other Parts of the Skull,' *Am. J. Phys. Anthrop.*, 1940, 26:211-28.

Hellman, M., 'Form of Talgai Palate,' *Am. J. Phys. Anthrop.*, 1934, 19:1-15.

———, 'Factors Influencing Occlusion,' *Angle Orthodontist*, 1942, 12:3-27.

Košir, A., 'Caries dentium in naše muzejske lobanje. Primer četrtega molarja,' *Glasnik Mus. Društva Slovenijo*, 1926-7, 7-8:44-50.

Krogman, W. M., 'Missing Teeth in Skulls and Dental Caries,' *Am. J. Phys. Anthrop.*, 1935, 20:43-9.

———, 'Dental Arch Form and Facial Growth Pattern in Healthy Children from Prehistoric Populations,' *J. Am. Dent. Ass.*, 1938, 25:1278-89.

———, 'The Skeletal and Dental Pathology of an Early Iranian Site,' *Bull. Hist. Med.*, 1940, 8:28-48.

Leigh, R. W., 'Dental Pathology of Aboriginal California,' *Univ. California Publ. Amer. Archaeol. & Ethnol.*, 1928, 23:399-440.

———, 'Dental Pathology of Aboriginal California,' *Dental Cosmos*, 1929, 71:756-67, 878-89.

———, 'Dental Morphology and Pathology of Prehistoric Guam,' *J. Dent. Res.*, 1930, 10:451-79.

Leigh, R. W., 'Dental Morphology and Pathology of Pre-Spanish Peru,' *Am. J. Phys. Anthrop.*, 1937, 22:267-96.

Markley, M. C., 'Toothaches of Primitive Man,' *Mouth Health Quart.*, 1936, 5:5-8.

Mathis, H. and Clementschitsch, F., 'Bericht über eine Untersuchung an Zähnen u. Kiefern der prähistorischen, historischen u. gegenwärtigen Bevölkerung im Gebiete des Gaues Niederdonau,' *Ztschr. f. Stomatol.*, 1939, 37:1418, 1470.

Moodie, R. L., 'Studies in Paleodontology; Edentulous Palates from Prehistoric Peru,' *Pacific Dent. Gaz.*, 1929, 37:461-8.

——, 'Teeth and Jaws of Nothroterium,' *Pacific Dent. Gaz.*, 1929, 37: 677-80.

——, 'What Bad Teeth Did to the Prehistoric Indian,' *Hygeia*, 1930, 8:551-2.

——, 'Apical Closure of Root Canals in Adult Pleistocene Carnivora,' *Pacific Dent. Gaz.*, 1930, 38:1-4.

——, 'Teeth, Jaws and Palates of Pre-Pueblo Indians from New Mexico,' *Pacific Dent. Gaz.*, 1930, 38:127-45.

——, 'Teeth of the Piros,' *Pacific Dent. Gaz.*, 1930, 38:795-807.

——, 'Prehistoric Maxillofacial Diseases in American Indians,' *Biol. med.*, Milano, 1931, 7:373-6.

——, 'Excessive Deposits of Salivary Calculus on Teeth of Pre-Columbian Peruvians,' *Pacific Dent. Gaz.*, 1931, 39:24-9.

Morton, F., Wolf, H., and Goll, H., 'Kiefer und Zähne in der La-Tène-Periode. Bericht über eine anatomisch-histologische Untersuchung von Kiefern und Zähnen neuer Grabfunde am Hallstädter Salzberg,' *Ztschr. f. Stomatol.*, 1939, 37:1067-80.

Proell, F., 'Untersuchungen an fossilen Funden und primitiven Völkern in ihrer Auswirkung für die praktische Medizin und Zahnheilkunde,' *Forsch. u. Fortschr.*, 1932, 8:360-61.

Rabkin, S., 'Dental Conditions among Prehistoric Indians of Northern Alabama,' *J. Dent. Res.*, 1942, 21:211-22.

——, 'Dental Conditions among Prehistoric Indians of Kentucky (Indian Knoll Collection),' *J. Dent. Res.*, 1943, 22:355-66.

Rihan, H. Y., 'Dental and Orthodontic Observations on 289 Adult and 53 Immature Skulls from Pecos, New Mexico,' *Internat. J. Orthodontia*, 1932, 18:708-12.

Rusconi, C., 'Tooth of Giant Prehistoric Crocodile Found in Bolivia,' *Semana méd.*, 1931, 1:531-3.

Schwarz, R., 'Anthropologie,' *Fortschr. d. Zahnh.*, 1930, 6:697-714.

Shaw, J. C. M. and Hayward, S. S., 'Fossil Teeth of Sharks from Cape Province of South Africa,' *J. Dent. Res.*, 1930, 10:439-42.

'Sixty thousand years of dentistry,' *Mouth Health Quart.*, 1934, 3:4-9.

Steadman, F. St. J., 'Teeth of Australian Aborigines,' *Proc. Roy. Soc. Med.*, 1939, 33:29-49.

Stewart, T. D., 'Dental Caries in Peruvian Skulls,' *Am. J. Phys. Anthrop.*, 1931, 15:315-26.

Webb, C. H., 'Dental Abnormalities as Found in the American Indian,' *Am. J. Orthodontics*, 1944, 30:474-86.

Weidemann, R., *Morphologische Betrachtung von prähistorischen Zähnen aus schlesischen steinzeitlichen Gräberfunden*, Würzburg, 1937, 21 pp.

Index